SPORTS NUTRITION

A Guide for the Professional Working with Active People

THIRD EDITION

Christine A. Rosenbloom, PhD, RD, Editor

Sports, Cardiovascular, and Wellness Nutritionists
Dietetic Practice Group

THE AMERICAN DIETETIC ASSOCIATION
Chicago, Illinois

Library of Congress Cataloging-in-Publication Data

Sports Nutrition : a guide for the professional working with active people / Christine Rosenbloom, editor ; Sports, Cardiovascular, and Wellness Dietetic Practice Group, The American Dietetic Association.— 3rd ed.

   p. cm.

   Includes bibliographical references and index.

   ISBN 0-88091-176-X (Softbound)

   1. Athletes—Nutrition. 2. Exercise—Physiological aspects. I. Rosenbloom, Christine 1951- II. American Dietetic Association. Sports, Cardiovascular, and Wellness Dietetic Practice Group.

TX361.A8 S673 1999
613.2'088'796—dc21

99-052142

The views expressed in this publication are those of the authors and do not necessarily reflect policies and/or official positions of The American Dietetic Association. Mention of product names in this publication does not constitute endorsement by the authors or The American Dietetic Association. The American Dietetic Association disclaims responsibility for the application of the information contained herein.

First edition 1986. Second edition 1993.

10 9 8 7 6 5 4 3 2

CONTRIBUTING WRITERS

Katherine A. Beals, PhD, RD
Assistant Professor
Ball State University
Muncie, Indiana

Leslie J. Bonci, MPH, RD
Director of Sports Medicine
    Nutrition Program
University of Pittsburgh
Nutrition Consultant to Pittsburgh Steelers
Pittsburgh, Pennsylvania

Kyra M. Bramble, MS, RD
Nutrition Consultant
Atlanta, Georgia

Julie H. Burns, MS, RD
SportFuel, Inc
Nutrition Consultant to the Chicago Bulls
Western Springs, Illinois

Cindy Carroll, MS, RD
Nutrition Coordinator
Harvard Pilgrim Health Plan
Boston, Massachusetts

Nancy Clark, MS, RD, FADA, FACSM
Director of Nutrition Services
SportsMedicine Brookline
Brookline, Massachusetts

Ellen Coleman, MA, MPH, RD
Nutrition Consultant
The Sport Clinic
Riverside, California

Josephine Connolly-Schoonen, MS, RD
Clinical Assistant Professor
University Hospital and Medical Center
State University of New York at
Stony Brook

Brenda Davy, MS, RD
Research Dietitian
Colorado State University-Fort Collins

Lisa Dorfman, MS, RD
Food Fitness International, Inc
Miami, Florida

Lynn D. Dugan, MS, RD
Nutrition Consultant
Glen Ellyn, Illinois

Marie Dunford, PhD, RD
Associate Professor and Chair
California State University-Fresno

Kathy Engelbert-Fenton, MPH, RD
Consulting Nutritionist
Park City, Utah

Shirley Gerrior, PhD, RD
Nutritionist
Master Fitness Trainer,
US Army Reserves
Fairfax Station, Virginia

Ann Grandjean, EdD
Director
International Center for Sports Nutrition
Omaha, Nebraska

Diane Habash, PhD, RD
Director of Nutrition Research
The Ohio State University Medical Center
Columbus, Ohio

Charlene Harkins, MEd, RD, FADA
Instructor
University of Minnesota-Duluth

Charlotte Hayes, MMSc, MS, RD, CDE
Diabetes Nutrition and Exercise Specialist
Atlanta, Georgia

Satya S. Jonnalagadda, PhD
Assistant Professor
Georgia State University-Atlanta

Jayanthi Kandiah, PhD, RD
Associate Professor
Ball State University
Muncie, Indiana

Susan M. Kleiner, PhD, RD
Owner, High Performance Nutrition
Affiliate Assistant Professor
University of Washington-Seattle

Kelly Kullick, RD
Owner and Founder
HealthyMoms, LLC
Atlanta, Georgia

Susan Kundrat, MS, RD
Nutrition On The Move
Champaign, Illinois

Susie Langley, MS, RD
Sport Nutrition Consultant
Nutrition Consultant to the
Toronto Maple Leafs
Toronto, Ontario, Canada

Kim LaPiana, MS, RD
Sports Nutritionist
Corona del Mar, California

D. Enette Larson, PhD, RD
Instructor and Sports Nutritionist
University of Alabama-Birmingham

Richard D. Lewis, PhD, RD
Associate Professor
University of Georgia-Athens

Julie Ann Lickteig, MS, RD, FADA
Associate Professor
Cardinal Stritch University
Milwaukee, Wisconsin

Michele Macedonio, MS, RD
Nutrition Consultant
Loveland, Colorado

Melinda M. Manore, PhD, RD
Professor
Arizona State University-Tempe

Christopher M. Modlesky, MA
Research Coordinator
University of Georgia-Athens

Robert Murray, PhD
Director
Gatorade Exercise Physiology Laboratory
Barrington, Illinois

Kristen J. Reimers, MS, RD
Associate Director
International Center for Sports Nutrition
Omaha, Nebraska

Christine A. Rosenbloom, PhD, RD
Associate Professor
Georgia State University
Nutrition Consultant
Georgia Tech Athletic Association
Atlanta, Georgia

Jaime S. Ruud, MS, RD
Nutrition Consultant
Lincoln, Nebraska

Rob Skinner, RD, CSCS
Director of Sports Nutrition
Georgia Tech Athletic Association
Atlanta, Georgia

Karen Sossin, MS, CDN
Nutrition Consultant
West Islip, New York

Suzanne Nelson Steen, DSc, RD
The University of Washington
Huskies Sports Nutrition Services
Seattle, Washington

Jean Storlie, MS, RD
Senior Research Nutrition Scientist
General Mills, Inc
Minneapolis, Minnesota

Debra Vinci, DrPH, RD
Director, Health Education Program
University of Washington-Seattle

Stella L. Volpe, PhD, RD, FACSM
Assistant Professor
University of Massachusetts-Amherst

Julie Walsh, MS, RD
Sports Nut Communications
New York, New York

Monika M. Woolsey, MS, RD
President/CEO
A Better Way Health Consulting, Inc
Glendale, Arizona

Paula J. Ziegler, PhD, RD, CFCS
Chief Dietitian, National Governing Body
    of United States Figure Skating
Manager, Nutrition Sciences
Gerber Products Company
Fremont, Michigan

CONTENTS

FOREWORD

During my high school and college athletic career, it was usually forbidden to drink water at practices. The pregame meal was the traditional steak. How far we have advanced in the field of sports nutrition in the past 40 years!

At Georgia Tech, sports nutrition is given major emphasis. The preseason physicals include individual consultations with a nutritionist. Body composition is carefully assessed to keep the athletes' body fat in the desirable range.

I also work as a team physician for the Atlanta Braves. In the late 1980s, the national media made fun of several of our players, calling one "a tub of goo." A different atmosphere has existed in the 1990s, thanks to a new general manager. A strength coach travels with the team. Body mass index (BMI) and blood fats are followed. The players are much more fit and have performed accordingly.

The Braves' trainers are inundated with information from various vendors, trying to get them to use a certain sports drink, vitamin, or performance enhancer. I usually pass such information under the critical eye of my colleague, Chris Rosenbloom, PhD, RD, who has a unique ability to sift out the wheat from the chaff.

The 3rd edition of *Sports Nutrition: A Guide for the Professional Working with Active People* is a valuable asset to all medical personnel who work with athletes. It is authoritative, up-to-date, and well designed, under the guiding influence of Dr. Rosenbloom. It will also be of value to athletes who are trying to become the best they can be. This book is an important step in that direction.

John Davis Cantwell, MD
Medical Director,
    The Homer Rice Center for Sports Performance,
    Georgia Tech
President-Elect 2000,
    Association of Major League Baseball Team Physicians
Chief Medical Officer,
    1996 Olympic Games

PREFACE

Congratulations on your purchase of the third edition of *Sports Nutrition: A Guide for the Professional Working with Active People*. Developed under the able leadership of Christine A. Rosenbloom for the Sports, Cardiovascular, and Wellness Nutritionists (SCAN) dietetic practice group of The American Dietetic Association, this manual is an essential reference for food, nutrition, and other health professionals who work with active people of all ages and ability levels.

SCAN is proud to have brought together many of the field's most noted authors, educators, and researchers to contribute to this manual. Most of our authors and reviewers are SCAN members who dedicated many hours to bring you the most up-to-date research in the field of sports nutrition. You will read chapters written by Ironman triathletes, former elite figure skaters, USA gymnastics competitors, respected educators, and nutritionists who work directly with professional athletes, as well as by those who have years of experience counseling both elite and recreational athletes.

The science of sports nutrition is relatively new and ever changing. For that reason, this 3rd edition of *Sports Nutrition* is greatly expanded. It now offers more in-depth information on macronutrient requirements, an expanded section on assessment, and much more detail about working with special populations. Because it is so important to the longevity of our field, we have added a chapter on documenting sports nutrition outcomes. New chapters on nutrition through the life cycle—from elementary athletes through masters competitors, and a section on sports-specific nutrition recommendations make this book a resource that will not collect dust on your bookshelf.

Section 5, Tools and Resources for the Sports Nutritionist has replaced the traditional appendixes. It includes guidelines for evaluating sports nutrition information on the Internet, nutrition screening forms, glycemic indexes of commonly consumed foods, helpful Web site addresses, and much more. You will refer to this very useful section often.

Whether you are working with a professional athlete, a client in an employee fitness center, a recreational athlete with diabetes, or a youth soccer club, you will find your questions on fluids, vitamins/minerals, carbohydrates, protein, ergogenic aids, eating disorders, weight control, and more answered here. We hope that you find this manual helpful and easy to use.

We extend a special thanks to Editor Rosenbloom, PhD, RD for her time and talents devoted to this edition of *Sports Nutrition*. Her focus on research, her organizational skills, and her professional tenacity brought this edition to fruition. We also thank all of the authors and reviewers whose contributions are invaluable. As always, we thank The American Dietetic Association for its support of this project.

Ruth Carey, RD
SCAN Chair 1998-1999

Rita M. Johnson, PhD, RD, FADA
SCAN Chair 1999-2000

ACKNOWLEDGEMENTS

An editor is like a coach. And as the coach of the team that compiled the 3rd edition of *Sports Nutrition: A Guide for the Professional Working with Active People,* I want to acknowledge everyone who contributed to this project. Special thanks to:

- The SCAN leadership who, like a team's general manager, recognized the need for a revised manual and who eagerly shared their vision for the final product.
- The authors, or players, who shared their time, expertise, and talent. A scan of the names of contributors reveals a real "dream team" of sports nutrition professionals.
- My Georgia State University colleagues, Dea Baxter, Barbara Hopkins, Satya Jonnalagadda, and Jana Kicklighter; and my Georgia Tech colleagues, Rob Skinner and Mindy Millard-Stafford, who provided advice and support at all stages of the project.
- The athletes, coaches, and administrators of the Georgia Tech Athletic Association who have allowed me to be a part of their team for the past ten years.
- The Gatorade Company, which provided financial support for this edition.
- My husband, Rob, for his role as volunteer administrative assistant, fixer of all computer problems, and biggest fan.
- My editors at ADA, Betsy Hornick and Jude Clayton, who guided the project to completion.
- And lastly, the reviewers, our team's critics, whose watchful eye helped to shape the final product. Special thanks to Lyn Almon, Ellen Coleman, Suzanne Nelson Steen, and Patti Steinmuller who reviewed the entire manuscript, working diligently to assure high-quality information.

Christine A. Rosenbloom, PhD, RD
Associate Professor
  Georgia State University-Atlanta
Nutrition Consultant
  Georgia Tech Athletic Association

REVIEWERS

Lyn Almon, MSPH, RD
American Cancer Society
Atlanta, Georgia

Ellen Coleman, MA, MPH, RD
Nutrition Consultant
The Sport Clinic
Riverside, California

Sandra J. Gillespie, MMSc, RD
Diabetes Nutrition Specialist
Piedmont Hospital-Promina
Atlanta, Georgia

Craig A. Horswill, PhD
Senior Research Scientist
Gatorade Research and Development
Barrington, Illinois

Satya S. Jonnalagadda, PhD
Department of Nutrition
Georgia State University
Atlanta, Georgia

Susan M. Kleiner, PhD, RD
High Performance Nutrition
Mercer Island, Washington

D. Enette Larson, PhD, RD
Department of Nutrition Sciences
University of Alabama
Birmingham, Alabama

Amy Ogle, MS, RD
Nutrition Consultant
San Diego, California

Suzanne Nelson Steen, DSc, RD
Sports Nutritionist
University of Washington
Seattle, Washington

Patti Steinmuller, MS, RD
Department of Health and
  Human Development
Montana State University
Bozeman, Montana

Lynn Umbreit, MS, RD
Nutrition Consultant
Denver, Colorado

SECTION 1 NUTRIENT AND FLUID NEEDS OF ACTIVE PEOPLE

Understanding the physiology of exercise and the role of nutrients in exercise performance is essential for nutrition and fitness professionals working with active people. This knowledge has led to food and nutrition recommendations for active people to sustain exercise and even enhance performance. The challenge for nutrition professionals is translating this knowledge to help athletes obtain energy, fluid, and associated nutrients in the right amounts and at the right times. While this may seem like a relatively easy task, it is not. Actual nutrient requirements are influenced by many factors, including sport, body size and composition, gender, exercise intensity and duration, age, ambient temperature and humidity, conditioning level of the athlete, altitude, muscle type predominance, and individual genetic variability. This section lays the foundation for this book. It presents an overview of our current knowledge about exercise physiology and provides a concise look at the role of carbohydrate, protein, fat, vitamins, minerals, and fluids in exercise performance. Because of increasing popularity and interest in ergogenic aids, Section 1 closes with a review of twenty of the most popular dietary supplements and offers prudent recommendations for their use.

SECTION 1 CONTENTS

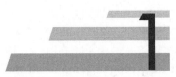

PHYSIOLOGY OF ANAEROBIC AND AEROBIC EXERCISE

Josephine Connolly-Schoonen, MS, RD

The energy to fuel physical movement and activity has its origin in the chemical bonds of food. This energy is stored and transferred within the body in many different ways. Eventually it is used to fuel all of the cells' activities, such as shortening or contracting muscle fibers, to facilitate physical movement. Physical performance, based on such factors as speed of muscle fiber contraction and number of muscle fibers contracted, depends largely on the energy available to the muscle fibers. Therefore, how the energy is stored and transferred is an essential determinant of physical performance. Dietary intake, as well as level of conditioning, genetic endowment, and type of physical activity performed, affects these processes. It is important to be aware of these processes and what affects them in order to develop individualized diets and training programs to optimize performance and overall health. This chapter focuses on the processes of energy storage and transfer.

ENERGY STORAGE

Energy is stored in the chemical bonds of macronutrients, dietary carbohydrates, fats, or proteins. However, the chemical energy in protein is not readily used as a fuel source for physical activity. The primary suppliers of chemical-bond energy reside in fats and carbohydrates. Dietary fats are digested to fatty acids and absorbed into the body. They may be used for a variety of synthetic processes or used immediately for energy. Excess fatty acids are converted back to triglycerides and largely stored in fat or adipose tissue, although some are stored in muscle tissue. There is essentially no limit to the amount of fat that can be stored, and there is, of course, large variability in people's fat storage levels. Fat stores represent at least 100 times the carbohydrate energy reserves.

Dietary carbohydrates are digested to glucose and other simple sugars and absorbed into the body. The simple sugars are converted into glucose. Glucose may be used for synthetic processes or for energy. Excess glucose molecules are then rearranged into long chains of glycogen and stored in liver and muscle tissue. The amount of glycogen that can be stored is limited to approximately 100 g in the adult liver and 375 g in muscles. Aerobic conditioning can increase muscle storage levels five-fold (1). Dietary carbohydrates eaten in excess of the amount necessary to maximally fill potential glycogen sites are converted into fatty acids and stored in adipose tissue.

By weight, fats provide more than twice the amount of energy, measured in kilocalories, than either carbohydrates or proteins. Therefore, fat is an efficient way to store energy while minimizing body weight that has to be carried—an evolutionary advantage. The energy in stored fat or glycogen remains in the chemical bonds of these substances.

One other storage form of energy that is readily used to fuel physical activity is indirectly derived from chemical-bond energy in food. It is called creatine phosphate or phosphocreatine. The body makes creatine phosphate and stores small amounts of this compound in the muscle. Creatine supplements increase intramuscular levels of creatine and creatine phosphate significantly (2). Supplemental creatine as an ergogenic aid is discussed in detail in Chapter 7, Ergogenic Aids.

THE ENERGY CURRENCY OF THE CELL

Adenosine triphosphate (ATP) is the energy currency of the cell. It is the intermediary between all forms of stored energy and cellular work. It is the only form of fuel a cell can use for all of the biological work it must do, such as contract muscle fibers, build new tissue, and transport minerals. Therefore, the chemical-bond energy that is stored in various forms is first transferred to ATP. ATP then directly transfers the energy to the structure or compound within the cell that requires it and the work is completed. During this process ATP loses energy. The high-energy ATP is reformed, again using chemical-bond energy from dietary fats or carbohydrates stored as fatty acids or glycogen, respectively. ATP is continuously formed, used, and reformed. The body stores only small amounts of ATP—about 80 to 100 g—enough energy to sustain maximum physical effort for a few seconds (3).

When the rate of energy metabolism increases, and therefore the demand for energy and ATP increases, the body immediately begins to break down energy stores. Different stored forms of energy can be used at the same time. The mix of stored energy forms used, as well as the method used to transfer the energy to ATP, depends on the availability of stored fuels, duration of the activity, type of activity, intensity of the activity, conditions in the cell, and training level of the individual.

ENERGY TRANSFER

There are three systems used to transfer stored energy to ATP:

1. The phosphagen system
2. The anaerobic glycolysis system (sometimes called the lactic acid system)
3. The aerobic system

The Phosphagen System

The phosphagen system is the first system used to transfer energy to ATP when there is an increase in energy demand. This system does not require that oxygen be present. It is a direct, quick process. The chemical bond energy in the creatine phosphate molecule is transferred directly to an ATP molecule through an enzyme-catalyzed reaction. The amount of creatine phosphate stored in the body is about 4 to 6 times greater than the amount of ATP stored (3). The combined energy stores of ATP and creatine phosphate are able to fuel muscle contraction for only a short time, depending on the intensity of exercise. For a 70-kg person, it is enough to fuel a 1-minute brisk walk or perform a maximum-effort sprint for 5 to 6 seconds (3). This system is also important to fuel short-burst, all-out efforts in many sporting events, such as weightlifting, track and field events, a slam-dunk in basketball, and a serve in tennis. When the demand for energy persists and the ATP and creatine phosphate stores are depleted, the accumulation of the byproducts of ATP breakdown initiates the anaerobic glycolysis system. This system provides energy at a slower rate and, therefore, the sustainable level of effort is somewhat decreased.

The Anaerobic Glycolysis System

The anaerobic glycolysis system allows for the continued production of ATP for several minutes (60 to 180 seconds), when adequate oxygen for aerobic metabolism is not available in the active muscles (3). Three scenarios when this may occur include the following.

1. At the start of an event, some time is required for the cardiovascular system to operate at full capacity to bring oxygenated blood to working cells. For example, this occurs at the beginning of a 10-km race or marathon.
2. During a short, high-intensity event, the cardiovascular system may not have adequate time to increase its capacity sufficiently to provide adequate oxygen to the cells and facilitate aerobic metabolism. Therefore, the anaerobic glycolysis system provides the majority of energy for the working muscles, such as in a 400-meter sprint.
3. Another reason for an inadequate oxygen supply may be a temporary increase in the intensity of the activity that exceeds the capacity of the cardiovascular- and aerobic-energy production systems. In such cases the anaerobic glycolysis system can play an important role in briefly boosting ATP production. Examples include a basketball player stealing a ball, dribbling down the court, and dunking the ball for a basket. Another example would be the end of a long aerobic event, such as a sprint to the finish line at the end of a 10-km race.

The anaerobic glycolysis system uses only glucose for fuel. The glucose may be derived from locally stored glycogen or from glucose in the bloodstream. During this process, glucose is partially broken down to two molecules of pyruvate. This is a 10-step, rapid process that results in the direct production of two or three ATP molecules. If the glucose is derived from the bloodstream, an additional ATP is required early in the process. Therefore, the net gain is only two ATPs. In addition to ATPs, two nicotinamide adenine dinucleotide (NAD^+) molecules are reduced to $NADH + H^+$. These molecules can be processed later in the aerobic system when oxygen is available to yield three additional ATPs each. Pyruvate can be converted to lactic acid, and this process allows for the continuation of the anaerobic-glycolytic pathway by resupplying necessary intermediate compounds. However, the build-up of lactic acid eventually decreases the pH within the cell and hinders anaerobic energy production. The accumulation of lactic acid also prevents the use of fatty acids for energy by the aerobic system and is associated with fatigue. See *Figure 1.1* for an abbreviated schematic.

FIGURE 1.1   The Anaerobic Glycolytic Energy System

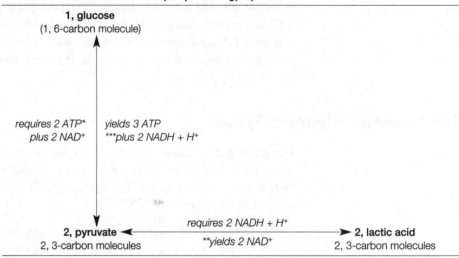

1, glucose
(1, 6-carbon molecule)

requires 2 ATP*   *yields 3 ATP*
plus 2 NAD⁺   ****plus 2 NADH + H⁺*

2, pyruvate ←   *requires 2 NADH + H⁺*   → **2, lactic acid**
2, 3-carbon molecules   ***yields 2 NAD⁺*   2, 3-carbon molecules

* If the original glucose source is locally stored glycogen, then only 1 ATP is required.

** This regenerates the NAD+ necessary for glycolysis.

*** The NADH + H⁺ can be used later in the aerobic pathways when oxygen is available to produce more ATPs.

Much of the lactic acid formed during exercise is released into the bloodstream, cleared, and rapidly metabolized by cells with high-oxidative capacity such as the heart. Lactic acid production increases as the intensity of exercise increases. When the lactic acid is produced faster than it can be cleared, it accumulates rapidly in the blood. This lactic acid build-up is called the blood lactate threshold. For trained athletes this build-up does not occur until approximately 70% to 80% of their maximum aerobic exercise capacity. For untrained individuals this build-up occurs at approximately 50% to 60% of their maximum aerobic exercise capacity. With training, athletes are able to use their aerobic metabolic system more readily, thereby delaying the production of lactic acid. They are also better able to clear lactic acid.

At rest virtually all of the body's energy needs are met aerobically. With the initiation of physical activity, energy needs rapidly increase, and the oxygen supply to the active muscles is not adequate to support this increased demand for energy through aerobic pathways. Therefore, until the rate of oxygen delivery increases, more energy is derived from anaerobic glycolysis than from aerobic metabolism in active muscles. As activity continues, however, the proportion of energy derived from aerobic metabolism increases. Short-burst sprint activities lasting approximately 1 to 2 minutes, such as 50-meter and 100-meter swimming events, are fueled primarily by anaerobic ATP production. In addition, this system is important to fuel intermittent, high-intensity bursts of activity important in sports such as football, basketball, and soccer. The aerobic system is much more efficient than the anaerobic system with regard to ATP production. However, the rate of ATP production is slower and, therefore, the sustainable level of effort is again somewhat decreased.

The Aerobic System

The aerobic system can use stored energy in the form of carbohydrates (glucose), fats (fatty acids), or proteins (amino acids) as energy sources. This system requires that adequate oxygen be available within the cell to participate in the final reaction of this system. This system has two parts—the Krebs Cycle and the electron transport chain. In the Krebs Cycle, ATP is formed directly. In addition, electrons are generated and carried to the electron transport chain by carriers, either by the reduction of nicotinamide adenine dinucleotide (NAD^+ to $NADH + H^+$) or flavin adenine dinucleotide (FAD to $FADH_2$). The electron transport chain consists of a series of coordinated oxidation-reduction reactions. During these reactions energy is released and captured in the formation of ATP molecules. Ultimately, oxygen accepts the electrons and is reduced to form water. Each $NADH + H^+$ is associated with the production of three ATPs. Since $FADH_2$ enters the electron transport chain midway through the chain, it is associated only with the production of two ATPs.

When using carbohydrate as an energy source, this system is a continuation of the anaerobic glycolysis system.

1. The two pyruvate molecules formed at the end of the glycolytic pathway are converted to acetyl-CoA and funneled into the Krebs Cycle. During this conversion one NAD per pyruvate is reduced to one $NADH + H^+$, and shuttles electrons over to the electron transport chain to yield three ATPs.
2. Within the Krebs Cycle, the following high-energy compounds are formed per pyruvate: three other $NADH + H^+$, one $FADH_2$, and one ATP. The three $NADH + H^+$ per pyruvate lead to production of nine ATPs in the electron transport chain, and the one $FADH_2$ per pyruvate is associated with two ATPs.
3. Therefore, the complete breakdown of pyruvate leads to 15 ATPs.
4. Since two pyruvate molecules are generated from one glucose molecule, this is doubled to 30 ATPs.
5. In addition, the anaerobic breakdown of glucose yields two ATPs directly and six additional ATPs from the complete aerobic metabolism of the two $NADH + H^+$ produced in the glycolytic pathway.
6. Therefore, the complete aerobic metabolism of a glucose molecule yields 38 ATP molecules.

Figure 1.2 illustrates these steps.

FIGURE 1.2   The Aerobic Energy System

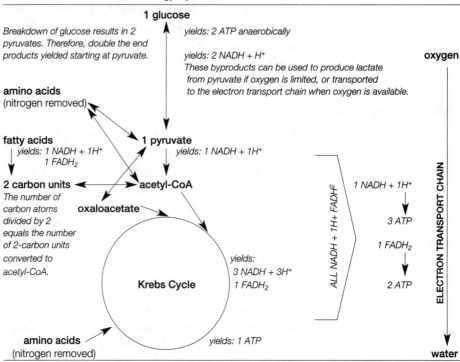

Fatty acids can also be used in the aerobic system, and stored fats represent an almost unlimited supply of energy—90,000 to 120,000 kcal at the lower range. This is in contrast to the approximate 1,000 to 2,000 kcal of stored carbohydrate energy, about 1% to 2% of the energy stored as fat (3,4). The majority of fatty acids are stored in fat cells, although fat is also stored directly in muscles and circulates in the bloodstream.

When using fat as the energy source for aerobic metabolism, stored triglycerides are first broken down to three fatty acids and a glycerol molecule. If the fatty acids are in fat cells, they diffuse into the bloodstream and attach to transporter albumin molecules. They are then carried in the bloodstream to active tissue. The initiation of exercise leads to the release of hormones such as epinephrine and glucagon. Such hormones activate the breakdown of triglycerides and facilitate the delivery of fatty acids to active muscles. The use of fatty acids in the aerobic energy pathways spares glycogen. This is important because glycogen energy stores are relatively small compared to fat energy stores. Therefore, the primary use of fat allows cells to save glycogen stores for periods of exercise when oxygen delivery is inadequate and the cell must switch to anaerobic energy metabolism. (Recall that only glucose can be used for anaerobic metabolism.)

Fatty acids consist of long chains of carbon molecules, typically 16 to 18 carbon atoms, although chains can be as long as 24 carbon atoms. These long chains are first broken down to 2-carbon acetyl units through the process of beta-oxidation.

1. A fatty acid molecule is first activated to begin the process of beta-oxidation, which requires one ATP.
2. For each 2-carbon unit cleaved off the fatty acid molecule, one $NADH + H^+$ and one $FADH_2$ are produced and shuttled to the electron transport chain to yield three ATPs and two ATPs, respectively.
3. The acetyl unit is converted to an acetyl-CoA and enters the Krebs cycle to yield the following high-energy compounds: one ATP, three $NADH + H^+$, and one $FADH_2$. The three $NADH + H^+$ lead to production of nine ATPs in the electron transport chain, and the one $FADH_2$ is associated with two ATPs.
4. Therefore, there are 17 ATPs generated per 2-carbon unit cleaved off the long-chain fatty acid molecule.
5. Since cleavage of the last 4-carbon unit yields two 2-carbon units, there are five less ATPs produced from the last 2-carbon unit since it is not cleaved from a chain.
6. Therefore, the number of ATPs produced from a fatty acid can be calculated using this formula: [(total number of carbon units/2 − 1)17 + 12] − 1. As an example, an 18-carbon fatty acid would yield 147 ATPs − [(18/2 − 1)17 + 12] − 1 = 147.

The glycerol molecule resulting from the breakdown of a triglyceride also yields energy. It is a 3-carbon unit that is funneled into the anaerobic glycolytic pathway approximately midway down, and yields one acetyl-CoA that enters into the Krebs cycle. It is associated with the production of the following high-energy compounds: three ATPs, five $NADH + H^+$, and one $FADH_2$. The five $NADH + H^+$ lead to the production of 15 ATPs in the electron transport chain, and the one $FADH_2$ is associated with two ATPs. Therefore, a glycerol molecule yields 20 ATPs, and a triglyceride with three 18-carbon fatty acids and a glycerol molecule would yield 461 ATPs. (See *Figure 1.2.*) Fats are obviously a rich energy source to fuel physical activity, but it is important to note that they can only be metabolized aerobically. If adequate oxygen is not available, cells revert to carbohydrate metabolism for energy production.

Protein is usually spared from entering energy production pathways and is conserved for tissue maintenance, repair, and growth. However, it can be used for the production of glucose or energy when glycogen stores are reduced, since it occurs with limited carbohydrate or total calorie intake or with prolonged exercise. Athletes may not fully replenish glycogen stores after training sessions, leading to a gradual depletion of glycogen stores. In these cases, protein stored in muscles can be called upon to synthesize glucose and to provide energy substrates. This is not desirable because it leads to decreased muscle mass and an increased workload on the kidneys, which must handle the byproducts of protein breakdown.

Protein is made up of amino acids. Some amino acids have long carbon chains, which can yield energy. They are referred to as branched-chain amino acids and include leucine, isoleucine, and valine. Two other amino acids are involved with energy pathways—glutamine and aspartate. Before amino acids can be funneled into energy pathways, their nitrogen-containing groups must be removed. Excess nitrogen is eventually removed from the body by the kidney as urine. Since the formation of urine requires water, excess breakdown of protein increases the risk for dehydration. Different amino acids are funneled into the energy pathways at different points. The highest point they can enter is at the level of pyruvate. Therefore, the most ATPs that can be produced is 15 ATPs. (See *Figure 1.2.*) However, there is a metabolic cost of excreting the nitrogen and the physiological cost of decreased muscle protein.

CARBOHYDRATE, FAT, AND PROTEIN ENERGY METABOLISM

The storage of energy-containing nutrients—carbohydrates (glucose), proteins (amino acids), and fats (fatty acids)—is integrated. Excesses of all these nutrients are stored as fats; however, stored fats cannot be turned back into carbohydrates or proteins. Glucose can be used to synthesize amino acids and some amino acids can be used to synthesize glucose; however, there are energy costs for these processes. For example, there is a 5% loss of energy when storing glucose as glycogen in muscles instead of using it immediately to produce ATP. This cost increases to 28% when converting glucose to fatty acids for storage (5).

The energy systems using these nutrients are not simply used sequentially, with the ATP-CP system first, anaerobic glycolysis second, and aerobic metabolism last. All systems and energy substrates are used simultaneously, with relative contributions varying according to such factors as storage levels, the cellular environment, and the activity level. For example, oxygen availability strongly influences what substrates are used for energy. There are 8.2 ATPs produced per carbon atom of a fatty acid, and only 6.2 ATPs produced per carbon atom of a glucose molecule. However, only 5.7 ATPs are produced per oxygen when metabolizing fatty acids, compared with 6.3 ATPs produced per oxygen when metabolizing glucose. Therefore, when oxygen is limited, glucose is the preferred fuel for aerobic metabolism and the only fuel used for energy metabolism anaerobically. Hormonal changes due to diet and exercise strongly influence flow through the energy pathways.

Fatty acids are metabolized aerobically to produce energy. However, the use of fatty acids depends on the simultaneous flow of carbohydrates through the energy pathways to regenerate the necessary intermediate compounds in the Krebs Cycle. Without adequate dietary carbohydrates, fatty acids are rerouted to a different metabolic pathway. Therefore, instead of leading to ATP production, fatty acids lead to the production of ketones. Only some tissues, such as the brain, can use ketones for subsequent energy production. If carbohydrate stores are low, ketones can build up and cause fatigue and metabolic imbalances.

MUSCLE FIBER TYPE

There are two basic types of muscle fibers. Type I, or slow-twitch, muscle fibers have a relatively slow speed of contraction and primarily use aerobic metabolic pathways. They have a lot of mitochondria with high levels of enzymes necessary for the aerobic energy production pathways (ie, the enzymes necessary in the Krebs Cycle and the electron transport chain). They also have a higher density of capillaries to supply them with oxygen and energy substrates, and to remove byproducts such as lactic acid. Athletes with a large amount of type I muscle fibers have higher blood lactate thresholds because they can more readily funnel pyruvate into the Krebs cycle and less pyruvate is converted into lactic acid. Therefore, they facilitate long duration activities and take longer to fatigue. Type II, or fast-twitch, muscle fibers have a relatively fast speed of contraction and have a high capacity for fast anaerobic energy production. Type II muscle fibers are subdivided into categories, two of which are well defined. Type IIa muscle fibers have a high speed of contraction and fairly well developed aerobic and anaerobic energy production systems. The type IIb muscle fiber types are the fastest, most glycolytic fiber types. Most activities require a combination of fast- and slow-twitch muscle fibers, sustainable relatively slow muscle contractions with occasional short bursts of fast muscle contraction. Activities that require the recruitment of more type II muscle fibers, such as sprinting and high-intensity stop and go movements, depend more heavily on stored carbohydrate energy substrates. Therefore, these activities are associated with a more rapid depletion of glycogen stores. The ratio of slow-twitch to fast-twitch muscle fibers depends largely on genetic predisposition. On average 45% to 55% of people's muscle fibers are slow-twitch fibers. However, training can affect the distribution of muscle fiber types. Athletes trained in sports requiring a high aerobic energy production, such as long-distance running, have up to 90% to 95% slow-twitch muscle fibers in the muscles engaged in the activity (3).

The chemical bond energy of food is stored as fats and carbohydrates, and to a lesser extent as protein. This chemical bond energy is transferred to ATP, which directly transfers energy to the structure or compound in the cell that needs it. Three different systems can be used to transfer energy to ATP: the phosphagen system, the anaerobic system, and the aerobic system. The phosphagen system transfers energy most quickly, but it has a very limited capacity. The anaerobic system can also transfer energy relatively quickly; however, the end products of this pathway decrease the pH within the cell and limit its continuation. The aerobic system transfers energy the most slowly, but it has the greatest transfer capacity due to the fact that it can use carbohydrate or fat as energy substrates. These systems may be used simultaneously within different cells in the body, and the cellular environment and energy demands determine the preferred energy transfer system. Oxygen availability and energy substrate availability are two important factors in the cellular environment. For muscle cells, the type of muscle fiber and its inherent characteristics are also key factors in the determination of the energy transfer system. Dietary manipulations and training can change the cellular environment and strongly influence the capacity of the energy transfer systems, as well as the storage of energy substrates.

REFERENCES

1. Williams MH. *Nutrition for Health, Fitness, and Sport*. 5th ed. Boston, Mass: McGraw-Hill; 1999.
2. Plisk SS, Kreider RB. Creatine controversy. *J Strength and Cond Res*. 1999;21:14-23.
3. McArdle W, Katch F, Katch V. *Exercise Physiology*. Baltimore, Md: Williams and Wilkins; 1996.
4. Linscheer WG, Vergroesen AJ. Lipids. In: Shils ME, Olson JA, Shike M, eds. *Modern Nutrition in Health and Disease*. 8th ed. Philadelphia, Penn: Lea & Febiger; 1994:47-88.
5. Macdonald I. Carbohydrates. In: Shils M, Olson JA, Shike M, eds. *Modern Nutrition in Health and Disease*. 8th ed. Philadelphia, Penn: Lea & Febiger; 1994:36-46.

CARBOHYDRATE AND EXERCISE

Ellen Coleman, MA, MPH, RD

Adequate carbohydrate stores (muscle and liver glycogen and blood glucose) are critical for optimum athletic performance. Consuming adequate carbohydrate on a daily basis is necessary to replenish muscle and liver glycogen between daily training sessions or competitive events. Consuming carbohydrate prior to exercise can help performance by "topping off" muscle and liver glycogen stores. Furthermore, consuming carbohydrate during exercise can improve performance by maintaining blood glucose levels and carbohydrate oxidation.

GENERAL CONSIDERATIONS

A high-carbohydrate food may be classified by the type of carbohydrate (simple versus complex), by the form of carbohydrate (liquid versus solid), or by the glycemic index of the carbohydrate (low, moderate, or high). The "simple" versus "complex" classification and "liquid" versus "solid" classifications do not indicate the effect of carbohydrate-rich foods and fluids on blood glucose and insulin levels. The glycemic index classification, however, does indicate the actual effects of carbohydrate-rich foods and fluids on blood glucose and insulin levels (1).

The glycemic index is a ranking of foods based on their measured blood glucose response compared to a reference food, either glucose or white bread. The glycemic index is calculated by measuring the incremental area under the blood glucose curve following ingestion of a test food providing 50 g of carbohydrate, compared with the area under the blood glucose curve following an equal carbohydrate intake from the reference food. All tests are conducted after an overnight fast (1).

Generally, foods are divided into those that have a high glycemic index (glucose, bread, potatoes, breakfast cereal, sports drinks), a moderate glycemic index (sucrose, soft drinks, oats, tropical fruits such as bananas and mangos), or a low glycemic index (fructose, milk, yogurt, lentils, pasta, cold climate fruits such as apples and oranges). Tables of the glycemic index of a large number of foods have been published internationally (2). (See the Tools section for a listing of the glycemic index of commonly consumed foods.)

The glycemic index reflects the rate of digestion and absorption of a carbohydrate-rich food. Thus, the glycemic index is influenced by the food form (including particle size, presence of intact grains, texture, and viscosity), the degree of food processing and cooking, the presence of fructose or lactose (both have a low glycemic index), the ratio of amylopectin and amylose in starch (amylose has a slower rate of digestion), starch-protein or starch-fat interactions, and the presence of antinutrients such as phytates and lectins (1).

It has been suggested that manipulating the glycemic index of foods and meals may enhance carbohydrate availability and improve athletic performance. For example, low glycemic index carbohydrate-rich foods may be recommended before exercise to promote sustained carbohydrate availability. Moderate to high glycemic index carbohydrate-rich foods may be recommended during exercise to promote carbohydrate oxidation and following exercise to promote glycogen repletion.

The glycemic index concept has limitations. The glycemic index is based on equal grams of carbohydrate (50 g), not average serving sizes. The numbers that are available are also largely based on tests using single foods. The blood glucose response to high glycemic foods may be blunted when combined with low glycemic foods in the meal. However, the glycemic index can be applied to mixed meals by taking a weighted mean of the glycemic index of the carbohydrate-rich foods that make up the meal (1).

The glycemic index may be useful in sports by helping to fine-tune food choices. However, further studies are warranted. The glycemic index should not be used exclusively to provide guidelines for carbohydrate and food intake before, during, and after exercise. There are other features of foods that are important to the athlete, such as the food's nutritional content and the practical issues of palatability, portability, cost, gastric comfort, and ease of preparation. Since food choices are specific to the individual athlete and exercise situation, athletes should choose foods according to their nutrition goals (1).

CARBOHYDRATE AVAILABILITY DURING EXERCISE

Muscle glycogen represents the major source of carbohydrate in the body (300 to 400 g or 1,200 to 1,600 kcal), followed by liver glycogen (75 to 100 g or 300 to 400 kcal) and, lastly, blood glucose (25 g or 100 kcal). These amounts vary widely among individuals, depending on factors such as dietary intake and state of training. Untrained individuals have muscle glycogen stores that are roughly 80 to 90 mmol/kg of wet muscle weight. Endurance athletes have muscle glycogen stores of 130 to 135 mmol/kg of wet muscle weight. Carbohydrate loading increases muscle glycogen stores to 210 to 230 mmol/kg of wet muscle weight (3).

Exercise energetics dictate that carbohydrate is the preferred fuel for exercise intensities at and above 65% of VO_2max—the levels at which most athletes train and compete. Fat oxidation cannot supply adenosine triphosphate (ATP) rapidly enough to support such high-intensity exercise. While it is possible to exercise at light to moderate levels (<60% of VO_2max) with low levels of muscle glycogen and blood glucose, it is impossible to meet the ATP requirements necessary for heavy exercise when these fuels are depleted. The utilization of muscle glycogen is most rapid during the early stages of exercise and is exponentially related to exercise intensity (3).

There is a strong relationship between the pre-exercise muscle glycogen content and the length of time that exercise can be performed at 70% of VO_2max. The greater the pre-exercise glycogen content, the greater the endurance potential. Bergstrom et al (4) compared the exercise time to exhaustion at 75% of VO_2max after 3 days of three diets varying in carbohydrate content. A mixed diet (50% calories from carbohydrate) produced a muscle glycogen content of 106 mmol/kg and enabled the subjects to exercise 115 minutes. A low-carbohydrate diet (less than 5% of calories from carbohydrate) produced a muscle glycogen content of 38 mmol/kg and supported only 1 hour of exercise. However, a high-carbohydrate diet (≥82% of calories from carbohydrate) provided 204 mmol/kg of muscle glycogen and enabled the subjects to exercise for 170 minutes.

Liver glycogen stores maintain blood glucose levels both at rest and during exercise. At rest, the brain and central nervous system (CNS) utilize most of the blood glucose, and the muscle accounts for less than 20% of blood glucose utilization. During exercise, however, muscle glucose uptake can increase 30-fold, depending on exercise intensity and duration. Initially, the majority of hepatic glucose output comes from glycogenolysis; however, as the exercise duration increases and liver glycogen declines, the contribution of glucose from gluconeogenesis increases (3).

At the beginning of exercise, hepatic glucose output matches the increased muscle glucose uptake so that blood glucose levels remain near resting levels. Although muscle glycogen is the primary source of carbohydrate during exercise intensities above 65% of VO_2max, blood glucose becomes an increasingly important source of carbohydrate as muscle glycogen stores decline. When hepatic glucose output can no longer keep up with muscle glucose uptake during prolonged exercise, the blood glucose drops. While a few athletes experience central nervous system symptoms typical of hypoglycemia, most athletes note local muscular fatigue and have to reduce their exercise intensity (3).

Liver glycogen stores can be emptied by a 15-hour fast and can fall from a typical level of 490 mmol on a mixed diet to 60 mmol on a low-carbohydrate diet. A high-carbohydrate diet can increase liver glycogen content to about 900 mmol (3).

TRAINING RECOMMENDATIONS

Building up and maintaining glycogen stores during training require a carbohydrate-rich diet. When adequate carbohydrate is not consumed on a daily basis between training sessions, the pre-exercise muscle glycogen content gradually declines and training or competitive performance may be impaired. Daily restoration of the body's carbohydrate reserves should be a priority for athletes involved in intense training.

Costill et al evaluated glycogen synthesis on a 45% carbohydrate diet during 3 successive days of running 16.1 km at 80% of VO_2max (5). pre-exercise muscle glycogen levels started at 110 mmol/kg and fell to 88 mmol/kg on Day 2 and 66 mmol/kg on Day 3. Another study out of Costill's lab found that a diet providing 525 to 648 g of carbohydrate promoted glycogen synthesis of 70 to 80 mmol/kg and provided near maximal repletion of muscle glycogen within 24 hours (6).

Fallowfield and Williams (7) also evaluated the importance of a high-carbohydrate intake on recovery from prolonged exercise. Their subjects ran at 70% of VO_2max for 90 minutes or until volitional fatigue, whichever came first. During the next 22.5 hours, the runners consumed isocaloric diets containing either 5.8 or 8.8 g of carbohydrate/kg. After the rest period the runners ran at the same intensity to assess endurance capacity. Those who consumed 8.8 g of carbohydrate/kg were able to match their running time from the first race. Even though the two diets were isocaloric, the running time of those who consumed only 5.8 g of carbohydrate/kg decreased by more than 15 minutes.

For many athletes the energy and carbohydrate needs of training are greater than the requirements of competition. Some athletes involuntarily fail to increase caloric intake to meet the energy demands of increased training. Costill et al (8) studied the effects of 10 days of increased training volume at a high intensity on muscle glycogen and swimming performance. Six swimmers self-selected a diet containing 4,700 calories per day and 8.2 g of carbohydrate/kg per day, while four swimmers self-selected a diet containing only 3,700 calories per day and 5.3 g of carbohydrate/kg per day. These four swimmers could not tolerate the heavier training demands and swam at significantly slower speeds, presumably due to a 20% decline in muscle glycogen.

The feeling of sluggishness associated with muscle glycogen depletion is often referred to as "staleness" and blamed on overtraining. Athletes who train exhaustively on successive days must consume adequate carbohydrate and energy to decrease the threat of fatigue caused by the cumulative depletion of muscle glycogen.

Glycogen depletion associated with training can occur during training in sports which require repeated, near-maximal bursts of effort (such as football, basketball, and soccer) as well as during endurance exercise. A revealing sign of glycogen depletion is when the athlete has difficulty maintaining a normal exercise intensity. A sudden weight loss of several pounds (due to glycogen and water loss) may accompany glycogen depletion.

A review of the literature by Sherman and Wimer (9) questions the assumption that a high-carbohydrate diet optimizes training adaptation and athletic performance. They report that the relationship between muscle glycogen depletion and exhaustion is strongest at moderate training intensities (65% to 85% of VO_2max). However, Sherman and Wimer note that it is well established that low blood glucose, and muscle and/or liver glycogen concentrations can contribute to fatigue during other types of exercise. Because dietary carbohydrate contributes directly to maintenance of body carbohydrate reserves, Sherman and Wimer recommend continuing to advise athletes to eat a high-carbohydrate diet. They also recommend watching for signs of staleness during training and taking note of those athletes whose dietary habits make them more prone to glycogen depletion (9).

It is suggested that athletes who train heavily consume 7 to 10 g of carbohydrate/kg per day (10). The typical American diet supplies about 4 to 5 g of carbohydrate/kg per day. An intake of 6 to 7 g of carbohydrate/kg per day is sufficient when the athlete exercises hard (≥70% of VO_2max) for about 1 hour per day. An intake of 8 to 10 g of carbohydrate/kg per day is recommended when the athlete exercises hard for several hours or more per day. See *Box 2.1*.

BOX 2.1   Carbohydrate Recommendations for Athletes

The typical US diet supplies 4 to 5 g of carbohydrate/kg per day.

Recommended intake for most athletes:

- 7 to 10 g of carbohydrate/kg per day
- 6 to 7 g/kg for 1 hour of training per day
- 8 g/kg for 2 hours of training per day
- 10 g/kg for 3 hours of training per day
- 12 to 13 g/kg for 4 hours or more of training per day

Some athletes may need to reduce fat intake to below 30% of total calories to obtain 8 to 10 g of carbohydrate/kg per day. Sugar intake may be increased to meet the increased carbohydrate requirement, but the majority of the carbohydrate should come from complex carbohydrates. They are more nutrient-dense and compared to sugary foods provide more B vitamins necessary for energy metabolism as well as more fiber and iron. Sugar, however, contributes to tooth decay and many products that are high in sugar are also high in fat.

Athletes should consume sufficient calories in addition to carbohydrate. Consumption of a reduced-energy diet will impair endurance performance due to muscle and liver glycogen depletion. Adequate carbohydrate intake is also important for athletes in high-power activities (eg, wrestling, gymnastics, and dance) who have lost weight due to negative energy balances (10).

Desire for weight loss and consumption of low-energy diets are prevalent among athletes in high-power activities. Negative-energy balance can harm high-power performance due to impaired acid-base balance, reduced glycoloytic enzyme levels, selective atrophy of Type II muscle fibers, and abnormal sarcoplasmic reticulum function. Adequate dietary carbohydrate may ameliorate some of the damaging effects of energy restriction on the muscle (10).

Athletes participating in ultraendurance events (those lasting over 4 hours) have the highest carbohydrate requirements. (See Chapter 48, Ultraendurance Sports.) Saris et al studied food intake and energy expenditure during the Tour de France (11). In this demanding 22-day, 2,400-mile race, the cyclists consumed an average of 850 g of carbohydrate per day or 12.3 g/kg per day. About 30% of the total energy consumed was provided by high-carbohydrate beverages. Brouns et al (12,13) evaluated the effect of a simulated Tour de France study on food and fluid intake, energy balance, and substrate oxidation. Although the cyclists consumed 630 g of carbohydrate (8.6 g/kg per day), they oxidized 850 g of carbohydrate per day (11.6 g/kg per day). In spite of ad libitum intake of conventional foods, the cyclists were unable to ingest sufficient carbohydrate and calories to compensate for their increased energy expenditure. When the diet was supplemented with a 20% carbohydrate beverage, carbohydrate intake increased to 16 g/kg per day and carbohydrate oxidation rose to 13 g/kg per day.

Ultraendurance athletes who require over 600 g of carbohydrate per day should consider supplementing their dietary intake with high-carbohydrate beverages if they cannot eat enough conventional foods to meet their carbohydrate and energy requirements (13). Both Saris and Brouns recommend that ultraendurance athletes in training or competition consume 12 to 13 g of carbohydrate/kg per day. They also suggest that this range represents the maximum contribution of carbohydrate to energy metabolism during extreme ultraendurance exercise (11).

MUSCLE GLYCOGEN SUPERCOMPENSATION

During endurance exercise lasting 90 to 120 minutes at 70% of VO_2max (eg, running a marathon), muscle glycogen stores become progressively lower. When they drop to critically low levels (the point of glycogen depletion), high-intensity exercise cannot be maintained. In practical terms the athlete is exhausted and must either stop exercising or drastically reduce the intensity of exercise. Muscle glycogen depletion is a well-recognized limitation to endurance exercise. Athletes using glycogen supercompensation techniques (carbohydrate loading) can nearly double their muscle glycogen stores.

The carbohydrate-loading sequence was originally a week-long regimen starting with an exhaustive training session 1 week before competition. For the next 3 days, the athlete consumed a low-carbohydrate diet, yet continued exercising to lower muscle glycogen stores even further. On the 3 days prior to competition, the athlete rested and ate a high-carbohydrate diet to promote glycogen supercompensation. This regimen had many drawbacks. Three days of reduced carbohydrate intake often caused hypoglycemia and ketosis with associated nausea, fatigue, and irritability. The dietary manipulations also proved to be too cumbersome for many athletes.

The revised method of carbohydrate loading proposed by Sherman et al eliminates many of the problems associated with the old regimen (14). On the sixth day before the event, the athlete trains at 70% of VO_2max for 90 minutes. On the fifth and fourth days before the event, the athlete trains for 40 minutes at 70% of VO_2 max. The athlete trains for 20 minutes at 70% of VO_2max on the third and second day before the event, and rests the day before the event. During the first 3 days, the athlete consumes a normal diet providing about 5 g of carbohydrate/kg per day. During the last 3 days, the athlete consumes a high-carbohydrate diet providing 10 g of carbohydrate/kg per day. (See *Table 2.1* for some guidelines related to carbohydrate loading.) It is essential that training be reduced prior to competition. The final 3 days, when the athlete tapers and eats a high-carbohydrate diet, is the real "loading" phase of the regimen. This modified regimen results in muscle glycogen stores equal to those provided by the classic carbohydrate-loading regimen.

TABLE 2.1   Carbohydrate-loading Guidelines

Day	Training (70% of VO_2max)	Diet
1	90 minutes	5 g of carbohydrate/kg
2	40 minutes	5 g of carbohydrate/kg
3	40 minutes	5 g of carbohydrate/kg
4	20 minutes	10 g of carbohydrate/kg
5	20 minutes	10 g of carbohydrate/kg
6	Rest	10 g of carbohydrate/kg
7	Competition	

In a field study conducted by Karlsson and Saltin, runners participated in a 30-km race after eating a normal diet or high-carbohydrate diet (15). The high-carbohydrate diet provided muscle glycogen levels of 193 mmol/kg, compared to 94 mmol/kg for the normal diet. All runners covered the 30-km distance faster (by about 8 minutes) when they began the race with high muscle glycogen stores. Carbohydrate loading enables the athlete to maintain high-intensity exercise longer but will not affect pace for the first hour of the event.

Endurance training promotes muscle glycogen supercompensation by increasing the activity of glycogen synthase—the enzyme responsible for glycogen storage. The athlete must be endurance-trained or the regimen will not be effective. Since glycogen stores are specific to the muscle groups used, the exercise to deplete the stores must be the same as the athlete's competitive event.

A commercial, high-carbohydrate liquid supplement can be added if the athlete has difficulty consuming enough carbohydrate through food. Athletes who have diabetes or hypertriglyceridemia may have medical complications if they carbohydrate load and should obtain medical clearance before attempting the regimen.

For each gram of glycogen stored, additional water is stored. While some athletes note a feeling of stiffness and heaviness associated with the increased glycogen storage, these sensations usually dissipate with exercise.

Carbohydrate loading will help only athletes engaged in intense, continuous endurance exercise lasting longer than 90 minutes. Above-normal muscle glycogen stores will not enable the athlete to exercise harder during shorter duration exercise. The stiffness and heaviness associated with the increased glycogen stores may actually hurt performance during shorter events such as 5- and 10-km runs.

HIGH-CARBOHYDRATE LIQUID SUPPLEMENTS

Some athletes train so heavily that they have difficulty eating enough food to obtain the amount of carbohydrate needed for optimum performance. Athletes who have this problem can consider using a commercial, high-carbohydrate liquid supplement (13). Most products are 18% to 24% carbohydrate and contain glucose polymers (maltodextrins) to reduce the solution's osmolality and potential for gastrointestinal distress.

High-carbohydrate supplements do not replace regular food but are designed to supply supplemental calories, carbohydrate, and liquid when needed, as during heavy training or carbohydrate loading. Compared to conventional high-carbohydrate foods, high-carbohydrate liquid supplements are fiber free and produce a low stool residue.

High-carbohydrate supplements can be consumed before or after exercise (eg, with meals or in between meals). Though ultraendurance athletes may also utilize them during exercise to obtain energy and carbohydrate, they are too concentrated in carbohydrate to double for use as a fluid replacement beverage. If the athlete has no difficulty eating enough conventional food, these products are unnecessary and offer only the advantage of convenience.

CARBOHYDRATE BEFORE EXERCISE

Athletes have been warned not to eat large amounts of carbohydrate prior to exercise. This admonition was based on results of a study conducted by Foster et al (16) in the late 1970s that indicated that consuming 75 g of glucose 30 minutes prior to exercise reduced endurance by causing accelerated muscle glycogen depletion and hypoglycemia. The high blood insulin levels induced by the pre-exercise carbohydrate feeding were blamed for this chain of events.

As a result of this early research, some practitioners have advised athletes to either avoid carbohydrates entirely or to consume low glycemic index foods before exercise. The rationale is that low glycemic index foods such as beans, milk, and pasta provide a slow but sustained release of glucose to the blood, without an accompanying insulin surge. By comparison, sugar and high glycemic index foods such as bread, potato, sports drinks, and many breakfast cereals rapidly increase blood glucose and blood insulin levels.

A 1987 study by Hargreaves et al (17) contradicted Foster's earlier findings. The subjects consumed 75 g of glucose (high glycemic index), 75 g of fructose (low glycemic index), or water 45 minutes prior to bicycling to exhaustion. Although the glucose feeding caused high blood insulin and low blood glucose levels, there were no differences in the exercise time to exhaustion among the rides taken with glucose, fructose, or water.

Consuming a high glycemic index carbohydrate 1 hour before exercise may actually improve performance, particularly if the athlete has fasted overnight. Sherman et al (18) compared the ingestion of 1.1 g/kg and 2.2 g/kg of a carbohydrate beverage 1 hour prior to exercise. The subjects cycled at 70% of VO_2max for 90 minutes and then underwent a performance trial. Serum insulin was initially elevated at the start of and during exercise and blood glucose initially decreased. However, time-trial performance was significantly increased 12.5% by the carbohydrate feedings, presumably via increased carbohydrate oxidation.

The hypoglycemia and hyperinsulinemia following pre-exercise carbohydrate feedings are transient and probably will not harm performance unless the athlete is sensitive to a decrease in blood glucose and experiences premature muscular fatigue or central nervous system symptoms indicative of hypoglycemia. Athletes should evaluate their responses to high-carbohydrate foods with both low and high glycemic indexes in training to find what works the best.

A low glycemic index carbohydrate may be an option for those athletes who are sensitive to decreases in blood glucose. Thomas et al (19) compared the consumption of 1 g of carbohydrate/kg of lentils (low glycemic index), potato (high glycemic index), glucose (high glycemic index), and water 1 hour prior to exercise. The subjects cycled to exhaustion at 65% to 70% of VO_2max. Compared to the potato, glucose, and water trials, the lentil feeding provided a more gradual rise and fall in blood glucose. The endurance time for the low glycemic index lentils was 20 minutes longer than for all other trials, which were not different from each other.

Athletes who are sensitive to having their blood glucose decreased can choose from several strategies.

1. Consume a low glycemic index carbohydrate before exercise.
2. Take in carbohydrate a few minutes before exercise.
3. Wait until exercising to consume carbohydrate.

The exercise-induced rise in the hormones epinephrine, norepinephrine, and growth hormone inhibit the release of insulin and thus counter insulin's effect in lowering blood glucose. See *Box 2.2*.

BOX 2.2   Considerations in Using the Glycemic Index

- High-glycemic carbohydrates are recommended before exercise for athletes who are not sensitive to having their blood glucose lowered.
- Low-glycemic carbohydrates are recommended before exercise for athletes who are sensitive to having their blood glucose lowered and experience symptoms of early fatigue or hypoglycemia.
- High-glycemic carbohydrates are recommended during exercise to raise blood glucose and promote carbohydrate oxidation.
- High-glycemic carbohydrates are recommended following exercise to enhance glycogen repletion.

Consuming a high glycemic index carbohydrate (eg, glucose) immediately before anaerobic exercise, such as sprinting or weightlifting, will not improve performance. There is already enough ATP, CP (creatine phosphate), and muscle glycogen stored for these anaerobic tasks. The high-glycemic carbohydrate will not provide athletes with a quick burst of energy, allowing them to exercise harder. In fact, eating too much carbohydrate before exercise can increase the risk of gastrointestinal distress in the form of cramps, nausea, diarrhea, and bloating.

The Pre-exercise Meal

Athletes are often advised to eat 2 to 3 hours before exercise to allow adequate time for gastric emptying. The rationale is that if any food remains in the stomach at the start of exercise, the athlete may become nauseated or uncomfortable when blood is diverted from the gastrointestinal tract to the exercising muscles. So, rather than getting up at the crack of dawn to eat, many athletes who train or compete in the morning simply forgo food prior to exercise. This overnight fast lowers liver glycogen stores and can impair performance, especially if the athlete engages in prolonged endurance exercise that relies heavily on blood glucose.

During exercise athletes rely primarily on their preexisting glycogen and fat stores. Although the pre-exercise meal does not contribute immediate energy for exercise, it can provide energy when the athlete exercises hard for 1 hour or longer. It can also prevent athletes from feeling hungry, which in itself may impair performance. The carbohydrate in the meal can elevate blood glucose to provide energy for the exercising muscles.

Consuming carbohydrate 2 to 4 hours prior to morning exercise helps to restore suboptimal liver glycogen stores, which will help endurance events that rely heavily on blood glucose. If muscle glycogen levels are also low, consuming carbohydrate several hours before exercise can help to increase them as well. If delayed gastric emptying is a concern, liquid meals should be considered.

Sherman et al (20) evaluated the effect of a 312-g, 156-g, and 45-g liquid carbohydrate feeding 4 hours prior to exercise. The high glycemic index carbohydrate feedings provided 4.5 g/kg, 2 g/kg, and 0.6 g/kg, respectively. Interval cycling was undertaken for 95 minutes, followed by a performance trial after a 5-minute rest. The 312-g carbohydrate feeding improved performance by 15%, despite elevated insulin levels at the start of exercise.

Nuefer et al (21) found that endurance performance was also improved when a mixed meal (cereal, bread, milk, and fruit juice) supplying 200 g of carbohydrate was consumed 4 hours before exercise.

The ideal pre-exercise meal is high in carbohydrate, palatable, and well tolerated. The research by Sherman et al (18,20) suggests that the pre-exercise meal contain 1.0 to 4.5 g of carbohydrate/kg, consumed 1 to 4 hours prior to exercise. To avoid potential gastrointestinal distress, the carbohydrate and calorie content of the meal should be reduced the closer to exercise the meal is consumed. For example, a carbohydrate feeding of 1 g/kg is appropriate 1 hour before exercise, whereas 4.5 g/kg can be consumed 4 hours before exercise.

Liquid Meals

A number of commercially formulated liquid meals are available to the athlete. Some of these were initially designed for hospital patients (eg, Sustacal and Ensure), while others have been specifically created for and marketed to the athlete (eg, GatorPro, Nutrament, and Exceed Nutritional Beverage).

These products satisfy the requirements for pre-exercise food—they are high in carbohydrate, palatable, and provide both energy and fluid. Liquid meals can often be consumed closer to competition than regular meals due to their shorter gastric emptying time. This may help to avoid precompetition nausea for those athletes who are tense and have an associated delay in gastric emptying.

Liquid meals also produce a low stool residue and so help to keep immediate weight gain following the meal to a minimum. This is especially advantageous for wrestlers who need to "make weight." Liquid meals are also convenient for athletes competing in day-long competitions, tournaments, and multiple events (eg, triathlons).

Liquid meals can also be used for nutritional supplementation during heavy training when caloric requirements are extremely elevated. They supply a significant amount of calories and contribute to satiety.

CARBOHYDRATE INTAKE DURING EXERCISE

Carbohydrate feedings during exercise lasting at least 1 hour enable athletes to exercise longer and/or sprint harder at the end of exercise. Coyle et al (22,23) have demonstrated that consuming carbohydrate during cycling exercise at 70% of VO_2max can delay fatigue by 30 to 60 minutes.

Coyle et al (22) compared the effects of carbohydrate feedings on the onset of fatigue and decrease in work capacity of cyclists. The carbohydrate feedings enabled the cyclists to exercise an average of 33 minutes longer (159 minutes compared to 126 minutes) before reaching the point of fatigue. The carbohydrate feedings maintained blood glucose at higher levels, thereby increasing the utilization of blood glucose for energy.

Coyle et al (23) also measured performance during prolonged strenuous bicycling with and without carbohydrate feedings. During the ride without carbohydrate, fatigue occurred after 3 hours and was preceded by a drop in blood glucose. During the ride where they were fed carbohydrate, blood glucose levels were maintained and the cyclists were able to ride an additional hour before reaching the point of fatigue. Both groups utilized muscle glycogen at the same rate, indicating that endurance was improved by maintaining blood glucose levels rather than by glycogen sparing.

Carbohydrate feedings maintain blood glucose levels at a time when muscle glycogen stores are diminished. Thus, carbohydrate oxidation (and, therefore, ATP production) can continue at a high rate and endurance is enhanced.

Running performances with and without carbohydrate feedings have also been evaluated. During a 40-km run in the heat, Millard-Stafford et al (24) found that a carbohydrate feeding (55 g per hour) increased blood glucose levels and enabled runners to finish the last 5 km significantly faster compared to the run without carbohydrate. In a treadmill run at 80% of VO₂max, Wilber and Moffatt (25) found that the run time when fed carbohydrate (35 g per hour) was 23 minutes longer (115 minutes) compared to the run without carbohydrate (92 minutes).

Carbohydrate feedings may also improve performance in stop-and-go sports, such as football and basketball, that require repeated bouts of high-intensity, short-duration effort. Davis et al (26) evaluated the effect of carbohydrate feedings on performance during intermittent, high-intensity cycling. The subjects performed repeated 1-minute sprints at 120% to 130% of VO₂max separated by 3 minutes of rest until fatigue. Before and every 20 minutes during the exercise, the subjects drank a placebo or a 6% carbohydrate-electrolyte drink that provided 47 g of carbohydrate per hour. The average time to fatigue in the carbohydrate trial was 89 minutes (21 sprints) compared to 58 minutes (14 sprints) for the placebo. The results of this study suggest that the benefits of carbohydrate feedings are not limited to prolonged endurance exercise.

The performance benefits of a pre-exercise carbohydrate feeding appear to be additive to those of consuming carbohydrate during exercise. In a study by Wright et al (27), cyclists who received carbohydrate both 3 hours before exercise and during exercise were able to exercise longer (289 minutes) than when receiving carbohydrate either before exercise (236 minutes) or during exercise (266 minutes).

Combining carbohydrate feedings improved performance more than either feeding alone. However, the improvement in performance with the pre-exercise carbohydrate feedings was less than when smaller quantities of carbohydrate were consumed during exercise. When the goal is to provide a continuous supply of glucose during exercise, as during endurance events, the athlete should consume carbohydrate during exercise.

Carbohydrate's primary role in fluid replacement drinks is to maintain blood glucose concentration and enhance carbohydrate oxidation (28). Carbohydrate feedings enhance performance during exercise lasting 1 hour or longer, especially when muscle glycogen stores are low. In fact, carbohydrate ingestion and fluid replacement independently improve performance and their beneficial effects are additive.

Below and Coyle (29) evaluated the effects of fluid and carbohydrate ingestion, alone or in combination, during 1 hour of intense cycling exercise. In the four trials, the subjects ingested either 1,330 mL of water which replaced 79% of sweat loss, 1,330 mL of fluid with 79 g of carbohydrate, 200 mL of water which replaced 13% of sweat losses, or 200 mL of fluid with 79 g of carbohydrate. When a large volume of fluid or 79 g of carbohydrate was ingested individually, each improved performance by about 6% compared to the placebo trial. When both the large volume of fluid and carbohydrate were combined, performance was improved by 12%.

Coyle and Montain (30) suggest that athletes take in 30 to 60 g (120 to 240 kcal) of carbohydrate every hour to improve performance. This amount can be obtained through either carbohydrate-rich foods or fluids.

Liquid versus Solid Carbohydrate

The benefits of consuming beverages containing carbohydrate during exercise are well established. However, endurance athletes often consume high-carbohydrate foods such as energy bars, fig bars, cookies, and fruit. Solid food empties from the stomach more slowly than liquids, and the protein and fat found in many high-carbohydrate foods can further delay gastric emptying. Despite this, liquid and solid carbohydrate feedings are equally effective in increasing blood glucose and improving performance.

Lugo et al (31) evaluated the metabolic effects of consuming liquid carbohydrate, solid carbohydrate, or both during 2 hours of cycling at 70% of VO_2max followed by a time trial. The liquid was a 7% carbohydrate-electrolyte beverage and the solid carbohydrate was an energy bar that provided 76% of calories from carbohydrate, 18% from protein, and 6% from fat. Each feeding provided 0.4 g of carbohydrate/kg (an average of 28 g per feeding and 56 g per hour) and was consumed immediately before and every 30 minutes during the first 120 minutes of exercise.

While the caloric content of the treatments varied, they were isoenergetic with respect to carbohydrate. Carbohydrate availability and time trial performance were similar when equal amounts of carbohydrate were consumed as liquid, solid, or in combination. Regardless of carbohydrate form, there were no differences in blood glucose, insulin, or total carbohydrate oxidized during 120 minutes of cycling at 70% of VO_2max (31).

Robergs et al (32) at the University of New Mexico in Albuquerque compared blood glucose and glucoregulatory hormone (insulin and glucagon) responses to solid and liquid carbohydrate feedings during 2 hours of cycling at 65% of VO_2max, followed by a 30-minute maximal isokinetic ride. The liquid was a 7% carbohydrate-electrolyte beverage and the solid carbohydrate was a meal replacement bar that provided 67% of calories from carbohydrate, 10% from protein, and 23% from fat. Each feeding provided 0.6 g of carbohydrate/kg body weight per hour (an average of 20 g per feeding and 40 g per hour) and was consumed at 0-, 30-, 60-, 90-, and 120-minutes of exercise. Two resting glycemic response trials were also conducted. Following consumption of 75 g of either liquid or solid carbohydrate, blood glucose and insulin levels were measured every 20 minutes for 2 hours.

The resting glycemic response study found that the liquid carbohydrate feeding was associated with greater insulin-dependent glucose disposal than the solid carbohydrate feeding for the same total carbohydrate intake. This was attributed to the combined protein, fat, and fiber in the solid carbohydrate, which are known to delay gastric emptying and so blunt the insulin response to a given amount and type of carbohydrate in the food. However, there were no differences between liquid and solid carbohydrate feedings on blood glucose, glucoregulatory hormones, and exercise performance during prolonged cycling (32).

Each carbohydrate form (liquid versus solid) holds certain advantages for the athlete (33). Sports drinks and other liquids encourage the consumption of water needed to maintain hydration during exercise. However, compared to liquids, high-carbohydrate foods, energy bars, and gels can be easily carried by the athlete during exercise and provide both variety and satiety. See *Table 2.2* for the pros and cons of liquid versus solid carbohydrates.

TABLE 2.2   Pros and Cons of Liquid versus Solid Carbohydrates

Liquid Pros:	Liquid Cons:
Replace sweat losses	Large volume, difficult to carry
Empty rapidly from stomach	Do not provide variety or satiety
Solid Pros:	**Solid Cons:**
Compact, easy to carry	Require additional water for digestion
Provide variety and satiety	Do not replace sweat losses

Drinking 5 to 10 oz (150 to 300 mL) of a sports drink containing 4% to 8% carbohydrate (eg, Gatorade, Allsport, and Powerade) every 15 to 20 minutes can provide the proper amount of carbohydrate. For example, drinking 20 oz each hour of a sports drink that contains 6% carbohydrate provides 36 g of carbohydrate. Drinking the same quantity each hour of a sports drink containing 8% carbohydrate provides 48 g of carbohydrate. Eating one banana (30 g), one Power Bar (47 g), two gels (about 50 g) or three large graham crackers (66 g) every hour also supplies an adequate amount of carbohydrate.

The American College of Sports Medicine suggests that both fluid and carbohydrate requirements can be met by consuming 600 to 1,200 mL per hour (20 to 40 oz) of beverages containing 4% to 8% carbohydrate (28).

Fructose during Exercise

Some athletes take fructose tablets during exercise. Since fructose has a low glycemic index (it causes a lower blood glucose and insulin response) than glucose, athletes may mistakenly believe that fructose is a superior energy source.

Murray et al (34) compared the physiological, sensory, and exercise performance responses to the ingestion of 6% glucose, 6% sucrose, and 6% fructose solutions during cycling exercise. Blood insulin levels were lower with fructose as expected. However, fructose was associated with greater gastrointestinal distress, higher perceived exertion ratings, and higher serum cortisol levels (indicating greater physiological stress) than glucose or sucrose. Cycling performance times were also significantly better with sucrose and glucose than with fructose.

The lower blood glucose levels associated with fructose ingestion may explain why fructose does not improve performance. Fructose metabolism occurs primarily in the liver, where it is converted to liver glycogen. Fructose probably cannot be converted to glucose and released fast enough to provide adequate energy for the exercising muscles. In contrast, blood glucose is maintained or elevated by feedings of glucose, sucrose, or glucose polymers. These have been shown to enhance performance and are the predominant carbohydrates in sports drinks.

The greater incidence of gastrointestinal distress (bloating, cramping, and diarrhea) often reported with high-fructose intakes may be due to the slower intestinal absorption of fructose compared to glucose.

CARBOHYDRATE FOLLOWING EXERCISE

The restoration of muscle and liver glycogen stores following strenuous training is important to minimize fatigue associated with repeated days of heavy training. Athletes who consume 7 to 10 g of carbohydrate/kg per day will nearly replace their muscle glycogen stores during consecutive days of hard workouts.

The time period in which carbohydrate is consumed following exercise is also important for glycogen repletion. Ivy et al (35) evaluated glycogen repletion following 2 hours of hard cycling exercise that depleted muscle glycogen. When 2 g of carbohydrate/kg was consumed immediately after exercise, muscle glycogen synthesis was 15.4 mmol/kg 2 hours after exercise. When the same carbohydrate feeding was delayed for 2 hours, muscle glycogen synthesis was cut by 66% to 5.0 mmol/kg 2 hours after exercise. By 4 hours after exercise, total muscle glycogen synthesis for the delayed feeding was still 45% less (13.2 mmol/kg) than for the feeding given immediately after exercise (24.0 mmol/kg).

Providing liquid or solid carbohydrate with equal carbohydrate contents after exercise produces similar rates of glycogen repletion. Reed et al (36) evaluated the effect of the carbohydrate form on glycogen repletion following exercise. The researchers provided 3 g of carbohydrate/kg in liquid or solid form following 2 hours of cycling exercise at 60% to 75% of VO_2max. The subjects received half of the feeding immediately after exercise and half at 2 hours following exercise. There was no difference in muscle glycogen storage rates between the liquid and solid feedings at 2 hours postexercise or at 4 hours postexercise.

Delaying carbohydrate intake for too long after exercise may reduce muscle glycogen storage and impair recovery. Athletes who are not hungry after exercising can consume a high-carbohydrate drink (eg, sports drink, fruit juice, or a commercial high-carbohydrate beverage). This will also aid in rehydration.

Athletes who exercise hard for ≥90 minutes daily should consume 1.5 g of carbohydrate/kg immediately after exercise, followed by an additional 1.5 g of carbohydrate/kg feeding 2 hours later (37). The first carbohydrate feeding can be a high-carbohydrate beverage and the following feeding can be a high-carbohydrate meal. Replenishing muscle glycogen stores after exercise is particularly beneficial for athletes who train hard several times a day. This will enable them to get the most out of their second workout.

There are several reasons that glycogen repletion occurs faster following exercise.

1. The blood flow to the muscles is much greater immediately after exercise.
2. The muscle cell is more likely to take up glucose.
3. The muscle cells are more sensitive to the effects of insulin during this time period, which promotes glycogen synthesis (35).

Glucose and sucrose are twice as effective as fructose in restoring muscle glycogen after exercise (38). Most fructose is converted to liver glycogen, whereas glucose appears to bypass the liver and is stored as muscle glycogen.

The type of carbohydrate consumed (simple versus complex) does not appear to influence glycogen repletion following exercise. Roberts et al (39) compared simple and complex carbohydrate intake during both glycogen-depleted and nondepleted states. The researchers found that significant increases in muscle glycogen could be achieved with a diet high in simple or complex carbohydrates.

The most rapid increase in muscle glycogen content during the first 24 hours of recovery may be achieved by consuming foods with a high glycemic index. Burke et al (40) investigated the effect of glycemic index on muscle glycogen repletion following exercise. The subjects cycled for 2 hours at 75% of VO_2max to deplete muscle glycogen, then consumed foods with either a high glycemic index or a low glycemic index. The total carbohydrate feeding over 24 hours was 10 g of carbohydrate/kg, evenly distributed at meals eaten at 0, 4, 8, and 21 hours after exercise. The increase in muscle glycogen content after 24 hours was greater with the high glycemic index diet (106 mmol/kg) than with the low glycemic index diet (71.5 mmol/kg).

Athletes may have impaired muscle glycogen synthesis following unaccustomed exercise that results in muscle damage and delayed onset muscle soreness. The muscular responses to such damaging exercise appear to decrease both the rate of muscle glycogen synthesis and the total muscle glycogen content (41). While a diet providing 8 to 10 g of carbohydrate/kg will usually replace muscle glycogen stores within 24 hours, the damaging effects of unaccustomed exercise significantly delay muscle glycogen repletion. Also, Sherman (41) notes that even the normalization of muscle glycogen stores does not guarantee normal muscle function after unaccustomed exercise. See *Box 2.3*.

BOX 2.3   Summary of Carbohydrate Recommendations

- Consume 1 to 4 g of carbohydrate/kg, 1 to 4 hours before exercise.
- Consume 30 to 60 g of carbohydrate every hour during exercise.
- Consume 1.5 g of carbohydrate/kg immediately after exercise followed by an additional 1.5 g of carbohydrate/kg feeding 2 hours later.

THE ZONE DIET

Barry Sears, PhD, author of *Enter the Zone* and *Mastering the Zone*, claims that high-carbohydrate diets impair athletic performance and cause obesity. The Zone books treat carbohydrates and insulin as villains and recommend a complicated, carbohydrate-restricted diet. Sears tells people to eat exactly 40% of calories as carbohydrate, 30% as protein, and 30% as fat at each meal and snack.

Athletes must supposedly follow the Zone diet to reach their maximum athletic performance. The diet allegedly promotes optimal athletic performance by altering the production of eicosanoids so that the body makes more "good" eicosanoids than "bad" ones. Sears claims that eicosanoids are the most powerful hormones and control all physiological functions.

Zone diet proponents recommend limiting carbohydrate to keep the body from producing too much insulin because high insulin levels allegedly increase the production of "bad" eicosanoids. "Bad" eicosanoids purportedly impair athletic performance by reducing oxygen transfer to the cells, lowering blood glucose levels, and interfering with body fat utilization. According to Sears, insulin also makes people fat by causing carbohydrates to be stored as body fat.

The protein content of the Zone diet supposedly increases glucagon levels and helps to increase the production of "good" eicosanoids by opposing the effect of insulin. "Good" eicosanoids supposedly increase endurance by increasing oxygen transfer to the cells, promoting the utilization of stored fat and maintaining blood glucose levels.

Athletes must be impressed and intimidated by such scientific-sounding information. However, the scientific basis for this diet can be faulted on many fronts. Eicosanoids do not cause disease—they are the biologically active, hormone-like compounds known as prostaglandins, thromboxanes, and leukotrienes. Eicosanoids help to regulate inflammation, the blood's tendency to clot, and the immune system. The claim that eicosanoids are all-powerful is ridiculous—the body's physiology is just not that simple. There is also no evidence that insulin even makes "bad" eicosanoids or that glucagon makes "good" eicosanoids (42).

The metabolic pathways which supposedly connect diet, insulin and glucagon, and eicosanoids do not appear in standard nutrition or biochemistry texts. The idea that this diet (or any diet) completely regulates insulin and glucagon is not supported by endocrinology. Next, the notion that insulin and glucagon control the production of eicosanoids is not supported by biochemistry. And finally, the belief that eicosanoids control all physiological functions (including athletic performance) is not only unfounded and ridiculous, but also an appalling oversimplification of complex physiological processes (42).

Athletes need carbohydrates to perform at their best. Contrary to what the Zone books claim, eating a high-carbohydrate meal 1 to 4 hours before exercise improves performance by raising blood glucose and "topping off" glycogen stores (18-21,27). Consuming carbohydrate during exercise lasting 1 hour or more aids endurance by providing glucose for the muscles when muscle glycogen stores are low (22-27,29). And, taking in carbohydrate right after hard training enhances muscle glycogen storage (35-37).

In reality, what matters for weight loss is not carbohydrates or insulin, but energy. Body weight depends on how many kcal are consumed compared to how many are burned off. There is also no evidence that insulin makes people fat (43).

The Zone diet is merely a low-energy diet. The Zone books attempt to disguise this by having people count protein and carbohydrate blocks instead of kilocalories. Although Sears does not emphasize energy intake, the Zone diet provides only about 1,200 kcal (120 g of carbohydrate) for the average woman and 1,700 kcal a day (170 g of carbohydrate) for the average man. The diet is also inadequate in thiamin, pyridoxine, magnesium, copper, and chromium (44).

The Zone diet does not increase the ability to burn fat during exercise. It also does not change the body's preference for carbohydrate over fat as fuel for exercise. The best way for athletes to increase their fat-burning ability is to keep exercising. And as for gradual loss of body fat, that comes from burning more kilocalories during exercise than are eaten at the table, not from some special dietary ratio (43).

Lastly, athletes cannot train or compete well for very long on this low-energy, low-carbohydrate diet. Athletes require adequate calories and carbohydrate to maintain their glycogen stores and muscle tissue. Those who follow the Zone diet will eventually find themselves in a twilight zone of near starvation and impaired performance (43). See *Box 2.4.*

BOX 2.4   Dangers of the Zone Diet for Athletes

- Inadequate kilocalories (approximately 1,700 for men and 1,200 for women)
- Inadequate dietary carbohydrate (approximately 170 g for men and 120 g for women)
- Inadequate micronutrients (thiamin, pyridoxine, magnesium, copper, and chromium)
- False hope that Zone diet will enhance athletic performance

---

SUMMARY

Carbohydrate is the preferred fuel for most sports. Since the depletion of endogenous carbohydrate stores (muscle and liver glycogen and blood glucose) impairs athletic performance, athletes should strive to optimize their carbohydrate stores before, during, and after exercise.

Athletes should consume 7 to 10 g of carbohydrate/kg per day to replenish muscle and liver glycogen following training sessions or competitive events. One to 4 hours prior to exercise, athletes should consume 1 to 4 g of carbohydrate/kg to "top off" muscle and liver glycogen stores. During exercise lasting 1 hour or longer, athletes should consume 30 to 60 g of carbohydrate per hour to maintain blood glucose levels and carbohydrate oxidation. To optimize glycogen repletion following exercise lasting 90 minutes or longer, athletes should consume 1.5 g of carbohydrate/kg within 30 minutes, followed by an additional 1.5 g of carbohydrate/kg feeding 2 hours later.

REFERENCES

1. Burke LM, Collier GR, Hargreaves M. The glycemic index—a new tool in sport nutrition? *Int J Sport Nutr*. 1998;8:401-415.
2. Foster-Powell K, Brand Miller J. International tables of glycemic index. *Am J Clin Nutr*. 1995;62(suppl):S871-S893.
3. Frail H, Burke L. Carbohydrate needs for training. In: Burke L, Deakin V, eds. *Clinical Sports Nutrition*. Roseville, Australia: McGraw Hill; 1994:151-173.
4. Bergstrom J, Hermansen L, Saltin B. Diet, muscle glycogen, and physical performance. *Acta Physiol Scand*. 1967;71:140-150.
5. Costill DL, Bowers R, Branam G, Sparks K. Muscle glycogen utilization during prolonged exercise on successive days. *J Appl Physiol*. 1971;31:834-838.
6. Costill DL, Sherman WM, Fink WJ, Maresh C, Whitten M, Miller JM. The role of dietary carbohydrate in muscle glycogen resynthesis after strenuous running. *Am J Clin Nutr*. 1981;34:1831-1836.

7. Fallowfield JL, Williams C. Carbohydrate intake and recovery from prolonged exercise. *Int J Sport Nutr*. 1993;3:150-164.

8. Costill DL, Flynn MJ, Kirwan JP, et al. Effect of repeated days of intensified training on muscle glycogen and swimming performance. *Med Sci Sports Exerc*. 1988;20:249-254.

9. Sherman WM, Wimer GS. Insufficient dietary carbohydrate during training: does it impair athletic performance? *Int J Sport Nutr*. 1991;1:28-44.

10. Walberg-Rankin J. Dietary carbohydrate as an ergogenic aid for prolonged and brief competitions in sport. *Int J Sport Nutr*. 1995;5(suppl):S13-S28.

11. Saris WHM, van Erp-Baart MA, Brouns F, Westerterp KR, ten Hoor F. Study of food intake and energy expenditure during extreme sustained exercise: the Tour de France. *Int J Sport Med*. 1989;10(suppl):26-31.

12. Brouns F, Saris WHM, Stroecken J, et al. Eating, drinking, and cycling: a controlled Tour de France simulation study, Part I. *Int J Sport Med*. 1989;10(suppl):S32-S40.

13. Brouns F, Saris WHM, Stroecken J, et al. Eating, drinking, and cycling: a controlled Tour de France simulation study, Part II. Effect of diet manipulation. *Int J Sport Med*. 1989;10(suppl):S41-S48.

14. Sherman WM, Costill DL, Fink WJ, Miller JM. The effect of exercise and diet manipulation on muscle glycogen and its subsequent use during performance. *Int J Sport Med*. 1981;2:114-118.

15. Karlsson J, Saltin B. Diet, muscle glycogen, and endurance performance. *J Appl Physiol*. 1971;31:203-206.

16. Foster C, Costill DL, Fink WJ. Effects of pre-exercise feedings on endurance performance. *Med Sci Sports Exerc*. 1979;11:1-5.

17. Hargreaves M, Costill DL, Fink WJ, King DS, Fielding RA. Effects of pre-exercise carbohydrate feedings on endurance cycling performance. *Med Sci Sports Exerc*. 1987;19:33-36.

18. Sherman WM, Peden MC, Wright DA. Carbohydrate feedings 1 hour before exercise improves cycling performance. *Am J Clin Nutr*. 1991;54:866-870.

19. Thomas DE, Brotherhood JR, Brand JC. Carbohydrate feeding before exercise: effect of glycemic index. *Int J Sport Med*. 1991;12:180-186.

20. Sherman WM, Brodowicz G, Wright DA, Allen WK, Simonsen J, Dernbach A. Effects of 4 hour pre-exercise carbohydrate feedings on cycling performance. *Med Sci Sports Exerc*. 1989;12:598-604.

21. Nueffer PD, Costill DL, Flynn MG, Kirwan JP, Mitchell JB, Houmard J. Improvements in exercise performance: effects of carbohydrate feedings and diet. *J Appl Physiol*. 1987;62:983-988.

22. Coyle EF, Hagberg JM, Hurley BF, Martin WH, Ehsani AA, Holloszy JO. Carbohydrate feeding during prolonged strenuous exercise can delay fatigue. *J Appl Physiol*. 1983;55:230-235.

23. Coyle EF, Coggan AR, Hemmert WK, Ivy JL. Muscle glycogen utilization during prolonged strenuous exercise when fed carbohydrate. *J Appl Physiol*. 1986;61:165-172.

24. Millard-Stafford ML, Sparling PB, Rosskopf LB, Hinson BT, Dicarlo LJ. Carbohydrate-electrolyte replacement improves distance running performance in the heat. *Med Sci Sports Exerc*. 1992;24:934-940.

25. Wilber RL, Moffatt RJ. Influence of carbohydrate ingestion on blood glucose and performance in runners. *Int J Sport Nutr*. 1994;2:317-327.

26. Davis JM, Jackson DA, Broadwell MS, Queary JL, Lambert CL. Carbohydrate drinks delay fatigue during intermittent high intensity cycling in active men and women. *Int J Sport Nutr*. 1997;7:261-273.

27. Wright DA, Sherman WM, Dernbach AR. Carbohydrate feedings before, during, or in combination improves cycling performance. *J Appl Physiol*. 1991;71:1082-1088.

28. American College of Sports Medicine. Position stand: exercise and fluid replacement. *Med Sci Sports Exerc*. 1996;28:i-vii.

29. Below PR, Coyle EF. Fluid and carbohydrate ingestion independently improve performance during 1 hour of intense exercise. *Med Sci Sports Exerc*. 1995;27:200-210.

30. Coyle EF, Montain SJ. Benefits of fluid replacement with carbohydrate during exercise. *Med Sci Sports Exerc*. 1992;24(suppl):S324-330.

31. Lugo M, Sherman WM, Wimer GS, Garleb K. Metabolic responses when different forms of carbohydrate energy are consumed during cycling. *Int J Sport Nutr*. 1993;3:398-407.

32. Robergs RA, McMinn SB, Mermier C, Leabetter G, Ruby B, Quinn C. Blood glucose and glucoregulatory hormone responses to solid and liquid carbohydrate ingestion during exercise. *Int J Sport Nutr*. 1998;8:70-83.

33. Coleman E. Update on carbohydrate: solid versus liquid. *Int J Sport Nutr*. 1994;4:80-88.

34. Murray R, Paul GL, Seifert JG, Eddy DE, Halby GA. The effects of glucose, fructose, and sucrose ingestion during exercise. *Med Sci Sports Exerc*. 1989;21:275-282.

35. Ivy JL, Katz AL, Cutler CL, Sherman WM, Coyle EF. Muscle glycogen synthesis after exercise: effect of time of carbohydrate ingestion. *J Appl Physiol*. 1988;6:1480-1485.

36. Reed MJ, Broznick JT, Lee MC, Ivy JL. Muscle glycogen storage postexercise: effect of mode of carbohydrate administration. *J Appl Physiol*. 1989;75:1019-1023.

37. Ivy JL, Lee MC, Broznick JT, Reed MJ. Muscle glycogen storage after different amounts of carbohydrate ingestion. *J Appl Physiol*. 1988;65:2018-2023.

38. Blom PCS, Hostmark AT, Vaage O, Kardel KR, Maehlum S. Effect of different postexercise sugar diets on the rate of muscle glycogen synthesis. *Med Sci Sports Exerc*. 1987;19:471-496.

39. Roberts KM, Noble EG, Hayden DB, Taylor AW. Simple and complex carbohydrate-rich diets and muscle glycogen content of marathon runners. *Eur J Appl Physiol*. 1988; 57:70-74.

40. Burke LM, Collier GR, Hargreaves M. Muscle glycogen storage after prolonged exercise: effect of glycemic index. *J Appl Physiol*. 1993;75:1019-1023.

41. Sherman WM. Recovery from endurance exercise. *Med Sci Sports Exerc*. 1992;24(suppl):S336-339.

42. Coleman E. The biozone nutrition system—a dietary panacea? *Int J Sport Nutr*. 1996;6:69-71.

43. Coleman E. Carbohydrate unloading. *Phys Sportsmed*. 1997;25:97-98.

44. Rosenbloom C. Mastering the Zone (book review). *SCAN's Pulse*. 1997;16(3)25-26.

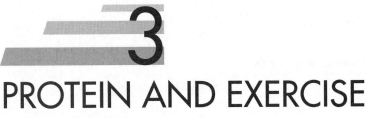

3

PROTEIN AND EXERCISE

Cindy Carroll, MS, RD

Most athletes have almost an instinctive belief that protein is good and a key nutrient for sports performance. The ever-increasing interest in the science of nutrition has many athletes following one of two extreme paths when it comes to eating protein. Some athletes are choosing to eat a diet composed of high levels of carbohydrate with inadequate fat and protein or, conversely, eating excessive protein believing that "more is better" (1-4). Such a polarized reaction to protein leaves many athletes wondering how much is necessary, is more protein better, and what constitutes a safe intake.

HISTORICAL PERSPECTIVE

Well over 100 years ago, protein was believed to be the major fuel for exercise (5). This belief changed in the 1900s as carbohydrate and fat became recognized as major fuels for exercise (6). Many bodybuilders and weightlifters still hold fast to the idea that calories from steak and eggs are the most important calories (3). Although carbohydrate and fat are the major fuel sources for exercise, a number of studies have suggested that regular physical exercise has dramatic effects on protein metabolism (4,7-12). The Recommended Dietary Allowance (RDA) set by the Food and Nutrition Board of the National Research Council does not recognize this potential need for increased dietary protein for active people. The RDAs are based on sedentary people, although they provide a large allowance (twice the standard deviation of the mean) that is adequate for many active people (13).

AMINO ACIDS

The need for protein is based on the need for individual amino acids, which when put together make various proteins in the body. An amino acid is comprised of a central carbon atom to which is attached a hydrogen, an acid group (COOH), a nitrogen-containing amino group (NH_2), and a distinguishing side group that is different for each amino acid, as illustrated. (See *Figure 3.1.*) There are 20 different amino acids, nine of which are indispensable or essential, meaning they must be obtained from food because the body cannot synthesize them. Both the indispensable (essential) and the dispensable (nonessential) amino acids are listed in *Box 3.1.*

FIGURE 3.1   Structure of Amino Acids

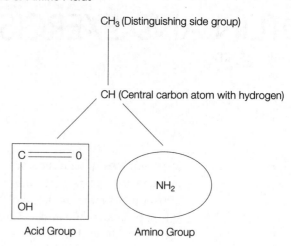

BOX 3.1   Amino Acids

Below are the nine essential amino acids that must be obtained in the diet. Histidine is an essential amino acid for infants; adults can synthesize it.

Histidine	Phenylalanine
Isoleucine	Threonine
Leucine	Tryptophan
Lysine	Valine
Methionine	

Below are the remaining nonessential amino acids that humans can synthesize. Cysteine can be produced from methionine and tyrosine can be produced from phenylalanine.

Alanine	Glutamine
Arginine	Glycine
Asparagine	Proline
Aspartic acid	Serine
Cysteine	Tyrosine
Glutamic acid	

ROLE OF PROTEIN IN THE BODY FOR EXERCISE

Protein comprises up to 45% of the body by weight (14). The uniqueness of amino acids is that they can link together with other amino acids to form complex structures that comprise all of the proteins in the body. These include enzymes that catalyze reactions; hormones, such as insulin and glucagon; hemoglobin and myoglobin that carry oxygen and serve as reservoirs for oxygen in muscles; and all structural tissue including myosin and actin that form muscle protein. All of these are essential for physical activity. Research shows that protein also contributes as an energy source during starvation and intense exercise, possibly by as much as 15% of total kilocalories during intense exercise (15). This is largely influenced by the adequacy of energy and carbohydrate in the diet (16). If the diet is inadequate in calories or carbohydrate to support the energy expended in the exercise, protein contributes as an energy source; hence, carbohydrates are referred to as "protein sparing." Protein's contribution as an energy source decreases to about 5% when energy intake is adequate (15,16).

PROTEIN METABOLISM

Dietary protein combines with endogenous protein from gastrointestinal secretions in the gut and is digested and absorbed as amino acids. About 10% of protein is excreted in the feces, leaving 90% of amino acids to cross the intestinal lining to form an amino acid pool (14). This "pool" of amino acids also includes body protein broken down from fluid and tissue. When the body is in equilibrium during protein synthesis, it recruits amino acids from the pool to keep up with protein degradation. If amino acids are not available to join the pool (ie, inadequate dietary protein intake), then protein synthesis cannot keep up with protein breakdown and body proteins are broken down to fulfill the pool's requirement for amino acids (14). Ultimately, tissue repair slows and muscle size and strength diminish, resulting in decreased physical performance (17). Conversely, if dietary intake of protein exceeds need, amino acids are deaminated (removal of amine group) and the excess nitrogen is excreted mainly as urea but also as ammonia, uric acid, and creatinine. The structure remaining after deamination is called an alpha-keto acid and it can be oxidized for energy or stored as body fat in the form of triglycerides. *Figure 3.2* illustrates whole-body protein metabolism.

FIGURE 3.2   Whole-body Protein Metabolism

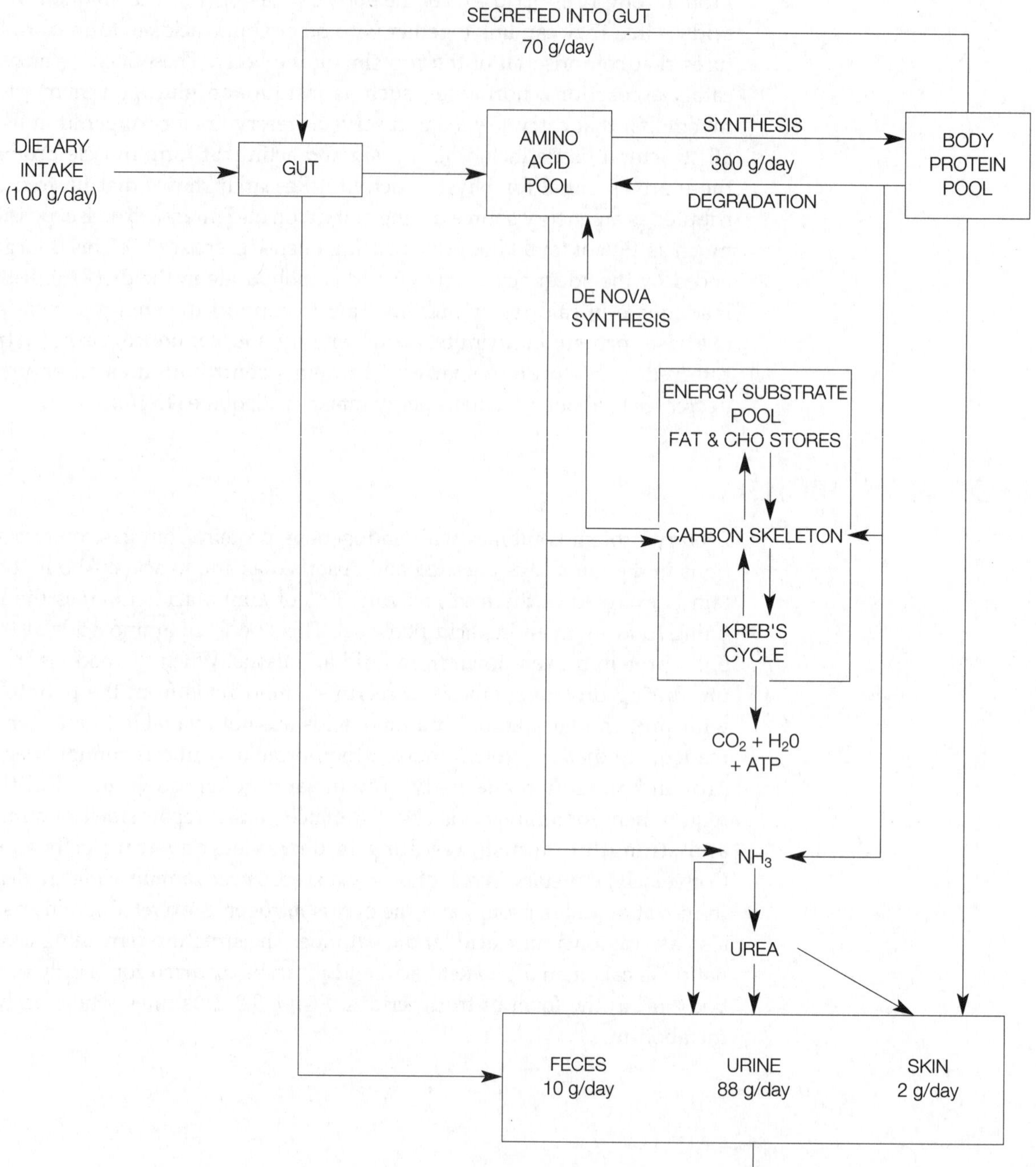

Used with permission. Butterfield G. Amino acids and high protein diets. In: Lamb D, Williams M, eds. *Perspectives in Exercise Science and Sports Medicine*. Carmel, Ind: Cooper Publishing Group; 1991.

Nitrogen Balance

The controversy over protein requirements remains partly because of the inconsistencies in measuring protein turnover in the body. Nitrogen balance is one of the most commonly used measures of assessing protein metabolism; however, it is not a perfect measure. Nitrogen balance measures nitrogen leaving the body versus nitrogen coming into the body (dietary protein) (13). Negative nitrogen balance occurs when nitrogen excretion exceeds nitrogen intake. Positive nitrogen balance occurs when intake exceeds protein excretion, usually during times of growth (eg, adolescence, pregnancy). Normally, the body is in nitrogen balance or equilibrium when intake equals excretion. Nitrogen balance measurements are not thought to be definitive because measurements account only for urinary and some fecal nitrogen losses (13,16,17). Nitrogen can also be lost in sweat and other body secretions such as sloughed skin, hair, and nails. Since protein is not truly being traced and measured after it enters the body, nitrogen balance does not account for all aspects of protein metabolism and utilization before excretion. Nitrogen balance assumes that what is not being excreted is being used for protein synthesis (17). Thus, when protein intake is altered (either an increase or decrease in protein intake), it is important to consider that there is a mandatory period of adaptation to the new dietary intake during which daily nitrogen excretion will be unreliable (16). This is an important point to keep in mind when assessing the reliability and validity of protein studies using nitrogen balance as a measure of protein status. The Food and Agriculture Organization (FAO) and the World Health Organization (WHO) specify a minimum of 10 days adaptation for determining protein requirements when nitrogen intake is changed (16,18).

WHAT DETERMINES PROTEIN NEEDS?

Various factors influence how much protein the body uses at any given time. The need for protein is based on the requirements for each essential amino acid. The requirements of the nine essential amino acids set by the WHO are based on nitrogen balance studies, but this method has been challenged by several researchers claiming that it grossly underestimates needs, particularly for certain populations such as young adults and athletes (16,19-22). Various tissues utilize amino acids at different rates. The muscles use the branched chain amino acids, especially leucine, during exercise. One study showed that the amount of leucine oxidized during a 2-hour exercise bout at 50% VO_2max was about 90% of the total daily requirement as determined by nitrogen balance estimates (19).

Although oxidized amino acids in the muscles reflect increased protein utilization, this is not reflective of whole-body total-protein turnover (16). The differences among research techniques employed in various studies on the amounts of individual amino acids needed could alter the amount of total protein needed. But, even though the need for some amino acids is theorized to be higher for active people, obtaining them from food is not difficult. *Table 3.1* gives estimated requirements of essential amino acids based on nitrogen balance studies and an estimation of increased needs.

TABLE 3.1 Summary of Estimated Requirements and Intake of
Indispensable Amino Acids (mg/kg per day)

Amino Acid	Estimated Requirement		Estimated Intake	
	WHO/FAO*	Young et al **	Dietary†	Dietary††
Leucine	14	39	100	57
Isoleucine	10	23	63	36
Valine	10	24	70	40
Threonine	9	21	50	29
Phenylalanine and Tyrosine	19	39	55	31
Tryptophan	3.5	6	14	8
Methionine and Cysteine	13	16	30	17
Lysine	12	42	84	48
Histidine	8-10	—	31	17

* Source: World Health Organization, 1985

** Source: Young et al, 1989 (19)

† Source: Butterfield et al, 1990. Estimated from 4-day weighed food records of six women who ran 44.8 km (27.8 miles) per week and consumed 77.8 g protein and 8.28 MJ (1,980 kcal) per day.

†† Estimated from amino acid composition of diets selected by physically active women, assuming a protein intake equivalent to that recommended by the National Research Council, Food and Nutrition Board (1989).

The following is a summary of the factors that influence individual amino acid turnover and ultimate total protein utilization:

- Body composition. The RDAs for adults are based on body weight (13). Protein is required to maintain muscle size and mass, and research suggests that protein in excess of the RDA must be allowed for muscle growth (8,11). Increased dietary protein alone will not increase muscle mass. Excess dietary protein will be stored as fat without the stimulus of strength training (6,11).
- Activity level. Both intensity and duration of exercise increase protein utilization. Resistance exercise and endurance exercise also influence protein utilization (6-11,15-17). Specifically, the initiation of an endurance program may increase protein needs for about a 2-week period (16). Conditioning also affects protein needs. Some evidence shows that leucine oxidation is higher in untrained athletes versus trained athletes and with training comes a period of adaptation, possibly lowering protein needs (16,18).
- Energy and carbohydrate adequacy. If energy is inadequate because of dieting or increased energy expenditure, then protein needs increase. It is well established that increasing kilocalories improves nitrogen balance. This is a recurring theme in much of the research literature: When adequate energy is present, protein needs do not increase (5,6,12,16,18).

- Protein quality. "High-quality proteins," such as found in egg albumin and casein and contain all of the essential amino acids, improve protein utilization, and cause minimal nitrogen to be excreted. Protein in a mixed diet produces slightly higher protein needs (13,16).
- Hormones. During times of growth, such as adolescence and pregnancy, protein needs are higher (13,14).
- Illness and injury. Individual diseases affect protein needs differently and each person's response may vary. Conditions such as burns, fever, fracture, and surgical trauma can produce extensive loss of body protein. An athlete convalescing in bed for a short time with a bone fracture can lose 0.3 to 0.7 kg of body protein (14).

EXERCISE AND PROTEIN NEEDS

Research shows that protein needs during various types of exercise are greater than the RDA of 0.8g/kg per day.

Endurance Exercise

Endurance exercise causes training adaptations that alter protein metabolism (7,9,10,17). Increased amino acid oxidation leads to an increase in mitochondrial protein content, which may require protein in excess of the RDA (17). Both exercise intensity and duration of training contribute to increased amino acid oxidation. It may be helpful to identify endurance athletes who participate in high- versus low-intensity training because their protein needs will differ (16,18).

- Low intensity. People who regularly exercise at less than 50% of VO_2max (leisurely walking, cycling, dancing) do not need additional protein. In fact, this level of exercise may provide a positive stimulus for protein utilization without increasing the body's demand for it (18).
- High intensity. Athletes who regularly engage in vigorous activities including running, swimming, and bicycling need slightly more protein than the RDA. The current research recommends a range of protein from 1.2 to 1.4 g/kg per day (140% to 160% of the RDA) (7,9,18). Research suggests that this increased need may be most important during the first 2 weeks of an intense endurance program (16,18).

Resistance Exercise

It is probably not surprising that the research shows weight training increases protein needs, but it always comes as a surprise to weightlifters or bodybuilders that it is not nearly as high as the amount they believe they need or are usually getting through their diets (3,4). Maintaining muscle mass requires significantly less protein than increasing muscle mass. In fact, providing energy intake is adequate, studies have shown that muscle mass can be maintained at protein levels of 0.5 to 1.0 g/kg per day. Bodybuilders and weightlifters, however, seldom want to just maintain their current muscle mass. Most go through training periods where they are trying to build additional muscle mass.

The current recommendations for increasing muscle mass for resistance training range from 1.4 to 1.8 g/kg per day (160% to 200% of the RDA) (8,11,17,23). There appears to be diminishing returns with levels higher than this and levels above 2 g/kg per day show little benefit (16,17). Adequate energy also helps improve protein utilization when increasing muscle mass. Energy must be at least adequate and even slightly exceed that needed to maintain weight (by 200 kcal per day or 3 kcal/kg per day) (16).

Timing of Protein Intake

Studies show that some protein with carbohydrate after exercise helps enhance glycogen resynthesis by helping to stimulate insulin. A 1:3 ratio of protein to carbohydrate is recommended (24-26). The combination of eating protein with carbohydrate after strength training may also help stimulate muscle growth by the release of insulin and growth hormone (27). A recent abstract (28) suggests that a carbohydrate supplement ingested immediately after or within 1 hour after resistance exercise resulted in a more positive nitrogen balance than when eaten several hours after exercise.

An important point to consider is advances in training techniques. Resistance training and endurance training are rarely mutually exclusive. Bodybuilders and weightlifters are participating in aerobic exercise, although certainly not at the levels of endurance athletes, and endurance athletes are recognizing the benefits of weight training, particularly in swimming and soccer (29). Since many athletes are engaging in both resistance training and endurance training, their protein requirements probably fall somewhere between 1.2 to 1.8 g/kg per day. Each athlete should be assessed individually to determine the most appropriate protein level.

CALCULATING PROTEIN NEEDS

By identifying a person's level of physical activity, protein needs can be assessed. *Table 3.2* gives recommendations for protein needs for active adults. It is important to consider if the athlete is just starting a training program and/or if he or she is involved in both weight training and endurance exercise. These recommendations are not minimum recommendations but include an adequate margin of safety. For example, a soccer player involved in both endurance training and regular weightlifting would be considered an adult competitive athlete and may have protein needs on the higher end of the range. Someone who is involved only in aerobic exercise without weight training may have protein needs on the lower range. *Box 3.2* illustrates the calculations for protein needs for two "sample" athletes.

Protein and Exercise 41

TABLE 3.2 Protein Needs for Active People Compared to Sedentary Adults

	Grams of protein per kg of body weight
Current RDA for sedentary adult	0.8 (0.4 g/lb)
Recreational exerciser, adult	1.0-1.5 (0.5-0.75 g/lb)
Competitive athlete, adult	1.2-1.8 (0.6-0.9 g/lb)
Growing teenage athlete	1.8-2.0 (0.9-1.0 g/lb)
Adult building muscle mass	1.4-1.8 (0.7-0.9 g/lb)
Athlete restricting calories	1.4-2.0 (0.7-1.0 g/lb)
Maximum usable amount for adults	2.0 (1.0 g/lb)

Adapted from: Clark N. *Nancy Clark's Sport Nutrition Guidebook.* 2nd ed. Champaign, Ill: Human Kinetics; 1997. Used with permission.

BOX 3.2 "Sample" Athletes' Protein Needs

Sample Athlete #1:

A 91-kg man (200 lb) who plays quarterback in football and participates in minimal aerobic exercise but wants to increase muscle mass.

Recommendation: 1.4-1.8 g/kg per day = 128-164 g of protein per day (adult building muscle mass)

Sample Athlete #2:

A 68-kg runner (150 lb) who participates in minimal weight training but extensive endurance training.

Recommendation: 1.2-1.4 g/kg per day or 82-95 g per day, the lower end of the adult competitive athlete range

---

DIET

Research shows that athletes who are engaging in regular, strenuous exercise need more protein than the RDA, most athletes are eating adequate amounts of protein, and many are eating in excess of their needs. Food can easily provide all the essential amino acids and total protein required to meet estimated needs. However, some athletes (eg, gymnasts, dancers, runners, wrestlers) who attempt to maintain a low body weight may have inadequate intakes of both total kilocalories and protein (30-34). When protein is restricted, intake of nutrients such as calcium, iron, and zinc may be inadequate. At the other extreme, some athletes consume excess protein and can be compromising their carbohydrate intake. The protein recommendations made in this chapter usually fall within 12% to 15% of an athlete's total calories, emphasizing the importance of maintaining adequate energy and carbohydrate. *Box 3.3* illustrates sample menus showing how food can provide the protein for those with higher protein needs and *Table 3.3* lists the protein content of common foods. *Figure 3.3* illustrates how much dietary protein is needed to build muscle.

BOX 3.3   Sample Menus Illustrating How to Obtain Protein from Diet

Sample Menu One (approximately 75 g of protein and 2,000 kcal; protein providing 15% of total energy)

Breakfast
- 1 cup orange juice
- 1 cup cereal
- 1 banana
- 1 cup low-fat milk
- 1 slice whole-wheat toast
- 1 T peanut butter

Lunch
- 1 tuna fish sandwich containing 2 slices whole-wheat bread, 1/2 can tuna (6 oz) with 2 T mayonnaise
- 2 medium carrots

Snack
- 1 medium apple

Dinner
- 2 cups cooked pasta
- 1 cup tomato sauce
- 1 cup salad greens with 1 T salad dressing
- 1 cup low-fat milk

Snack
- 1/2 cup fruit sorbet

Sample Menu Two (approximately 150 g of protein and 3,000 kcal; protein providing 20% of total energy)

Breakfast
- 1 cup orange juice
- 1 cup cereal
- 1 cup low-fat milk
- 1 banana
- 2 slices whole-wheat toast with 2 T peanut butter

Lunch
- Tuna fish sandwich containing 2 slices whole-wheat bread, 1/2 can tuna (6 oz) with 2 T mayonnaise and 1 oz cheese
- 2 medium carrots
- 1 cup low-fat milk
- 2 chocolate chip cookies

Snack
- 1 medium apple
- 2 crackers

Dinner
- 6 oz chicken breast
- 2 cups pasta
- 1 cup tomato sauce
- 1 cup salad with low-fat dressing
- 1 cup low-fat milk

Snack
- 1 cup low-fat yogurt

TABLE 3.3   Protein Content of Common Foods

Food	Serving Size	Grams of Protein
Egg, whole	1 large	6
Milk, 1%	1 cup	8
Yogurt, low-fat	1 cup	12.8
Cottage cheese, 1%	1/2 cup	14
Cheese, cheddar	1 oz	7
Ice cream, vanilla	1/2 cup	2
Frozen yogurt, vanilla, soft	1/2 cup	3
Beef, ground, lean	3 oz	21
Fish, cod, Atlantic	3 oz	19
Chicken breast	3 oz	27
Peanut butter, smooth	2 T	8
Hummus, commercial	1 T	1
Bread, whole-wheat	1 slice	3
Spaghetti, enriched, cooked	1 cup	7
Banana, raw	1 medium	3
Apple, raw with skin	1 medium	<1
Pizza, cheese	1 slice	8
Orange juice, frozen, diluted	1 cup	2
Beans, pinto, canned	1 cup	12
Beans, soy, mature, cooked	1 cup	29
Cereal	1 cup	3

Source: Food and Information Center. USDA Nutrient Database for Standard Reference on the World Wide Web. http://www.nal.usda.gov/fnic/cgi-bin/nut_search.pl. Accessed September 25, 1998.

FIGURE 3.3   How much protein does it take to build muscle?

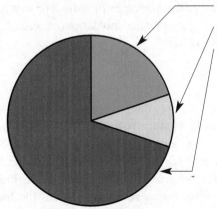

15%-20% Protein

5%-7% Fat, glycogen, minerals

70%-75% Water

One pound of muscle contains 70-105 g of protein.

To add 1 lb of pure muscle in a week:

• Body needs 10 to 14 g of additional protein a day.

• Body can add only 2 lb of muscle a week.

Protein intake alone will not build muscle. Muscle-building requires strength training and extra calories.

Adapted from: *Performance Power: The Nutrition Connection.* Natick, Mass: Military Division of the US Army Research Institute of Environmental Medicine; 1999. Modules 1-6.

SUPPLEMENTS

Manufacturers aggressively market protein supplements to the many athletes who still value protein as the most important nutrient (35). Although some athletes overuse protein supplements, there is a place for them within the athletic community. Protein supplements can be divided into two categories but often overlap. Whole-protein supplements contain egg, milk, or soy protein and other products contain individual or combinations of free amino acids.

Whole-protein

Whole-protein supplements are used to increase the total amount of protein in the diet. Whole-protein supplements are often fortified with additional individual amino acids. In general, whole-protein supplements are not needed to meet protein requirements because protein is readily available in food (36); however, these products can be convenient, especially for athletes with high calorie needs and little time for meal preparation or eating meals. Some of the products are portable, require no refrigeration, and are easy to eat during a hectic day. Some of these products are not the bargains they may seem to be because they may need to be mixed with milk, providing up to half of the protein. Some protein powders can be mixed with water and are appropriate for the lactose-intolerant athlete. Protein tablets or pills generally contain less protein than powders. Instant breakfast mixes are good alternatives to expensive protein powders. Energy bars containing at least 7 to 14 g of protein, equal to 1 to 2 oz of protein, can help contribute to protein requirements and are convenient to use. Athletes should be aware that some products contain excessive amounts of protein per serving (over 50 g) and are generally unnecessary.

Individual Amino Acids

Some research has shown that supplementation with low levels of some individual amino acids can improve performance by reducing muscle and blood lactate concentrations (37). Larger doses of these supplements have not been shown to enhance exercise performance. Supplementation with individual amino acids carries risk including metabolic imbalances, altered neurotransmitter activity, and even toxicity (16,17,38).

Branched-chain Amino Acids

Central nervous system fatigue. The branched-chain amino acids (BCAA) leucine, isoleucine, and valine have been studied in connection with central fatigue (39-41). Fatigue in exercise is usually thought to be of muscular origin, but central fatigue is recognized as originating in the brain. It is theorized that during prolonged exercise, excess serotonin crosses the blood-brain barrier and causes fatigue; some research even characterizes this as overtraining (39). The amino acid tryptophan is a precursor to serotonin. During exercise, BCAAs from skeletal muscle are oxidized, decreasing their availability (40). It is also theorized that during exercise plasma-free fatty acids increase in the blood, displacing tryptophan from its usual binding site on plasma albumin and allowing more tryptophan to be available to the brain (40). When the ratio of tryptophan to BCAAs increases, more serotonin enters the brain. Altering the ratio by increasing BCAAs or carbohydrates allows less tryptophan into the brain. The research is not consistent in demonstrating the efficacy of BCAAs in preventing fatigue. Research does support the use of carbohydrate to alter serotonin levels (42-44).

Growth hormone. The amino acids arginine and lysine have been hypothesized to increase growth hormone, thereby exerting an anabolic effect that enhances muscle growth. The research does not consistently support this theory (41,45).

Glutamine. Although glutamine is not recognized as an essential amino acid, it is believed by some researchers to be needed in higher amounts during strenuous exercise. Glutamine is important for immune function and the integrity of the gut (46,47). Some studies demonstrated that athletes who suffer from overtraining syndrome have reduced plasma glutamine levels, which may lead to poor immunity (46-48). Strenuous exercise without adequate recovery may deplete glutamine reserves and the body cannot synthesize glutamine at an appropriate rate to reach pre-exercise levels. Glutamine may also have a role in muscle glycogen synthesis. Adequate glutamine may enhance protein synthesis after exercise. Studies are inconclusive to support glutamine supplementation (46-48).

Two other protein-like supplements receiving attention are creatine and HMB (see Chapter 7, Ergogenic Aids). Both show promise to increase muscle mass and strength, but their long-term safety is unknown (35,36,49-51).

RISKS OF EXCESS PROTEIN CONSUMPTION

The popularity of high dietary protein intake is not new. Researchers have examined whether overconsumption of protein is a health risk. Some researchers believe that the potential adverse effects of excessive protein have been exaggerated (17).

Kidney Damage

Much of the concern about excess protein and kidney damage was based on studies of people with impaired kidney function (17). Excess protein does place an additional load on the kidney to process nitrogen excretion, so one might expect to see a higher rate of kidney problems in strength and power athletes, but the research does not support this idea (17). Animal studies do not support the idea that high protein intake causes kidney problems even when animals are fed a high-protein diet throughout life (17). Some researchers still remain cautious and warn against excessive protein intake (> 2 g/kg per day) to prevent kidney problems in an otherwise healthy kidney (52).

Dehydration

What seems to be clearer about excess protein is the risk for dehydration. Water is lost during the excretion of nitrogen, and athletes with high fluid needs may be placing themselves at increased risk for dehydration (16,17). Athletes must drink adequate fluids and monitor urine concentration especially when consuming a high-protein diet. Chapter 6, Fluid and Electrolytes provides details on monitoring fluid intake.

Calcium Loss

Calcium loss has been hypothesized to be the result of high-protein diets, creating an increased risk for osteoporosis. Calciuria may occur as dietary protein increases (53). Acid is generated when high-protein foods are eaten and the kidney excretes this acid. Calcium is released from bone as a buffer to the increased acid load. The high phosphate content of foods in a mixed diet may counteract this effect (17,54-56). However, it is also possible that the body adapts and decreases calcium losses if dietary calcium intake is adequate (55,56). Frequently, studies do not last long enough to see this adaptation period. A dietary calcium-to-protein ratio ≥20:1 (mg:g) may provide adequate protection to the skeleton (56).

Unbalanced Diet

The biggest risk of excessive protein may be that the athlete is eating inadequate carbohydrate to maintain and/or replenish muscle glycogen stores. The consumption of a high-protein diet may limit food choices, thus increasing the risk for vitamin and mineral deficiences (57-59).

RISKS OF CONSUMING INADEQUATE PROTEIN

Although many athletes focus on protein, some athletes do not eat enough protein (32). This is more of a problem for athletes participating in endurance sports such as running (32). Endurance athletes may not be focused on muscle-building and may be more concerned with excessive calories and weight gain. Some of the most common protein sources in North American diets are also high in fat, so some athletes may exclude them in favor of carbohydrates. Eating inadequate protein may place an athlete at risk for decreased muscle mass (17). Over time, the inadequate protein intake means essential amino acids are not available for tissue repair or synthesis, placing the athlete at risk for injury. Chronic fatigue may also be evident in these athletes because of poor muscle strength.

Female Athlete Triad

The female athlete triad (see Chapter 28, Eating Disorders in Athletes) is now a recognized syndrome in female athletes. It is characterized first by inadequate calorie intake, followed by loss of menstrual cycle (amenorrhea), and finally osteoporosis (60). Research suggests that inadequate protein intake may be linked to the onset of amenorrhea (61,62). Studies clearly show that the lack of a normal menses and estrogen leads to inadequate calcium deposition and bony defects including stress fractures and osteoporosis (61). Clark et al (63) found that amenorrheic runners consumed 300 to 500 fewer kcal per day than eumenorrheic women. Nelson et al (62) found protein intake was less than the RDA in 82% of the amenorrheic women but only 35% of the eumenorrheic women in her study had less protein than the RDA. Calcium intake did not differ between the two groups. The diets of runners, dancers, and gymnasts have shown to be inadequate in many nutrients including total calories and protein (63,64). The connection between protein and menstrual function is still unclear, but there is concern that athletes who have inadequate protein may be at risk for amenorrhea. Whether or not the quality of the protein is also related to amenorrhea risk is also of interest. *Box 3.4* highlights populations at risk for inadequate protein intake.

BOX 3.4   Special Populations at Risk for Inadequate Protein

Vegetarians: Quality of Protein

Protein utilization is more efficient with higher quality protein (13). Egg protein is used by FAO/WHO as a standard against which to measure the quality of other proteins. Exercisers should be reminded that a little animal protein goes a long way in meeting individual amino acid requirements. A diet that contains no animal products makes it more of a challenge to get all of the essential amino acids. The less animal protein in an athlete's diet, the greater volume of plant protein that is needed to meet his or her amino acid needs. The exception to this may be with soy products. The "amino acid score," an alternative procedure to the older Protein Efficiency Ratio (PER), is used by FAO/WHO to evaluate protein quality (65). This measurement gives soy protein isolates and soy protein concentrates equivalent scores to animal protein in the ability to meet long-term essential amino acid needs of children (65). Vegetarians who include dairy products, eggs, and soy products should have no difficulty meeting individual amino acid requirements as well as total protein needs. (See Chapter 26, Vegetarian Athletes for more detailed information.)

Weight-conscious Women

In an effort to reduce calories to lose weight, many women may eat inadequate protein. As energy levels decrease below energy expenditure, protein utilization decreases.

Pregnant Athletes

Pregnancy increases protein requirements. The average pregnant women needs 60 g per day compared to the RDA of 45 g per day for the average nonpregnant woman (13). Although research on exercise during pregnancy is relatively new, many women are engaging in exercise throughout pregnancy. The intensity and duration of exercise and its effects on the pregnancy depend on many factors including the fitness level of the woman. A pregnant woman's exercise program should be discussed with her physician. The protein needs of an exercising pregnant woman are unclear. Safe recommendations are in the range of 1.0 to 1.4 g/kg of prepregnant weight. (See Chapter 29, Pregnancy and Exercise for more information.)

Elderly

Protein utilization changes with aging, becoming less efficient (66-68). As the aging population becomes more active, the protein requirements of this population need more study. (See Chapter 20, Masters Athletes for more information.)

Diabetes

The American Diabetes Association recommends that people with diabetes not exceed the daily RDA for protein. People with diabetes who exercise to the levels described in this chapter should meet their slightly increased need for protein as long as they have no kidney damage and are consulting with their physician. (See Chapter 25, Diabetes Mellitus and Exercise for more information.)

REFERENCES

1. Grandjean AC. Diets of elite athletes: has the discipline of sports nutrition made an impact? *J Nutr*. 1998;127(suppl 5):874-877.
2. Hawley JA, Dennis SC, Lindsay FH, Noakes TD. Nutritional practices of athletes: are they sub-optimal [abstract]? *J Sports Sci*. 1995;13:75S-81S.
3. Kleiner SM, Bazzarre TL, Ainsworth BE. Nutritional status of nationally ranked elite bodybuilders. *Int J Sport Nutr*. 1994;4:54-69.
4. Lemon PW, Proctor DN. Protein intake and athletic performance. *Sports Med*. 1991;12:313-325.
5. Snyder AC, Naik J. Protein requirements of athletes. In: Berning JR, Steen SN, eds. *Nutrition for Sport and Exercise*. 2nd ed. Gaithersburg, Md: Aspen Publishers; 1998:45-55.
6. Astrand P, Rodahl K. *Textbook of Work Physiology*. 3rd ed. New York, NY: McGraw-Hill Book Co; 1986:523-576.
7. Lemon PW, Dolny DG, Yarasheski KE. Moderate physical activity can increase dietary protein needs [abstract]. *Can J Appl Physiol*. 1997;22:494-503.
8. Lemon PW, Tarnopolsky MA, MacDougall JD, Atkinson SA. Protein requirements and muscle mass/strength changes during intensive training in novice bodybuilders. *J Appl Physiol*. 1992;73:767-775.
9. Meredith CN, Zackin MJ, Frontera WR, Evans WJ. Dietary protein requirements and body protein metabolism in endurance-trained men. *J Appl Physiol*. 1989;66:2850-2856.
10. Friedman JE, Lemon PW. Effect of chronic endurance exercise on retention of dietary protein. *Int J Sports Med*. 1989;10:118-123.
11. Tarnopolsky MA, Atkinson SA, MacDougall JD, Chesley A, Phillips S, Schwarcz HP. Evaluation of protein requirements for trained strength athletes. *J Appl Physiol*. 1992;73;1986-1995.
12. Lemon PW. Effect of initial muscle glycogen levels on protein catabolism during exercise. *J Appl Physiol*. 1980;48:624-629. Abstract.
13. Food and Nutrition Board. *Recommended Dietary Allowances*. 10th ed. Washington, DC: National Academy Press; 1989.
14. Crim MC, Hamish MN. Proteins and amino acids. In: Shils ME, Olson JA, Shike M, eds. *Modern Nutrition in Health and Disease*. 8th ed. Philadelphia, Penn: Lea & Febiger; Waverly Co; 1994:3-35.
15. Paul GL. Dietary protein requirements of physically active individuals [abstract]. *Sports Med*. 1989;8:154-176.
16. Butterfield G. Amino acids and high protein diets. In: Lamb D, Williams M, eds. *Perspectives in Exercise Science and Sports Medicine*. Carmel, Ind: Cooper Publishing Group; 1991:87-122.
17. Lemon PW. Is increased dietary protein necessary or beneficial for individuals with a physically active lifestyle? *Nutr Rev*. 1996;54:S169-S175.
18. Butterfield GE. Whole-body protein utilization in humans. *Med Sci Sports Exerc*. 1987;119(suppl 5):157S-165S.
19. Young VR, Bier DM, Pellet PL. A theoretical basis for increasing current estimates of the amino acids requirements in adult men with experimental support [abstract]. *Am J Clin Nutr*. 1989;50:80-92.
20. Lemon PW, Benevenga JP, Mullin JP, Nagle FJ. Effect of daily exercise and food intake on leucine oxidation [abstract]. *Biochem Med*. 1989;33:67-76.
21. Marchini JS, Cortiella J, Hiramatsu T, Chapman TE, Young VR. Requirements for indispensable amino acids in adult humans: longer-term amino acid kinetic study with support for the adequacy of the Massachusetts Institute of Technology amino acid requirement pattern. *Am J Clin Nutr*. 1993;58:670-683.
22. Young VR. Adult amino acid requirements: the case for a major revision in current recommendations. *J Nutr*. 1994;124(suppl 8):1517S-1523S.
23. Lemon PW. Protein and amino acid needs of the strength athlete. *Int J Sport Nutr*. 1991;1:127-145.

24. Tarnopolsky MA. Influence of differing macronutrient intakes on muscle glycogen resynthesis after resistance exercise. *J Appl Physiol*. 1998;84 890-896.

25. Burke LM, Collier GR, Beasley SK, et al. Effect of coingestion of fat and protein with carbohydrate feedings on muscle glycogen storage. *J Appl Physiol*. 1995;78:2187-2192.

26. Tarnopolsky MA, Bosman M, Macdonald JR, Vandeputte D, Martin J, Roy BD. Postexercise protein—carbohydrate supplements increase muscle glycogen in men and women. *J Appl Physiol*. 1997;83:1877-1883.

27. Chandler RM, Byrne HK, Patterson JG, Ivy JL. Dietary supplements affect the anabolic hormones after weight-training exercise. *J Appl Physiol*. 1994;76:839-845.

28. Roy BD, Tarnopolsky MA, MacDougall JD, Fowles J, Yarasheski KE. Effect of glucose supplement timing on protein metabolism after resistance training [abstract]. *J Appl Physiol*. 1997;82:1882-1888.

29. Lemon PW. Protein requirements of soccer. *J Sports Sci*. 1994;12(suppl):17-22. Abstract.

30. Burgen JS, Corbin CB. Eating disorders among female athletes. *Phys Sports Med*. 1987;15:89-95.

31. Rosen LW, McKeag DB, Hough DD, Curley V. Pathogenic weight control behaviors of female college gymnasts. *Phys Sports Med*. 1986;14:79-86.

32. Tanaka JA, Tanaka H, Landi W. An assessment of carbohydrate intake in collegiate distance runners. *Int J Sport Nutr*. 1995;5:206-214.

33. Hawley JA, Williams MM. Dietary intakes of age—group swimmers. *Br J Sports Med*. 1991;25:154-158.

34. Beals KA, Manore MM. Nutritional status of female athletes with subclinical eating disorders. *J Am Diet Assoc*. 1998;98:419-425.

35. Armsey TD, Green G. Nutrition supplements: science vs hype. *Phys Sport Med*. http://www.physsportmed.com/issues/1997/06jun/armsey.htm. Accessed April 8, 1998.

36. Clarkson P. Nutritional supplements for weight gain. *Sport Sci Exch*. 1998;11(1).

37. Hefler SK, Widemann L, Gaesser GA, Weltman A. Branched-chain amino acid (BCAA) supplementation improves endurance performance in competitive cyclists [abstract]. *Med Sci Sports Exerc*. 1995;27(suppl):149.

38. Henning KJ, Jean-Baptiste E, Singh T, Hill RH, Friedman SM. Eosinophilia-myalgia syndrome in patients ingesting a single source of L-tryptophan [abstract]. *J Rheumatol*. 1993;20:273-278.

39. Gastmann UA, Lehmann MJ. Overtraining and the BCAA hypothesis. *Med Sci Sports Exerc*. 1998;30:1173-1178.

40. Davis M. Carbohydrates, branched-chain amino acids and endurance: the central fatigue hypothesis. *Int J Sport Nutr*. 1995;5(suppl):29-38.

41. Suminski R, Robertson RJ, Goss FL, et al. Acute effect of amino acid ingestion and resistance exercise on plasma growth hormone concentration in young men. *Int J Sport Nutr*. 1997;7:48-60.

42. Mittleman KD, Ricci MR, Bailey SP. Branched-chain amino acids prolong exercise during heat stress in men and women. *Med Sci Sports Exerc*. 1998;30:83-91.

43. Blomstrand E, Hassmen P, Ekblom B, Newsholm EA. Administration of branched-chain amino acids during sustained exercise—effects on performance and on plasma concentration of some amino acids [abstract]. *Eur J Appl Physiol*. 1991;63:83-88.

44. Krieder RB, Miriel V, Bertun E. Amino acid supplementation and exercise performance. Analysis of the proposed ergogenic value. *Sports Med*. 1993;16:190-209.

45. Yarashesk KE, Campbell JA, Smith K, Rennie MJ, Holloszy JO, Bier DM. Effect of growth hormone and resistance exercise on muscle growth in young men [abstract]. *Am J Physiol*. 1992;262(3 pt 1):261E-267E.

46. Castell LM, Poortmans JR, Newsholme EA. Does glutamine have a role in reducing infections in athletes [abstract]? *Eur J Appl Physiol*. 1996;73:488-490.

47. Rohde T, MacLean DA, Pedersen BK. Effect of glutamine supplementation on changes in the immune system induced by repeated exercise. *Med Sci Sports Exerc*. 1998;30:856-862.

48. Castell LM, Poortman JR, Leclercq R, Brasseur M, Duchateau J, Newsholme EA. Some aspects of the acute phase response after a marathon race, and the effects of glutamine supplementation [abstract]. *Eur J Appl Physiol.* 1997;75:47-53.

49. Burke LM, Pyne DB, Telford RD. Effect of oral creatine supplementation on single-effort sprint performance in elite swimmers. *Int J Sport Nutr.* 1996;6:222-233.

50. Grindstaff PD, Kreider R, Bishop R, et al. Effects of creatine supplementation on repetitive sprint performance and body composition in competitive swimmers. *Int J Sport Nutr.* 1997;7:330-346.

51. Volek J, Kraemer WJ, Bush JA, et al. Creatine supplementation enhances muscular performance during high-intensity resistance exercise. *J Am Diet Assoc.* 1997;97:765-776.

52. Eichner ER, Mahan J, Painter P, Zambraski E. Roundtable: the kidney, exercise, and hydration. *Sports Sci Exch.* 1994;5(3).

53. Barzel US, Massey LK. Excess dietary protein can adversely affect bone. *J Nutr.* 1998;128:1051-1053.

54. Spencer H, Kramer L, Osis D. Do protein and phosphorous cause calcium loss [abstract]? *J Nutr.* 1988;118:657-660.

55. Spencer H, Kramer L, Osis D, Norris C. Effect of a high protein (meat) intake on calcium metabolism in man [abstract]. *Am J Clin Nutr.* 1978;31:2167-2180.

56. Heaney RP. Excess dietary protein may not adversely affect bone. *J Nutr.* 1998;128:1054-1057.

57. Costill DL. Carbohydrate for athletic training [abstract]. *Bol Asoc Med P R.* 1991;83:350-353.

58. Evans WJ, Hughes VA. Dietary carbohydrates and endurance exercise. *Am J Clin Nutr.* 1985;41(suppl):1146-1154.

59. Sherman WM, Wimer GS. Insufficient dietary carbohydrate during training: does it impair athletic performance? *Int J Sport Nutr.* 1991;1:28-44.

60. Otis C. Too slim, amenorrheic fracture-prone: the female triad. *ACSM Health Fitness Journal.* 1998;2:20-25.

61. Freudenheim JL, Johnson NE, Smith EL. Relationships between usual nutrient intake and bone-mineral content of women 35-65 years of age: longitudinal and cross-sectional analysis. *Am J Clin Nutr.* 1986;44:863-876.

62. Nelson ME, Fischer EC, Catsos PD, Meredith CN, Turksoy NR, Evans WJ. Diet and bone status in amennorheic runners. *Am J Clin Nutr.* 1986;43:910-916.

63. Clark N, Nelson M, Evans W. Nutrition education for elite female runners. *Phys Sports Med.* 1986;16:124-134.

64. Dueck CA, Manore MM, Matt KS. Role of energy balance in athletic menstrual dysfunction. *Int J Sport Nutr.* 1996;6:165-190.

65. Young VR. The nutritional role of plant protein. *The Soy Connection.* 1998;2:1-4.

66. Campbell WW, Crim MC, Young VR, Joseph LJ, Evans WJ. Effects of resistance training and dietary protein intake on protein metabolism in older adults [abstract]. *Am J Physiol.* 1995;268(6pt 1):11143E-1153E.

67. Fukagawa NK, Young VR. Protein and amino acid metabolism and requirements in older persons [abstract]. *Clin Geriatr Med.* 1987;3:329-341.

68. Young VR. Amino acids and proteins in relation to the nutrition of elderly people [abstract]. *Age Ageing.* 1990;19(suppl):10-24.

DIETARY FAT AND EXERCISE

Satya S. Jonnalagadda, PhD

DEFINITION AND TYPE

Lipids are important components of plants, animals, and microbial cell membranes. They are marginally soluble in water and greatly soluble in organic solvents such as chloroform or acetone. There are two major groups of lipids which include open-chained and closed-ringed molecules. The open-chain lipid compounds include:

- Fatty acids
- Triacylglycerol
- Sphingolipids
- Phosphoacylglycerols
- Glycolipids

The second major group of lipids consists of closed-ringed compounds, namely steroids. The main one in this group is cholesterol.

Fat is a major energy source, meeting daily energy needs but also providing energy when:

- Other sources are unavailable, such as during starvation.
- Cells are unable to utilize energy stores, such as during diabetes mellitus.
- There is inadequate energy intake, such as during illness.

Fat stores also help maintain body temperature and protect body organs from trauma. Additionally, fat aids in the delivery and absorption of fat-soluble vitamins, contributes to the sensory appeal of foods, and influences the texture of foods. Its high-energy density contributes to the satiety value of foods (see *Box 4.1*).

BOX 4.1 Major Functions of Dietary Fat

- Energy source
- Source of essential fatty acids
- An aid in absorption and transport of fat-soluble vitamins
- Protector for major organs, since it insulates against injury
- Structural constituent of cells

FATTY ACIDS

Fatty acids are the simplest lipids and consist of straight hydrocarbon chains (see *Figure 4.1*). Fatty acids are a component of the more complex lipids and provide most of the calories from dietary fat. The common dietary fatty acids and the major contributors of these fatty acids are listed in *Table 4.1*.

FIGURE 4.1   Structure of a Saturated Fatty Acid

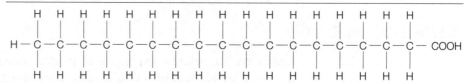

TABLE 4.1   Types and Sources of Fatty Acids

Fatty Acid Class	Fatty Acid	Common Abbreviation	Examples of Major Contributors to Intake
Saturated	Lauric acid	C12:0	Coconut oil
	Myristic acid	C14:0	Butterfat, coconut oil
	Palmitic acid	C16:0	Palm oil
	Stearic acid	C18:0	Cocoa butter
Monounsaturated	Oleic acid	C18:1 *cis* Ω-9*	Olive oil
	Elaidic acid	C18:1 *trans* Ω-9	Butterfat
Polyunsaturated	Linoleic acid	C18:2 Ω-6	Most vegetable oils (eg, safflower oil, corn oil)
	Arachidonic acid	C20:4 Ω-6	Lard, meats
	Linolenic acid	C18:3 Ω-3	Soybean oil, canola oil
	Eicosapentaenoic acid	C20:5 Ω-3	Fish oils, shellfish
	Docosahexaenoic acid	C22:6 Ω-3	Fish oils, shellfish

* Indicates position of double bond counting from the methyl end

Adapted from: Jonnalagadda SS, Mustad VA, Yu S, Etherton TD, Kris-Etherton PM. Effects of individual fatty acids on chronic diseases. *Nutr Today*. 1996;31:90-106.

Fatty acids are classified based on the number of carbons in the molecule (chain length). Fatty acids may be saturated (SFA) (ie, no double bond), with the common ones being lauric (C12:0), myristic (C14:0), palmitic (C16:0), and stearic (C18:0) acids. Monounsaturated fatty acids (MUFA), such as oleic acid (C18:1), contain one double bond. Polyunsaturated fatty acids (PUFA), such as linoleic acid (C18:2), contain more than one double bond. Some of these PUFA, namely linoleic and linolenic acid, cannot be synthesized in the body and are therefore considered essential fatty acids because they need to be provided in the diet. These essential fatty acids are used for the synthesis of other long-chain PUFA, which play a major role in the synthesis of eicosanoids. The unsaturated fatty acids are also classified according to the position of the double bond, ie, omega-9 (Ω-9 or n-9), omega-6 (Ω-6 or n-6), omega-3 (Ω-3 or n-3), based on the position of the first double bond from the methyl end (see *Figures 4.2A, 4.2B, 4.2C*). Additionally, these unsaturated fatty acids (UFA) are also classified based on the isomeric confirmation of the double bonds, namely *cis* and *trans* (see *Figure 4.3*), which determine the properties of these UFA. Therefore the type of fatty acid can influence the physical properties of the fat, its digestion, absorption, metabolism, utilization and consequently health.

FIGURE 4.2A Structure of a Monounsaturated Fatty Acid

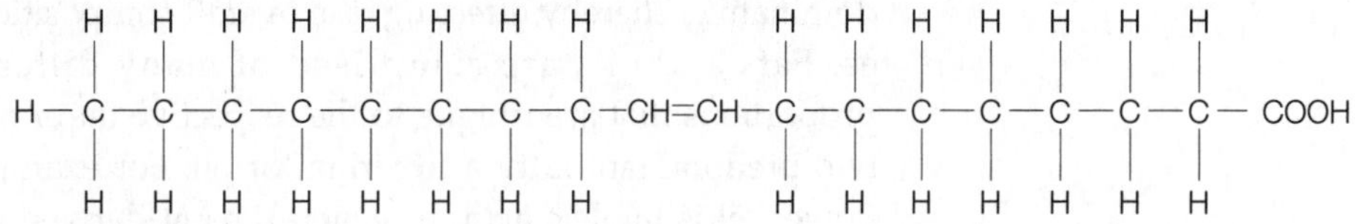

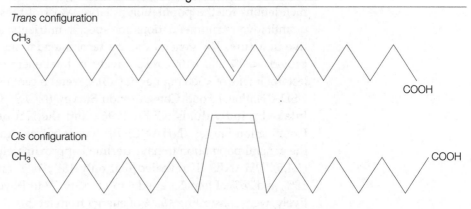

FIGURE 4.2B Structure of a Polyunsaturated Omega-3 Fatty Acid

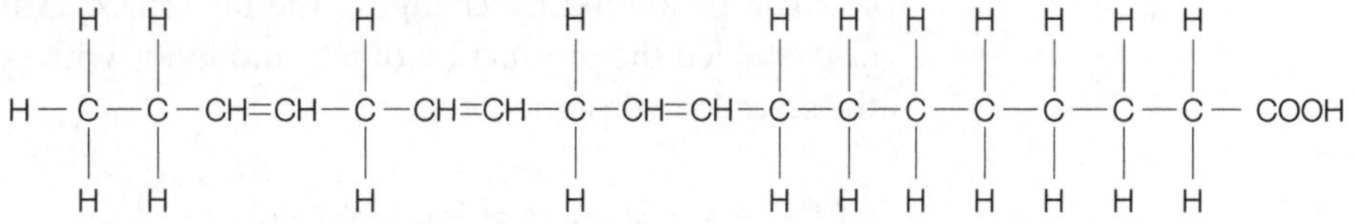

FIGURE 4.2C Structure of a Polyunsaturated Omega-6 Fatty Acid

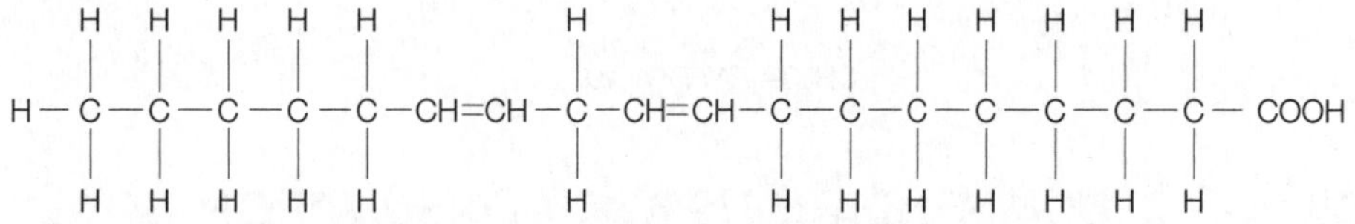

FIGURE 4.3 *Trans* and *Cis* Configurations of Double Bonds

Trans configuration

CH₃

COOH

Cis configuration

CH₃

COOH

Approximately 80% of the total fat intake in the American diet is provided by meat, poultry, fish, salad and cooking oils, shortening, and dairy products (1,2). Additionally, meat, poultry, fish, eggs, and dairy products are the major contributors of the SFA in the diet. Grain products, such as yeast breads, cakes, and cookies, make considerable contributions to the intake of MUFA and PUFA. Fish and shellfish are the main sources of the long-chain PUFA.

TRIACYLGLYCEROL

Dietary fats and oils are made up of triacylglycerol (TAG) in which three fatty acids are esterified to glycerol (see *Figure 4.4*) with a characteristic fatty acid predominating, thereby affecting the overall composition of the diet and food choices. Fats and oils are comprised of many different fatty acids present in proportions that are unique to the respective fat or oil. Typically, there are one or two predominant fatty acids in fat or oil. For example, 78% of fatty acids in safflower oil is linoleic acid. In general, plant-derived oils, except tropical oils such as coconut and palm oil, are rich sources of unsaturated fatty acids, while animal fats are rich sources of saturated fatty acids. Therefore, the fatty acid profile of the diet can be altered by changing the fat source. Additionally, biotechnology has also enabled the production of fats and foods with specific fatty acid composition, the so-called "designer foods."

FIGURE 4.4   Structure of Triacylglycerol

CH_2O—*FATTY ACID*

CHO—*FATTY ACID*

CH_2O—*FATTY ACID*

DIETARY RECOMMENDATIONS AND CONSUMPTION OF FAT IN THE UNITED STATES

In recognition of the role of diet in the development of chronic diseases, numerous federal agencies and professional organizations have made dietary recommendations for the population-at-large. Most of these dietary guidelines make quantitative recommendations for specific nutrients, although some are qualitative in nature. The general dietary recommendations are that total fat and SFA provide <30% and <10%, respectively, of total energy intake, with a dietary cholesterol intake of <300 mg per day (3). Several recent national surveys, such as the USDA National Food Consumption Survey (NCFS), Continued Survey of Food Intake by Individuals (CSFII 1996), and the National Health and Nutrition Examination Survey (NHANES III) have observed the total fat consumption of the general population to have declined approximately to 34% of calories in 1990 (1,4,5). NHANES III revealed that only 18%, 14%, and 21% of males and 18%, 18%, and 25% of females aged 6 to 11 years, 12 to 19 years, and >20 years, respectively, were consuming ≤30% of energy from fat (5).

DIETARY FAT INTAKE PATTERNS OF ATHLETES

The dietary fat intake patterns of athletes vary considerably depending on the sport, training, and performance level of the athlete. Although there are no sport-specific dietary recommendations, the dietary intake of an athlete is generally reflective of the energy demands of the sport during training and competition. In general, endurance athletes, such as runners and cyclists, have been observed to consume diets that meet the dietary fat guidelines (<30% energy from fat). Distance runners have been reported to consume between 27% to 35% of energy as fat, while professional cyclists, such as those competing in the Tour de France, were observed to consume approximately 27% of their total calories as fat (6). Likewise, rowers, basketball players, and nordic skiers were reported to consume diets that contained 30% to 40% of energy as fat (7). On the other hand, for athletes participating in sports where appearance plays a major factor in performance, such as gymnastics and figure skating, the dietary fat intake has been reported to range from 15% to 31% (8,9).

Consequences of a Low-fat Diet in Athletes

Most athletes' diets meet the general dietary guidelines of <30% energy from fat. However, to increase their competitiveness, such as endurance athletes, or improve their appearance, such as gymnasts and figure skaters, athletes may consume very low-fat diets (typically defined as <20% calories from fat) in order to keep their body weight and percent body fat down (10). Additionally, athletes, especially endurance athletes, tend to increase their dietary carbohydrate intake at the expense of dietary fat to increase their body glycogen stores. In either case, the resulting low-fat diets may not meet the energy demands for growth and development in the young athlete and the energy needs for endurance performance (6,10). Additionally, by subscribing to low-fat diets for prolonged periods of time, athletes are likely to develop deficiencies of essential fatty acids and fat-soluble vitamins. Intakes of micronutrients such as calcium and zinc may also be compromised. In female athletes these very low-fat diets can contribute to menstrual dysfunctions and may disrupt reproductive function in later life (10). Similarly, in male athletes low serum testosterone levels are observed with the intake of low-fat diets, which in turn can influence their reproductive functions (10). Therefore, the consumption of very low-fat diets by athletes is generally not recommended.

FAT REPLACERS AND SUBSTITUTES

In an attempt to decrease dietary fat intake, individuals have taken to the consumption of fat-modified foods. In 1996, approximately 88% of the US population was consuming low-fat, reduced-fat, or fat-free foods and beverages (11). To meet this high consumer demand, food manufacturers have developed various ingredients termed "fat substitutes" or "analogs" (see *Boxes 4.2A, 4.2B*). These fat replacers should be substituted for dietary fat (ie, replace dietary fat) in order to effectively observe a reduction in total fat intake. However, simply adding them to the diet without replacing dietary fat can defeat the purpose of these fat replacers and substitutes. Therefore, it is the position of The American Dietetic Association that "the fat content of foods may be safely reduced or replaced using appropriate processing methods and constituents. Individuals who choose such foods should do so within the context of a diet consistent with the Dietary Guidelines for Americans" (12).

BOX 4.2A   Definition of Fat Replacers and Substitutes

Fat substitutes or analogs
- No chemical similarities to fat
- Replicate functional and sensory properties of fat
- Provide less energy than fat
- Replace all or some fat in the product

Fat memetics
- Partially replicate a few properties of fat

Fat barriers
- Decrease fat absorption during frying process

Adapted from: Position of The American Dietetic Association. Fat replacers. *J Am Diet Assoc.* 1998;98:463-368.

BOX 4.2B   Types of Fat Replacers and Substitutes

Carbohydrate-based
- Cannot be used for frying
- Can withstand heat

Microparticulated protein
- Provide similar mouth feel as fat
- Cannot be used at high temperatures because of protein coagulation

Fat-based
- Mono and diglycerides
  1. Alter fatty acid composition
  2. Decrease total energy content
- Fatty acids bound to sugar molecules
  1. Not digested by intestinal enzymes
  2. Heat stable, can be used for frying

Adapted from: Position of The American Dietetic Association: Fat replacers. *J Am Diet Assoc.* 1998;98:463-368.

METABOLISM OF FAT DURING EXERCISE

Fat along with carbohydrate is oxidized in the muscle to supply energy to the exercising muscle. The extent to which these sources contribute to energy expenditure depends on the duration and intensity of exercise. Endurance (>90 minutes) athletes typically train at 65% to 75% VO_2max and are limited by the carbohydrate reserves in the body. After 15 to 20 minutes of endurance exercise, oxidation of fat deposits (lipolysis) is stimulated and glycerol and free fatty acids are released (see *Figure 4.5*). In the resting muscle, fatty acid oxidation provides a great extent of energy; however, this contribution decreases during light aerobic exercise. During high exercise intensities a shift in energy supply from fat to carbohydrate is observed, especially at intensities of 70% to 80% VO_2max suggesting that there might be limitations to the use of fatty acid oxidation as a means of energy to the exercising muscle. Abernethy et al (13) suggest the following mechanisms:

1. An increase in lactate production will lower catecholamine-induced lipolysis, thereby decreasing plasma fatty acid concentration and fatty acid supply to the muscle. It has been suggested that lactate may exhibit an antilipolytic effect in the adipose tissue. Additionally, lactate build-up can lead to a reduction in the blood pH, thereby lowering or destroying the activity of the various enzymes involved in the energy production process and resulting in muscle fatigue.

2. A lower rate of ATP production per unit time of fat oxidation compared to carbohydrate and the greater requirement for oxygen during fatty acid oxidation compared to carbohydrate oxidation. For instance, oxidation of one glucose molecule (6 carbon) produces 38 ATP, whereas the oxidation of an 18 carbon fatty acid molecules (stearic acid) produces 147 ATP (3.9 fold greater yield of ATP from one fatty acid molecule or 1.3 fold greater yield of ATP per carbon

FIGURE 4.5   Fatty Acid Metabolism

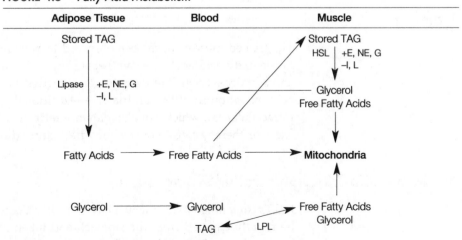

HSL = Hormone sensitive lipase; LPL = lipoprotein lipase; E = epinephrine; NE = norepinephrine; I = insulin; G = glucagon; L = lactate

Adapted from: Sherman WM, Leenders N. Fat loading: the next magic bullet? *Int J Sport Nutr.* 1995;5:S1-S12.

molecule). Additionally, the complete oxidation of one glucose molecule requires six oxygen molecules, whereas the complete oxidation of palmitic acid requires 26 oxygen molecules, which is 77% higher than that of glucose. Therefore, during prolonged exercise the higher oxygen requirements of fatty acid oxidation can increase the cardiovascular stress, which could be a limiting factor with regard to duration of activity (14,15).

3. Transport of long-chain fatty acids into mitochondria depends on the capacity of the carnitine transport system. This transport mechanism can be inhibited by other metabolic processes. An increase in glycogenolysis as seen during exercise can result in elevated concentrations in acetyl CoA, which tends to result in an increase in malonyl CoA, an important intermediate in fatty acid synthesis, which can inhibit the transport mechanism. Similarly, increased lactate formation can result in an elevation in acetylated carnitine concentrations and a reduction in free carnitine concentrations and further reduced transport of fatty acids and fatty acid oxidation.

Although fatty acid oxidation during endurance exercise yields greater amounts of energy when compared to carbohydrate, fatty acid oxidation requires more oxygen for oxidation when compared to carbohydrate (77% more O_2), thereby putting greater stress on the cardiovascular system. However, because of the limited carbohydrate storage capacity, high-intensity exercise performance can be impaired with glycogen depletion. Therefore, several interventions have been examined to spare muscle carbohydrate and increase fatty acid oxidation during endurance exercise (16). These include:

- Training
- Medium-chain triacylglycerol feedings
- Oral fat emulsion and fat infusion
- High-fat diets
- Supplements such as L-carnitine and caffeine

Training

The trained muscles have been observed to have high lipoprotein lipase, muscle lipase, fatty acid acyl CoA synthetase and reductase, carnitine acyl transferase, and 3-hydroxyl acyl CoA dehydrogenase activities, all of which can enhance fatty acid oxidation in mitochondria (11). Additionally, trained muscles store more intracellular fat, which can also enhance fatty acid supply and oxidation during exercise, thereby conserving carbohydrate stores during endurance exercise.

Medium-chain Triacylglycerol (MCT) Ingestion

MCTs contain fatty acids which have 6 to 10 carbon atoms. MCTs are believed to be rapidly emptied from the stomach and taken up by the intestine. MCTs are transported in the blood to the liver and can increase plasma medium-chain fatty acid and triacylglycerol levels. In the muscle these medium-chain fatty acids are rapidly taken up by the mitochondria because they do not require the carnitine transport system and can be oxidized faster and to a greater extent than long-chain triacylglycerol. However, studies examining the effect of MCT ingestion on exercise performance have been equivocal and the available data do not show a glycogen-sparing effect and/or improvement in endurance performance with MCT ingestion (17-20).

Oral Fat Ingestion and Fat Infusion

A reduction in the oxidation of endogenous carbohydrate during exercise could potentially be achieved by increasing plasma fatty acid concentrations through fat infusions (21). However, fatty acid infusions during exercise are impractical and impossible during competition and could be viewed as an artificial doping mechanism to enhance performance. Additionally, high oral fat emulsion intake could delay gastric emptying and can result in gastrointestinal discomfort (16).

High-fat Diets

It has been suggested that high-fat diets may enhance fatty acid oxidation and improve performance in endurance athletes. However, based on the current evidence, it is speculative to state that a high-fat diet could enhance performance potentially by down regulating carbohydrate metabolism and maintaining glycogen stores in muscle and liver (15,22,23). Additionally, the long-term adverse effects of high-fat intake on the cardiovascular system are well established and, therefore, this practice should be viewed with caution if being used by athletes to improve performance.

L-carnitine Supplements

The main function of L-carnitine is the transfer of long-chain fatty acids across the mitochondrial membrane to enter the oxidation pathway. Therefore, it has been speculated that consumption of oral L-carnitine supplements would enhance fatty acid oxidation in athletes. However, there is no substantial scientific evidence to validate this claim.

AEROBIC TRAINING AND SUBSTRATE OXIDATION

A carbohydrate-sparing effect of dietary fat has been suggested with aerobic training, implicating an increase in oxidation of fat and a decrease in oxidation of carbohydrates (24). This reduction in carbohydrate oxidation can enhance endurance performance with greater reliance on fat for energy. Therefore, it has been hypothesized that increasing dietary fat intake might increase fatty acid oxidation, spare carbohydrate, and improve performance. However, current evidence does not support this hypothesis.

Infusion of TAG emulsion or ingestion of SFA was not observed to influence muscle glycogen levels during exercise, work capacity, or exercise performance (21,24,25). Additionally, fasting has been used by some researchers in an attempt to increase fatty acid oxidation over carbohydrate during exercise. Although fasting appears to increase fatty acid availability for oxidation during exercise, it does not improve overall exercise performance (26). Additionally, studies have examined the influence of low-carbohydrate, high-fat diets on exercise performance and muscle glycogen stores. However, these dietary manipulations have not shown any consistent effects on muscle glycogen stores, exercise capacity, or performance (24). At the present time the effectiveness of short-term dietary manipulations that include fat-loading to enhance performance by increasing fat oxidation and lowering carbohydrate oxidation in endurance athletes is yet to be proven (15). On the other hand, long-term adaptation to fat-rich diets could potentially induce skeletal-muscle adaptations, metabolism and/or morphological changes which in turn could influence exercise performance (22). Lambert et al (27) observed that the consumption of a 76% fat diet versus a 74% carbohydrate diet for 14 days by endurance-trained cyclists did not impair maximal power output and time to exhaustion. However, muscle glycogen stores were two-fold lower on the high-fat diet compared to the high-carbohydrate diet, thus making it difficult to interpret the influence of this dietary manipulation on endurance performance. Similarly, Helge et al (23) observed in untrained male subjects fed a high-fat diet (62% energy) or a high-carbohydrate diet (65% energy) with training for 4 weeks a 9% increase in VO_2max, and endurance time to exhaustion was increased with both dietary treatments. This suggests that adaptation to a high-fat diet in combination with training for up to 4 weeks exercising at submaximal workload does not seem to impair endurance performance. However, consumption of a high-fat diet for 7 weeks was associated with a reduction in time to exhaustion compared to the high-carbohydrate diet group, suggesting that the duration of this high-fat dietary intake may have an impact on exercise performance (28).

This adaptation to dietary fat could be associated with fatty acid oxidation enzymes. A strong association has been demonstrated between b-hydroxyacyl CoA dehydrogenase activity and fatty acid uptake and oxidation in humans (29) and may also be associated with an increase in fatty acid binding protein in the cytosol and plasma membrane. Despite this adaptation, training-induced increase in endurance performance with high-fat ingestion is not comparable to that observed with a high-carbohydrate diet.

REFERENCES

1. Jonnalagadda SS, Egan SK, Heimbach JT, Harris SS, Kris-Etherton PM. Fatty acid consumption pattern of Americans: 1987-1988 USDA Nationwide Food Consumption Survey. *Nutr Res.* 1995;15:1767-1781.
2. Ernst ND. Fatty acid composition of present day diets. In: Nelson GJ, ed. *Health Effects of Dietary Fatty Acids.* Champaign, Ill: American Oil Chemists Society; 1991:1-11.
3. National Research Council. Diet and health: implications for reducing chronic disease risk. Committee on Diet and Health, Food and Nutrition Board, Commission on Life Sciences. Washington, DC: National Academy Press; 1989.

4. Wilson JW, Enns CW, Goldman JD, et al. Data tables: combined results from USDA's 1994 and 1995 Continuing Survey of Food Intakes by Individuals and 1994 and 1995 Diet and Health Knowledge Survey [online]. ARS Food Surveys Research Group. http://www.barc.usda.gov/bhnrc/foodsurvey/home.htm. Accessed August 28, 1997.

5. McDowell MA, Briefiel RR, Alaimo K, et al. Energy and macronutrient intakes of persons ages 2 months and over in the United States: Third National Health and Nutrition Examination Survey, Phase I, 1988-91. *Advanced Data from Vital and Health Statistics*, No: 255. Hyattsville, Md: National Center for Health Statistics; 1994.

6. Williams C. Dietary macro- and micronutrient requirements of endurance athletes. *Proc Nutr Soc.* 1998;57:1-8.

7. Burke LM. Nutrition for the female athlete. In: Krummel DA, Kris-Etherton PM, eds. *Nutrition in Women's Health.* Gaithersburg, Md: Aspen Publishers; 1996:263-298.

8. Jonnalagadda SS, Benardot D, Nelson M. Energy and nutrient intakes of the United States national women's artistic gymnastics team. *Int J Sport Nutr.* 1998;8:331-344.

9. Ziegler PJ, Khoo CS, Kris-Etherton PM, Jonnalagadda SS, Sherr B, Nelson JA. Nutritional status of nationally ranked junior US figure skaters. *J Am Diet Assoc.* 1998;98:809-811.

10. Brownell KD, Nelson-Steen S, Wilmore JH. Weight regulation practices in athletes: analysis of metabolic and health effects. *Med Sci Sports Exer.* 1987;18:546-556.

11. Calorie Control Council. Fat reduction in foods. *Calorie Control Council Commentary.* Atlanta, Ga; August 1996.

12. Position of The American Dietetic Association: Fat replacers. *J Am Diet Assoc.* 1998;98:463-468.

13. Abernethy PJ, Thayer R, Taylor AW. Acute and chronic responses of skeletal muscle to endurance and sprint exercise. *Sports Med.* 1990;10:365-389.

14. Ranallo RF, Rhodes EC. Lipid metabolism during exercise. *Sports Med.* 1990;26:29-42.

15. Sherman WM, Leenders N. Fat loading: the next magic bullet? *Int J Sport Nutr.* 1995;5:S1-S12.

16. Brouns F, van der Vusse GJ. Utilization of lipids during exercise in human subjects: metabolic and dietary constraints. *Br J Nutr.* 1998;79:117-128.

17. Jeukendrup AE, Saris WHM, Schrauwen P, Brouns F, Wagenmakers AJM. Metabolic availability of medium-chain triglycerides coingested with carbohydrates during prolonged exercise. *J Appl Physiol.* 1995;79:756-762.

18. Jeukendrup AE, Saris WHM, Brouns F, Halliday D, Wagenmakers AJM. Effects of carbohydrate (CHO) and fat supplements on CHO metabolism during prolonged exercise. *Metabolism.* 1996(a);45:915-921.

19. Jeukendrup AE, Saris WHM, Van Diesen R, Brouns F, Wagenmakers AJM. Effect of endogenous carbohydrate availability on oral medium-chain triglyceride oxidation during prolonged exercise. *J Appl Physiol.* 1996(b);80:949-954.

20. Jeukendrup AE, Thielen JJ, Wagenmakers AJ, Brouns F, Saris WH. Effect of medium-chain triacylglycerol and carbohydrate ingestion on substrate utilization and subsequent cycling performance. *Am J Clin Nutr.* 1998;67:397-404.

21. Vukovich MD, Costill DL, Hickey MS, Trappe SW, Cole KJ, Fink WJ. Effect of fat emulsion infusion and fat feeding on muscle glycogen utilization during cycle exercise. *J Appl Physiol.* 1993;75:1513-1518.

22. Kiens B, Helge JW. Effect of high-fat diets on exercise performance. *Proc Nutr Soc.* 1998;57:73-75.

23. Helge JW, Wulff B, Kiens B. Impact of a fat-rich diet on endurance in man: role of the dietary period. *Med Sci Sports Exer.* 1998;30:456-461.

24. Dyck DJ, Putman CT, Heigenhauser GJF, Hultman E, Spriet LL. Regulation of fat-carbohydrate interaction in skeletal muscle during intense aerobic cycling. *Am J Physiol.* 1993;265:E852-E859.

25. Hargreaves M, Kiens B, Richter EA. Effect of increasing plasma free fatty acid concentrations on muscle metabolism in exercising men. *J Appl Physiol*. 1991;70:194-201.
26. Loy SF, Conlee RK, Winder WW, Nelson AG, Arnall DA, Fisher AG. Effects of a 24-hour fast on cycling endurance time at two different intestines. *J Appl Physiol*. 1986;61:654-659.
27. Lambert EV, Speechly DP, Dennis SC, Noaks TD. Enhanced endurance in trained cyclists during moderate intensity exercise following 2 weeks adaptation to a high fat diet. *Eur J Appl Physiol*. 1994;69:287-283.
28. Helge JW, Richter EA, Kiens B. Interaction of training and diet on metabolism and endurance during exercise in man. *J Physiol*. 1996;492:293-306.
29. Kiens B. Effect of endurance training on fatty acid metabolism: local adaptations. *Med Sci Sports Exer*. 1997;29:640-645.

5

VITAMINS AND MINERALS FOR ACTIVE PEOPLE

Stella Volpe, PhD, RD, FACSM

Vitamins and minerals are necessary for many metabolic processes in the body, as well as to support growth and development (1). Vitamins and minerals are also required in a number of reactions involved with exercise and physical activity, such as energy, carbohydrate, fat and protein metabolism, oxygen transfer and delivery, and tissue repair (1).

The vitamin and mineral needs of individuals who are physically active have always been a subject of debate. Some reports state that those who exercise require more vitamins and minerals than their sedentary counterparts, while other studies do not report greater micronutrient requirements. The intensity, duration, and frequency of the physical activity, as well as the overall nutrient intake of the individual, all have an impact on whether or not micronutrients are required in greater amounts (1,2).

WATER-SOLUBLE VITAMINS

Vitamin B-6

There are three major forms of vitamin B-6: pyridoxine (PN), pyridoxal (PL), and pyridoxamine (PM). The active coenzyme forms of vitamin B-6 are pyridoxal 5'-phosphate (PLP) and pyridoxamine 5'-phosphate (PMP) (3). Vitamin B-6 is involved in about 100 metabolic reactions, including those of gluconeogenesis, niacin synthesis, and lipid metabolism (3).

Optimal vitamin B-6 intakes. Dietary Reference Intakes (DRIs), Adequate Intakes (AIs), and/or Recommended Dietary Allowances (RDAs) for several vitamins and minerals, including vitamin B-6, have been recently updated by the Food and Nutrition Board, Institute of Medicine-National Academy of Sciences (4). See the Tools section for the most recent DRIs for vitamin B-6. Note that the AIs, RDAs, Estimated Average Requirements (EARs), and the Tolerable Upper Intake Levels (ULs) are all under the heading "DRIs" (4). The RDA is the dietary intake level that is adequate for about 98% of healthy people (4). Adequate Intakes are recommendations "based on observed or experimentally determined approximations of nutrient intake by a group (or groups) of healthy people" and are used "when an RDA cannot be determined" (4). Estimated Average Requirements are values used to approximate the nutrient needs of half of the healthy people in a group (4). Tolerable Upper Intake Levels are the highest amount of a nutrient most individuals can consume without negative side effects (4).

Recommendations for individuals who are physically active. A number of research studies have reported that vitamin B-6 metabolism is affected by exercise and that poor vitamin B-6 status can impair exercise performance (5).

It appears that continuous aerobic exercise results in transient changes in vitamin B-6 status, and the intensity of the exercise may be related to the changes in vitamin B-6 status (5). However, Crozier et al (6) did not observe differences in plasma vitamin B-6 concentrations with varying intensities of bicycle ergometry. The transient effects of exercise on changes in plasma vitamin B-6 status make it difficult to ascertain whether individuals who are physically active require more vitamin B-6 in their diets than sedentary individuals. In an attempt to address this, Singh et al (7) supplemented 22 physically active men with either high doses of a vitamin-mineral supplement or a placebo. Blood concentrations of the B vitamins increased significantly, but subsequently decreased after supplementation was discontinued (7). Blood concentrations of vitamins A and C, zinc, magnesium, and calcium did not change, possibly suggesting an increased need for the B vitamins in individuals who are physically active. Singh et al (7) did not assess the effects of supplementation on exercise performance. Nonetheless, with the research conducted thus far, it appears that individuals who exercise do not need a greater amount of vitamin B-6, but if deficiencies exist, it may be necessary to supplement with vitamin B-6 at the level of the DRI or greater. Because limited research has been conducted in the area of vitamin B-6 and exercise, more research is required before more definitive recommendations about intake can be made to the individual who exercises. Dietary sources of vitamin B-6 can be found in *Table 5.1*.

TABLE 5.1   Dietary Sources of Vitamin B-6, Vitamin B-12, and Folate

Food	Vitamin B-6 Content (mg)*	Vitamin B-12 Content (µg)*	Folate Content (µg)*
3 oz beef liver, pan fried	1.2	95.1	187
1 cup skim milk	0.1	0.9	13
1/2 cup sunflower seeds, dried	0.6	0	164
1 cup spinach, fresh	0.1	0	109
3 oz chicken, giblets	0.5	11.3	322
3 oz raw oysters	0.1	13.8	15
3 oz bluefish, cooked, dry heat	0.4	5.3	2
3 oz wild Atlantic salmon	0.8	2.6	25
1 cup fortified oat flakes	0.9	2.5	169
3/4 cup orange juice, from concentrate	0.1	0	82

*Values do not reflect bioavailability.

Wardlaw GM. *Perspectives in Nutrition*. 4th ed. Boston, Mass: WCB McGraw-Hill; 1999. Used with permission.

Vitamin B-12 and Folate

Vitamin B-12, or cyanocobalamin, and folate (folic acid) are both necessary for DNA synthesis (8,9) and are interrelated in their synthesis and metabolism. Both are required for normal erythrocyte synthesis, and it is this function where these two vitamins may have an effect on exercise (10). The Tools section contains the most recent DRIs for vitamin B-12 and folate.

Requirements for individuals who are physically active. Although a number of researchers have reported adequate intakes of vitamin B-12 and folate in athletes, inadequate intakes of these two vitamins can lead to megaloblastic anemia. Because vitamin B-12 is secreted daily into the bile and then reabsorbed, it takes about 20 years for healthy people to show signs of vitamin B-12 deficiency (11). Nonetheless, it is recommended that vegan athletes supplement with vitamin B-12 (12). The adequate intake of vitamin B-12 is of special concern in vegetarian athletes because vitamin B-12 is almost exclusively found in animal products (8). Additionally, many athletes supplement with vitamins and minerals and megadoses (500 to 1,000 mg) of vitamin C which may decrease vitamin B-12 bioavailability from food and may also lead to vitamin B-12 deficiency (13,14). Athletes who consume adequate vitamin B-12 and folate in their diets are probably not at risk for vitamin B-12 or folate deficiencies. Telford et al (15) supplemented 82 male and female athletes from different sports with either a vitamin-mineral supplement or a placebo for 7 to 8 months. All athletes in the study consumed diets which met the recommended daily intakes of vitamins and minerals. Although Telford et al reported that vitamin-mineral supplementation did not improve performance in any of the sport-specific variables measured, they did report improved jumping ability, increased body weight, and increased sum of skinfolds in female basketball players. They were unable to ascertain if the increased body weight was solely due to an increase in fat mass or muscle mass, but speculated that most of the weight gain was probably due to an increase in fat mass because of the increased sum of skinfolds. However, they speculated that some of the weight gain may have been a result of increased muscle mass because of the improved jumping ability in the female basketball players. Certainly, the area of supplementation and athletic performance needs to be further studied; however, it appears that individuals who consume adequate intakes of vitamins and minerals do not benefit from supplementation. Nonetheless, Vitamin B-12 or folate deficiencies can lead to increased serum homocysteine levels which can lead to cardiovascular disease (16), pointing to the need of individuals who exercise to be concerned not only about nutrition and performance but also about nutrition and overall health. Dietary sources of folate and vitamin B-12 can be found in *Table 5.1*.

Thiamin

Thiamin participates in several energy-producing reactions as part of thiamin diphosphate (TDP) (also known as thiamin pyrophosphate (TPP)), including the citric acid cycle, branched-chain amino acid (BCAA) catabolism, and the pentose phosphate pathway (17). For example, thiamin is required for the conversion of pyruvate to acetyl-CoA during carbohydrate metabolism (1). This conversion is essential for the aerobic metabolism of glucose, and exercise performance and health will be impaired if this conversion does not occur (1). Thus, it is imperative that individuals who exercise consume the proper amount of both thiamin and carbohydrates. The Tools section contains the most recent DRIs for thiamin.

Recommendations for individuals who are physically active. There appears to be a strong correlation between high-carbohydrate intakes, physical activity, and thiamin requirements (17). This may be a concern for individuals who exercise because carbohydrates are needed in the highest amounts in the diet. However, some studies have not shown that individuals who exercise require more thiamin in their diets than sedentary individuals. Thus, it may be prudent to recommend that individuals who exercise obtain at least the DRI for thiamin to prevent depletion. However, some of the literature suggests that thiamin intakes of one to two times the RDA would be safe and sufficiently meet the requirements for individuals who are physically active (17). Weight et al (18) reported that 3 months of a multivitamin-mineral supplementation did not significantly increase serum thiamin levels in athletes. These researchers did not assess any performance measures of the supplementation (18). More research is required to definitively ascertain whether thiamin requirements are greater in individuals who exercise. Thiamin requirements may be greater for individuals who train several hours a day compared to individuals who are moderately physically active; however, more research is required to assess the different needs of athletes/exercisers. Dietary sources of thiamin are listed in *Table 5.2.*

TABLE 5.2   Dietary Sources of Thiamin, Riboflavin, and Niacin

Food	Thiamin Content (mg)*	Riboflavin Content (mg)*	Niacin Content (mg)*
1 cup skim milk	0.1	0.3	0.2
1/2 cup fresh hummus	0.1	0.1	0.5
1 white pita, enriched	0.4	0.2	2.8
1/2 cup black beans, cooked	0.2	0.1	0.4
3 oz beef liver, braised	0.2	3.5	9.1
1/2 cup bean sprouts	0.3	0.1	0.7
1 medium banana	0.1	0.1	0.6
1 3.5 in toasted egg bagel	0.3	0.1	2.2
1/2 cup enriched egg noodles	0.1	0.1	1.2
1 cup Corn Bran cereal	0.4	0.7	10.9

*Values do not reflect bioavailability.

Wardlaw GM. *Perspectives in Nutrition.* 4th ed. Boston, Mass: WCB McGraw-Hill; 1999. Used with permission.

Riboflavin

Riboflavin is involved in a number of key metabolic reactions which are important during exercise: glycolysis, the citric acid cycle, and the electron transport chain (19). Riboflavin is the precursor in the synthesis of the flavin coenzymes—flavin mononucleotide (FMN) and flavin-adenine dinucleotide (FAD)—which assist in redox reactions by acting as 1- and 2-electron transfers (19). See the Tools section for the most recent DRIs for riboflavin.

Recommendations for individuals who are physically active. Riboflavin status may be altered in individuals who are initiating an exercise program (19). However, it seems that individuals who are physically active and consume adequate amounts of dietary riboflavin are not at a risk for depletion of riboflavin and, thus, do not require levels above the DRI (19). In a crossover design study, Weight et al (18) investigated the effects of 3 months of vitamin-mineral supplementation in 30 athletes. They reported no significant increases in blood vitamin or mineral concentrations, except for increases in pyridoxine and riboflavin. These authors did not assess the effects of supplementation on exercise performance. Weight et al (18) concluded that vitamin-mineral supplementation is not necessary in individuals who exercise, if they consume diets adequate in vitamins and minerals. Nonetheless, studies of longer duration are necessary to evaluate the long-term effects of exercise on riboflavin status (19). Dietary sources of riboflavin are listed in *Table 5.2*.

Niacin

Niacin is sometimes referred to as nicotinic acid or nicotinamide (19). The coenzyme forms of nicotinamide are nicotinamide adenine dinucleotide (NAD) and NAD phosphate (NADP). Both are involved in glycolysis, the pentose pathway, the citric acid cycle, lipid synthesis, and the electron transport chain (19). See the Tools section for the most recent DRIs for niacin.

Recommendations for individuals who are physically active. Nicotinic acid is often prescribed and used in pharmacological doses to reduce serum cholesterol levels (19). It appears that pharmacological doses of nicotinic acid may augment the use of carbohydrate as a substrate during exercise by decreasing the availability of free fatty acids (19). Despite this very strong connection to exercise metabolism, no solid data presently exist to support increased niacin supplementation for individuals who exercise (19).

Because of niacin's role in vasodilation, several researchers have studied the effect of niacin supplementation on thermoregulation and reported mixed results (20,21). Nonetheless, it is important that individuals who exercise obtain the DRI for niacin to prevent alterations in fuel utilization that could possibly impair performance. Dietary sources of niacin are listed in *Table 5.2*.

Pantothenic Acid

Pantothenic acid, whose biologically active forms are coenzyme A (CoA) and acyl carrier protein, is involved in acyl group transfers such as the acylation of amino acids (22,23). Pantothenic acid coenzymes are also involved in lipid synthesis and metabolism and oxidation of pyruvate and α-ketoglutarate (23). Acetyl Co-A is an important intermediate in fat, carbohydrate, and protein metabolism (23). The Tools section contains the most recent DRIs for pantothenic acid.

Recommendations for individuals who are physically active. To date, only a few studies have looked at the effects of pantothenic acid supplementation on exercise performance (23). Nice et al (24) supplemented 18 trained men with pantothenic acid or a placebo for 2 weeks and reported no significant differences in time to exhaustion in running, pulse rate, or blood biochemical variables between the groups. Smith et al (25) reported that trained pantothenate-deficient mice had lower body weights and liver and muscle glycogen contents, as well as decreased running times to exhaustion, than trained pantothenate-supplemented mice. Nonetheless, it is difficult to extrapolate these results to humans. These research studies suggest that increased intakes of pantothenic acid provide no benefit to individuals who exercise, if they have adequate pantothenic acid status; however, more research is required with individuals who may be deficient in pantothenic acid to assess if they have the same adverse consequences as pantothenate-deficient animals.

Sources. Dietary sources for pantothenic acid include sunflower seeds, mushrooms, peanuts, brewer's yeast, yogurt, and broccoli (1).

Biotin

Biotin is an essential cofactor in four mitochondrial carboxylases (one carboxylase is in both the mitochondria and cytosol) (26). These carboxylase-dependent reactions are involved in energy metabolism and, thus, biotin deficiency could potentially result in impaired exercise performance. The Tools section contains the most recent DRIs for biotin.

Recommendations for individuals who are physically active. To date, no studies have been conducted on the role of biotin on exercise performance or biotin requirements for individuals who are physically active. Controlled, well-designed studies are necessary to establish if biotin is needed in greater amounts by individuals who exercise.

Sources. Good dietary sources of biotin include peanut butter, boiled eggs, toasted wheat germ, egg noodles, Swiss cheese, and cauliflower (1). It is hypothesized that biotin is synthesized by bacteria in the gastrointestinal tract of mammals; however, there are no published reports that this actually occurs (26).

Vitamin C

Vitamin C, also referred to as ascorbic acid, ascorbate, or ascorbate monoanion (27), is a vitamin that is often supplemented in very high amounts in the hope that it may prevent colds.

Although vitamin C supplementation does not prevent the common cold, some studies have shown decreased severity and duration with supplementation. However, megadosing with one vitamin and/or mineral can impair the functions of other vitamins and minerals. Vitamin C is involved in the maintenance of collagen synthesis, oxidation of fatty acids, and formation of neurotransmitters, and is an antioxidant (27,28).

Optimal intakes. To date, there are no new RDAs, DRIs, or AIs for vitamin C, so the 1989 RDAs for vitamin C are still in effect (29). These requirements may be increased based on new studies reviewed by the Food and Nutrition Board,

Institute of Medicine-National Academy of Sciences. The Tools section contains the 1989 RDAs for vitamin C.

Recommendations for individuals who are physically active. Several animal studies have shown that exercise decreases the content of vitamin C in various tissues in the body (28). Although some studies have shown an ergogenic effect of vitamin C supplementation on exercise performance, others have not. It appears that if an individual has an adequate vitamin C status, supplementation with vitamin C does not enhance exercise performance. However, individuals who exercise may require at least 100 mg per day of vitamin C to maintain normal vitamin C status and protect the body from oxidant damage as a result of exercise (28). Individuals who are competing in ultraendurance events may require up to 500 mg per day or more of vitamin C (28). Peters et al (30) studied the effects of 600 mg of vitamin C per day compared to a placebo on the occurrence of upper respiratory tract infections (URTI) in individuals who competed in ultramarathons. They found that the runners who took vitamin C had significantly less URTIs than those who took the placebo. Although some researchers have reported lower than normal vitamin C concentrations in athletes, others have reported normal values (15,31,32). Nonetheless, vitamin C levels in the blood can be increased up to 24 hours postexercise; thus, one must be cautious when blood measurements of vitamin C are used as assessment parameters in research studies (31,33,34). Dietary sources of vitamin C can be found in *Table 5.3*.

TABLE 5.3 Dietary Sources of Vitamin C

Food	Vitamin C Content (mg)*
1 cup tomato soup	68
3/4 cup fresh orange juice	93
1 medium orange	70
1 medium kiwi fruit	74
3/4 cup unsweetened apple juice	77
1 cup 100% Bran cereal	63
1/2 cup collards, cooked	22
1 medium grapefruit, pink and red	56
1 medium sweet red pepper	141
1 medium potato, baked, with skin	26

*Values do not reflect bioavailability.

Wardlaw GM. *Perspectives in Nutrition.* 4th ed. Boston, Mass: WCB McGraw-Hill; 1999. Used with permission.

Choline

Choline is a vitamin-like compound required for the synthesis of the inherent constituents of all cell membranes: phosphatidylcholine, lysophosphatidylcholine, choline plasmogen, and sphingomyelin (35). Choline can be synthesized from the amino acid methionine (36). Choline is involved in carnitine and very-low density lipoprotein cholesterol (VLDL-C) synthesis (35,37). Overt choline deficiencies have not been reported in humans (38).

Optimal intakes. Prior to the 1998 dietary recommendations, there were no recommended intakes for choline. The Tools section contains the most recent DRIs for choline.

Recommendations for individuals who are physically active. Because choline is a precursor of acetylcholine and phosphatidylcholine, it has been suggested that choline may affect nerve transmission, improve strength, and expedite the loss of body fat (36). Although there have been reports that plasma choline concentrations significantly decrease after long distance swimming, running, and triathlons (39,40), not all researchers observe this same decline (41). The reductions in plasma choline may be observed only following long-distance endurance events. Furthermore, choline supplementation, to date, has not been shown to enhance exercise performance, increase strength, or cause decreases in body fat (42).

Sources. Beef liver, peanuts, peanut butter, iceberg lettuce, cauliflower, and whole-wheat bread have some of the highest sources of choline (ranging from 5,831 μmoles/kg for beef liver to 968 μmoles/kg for whole-wheat bread) (35). Potatoes, grape juice, tomatoes, bananas, and cucumbers are also good sources of choline (35).

FAT-SOLUBLE VITAMINS

The fat-soluble vitamins include vitamins A, D, E, and K. Aside from vitamin E, data on the other fat-soluble vitamins and exercise are not as abundant as with other micronutrients.

Vitamin A

Vitamin A, which is considered a subset of the retinoids, is a fat-soluble vitamin well-known for the role it plays in the visual cycle (43). Other important functions of vitamin A include its role in cellular differentiation, reproduction, fetal development, bone formation, and gestation (43,44). The 1989 RDAs for vitamin A are still in effect (29) and can be found in the Tools section.

Recommendations for individuals who are physically active. Assessment of vitamin A intake in individuals who are physically active has shown varied results; however, some of these assessments are faulty in that they do not necessarily specify the source of vitamin A (plant versus animal) (44). Individuals with low fruit and vegetable consumption will typically have lower vitamin A intakes than those with high fruit and vegetable consumption. Because vitamin A is a fat-soluble vitamin and stored in the body, megadosing of vitamin A should be discouraged.

Vitamin A is also a well-known antioxidant. It may prove to be ergogenic for endurance athletes (44). More controlled studies are required to evaluate vitamin A's role in the prevention of oxidative damage as a result of endurance exercise.

It has recently been documented that excessive intakes of vitamin A may lead to reduced bone-mineral density and increased risk for hip fractures (45). Although this was a cross-sectional study, it underscores the fact that megadosing can have detrimental effects on the body.

Although vitamin A is a well-known antioxidant, beta-carotene has not been shown to be an effective antioxidant and may be a pro-oxidant (46). It appears that derivatives of beta-carotene may be manifest in the lungs and arterial blood, possibly encouraging tumor growth, especially in smokers and individuals exposed to second-hand smoke and automobile fumes (46). Thus, individuals who exercise, and especially those who exercise in cities where there are greater numbers of automobiles, may be wise not to supplement with beta-carotene. Omenn states, "... present knowledge indicates that beta-carotene is a weak or ineffective antioxidant in vivo. It may well be a pro-oxidant in lipid compartments or other microenvironments" (46). *Table 5.4* lists some dietary sources of vitamin A.

TABLE 5.4   Dietary Sources of Vitamin A and Vitamin E

Food	Vitamin A Content (RE)*	Vitamin E Content (mg)*
3 oz beef liver, pan-fried	9,125	0.5
1/2 cup toasted almonds, unblanched	0	11.4
3 oz European anchovies, canned in oil	18	4.3
3 medium apricots	277	0.9
1 T whipped butter	83	0.2
1 cup Total cereal	1,748	34.9
1.5 oz Muenster cheese	134	0.2
3 oz chicken liver, simmered	4,179	1.2
3 oz canned clams	145	0.9
1 T safflower oil	0	4.7

RE = retinol equivalents

* Values do not reflect bioavailability.

Wardlaw GM. *Perspectives in Nutrition.* 4th ed. Boston, Mass: WCB McGraw-Hill; 1999. Used with permission.

Vitamin D

Vitamin D is considered both a hormone and a vitamin (47). Its roles in maintaining calcium homeostasis and in bone remodeling are well established. Vitamin D can be obtained by foods as well as from sunlight, because conversion of 7-dehydrocholesterol is converted to previtamin D_3 on the skin (47). Conversion of vitamin D to its more active forms first begins in the liver, then in the kidney where the 1-alpha-hydroxylase adds another hydroxyl group to the first position on 25-hydroxyvitamin D, resulting in 1,25-dihydroxyvitamin D_3 (1,25-$(OH)_2$ D_3), also known as calcitriol, the most active form of vitamin D (47). The effects of calcitriol on calcium metabolism are discussed in more detail in the section on calcium. The Tools section contains the most recent DRIs for vitamin D.

Recommendations for individuals who are physically active. To date, very little research has been conducted on the effects of physical activity on vitamin D requirements and the effects of vitamin D on exercise performance (48). However, there have been reports that weightlifting may increase serum calcitriol and serum Gla-protein (indicator of bone formation) levels that may result in enhanced bone accretion (49). Bell et al (49) reported changes in serum calcitriol levels without observing changes in serum calcium, phosphate, and magnesium levels. Furthermore, there is convincing evidence that 1-25 dihydroxyvitamin D_3 affects muscle function; receptors for 1-25 dihydroxyvitamin D_3 have been found in cultured human muscle cells (50,51). However, 6 months of daily supplementation with 0.50 µg of 1-25 dihydroxyvitamin D_3 did not improve muscle strength in ambulatory men and women over the age of 69 years (52). Nonetheless, as with other nutrients, athletes who may be consuming lower or inadequate kilocalories should be evaluated for vitamin D status because long-term negative effects on calcium homeostasis and bone mineral density may occur. Furthermore, individuals who live at or above 42° latitude (eg, the New England states) may require more vitamin D during the winter months to prevent increases in parathyroid hormone secretion and decreased bone mineral density (53,54).

Sources. Vitamin D is not found in many foods. The best dietary sources of vitamin D include fortified milk, fatty fish, and fortified breakfast cereals (1). Exposure to only 15 minutes of sunlight a day will also result in sufficient amounts of vitamin D, but not all individuals obtain this amount of sunlight per day because of confinement to the indoors and/or location of residence.

Vitamin E

Vitamin E actually refers to a family of eight related compounds known as the tocopherols and the tocotrienols (55). Like vitamin A, vitamin E is well-known for its antioxidant function in the prevention of free radical damage to cell membranes (55). Vitamin E also plays a role in immune function (55). Vitamin E requirements at this time are still based on the 1989 RDAs (29) and can be found in the Tools section.

Recommendations for individuals who are physically active. Researchers have assessed the effects of exercise on vitamin E status. Duly et al (56) reported a significant relationship between levels of lifetime physical activity and vitamin E levels in males living in Northern Ireland. Swift et al (57) concluded that in rats there is an exercise-related decrease in vitamin E concentrations in skeletal muscle which needs more than 24 hours to return to pre-exercise levels and likely includes a liver-to-muscle redistribution of vitamin E. Conversely, Thomas et al (58) reported that habitual exercise or a single bout of exercise did not affect plasma vitamin E concentrations in individuals with different levels of exercise training.

In addition to assessing the effect of exercise on vitamin E status, a number of supplementation studies on vitamin E's role with exercise have been conducted. Because endurance exercise results in increased oxygen consumption and thus increased oxidant stress, it seems logical that vitamin E supplementation might be beneficial to individuals who are physically active. Additionally, exercise results in increased core temperature, increased catecholamine levels, increased lactic acid production, and increased transient hypoxia and tissue reoxygenation, which are all promoters of free radical production (59-62). Furthermore, one of the physiological responses to exercise is an increase in size and number of mitochondria. The mitochondria are the main sites of oxygen production, and also contain unsaturated lipids, iron, and unpaired electrons, making them key locations for free radical attack (63). Because vitamin E functions to protect the skeletal muscle from free radical damage (55), it may potentially be an ergogenic aid for athletes as well.

Many studies on vitamin E and exercise have evaluated the effects of exercise and vitamin E levels and supplementation on skeletal muscle oxidant damage as well as on antioxidant enzymes (64). A number of animal studies have reported that vitamin E supplementation decreased oxidative damage from exercise stress, but only a few human studies have been conducted (64). For example, Reddy et al (65) studied the effect of a single bout of exhaustive exercise in rats and reported that rats who were vitamin E- and selenium-deficient had greater free radical production than the vitamin E- and selenium-supplemented rats. In a human study Vasankari et al (66) investigated the effects of supplementing eight male endurance runners with 294 mg of vitamin E, 1,000 mg vitamin C, and 60 mg of ubiquinone. They reported that supplementation with vitamins E and C and ubiquinone increased the antioxidant potential of their subjects, and that when vitamin E is supplemented with other antioxidants, it may work synergistically to prevent low-density lipoprotein cholesterol (LDL-C) oxidation. Others have reported decreased serum creatine kinase levels, a measure of muscle damage, in marathoners supplemented with vitamins E and C (67). More recently, McBride et al (68) assessed whether resistance training would increase free radical production and whether supplemental vitamin E would affect free radical production. Twelve men who were recreational weight trainers were supplemented with 1,200 IU of vitamin E (RRR-d-alpha-tocopherol succinate) or a placebo for 2 weeks. Both the placebo- and vitamin E-supplemented groups showed increases in plasma creatine kinase and malondialdehyde levels pre- to postexercise; however, vitamin E diminished the rise in these variables postexercise, thus decreasing muscle membrane disruption (68). Additionally, vitamin E supplementation does not seem to be effective as an ergogenic aid (64). That is, although vitamin E has been shown to sequester free radicals in exercising individuals by decreasing membrane disruption (68), there have not been reports that vitamin E actually improves exercise performance. Nonetheless, vitamin E's role in prevention of oxidative damage due to exercise may be significant and more long-term research to assess its effects are necessary. Dietary sources of vitamin E are listed in *Table 5.4*.

Vitamin K

Vitamin K, a group of three related substances, is a fat-soluble vitamin. Phylloquinone or phytonadione (vitamin K_1) is found in plants (69). Menaquinone (MK), once referred to as vitamin K_2, is produced by bacteria in the intestines, supplying an undetermined amount of the daily requirement of vitamin K (70). Menadione (K_3) is the synthetic form of vitamin K (69).

All vitamin K variants are fat soluble and stable to heat. Alkalies, strong acids, radiation, and oxidizing agents can destroy vitamin K. It is absorbed from the upper small intestine with the help of bile or bile salts and pancreatic juices, and then carried to the liver for the synthesis of prothrombin, a key blood-clotting factor (71).

Vitamin K is necessary for normal blood clotting. It is required for the synthesis of prothrombin and other proteins (eg, Factors IX, VII, and X) involved in blood coagulation (72). Vitamin K also helps prothrombin convert to thrombin with the aid of potassium and calcium. Thrombin is the important factor needed for the conversion of fibrinogen to the active fibrin clot (71). Coumarin acts as an anticoagulant by competing with vitamin K at its active sites. Coumarin, or synthetic dicumarol, is used medically primarily as an oral anticoagulant to decrease prothrombin (72). The salicylates, such as aspirin often taken by patients who have had a myocardial infarction, increase the need for vitamin K (73).

Vitamin K is known to influence bone metabolism by facilitating the synthesis of osteocalcin (also known as bone gla protein (BGP) (74). Bone contains proteins with vitamin K-dependent gamma-carboxyglutamate residues (69). Impaired vitamin K metabolism is associated with undercarboxylation of the noncollagenous bone-matrix protein osteocalcin (which contains gamma-carboxyglutamate residues) (75). If osteocalcin is not in its fully carboxylated state, normal bone formation will be impaired (75).

Optimal intakes. The RDAs for vitamin K are based on the 1989 recommendations and are listed in the Tools section (29). An average diet will usually provide at least 75 to 150 μg per day of vitamin K, which is the suggested minimum, although 300 to 750 μg per day may be optimal (76). Absorption of vitamin K may vary from person to person but is estimated to be 20% to 60% of total intake (76). Toxicity rarely occurs from Vitamin K from its natural sources (vitamin K_1 or MK), but toxic side effects are more likely from the synthetic vitamin K used in medical treatment (77). However, a deficiency of vitamin K is more common than once previously thought. Western diets high in sugar and processed foods, megadoses of vitamins A and E, and antibiotics may contribute to a decrease in intestinal bacterial function, resulting in a decrease in the production and/or metabolism of vitamin K (78).

Recommendations for individuals who are physically active. No research on vitamin K and exercise or vitamin K as a potential for an ergogenic aid have been conducted (48). Because vitamin K may not be absorbed as efficiently as once was thought, its role in the prevention of bone loss has become more apparent, and this may establish a connection for research on vitamin K in athletes, especially female athletes.

Sources. The best dietary sources of vitamin K include green, leafy vegetables, liver, broccoli, peas, and green beans (1).

MAJOR MINERALS

The major minerals include calcium, phosphorus, magnesium, sulfur, potassium, sodium, and chloride (1).

Calcium

Calcium, one of the most well-studied minerals, is the fifth most common element in the human body (79,80). Ninety-nine percent of calcium exists in the bone and teeth, with the remaining 1% distributed in extracellular fluids, intracellular structures, cell membranes, and various soft tissues (29,79,81,82). The major functions of calcium include:

- Bone metabolism
- Blood coagulation
- Neuromuscular excitability
- Cellular adhesiveness
- Transmission of nerve impulses
- Maintenance and function of cell membranes
- Activation of enzyme reactions and hormone secretions

Calcium homeostasis. The level of calcium in the serum is tightly managed within a range of 2.2 to 2.5 mmol/L (divide mmol/L by 0.2495 to convert to mg/dL) by the hormones parathyroid hormone (PTH), vitamin D, and calcitonin (79,81-83). When serum calcium levels fall below the normal range, PTH responds by increasing the synthesis of calcitriol in the kidney (81,82). Calcitriol will then cause the following to occur:

- Increased calcium reabsorption in the kidney
- Increased calcium absorption in the intestines
- Increased osteoclastic activity in the bone (releasing calcium into circulation) (79,81,82)

When serum calcium levels are above normal values, the hormone calcitonin causes the following to occur:

- Greater renal excretion of calcium
- Reduced calcium absorption in the intestines
- Decreased osteoclastic activity (79,81,82)

Average calcium intakes. Calcium intakes are typically lower in females than in males.

- One-half of all teenage girls consume <2/3 of the recommended intake (84).
- One-half of adult women consume <70% of the recommended intake (84).
- Average intake of calcium for women 20 to 29 years of age is 778 mg per day (85).
- For women >65 years of age, 600 mg per day is the common daily intake (84).

If an individual is physically active, low calcium intakes will result in larger negative effects on the body because calcium is lost in the sweat and urine (86). The Tools section contains the most recent DRIs for calcium.

Recommendations for individuals who are physically active. Individuals who are physically active should strive to consume at least the DRI for calcium. If an individual has high sweat rates and/or exercises in hot conditions, he or she may need more calcium than the DRI, since it has been reported that there is a great amount of calcium lost in the sweat of individuals exercising in the heat (86).

Sources. Various sources of calcium are listed in *Table 5.5*. Dairy sources have the highest bioavailable form of calcium.

TABLE 5.5   Dietary Sources of Calcium and Phosphorus

Food	Calcium Content (mg)*	Phosphorus Content (mg)*
1 cup skim milk	302	247
1 large plain muffin	130	99
1.5 oz cheddar cheese	307	218
1.5 oz feta cheese	209	143
3/4 cup orange juice, with added calcium	224	30
1 oz fresh tofu, firm	58	54
1 cup, plain, low-fat yogurt	415	326
1 plain waffle	191	143
1/2 cup cooked broccoli	47	51
3 oz Atlantic sardines, canned in oil (with bones)	325	417

*Values do not reflect bioavailability.

Wardlaw GM. *Perspectives in Nutrition.* 4th ed. Boston, Ma: WCB McGraw-Hill; 1999. Used with permission.

If an individual is not consuming enough calcium in his or her diet, supplementation with calcium citrate or calcium carbonate is best. Individuals should avoid calcium supplements containing bone meal, oyster shell, and shark cartilage due to the increased lead content in these supplements, which can result in toxic effects in the body (1). Calcium supplements are best absorbed if taken in doses of 500 mg or less and when taken between meals (1). In older individuals who may suffer from achlorhydria, calcium carbonate is better absorbed with meals (1). Because calcium citrate does not require gastric acid for optimal absorption, it is considered the best calcium supplement for older women (87).

Factors affecting calcium absorption. A number of factors can inhibit or enhance calcium absorption. High-protein and sodium diets result in increased urinary calcium excretion (1,80). Although phosphorus can reduce urinary calcium loss, high levels of phosphorus may lead to hyperparathyroidism and result in bone loss (1). Fiber and caffeine have small negative effects on calcium loss; a cup of brewed coffee results in a 3.5 mg loss of calcium which can be compensated for by adding milk (80). Phytates, however, greatly decrease calcium absorption and oxalates greatly reduce calcium bioavailability (1,80). Conversely, vitamin D, lactose, glucose, a healthy digestive system, and higher dietary requirements (eg, pregnancy) all enhance calcium absorption (1).

Phosphorus

Phosphorous is the second most abundant mineral in the body, with about 85% of total body phosphorous in bone, mainly as hydroxyapatite crystals (79,88).

Phosphate is important in bone mineralization in both animals and humans (88). Even in the presence of a high amount of calcitriol, rickets can result from a phosphate deficiency in humans (88). Although phosphorous is required for bone growth, excessive amounts of phosphorous may actually harm the skeleton, especially when accompanied by a low calcium intake (88). Excessive phosphorus (and protein) intakes have been negatively correlated with radial bone mineral density (89).

High phosphorous intakes reduce serum calcium levels, especially when calcium intake is low, because phosphorous carries calcium with it into soft tissues (82,88). The resulting hypocalcemia activates PTH secretion, which results in increased bone loss (resorption) to maintain serum calcium homeostasis (88). High phosphorous intakes can also decrease vitamin D production, further affecting calcium absorption and producing secondary hyperparathyroidism (88).

Optimal intakes. The Tools section contains the most recent DRIs for phosphorus. Because of its ubiquitous nature, phosphorus intakes are usually above recommended intakes. Average phosphorus intakes of 1,137 mg per day have been reported for females 20 to 29 years of age (85).

Recommendations for individuals who are physically active. Because most individuals consume enough phosphorus in their diets, overconsumption is usually the concern, especially with the amount of soft drinks individuals consume because these contain high amounts of phosphate and generally replace milk. In a retrospective study Wyshak et al (90) reported that athletes who consumed carbonated beverages suffered more fractures than athletes who consumed few or no carbonated beverages. These researchers also reported a significant dose response: The greater the number of carbonated beverages consumed, the greater the number of fractures. These results may have important health implications due to the 300% increase in carbonated beverage consumption combined with a decrease in milk consumption over the past three decades (90).

Another way individuals who exercise, especially competitive athletes, may consume excessive phosphorus is via "phosphate-loading." Phosphate-loading is thought to decrease the build-up of hydrogen ions that increase during exercise and negatively affect energy production (91). Research on phosphate-loading as an ergogenic aid has shown equivocal results; however, individuals who perform high-intensity exercise may benefit with appropriate dosages (91). Regardless, the long-term negative consequences of phosphate-loading on bone-mineral density have not been documented. Phosphorus is highest in protein foods. *Table 5.5* lists some foods with varying amounts of phosphorus.

Magnesium

About 60% to 65% of the body's magnesium is present in bone, approximately 27% is present in muscle, 6% to 7% is found in other cells, and 1% is found in the extracellular fluid (92). Magnesium plays an important role in a number of metabolic processes required for exercise, such as mitochondrial function; protein, lipid and carbohydrate synthesis; energy-delivering processes; and neuromuscular coordination (93,94). The Tools section contains the most recent DRIs for magnesium.

Recommendations for individuals who are physically active Urinary and sweat magnesium excretion may be exacerbated in individuals who exercise (95). A female tennis player who suffered from hypomagnesemia was supplemented with 500 mg per day of magnesium gluconate, which dissipated her muscle spasms (96). If individuals are consuming inadequate kilocalories and are exercising intensely on a daily basis, especially in the heat, they may be losing a large amount of magnesium through sweat (1). Clinical signs of magnesium deficiency, such as muscle spasms, should be monitored. Nevertheless, hypomagnesemia during exercise is the exception rather than the norm. *Table 5.6* lists some food sources of magnesium.

TABLE 5.6 Dietary Sources of Magnesium

Food	Magnesium Content (mg)*
3 oz Chinook salmon, dry heat	104
1/2 cup black beans, cooked	60
1/2 cup Brazilnuts, dried, unblanched	158
1 whole-wheat pita bread	44
1 cup 100% Bran cereal	312
1.5 oz Parmesan cheese, shredded	22
3 oz Atlantic cod, dry heat	36
1 cup chocolate pudding	63
1 1/2 cup chocolate ice cream	57
1/2 cup Valencia peanuts, fresh	134

*Values do not reflect bioavailability.

Wardlaw GM. *Perspectives in Nutrition.* 4th ed. Boston, Mass: WCB McGraw-Hill; 1999. Used with permission.

Sulfur

Sulfur is present in the body in a nonionic form and is a constituent of some vitamins (eg, thiamin and biotin), amino acids (eg, methionine and cysteine), and proteins (1). Sulfur also assists with acid-base balance (1). If protein needs are met, sulfur is not required in the diet because it is present in protein foods (1). There are no dietary requirements for sulfur at this time.

Recommendations for individuals who are physically active. At present, research on the effects of sulfur on exercise performance or sulfur loss with exercise has not been reported. Because of sulfur's role with proteins, vitamins, amino acids, and acid-base balance, research with exercise may be warranted.

Sources Sulfur is present in protein-rich foods (1).

Potassium

One of the three major electrolytes, potassium is the most substantial intracellular cation (97,98). Total body potassium is about 3,000 to 4,000 mmol (1 g of potassium = 25 mmol) (98). The two major roles of potassium in the body are maintaining intracellular ionic strength and maintaining transmembrane ionic potential (97).

Optimal intakes. There is no RDA or DRI for potassium. The 1989 Estimated Minimum Requirements (EMR) are still being used (29). The EMR for potassium is 2,000 mg per day.

Recommendations for individuals who are physically active. A number of studies on electrolyte balance have been conducted. After a 42.2-km road race, runners' plasma potassium concentrations were significantly increased, which demonstrates a shift of potassium from intracellular to extracellular space (99). Additionally, Ljungberg et al (100) reported significant increases in saliva potassium concentrations in their subjects after a marathon, with a return to baseline 1 hour postmarathon. Millard-Stafford et al (101) found that female runners had a greater increase in serum potassium concentrations than did male runners following a simulated 40-km road race in a hot, humid environment. Therefore, it appears that serum potassium shifts into the extracellular space during and immediately postexercise. However, this shift appears to be transient because most researchers report a return to baseline in extracellular serum potassium concentrations at 1 hour or more after exercise. The transient shift in potassium may require that individuals who are physically active consume more potassium in their diets than the Estimated Minimum Requirements. If an individual becomes hyperkalemic or hypokalemic, cells may become nonfunctional (98). Thus, if the observed shift in potassium postexercise is not transient, serious consequences can ensue. However, because potassium is ubiquitous in foods, individuals who exercise may not require more in their diets than they already consume. Furthermore, individuals who exercise at lower levels (eg, walking, gardening, recreational jogging) may not experience significant shifts in serum potassium concentrations. *Table 5.7* lists some food sources of potassium.

TABLE 5.7 Dietary Sources of Potassium and Sodium

Food	Potassium Content (mg)*	Sodium Content (mg)*
3 oz European Anchovies, canned in oil	463	3,120
1 medium banana	451	1
1 cup barley	832	22
1/2 cup black beans, cooked	305	204
1 whole-wheat pita	109	340
1 cup All-Bran cereal	1,051	961
1.5 oz blue cheese	109	593
3 oz trout, dry heat	394	57
3/4 cup tomato juice with salt	403	661
2 T peanut butter, smooth style, with salt	233	154

*Values do not reflect bioavailability.

Wardlaw GM. *Perspectives in Nutrition.* 4th ed. Boston, Ma: WCB McGraw-Hill; 1999. Used with permission.

Sodium and Chloride

Sodium and chloride are the most abundant cations and anions, respectively, in the extracellular fluid (102). Sodium and chloride are the major ions in the extracellular fluid and assist in nerve transmission (1). In this respect they are important in exercise.

Optimal intakes. Sodium and chloride requirements are based on the 1989 Estimated Minimum Requirements (29). The EMR is 500 mg per day for sodium and 750 mg for chloride.

Requirements for individuals who are physically active. Sweat sodium is often measured during and after exercise to assess sodium changes. In a study of 14 women, sweat sodium was increased after 60 minutes of cycling in dry heat and the amount of sodium in the sweat was greater in the winter than in the summer (103). Millard-Stafford (101) reported that females had higher serum sodium concentrations than males following a 40-km run. Stachenfeld et al (104) reported similar results in sodium concentrations in their female subjects 120 minutes after cycling. As with potassium, this increase in serum sodium concentration appears to be transient. Nonetheless, it appears that increased dietary sodium is warranted in individuals who exercise, especially if they are exercising in hot, humid conditions. Increased sodium is required to maintain fluid balance and prevent cramping. The increase in dietary sodium may be met by consuming higher sodium foods and adding salt to foods. Because sodium also increases urinary calcium excretion, a good balance between sodium and calcium intake is required. *Table 5.7* lists some food sources of sodium. Foods high in sodium are typically salty (sodium chloride), and therefore, are also high in chloride.

TRACE MINERALS

The trace minerals include iron, zinc, copper, selenium, iodide, fluoride, chromium, manganese, molybdenum, boron, and vanadium (1).

Iron

Total body iron constitutes about 5.0 and 3.8 mg/kg body weight in men and women, respectively (105). Iron is utilized for many functions related to exercise, such as hemoglobin and myoglobin synthesis (106), as well as incorporation into mitochondrial cytochromes and nonheme iron compounds (107). Some iron-dependent enzymes (ie, NADH and succinate dehydrogenase) are involved in oxidative metabolism (107,108).

Optimal intakes. The 1989 RDAs are still the basis for iron recommendations (29) and are listed in the Tools section.

Recommendations for individuals who are physically active. The incidence of iron deficiency anemia among athletes and nonathletes alike is only about 5% to 6% (109,110); however, these percentages may be greater in adolescent female athletes due to growth requirements and menstruation (111). On the other hand, iron depletion is a relatively common occurrence among athletes, ranging between 30% and 50%, especially among female athletes and male and female athletes who participate in endurance sports (109,112-114).

Because female athletes often do not consume proper amounts of dietary iron (as a result of lower kilocalorie consumption and/or reduction in meat content of the diet), coupled with iron losses in sweat, gastrointestinal bleeding, myoglobinuria from myofibrillar stress, hemoglobinuria due to intravascular hemolysis, and menstruation (115-118), health and optimal exercise performance may be compromised. Decreased exercise performance is related not only to anemia and a decreased aerobic capacity, but also to tissue iron depletion and diminished exercise endurance (119). Dietary iron deficiency anemia negatively impacts the oxidative production of adenosine triphosphate (ATP) in skeletal muscle, as well as the capacity for prolonged exercise (120,121). A recent study reported that iron-depleted women had a reduction in their maximal oxygen consumption (VO$_2$max) as a result of decreased iron storage and not to a decreased oxygen-transport capacity of the blood (122). Others have reported alterations in metabolic rate, thyroid hormone status, and thermoregulation with iron depletion and iron deficiency anemia (123-125). Mild iron deficiency anemia has also been shown to negatively affect psychomotor development and intellectual performance (126). *Table 5.8* lists some dietary sources of iron.

TABLE 5.8 Dietary Sources of Iron and Zinc

Food	Iron Content (mg)*	Zinc Content (mg)*
3 oz Eastern oysters, canned	5.7	77.4
1/2 cup Spanish peanuts, fresh	2.9	1.5
3 oz beef liver, braised	5.8	5.2
1/2 cup toasted almonds, unblanched	3.5	3.5
1 cup barley	6.6	5.1
1/2 cup bean sprouts	0.3	1.4
1 meatless hamburger patty	1.5	7.5
3 oz Pacific herring, dry heat	1.2	0.6
1/2 cup fresh hummus	1.9	1.4
1 milk chocolate bar	0.4	0.6

*Values do not reflect bioavailability.

Wardlaw GM. *Perspectives in Nutrition*. 4th ed. Boston, Mass: WCB McGraw-Hill; 1999. Used with permission.

Iron supplementation. For individuals who are diagnosed with iron deficiency anemia, iron supplementation is the most prudent way to increase iron stores and prevent adverse physiological effects (127). Ferrous sulfate is the least expensive and most widely used form of iron supplementation (127,128). For adults diagnosed with iron deficiency anemia, a daily dose of at least 60 mg of elemental iron taken between meals is recommended (127). Nielsen and Nachtigall (129) "believe that there are sufficient arguments to support controlled iron supplementation in all athletes with low serum ferritin levels."

Factors affecting iron absorption. As with calcium, a number of factors inhibit and enhance iron absorption. Factors that inhibit iron absorption include (1):

- Phytates
- Oxalates
- Polyphenols (eg, tannins) in tea and coffee
- Adequate body stores of iron
- Excess intakes of other minerals (eg, zinc, calcium, manganese)
- A reduction in gastric acid production
- Certain antacids

Factors that enhance iron absorption include (1):

- Appropriate gastric acid secretion
- Heme iron
- High body demand for red blood cells (eg, blood loss, high altitude, exercise training, pregnancy)
- Low body stores of iron
- The meat protein factor (MPF)
- Ascorbic acid

Consuming vitamin C-containing foods or beverages with meals and consuming tea or coffee at least an hour before or after a meal will augment dietary iron absorption. These routines should be strongly recommended even if a person who has iron deficiency anemia is taking iron supplements (1).

Zinc

Zinc exists in all organs, tissues, fluids, and secretions. About 60% of total body zinc is present in muscle, 29% in bone, and 1% in the gastrointestinal tract, skin, kidney, brain, lung, and prostate (130). Zinc plays a role in over 300 metabolic reactions in the body (1). Alkaline phosphatase, carbonic anhydrase, and zinc-copper superoxide dismutase are just a few of the zinc metalloenzymes (1).

Optimal intakes. At present zinc requirements are still based on the 1989 RDAs (29) and can be found in the Tools section.

Recommendations for individuals who are physically active. Many individuals in the United States do not consume the recommended intakes of zinc. It has been reported that young women consume only 9.7 mg per day (85). Others have reported that about 50% of female distance runners consume less than the recommended intakes of zinc (131). More recent studies have reported zinc intakes greater than 70% of recommended intakes in female and male collegiate swimmers (132). It appears that when dietary zinc intakes are sufficient, zinc status is not negatively affected by exercise training (133).

The studies conducted on zinc and exercise also show a transient effect of exercise on zinc status. Zinc status has been shown to directly affect basal metabolic rate (BMR) and thyroid hormone levels in men (134), which can have a negative effect on exercise performance and health. Wada and King (134) studied the effects of zinc supplementation on BMR, thyroid hormone levels, and protein utilization in six young men who participated in a 75-day metabolic study. The study was a crossover design in which the subjects were first given 16.5 mg per day of zinc for 12 days. Next, the subjects received 5.5 mg per day of zinc for 54 days, which resulted in zinc deficiency. The researchers (134) reported a significant decrease in BMR, thyroid hormone levels (T4), and protein utilization. They also noted an increase in BMR and thyroid hormone levels during the zinc repletion phase of their study (134). Wada and King's investigation provides insight into the relationship between zinc status, BMR, and thyroid hormone levels. The long-term effects of daily exercise regimens on zinc status need to be researched so that more definitive recommendations for individuals who are physically active can be made. *Table 5.8* lists some dietary sources of zinc.

Copper

About 50 to 120 mg of copper exist in the human body (135). Some of the functions of copper include enhancing iron absorption (via metalloenzyme ceruloplasmin), forming collagen and elastin, participating in the electron transport chain (cytochrome C oxidase), and acting as an antioxidant (zinc-copper superoxide dismutase) (1,135).

Optimal intakes. There is no RDA for copper. The Estimated Safe and Adequate Daily Dietary Intakes (ESADDI) established for copper are based on the 1989 recommendations (29). The ESADDI for adults is 1.5 to 3.0 mg per day (29).

Recommendations for individuals who are physically active. Research findings on the copper status and requirements of individuals who exercise are equivocal. Deficiencies of copper are unlikely, but because copper plays a role in red blood cell maturation, anemia can ensue with copper deficiencies (1,135). Toxicity symptoms of copper include vomiting (1,135).

Sources. Because the copper content of food is greatly affected by soil conditions, it is rarely listed. Some good dietary sources of copper are organ meats (eg, liver), seafood (eg, oysters), cocoa, mushrooms, various nuts, seeds (eg, sunflower seeds), and whole-grain breads and cereals (1).

Selenium

Selenium is well-known for its role as an antioxidant in the body (metalloenzyme: glutathione peroxidase) (1). Selenium also functions in normal thyroid hormone metabolism (1).

Optimal requirements. The recommendations for selenium are based on the 1989 RDAs (29) and are listed in the Tools section.

Recommendations for individuals who are physically active. Limited data are available as to whether individuals who exercise require more selenium in their diets than sedentary individuals. Because of the increased oxidation with exercise, it seems that more selenium in the diet would be necessary for individuals who are physically active. In a double-blind study, Tessier et al (136) placed 12 men on 180 µg of selenomethionine and 12 men on a placebo for 10 weeks and reported that endurance training enhanced the antioxidant potential of glutathione peroxidase, but the selenium supplementation had no effect on performance. However, because little data are available, individuals who exercise should consume no more than the RDA for selenium.

Sources. Dietary sources of selenium, like copper, vary greatly with the soil content. Good sources of selenium in foods include fish, shellfish, meat, eggs, and milk (1).

Iodide

The thyroid hormones are synthesized from iodide and tyrosine (1). Thus, iodide is required for normal metabolic rate.

Optimal intakes. The 1989 RDAs are the basis for iodide recommendations (29) and are listed in the Tools section.

Recommendations for individuals who are physically active. No data on iodide requirements for individuals who are physically active have been reported. Nonetheless, inadequate intake of iodide may have an impact on performance because of its role in thyroid hormone synthesis.

Sources. Iodide is mainly found in saltwater fish, molasses, iodized salt, and seafood (1).

Fluoride

Fluoride's main function is to maintain teeth and bone health (1). It has long been known that fluoride in adequate amounts in the water can prevent tooth decay (1,137). Fluoride is important to bone health because it stimulates bone growth (osteoblasts), increases trabecular bone formation, and increases vertebral bone mineral density (138). The Tools section contains the most recent DRIs fluoride.

Recommendations for individuals who are physically active. To date, studies are lacking on the needs of fluoride for the individual who exercises. Most research on fluoride has been conducted to assess its effect on bone mineral density and prevention of osteoporosis. Because of fluoride's important role in bone metabolism, more studies with fluoride and female athletes are warranted.

Sources. Dietary sources of fluoride are limited to tea, seaweed, seafood, and fluoridated public water systems (1).

Chromium

Chromium is a well studied mineral. Chromium potentiates the action of insulin and thus influences carbohydrate, lipid, and protein metabolism (139). Chromium may also have antiatherogenic effects by lowering serum cholesterol levels, but these reports have not been well documented. More recently, chromium has been proposed to increase lean body mass and decrease body weight. However, a number of researchers have shown that chromium does not increase lean body mass or decrease body weight (140-142).

Optimal intakes. The ESADDI for chromium (29) is 50 to 200 µg per day for adults. Anderson and Kozlovsky (143) reported an average chromium intake of 25 µg per day and 33 µg per day for females and males, respectively, suggesting that the majority of Americans fail to consume the minimum ESADDI.

Recommendations for individuals who are physically active. Urinary chromium excretion has been reported to be greater during the days individuals exercise compared to days individuals do not exercise (144,145). Increased chromium excretion coupled with inadequate dietary intake suggests that individuals who exercise need more chromium in their diets. However, because chromium may alter the status of other minerals (eg, iron), intakes greater than the ESADDI are not recommended until more studies are completed (141).

Sources. Dietary sources of chromium include whole grains, organ meats, beer, egg yolks, mushrooms, and nuts (1).

Manganese

Manganese plays a role in antioxidant activity in the body because it is part of superoxide dismutase (1). Manganese also plays a role in carbohydrate metabolism and bone metabolism (1).

Optimal intakes. The ESADDI for manganese is 2 to 5 mg per day for adults (29).

Recommendatons for individuals who are physically active. There are no data on whether individuals who exercise require more manganese in their diets or if it contributes as an ergogenic aid.

Sources. Dietary sources of manganese include whole grains, leafy vegetables, nuts, beans, and tea (1).

Molybdenum

Molybdenum interacts with copper and iron. Excessive intakes of molybdenum may inhibit copper absorption (1). Molybdenum also plays a role in glucocorticoid metabolism (104).

Optimal intakes. The ESADDI for molybdenum is 74 to 250 µg per day for adults (29).

Minimum recommendations for individuals who are physically active. There are no data on molybdenum requirements for individuals who are physically active.

Sources. Beans, nuts, whole grains, milk, and milk products are all good dietary sources of molybdenum (1).

Boron

Presently, boron has not been found to be essential for humans but may play a role in bone metabolism by its interactions with calcitriol, estradiol, testosterone, magnesium, and calcium (146-149). Many athletes believe that boron will increase lean body mass and increase bone mineral density, but recent reports have not shown boron to have these effects (148,150).

Optimal intakes. There are presently no dietary requirements for boron. However, adults may need between 1 to 10 mg per day of boron (1).

Recommendations for individuals who are physically active. To date, most of the research on boron has been limited to its effect on bone-mineral density and lean body mass. Whether individuals who exercise require more boron in their diets has not been established. Chapter 7, Ergogenic Aids includes a discussion of boron as an ergogenic aid.

Sources. Dietary sources of boron include fruits and vegetables as well as nuts and beans (1).

Vanadium

Like chromium, vanadium has been shown to potentiate the effects of insulin (151). Also like chromium, supplements of vanadium, as vanadyl sulfate, have been proposed to increase lean body mass, but these anabolic effects have not been reported in research studies (151).

Optimal intakes. There are no dietary recommendations for vanadium. Vanadium requirements for adults is estimated to be between 10 and 100 µg per day (1).

Recommendations for individuals who are physically active. No reports of increased needs or ergogenic effects of vanadium have been documented. Supplementation with vanadium is not warranted. Chapter 7, Ergogenic Aids discusses vanadium in more detail.

Sources. Dietary sources of vanadium include grains, mushrooms, and shellfish (1).

SUMMARY

Overall, the vitamin and mineral needs of individuals who are physically active are similar to the requirements for healthy individuals, if dietary intakes are adequate. However, sweat and urinary losses, coupled with lower intakes by some athletes, may require these individuals to consume higher amounts of some micronutrients. Care must be taken so that individuals do not megadose, which could impair both exercise performance and health. Special attention must be given to individuals who are physically active to assess their micronutrient needs. In assessing these individuals, one must keep in mind the following: frequency, intensity, duration, and type(s) of physical activity; environment (hot or cold) in which exercise is performed; gender; and dietary intakes and food preferences. All of these components will assist the professional in helping individuals who are physically active consume adequate amounts of micronutrients for optimal health and performance.

REFERENCES

1. Wardlaw GM. *Perspectives in Nutrition.* 4th ed. Boston, Mass: WCB McGraw-Hill; 1999.

2. Burke L, Heeley P. Dietary supplements and nutritional ergogenic aids in sport. In: Burke L, Deakin V, eds. *Clinical Sports Nutrition.* Sydney, Australia: McGraw-Hill Book Co; 1994:227-284.

3. Leklem JE. Vitamin B-6. In: Ziegler EE, Filer LJ Jr, eds. *Present Knowledge in Nutrition.* 7th ed. Washington, DC: ILSI Press; 1996:174-183.

4. Yates AA, Schlicker SA, Suitor CW. Dietary reference intakes: the new basis for recommendations for calcium and related nutrients, B vitamins, and choline. *J Am Diet Assoc.* 1998;98:699-706.

5. Sampson DA. Vitamin B-6. In: Wolinsky I, Driskell JA, eds. *Sports Nutrition.* Boca Raton, Fla: CRC Press; 1997:75-84.

6. Crozier PG, Cordain L, Sampson DA. Exercise-induced changes in plasma vitamin B-6 concentrations do not vary with exercise intensity. *Am J Clin Nutr.* 1994;60:552-558.

7. Singh A, Moses FM, Deuster PA. Vitamin and mineral status in physically active men: effects of a high-potency supplement. *Am J Clin Nutr.* 1992;55:1-7.

8. Herbert V. Vitamin B-12. In: Ziegler EE, Filer LJ Jr, eds. *Present Knowledge in Nutrition.* 7th ed. Washington, DC: ILSI Press; 1996:191-205.

9. Selhub J, Rosenberg IH. Folic acid. In: Ziegler EE, Filer LJ Jr, eds. *Present Knowledge in Nutrition.* 7th ed. Washington, DC: ILSI Press; 1996:206-219.

10. McMartin K. Folate and Vitamin B-12. In: Wolinsky I, Driskell JA, eds. *Sports Nutrition.* Boca Raton, Fla: CRC Press; 1997:75-84.

11. Frail H. Special needs: the vegetarian athlete. In: Burke L, Deakin V, eds. *Clinical Sports Nutrition.* Sydney, Australia: McGraw-Hill Book Co; 1994:365-378.

12. American Dietetic Association. Position paper on vegetarian diets (technical support paper). *J Am Diet Assoc.* 1988;88(3):352-355.

13. Herbert V. Vitamin C supplements and disease: counterpoint (editorial). *J Am Coll Nutr.* 1995;14:112-113.

14. Herbert V. Folic acid and vitamin B$_{12}$. In: Rothfield B, ed. *Nuclear Medicine In Vitro.* Philadelphia, Penn: J B Lippincott; 1983:337-354.

15. Telford RD, Catchpole EA, Deakin V, Hahn AG, Plank AW. The effect of 7 to 8 months of vitamin/mineral supplementation on athletic performance. *Int J Sport Nutr.* 1992;2:135-153.

16. Green R, Jacobsen DW. Clinical implications of hyperhomocysteinemia. In: Bailey LB, ed. *Folate in Health and Disease.* New York, NY: Marcel Dekker; 1995:75-122.

17. Peifer JJ. Thiamin. In: Wolinsky I, Driskell JA, eds. *Sports Nutrition.* Boca Raton, Fla: CRC Press; 1997:47-55.

18. Weight LM, Noakes TD, Labadarios D, Graves J, Jacobs P, Berman PA. Vitamin and mineral status of trained athletes including effects of supplementation. *Am J Clin Nutr.* 1988;47:186-191.

19. Lewis RD. Riboflavin and niacin. In: Wolinsky I, Driskell JA, eds. *Sports Nutrition.* Boca Raton, Fla: CRC Press; 1997:57-73.

20. Murray R, Bartoli WP, Eddy DE, Horn MK. Physiological and performance responses to nicotinic-acid ingestion during exercise. *Med Sci Sports Exerc.* 1995;27:1057-1062.

21. Stephenson LA, Kolka MA. Increased skin blood flow and enhanced sensible heat loss in humans after nicotinic acid ingestion. *J Therm Biol.* 1995;20:409.

22. Plesofsky-Vig N. Pantothenic acid. In: Ziegler EE, Filer LJ Jr, eds. *Present Knowledge in Nutrition.* 7th ed. Washington, DC: ILSI Press; 1996:236-244.

23. Thomas EA. Pantothenic acid and biotin. In: Wolinsky I, Driskell JA, eds. *Sports Nutrition.* Boca Raton, Fla: CRC Press; 1997:97-100.

24. Nice C, Reeves AG, Brinck-Johnsen T, Noll W. The effects of pantothenic acid supplementation on human exercise capacity. *J Sports Med Phys Fitness*. 1984;24:26-29.

25. Smith CM, Narrow CM, Kendrick ZV, Steffen C. The effect of pantothenate deficiency in mice on their metabolic response to fast and exercise. *Metabolism*. 1987;36:115-121.

26. Mock DM. Biotin. In: Ziegler EE, Filer LJ Jr, eds. *Present Knowledge in Nutrition*. 7th ed. Washington, DC: ILSI Press; 1996:220-235.

27. Levine M, Rumsey S, Wang Y, et al. Vitamin C. In: Ziegler EE, Filer LJ Jr, eds. *Present Knowledge in Nutrition*. 7th ed. Washington, DC: ILSI Press; 1996:146-159.

28. Keith RE. Ascorbic acid. In: Wolinsky I, Driskell JA, eds. *Sports Nutrition*. Boca Raton, Fla: CRC Press; 1997:29-45.

29. Food and Nutrition Board. *Recommended Dietary Allowances*. 10th ed. Washington, DC: National Academy Press; 1989.

30. Peters EM, Goetzsche JM, Grobbelaar B, Noakes TD. Vitamin C supplementation reduces the incidence of postrace symptoms of upper-respiratory-tract infection in ultramarathon runners. *Am J Clin Nutr*. 1993;57:170-174.

31. Duthie GG, Robertson JD, Maughan RJ, Morrice PC. Blood antioxidant status and erythrocyte lipid peroxidation following distance running. *Arch Biochem Biophys*. 1990;282:78-83.

32. Cohen JL, Potosnak L, Frank O, Baker H. A nutritional and hematological assessment of elite ballet dancers. *Phys Sportsmed*. 1985;5:43.

33. Fishbaine B, Butterfield G. Ascorbic acid status of running and sedentary men. *Int J Vitam Nutr Res*. 1984;54:273.

34. Gleeson M, Robertson JD, Maughan RJ. Influence of exercise on ascorbic acid status in man. *Clin Sci*. 1987;73:501-505.

35. Zeisel SH. Choline. In: Shils ME, Olson JA, Shike M, eds. *Modern Nutrition in Health and Disease*. 8th ed. Philadelphia, Penn: Lea & Febiger; 1994:449-458.

36. Burke ER. Nutritional ergogenic aids. In: Berning JR, Steen SN, eds. *Nutrition for Sport & Exercise*. 2nd ed. Gaithersburg, Md: Aspen Publishers; 1998:119-142.

37. McChrisley B. Other substances in foods. In: Wolinsky I, Driskell JA, eds. *Sports Nutrition*. Boca Raton, Fla: CRC Press; 1997:205-219.

38. Kanter MM, Williams MH. Antioxidants, carnitine, and choline as putative ergogenic aids. *Int J Sport Nutr*. 1995;5:S120-S131.

39. Sandage BW, Sabounjian LA, White R, et al. Choline citrate may enhance athletic performance. *Physiologist*. 1992;35:236a.

40. Von Allworden HN, Horn S, Kahl J, Feldheim W, et al. The influence of lecithin on plasma choline concentrations in triathletes and adolescent runners during exercise. *Eur J Appl Physiol*. 1993;67:87-91.

41. Spector SA, Jackman MR, Sabounjian LA, Sakkas C, Landers DM, Willis WT. Effect of choline supplementation on fatigue in trained cyclists. *Med Sci Sports Exerc*. 1995;27:668-673.

42. Grunewald K, Bailey R. Commercially marketed supplements for body-building athletes. *Sports Med*. 1993;15:90-103.

43. Olson JA. Vitamin A, retinoids, and carotenoids. In: Shils ME, Olson JA, Shike M, eds. *Modern Nutrition in Health and Disease*. 8th ed. Philadelphia, Penn: Lea & Febiger; 1994:287-307.

44. Stacewicz-Sapuntzakis M. Vitamin A and carotenoids. In: Wolinsky I, Driskell JA, eds. *Sports Nutrition*. Boca Raton, Fla: CRC Press; 1997:101-109.

45. Melhus H, Michaelsson K, Kindmark A, et al. Excessive dietary intake of vitamin A is associated with reduced bone mineral density and increased risk for hip fracture. *Ann Intern Med*. 1998;129:770-778.

46. Omenn GS. An assessment of the scientific basis for attempting to define the Dietary Reference Intake for beta carotene. *J Am Diet Assoc*. 1998;98:1406-1409.

47. Norman AW. Vitamin D. In: Ziegler EE, Filer LJ Jr, eds. *Present Knowledge in Nutrition*. 7th ed. Washington, DC: ILSI Press; 1996:120-129.

48. Lewis NM, Frederick AM. Vitamins D and K. In: Wolinsky I, Driskell JA, eds. *Sports Nutrition*. Boca Raton, Fla: CRC Press; 1997:111-117.

49. Bell NH, Godsen RN, Henry DP, Shary J, Epstein S. The effects of muscle-building exercise on vitamin D and mineral metabolism. *J Bone Mineral Health*. 1988;3:369-373.

50. Simpson R, Thomas G, Arnold A. 1,25 dihydroxyvitamin D receptors in skeletal and heart muscle. *J Biol Chem*. 1985;260:8882-8884.

51. Costa E, Blau H, Feldman D. 1,25(OH)$_2$-D$_3$ receptors and humoral responses in cloned human skeletal muscle cells. *Endocrinology*. 1986;119:2214-2217.

52. Grady D, Halloran B, Cummings S, et al. 1,25-dihydroxyvitamin D$_3$ and muscle strength in the elderly: a randomized controlled trial. *J Clin Endocrin Metab*. 1991;73:1111-1117.

53. Krall EA, Sahyoun N, Tannenbaum S, Dallal GE, Dawson-Hughes B. Effect of vitamin D intake on seasonal variations in parathyroid hormone secretion in postmenopausal women. *N Engl J Med*. 1989;321:1777-1783.

54. Dawson-Hughes B, Dallal GE, Krall EA, Harris S, Sokoll LJ, Falconer G. Effects of vitamin D supplementation on wintertime and overall bone loss in healthy postmenopausal women. *Ann Intern Med*. 1991;115:505-512.

55. Sokol RJ. Vitamin E. In: Ziegler EE, Filer LJ Jr, eds. *Present Knowledge in Nutrition*. 7th ed. Washington, DC: ILSI Press; 1996:130-136.

56. Duly EB, Trinick TR, Kennedy DG, et al. Vitamin E and exercise in the Northern Ireland population. *Ann Clin Biochem*. 1996;33(pt 3):234-240.

57. Swift JN, Kehrer JP, Seiler S, Starnes JW. Vitamin E concentration in rat skeletal muscle and liver after exercise. *Int J Sport Nutr*. 1998;8:105-112.

58. Thomas TR, Ziogas G, Yan P, Schmitz D, LaFontaine T. Influence of activity level on vitamin E status in healthy men and women and cardiac patients. *J Cardiopulm Rehab*. 1998;18:52-59.

59. Cohen G, Heikkila R. The generation of hydrogen peroxide, superoxide and hydroxyl radical by 6-hydroxydopamine dialuric acid and related cytotoxic agents. *J Biol Chem*. 1974;249:2447.

60. Demopoulos HB, Santomier JP, Seligman ML, Pietronigro DD. Free radical pathology: rationale and toxicology of antioxidants and other supplements in sports medicine and exercise science. In: Katch FI, ed. *Sport, Health and Nutrition*. Champaign, Ill: Human Kinetics; 1986:139.

61. Salo DC, Donovan CM, Davies KJA. HSP70 and other possible heat shock or oxidative stress proteins are induced in skeletal muscle, heart and liver during exercise. *Free Radic Biol Med*. 1991;11:239-246.

62. Merry P, Grootveld M, Lunec J, Blake DR. Oxidative damage to lipids within the inflamed human joint provides evidence of radical-mediated hypoxic-reperfusion injury. *Am J Clin Nutr*. 1991;53(suppl):362S-369S.

63. Kanter MM. Nutritional antioxidants and physical activity. In: Wolinsky I, ed. *Nutrition in Exercise and Sport*. 3rd ed. Boca Raton, Fla: CRC Press, LLC; 1998:245-255.

64. Meydani M, Fielding RA, Fotouhi N. Vitamin E. In: Wolinsky I, Driskell JA, eds. *Sports Nutrition*. Boca Raton, Fla: CRC Press; 1997:119-135.

65. Reddy KV, Kumar TC, Prasad M, Reddanna P. Pulmonary lipid peroxidation and antioxidant defenses during exhaustive physical exercise: the role of vitamin E and selenium. *Nutrition*. 1998;14:448-451.

66. Vasankari TJ, Kujala UM, Vasankari TM, Vuorimaa T, Ahotupa M. Increased serum and low-density-lipoprotein antioxidant potential after antioxidant supplementation in endurance athletes. *Am J Clin Nutr*. 1997;65:1052-1056.

67. Rokitzi L, Logemann E, Sagredos AN, Murphy M, Wetzel-Roth W, Keul J. Lipid peroxidation and antioxidant vitamins under extreme endurance stress. *Acta Physiol Scand*. 1994;154:149-154.

68. McBride JM, Kraemer WJ, Triplett-McBride T, Sebastianelli W. Effect of resistance exercise on free radical production. *Med Sci Sports Exerc*. 1998;30(1):67-72.

69. Suttie JW. Vitamin K. In: DeLuca HF, ed. *The Fat Soluble Vitamins*. London, England: Plenum Press; 1978.

70. Binkley NC, Suttie JW. Vitamin K nutrition and osteoporosis. *J Nutr*. 1995;125:1812-1821.

71. Tortora G, Grabowski S. In: Tortora GJ, Grabowski SR. *Principles of Anatomy and Physiology*. 8th ed. New York, NY: John Wiley & Sons; 1996:569.

72. Brown WH, Foote CS. Vitamin K, blood clotting, and basicity. In: Brown WH, Foote CS, eds. *Organic Chemistry*. 2nd ed. Orlando, Fla: Saunders College Publishing; 1998:635,1026.

73. Mayers PA. Structure and function of the lipid-soluble vitamins. In: Murray RK, Granner DK, Mayers PA, Rodwell VW, eds. *Biochemistry*. Sydney, Australia: Prentice-Hall International; 1990.

74. Kanai T, Takagi T, Masuhiro K, Nakamura M, Iwata M, Saji F. Serum vitamin K level and bone mineral density in post-menopausal women. *Int J Gynecol Obstetr*. 1997;56:25-30.

75. Philip WJ, Martin JC, Richardson JM, Reid DM, Webster J, Douglas AS. Decreased axial and peripheral bone density in patients taking long-term warfarin. *QJM: Monthly Journal of the Association of Physicians*. 1995;88:635-640.

76. Booth SL, Suttie JW. Dietary intake and adequacy of vitamin K. *J Nutr*. 1998;128:785-788.

77. Shearer MJ, Bach A, Kohlmeier M. Chemical, nutritional sources, tissue distribution, and metabolism of vitamin K with specific reference to bone health. *J Nutr*. 1996;126(suppl):1181S-1186S.

78. Olson RE. Vitamin K. In: Shils ME, Olson JA, Shike M, eds. *Modern Nutrition in Health and Disease*. 8th ed. Philadelphia, Penn: Lea & Febiger; 1994:342-358.

79. Arnaud CD, Sanchez SD. Calcium and phosphorus. In: Ziegler EE, Filer LJ Jr, eds. *Present Knowledge in Nutrition*. 7th ed. Washington, DC: ILSI Press; 1996:245-255.

80. Heaney RP. Osteoporosis. In: Krummel DA, Kris-Etherton PM, eds. *Nutrition in Womens Health*. Gaithersburg, Md: Aspen Publishers; 1996:418-439.

81. Allen LH, Wood RJ. Calcium and phosphorous. In: Shils ME, Olson JA, Shike M, eds. *Modern Nutrition in Health and Disease*. 8th ed. Philadelphia, Penn: Lea & Febiger; 1994:144-163.

82. Clarkson PM, Haymes EM. Exercise and mineral status of athletes: calcium, magnesium, phosphorus, and iron. *Med Sci Sports Exerc*. 1995;27:831-843.

83. Zeman FJ, Ney DM. *Applications in Medical Nutrition Therapy*. 2nd ed. Upper Saddle River, NJ: Prentice Hall; 1996.

84. Looker AC, Bilezikian JP, Baily L, et al. Calcium intake in the United States. In: *Optimal Calcium Intake*. In: Program and abstracts of the NIH Consensus Panel Development Conference; June 6-8, 1994; Bethesda, Md.

85. Hendricks KM, Herbold NH. Diet, activity, and other health-related behaviors in college-age women. *Nutr Rev*. 1998;56:65-75.

86. Bergeron MF, Volpe SL, Gelinas Y. Cutaneous calcium losses during exercise in the heat: a regional sweat patch estimation technique [abstract]. *Clin Chem*. 1998;44(suppl):A-167.

87. Dawson-Hughes B, Dallal GE, Krall EA, Sadowski L, Sahyoun N, Tennenbaum S. A controlled trial of the effect of calcium supplementation on bone density in post-menopausal women. *N Engl J Med*. 1990;323:878-883.

88. US Dept Health and Human Services. *The Surgeon General's Report on Nutrition and Health*. Rocklin, Calif: Prima Publishing and Communications; 1988.

89. Metz JA, Anderson JJ, Gallagher PN Jr. Intakes of calcium, phosphorus, and protein, and physical activity level are related to radial bone mass in young adult women. *Am J Clin Nutr*. 1993;58:537-542.

90. Wyshak G, Frisch RE, Albright TE, Albright NL, Schiff I, Witschi J. Nonalcoholic carbonated beverage consumption and bone fractures among former college athletes. *J Orthopaedic Res*. 1989;7:91-99.

91. Horswill CA. Effects of bicarbonate, citrate, and phosphate loading on performance. *Int J Sport Nutr*. 1995;(suppl):S111-S119.

92. Shils ME. Magnesium. In: Ziegler EE, Filer LJ Jr, eds. *Present Knowledge in Nutrition*. 7th ed. Washington, DC: ILSI Press; 1996:256-264.

93. Haymes EM, Clarkson PC. Minerals and trace minerals. In: Berning JR, Steen SN, eds. *Nutrition for Sport & Exercise*. 2nd ed. Gaithersburg, Md: Aspen Publishers; 1998:77-107.

94. Konig D, Weinstock C, Keul J, Northoff H, Berg A. Zinc, iron, and magnesium status in athletes—influence on the regulation of exercise-induced stress and immune function. *Exerc Immunology Rev*. 1998;4:2-21.

95. McDonald R, Keen CL. Iron, zinc and magnesium nutrition and athletic performance. *Sports Med*. 1988;5:171-184.

96. Liu L, Borowski G, Rose LI. Hypomagnesemia in a tennis player. *Phys Sportsmed*. 1983;11:79-80.

97. Oh MS. Water, electrolyte, and acid-base balance. In: Shils ME, Olson JA, Shike M, eds. *Modern Nutrition in Health and Disease*. 8th ed. Philadelphia, Penn: Lea & Febiger; 1994:112-143.

98. Luft FC. Potassium and its regulation. In: Ziegler EE, Filer LJ Jr, eds. *Present Knowledge in Nutrition*. 7th ed. Washington, DC: ILSI Press; 1996:272-276.

99. Pastene J, Germain M, Allevard AM, Gharib C, Lacour JR. Water balance during and after marathon running. *European J Appl Physiol*. 1996;73:49-55.

100. Ljungberg G, Ericson T, Ekbolm B, Birkhed D. Saliva and marathon running. *Scand J Med Sci Sports*. 1997;7:214-219.

101. Millard-Stafford M, Sparling PB, Rosskopf LB, Snow TK, DiCarlo LJ, Hinson BT. Fluid intake in male and female runners during a 4-km field run in the heat. *J Sports Sci*. 1995;13:257-263.

102. Luft FC. Salt, water, and extracellular volume regulation. In: Ziegler EE, Filer LJ Jr, eds. *Present Knowledge in Nutrition*. 7th ed. Washington, DC: ILSI Press; 1996:265-271.

103. Keatisuwan W, Ohnaka T, Tochihara Y. Physiological responses of women during exercise under dry-heat condition in winter and summer. *Appl Human Sci*. 1996;15:169-176.

104. Stachenfeld NS, Gleim GW, Zabetakis PM, Nicholas JA. Fluid balance and renal response following dehydrating exercise in well-trained men and women. *Eur J Appl Physiol*. 1996;72:469-477.

105. Huebers H, Finch CA. Transferrin: physiologic behavior and clinical implications. *Blood*. 1984;64:763-767.

106. Finch CA, Lenfant L. Oxygen transport in men. *N Engl J Med*. 1972;286:407-410.

107. Dallman PR. Tissue effects of iron deficiency. In: Jacobs A, Worwood M, eds. *Iron in Biochemistry and Medicine*. London, England: Academic Press; 1974:437-476.

108. Dallman PR. Biochemical basis for the manifestations of iron deficiency. *Ann Rev Nutrition*. 1986;6:13-40.

109. Balaban EP, Cox JV, Snell P, Vaughan RH, Frenkel EP. The frequency of anemia and iron deficiency in the runner. *Med Sci Sports Exerc*. 1989;21:643-648.

110. Fogelholm GM, Himber JJ, Alopaeus K, et al. Dietary and biochemical indices of nutritional status in male athletes and controls. *J Am Coll Nutr*. 1992;11:181-191.

111. Brown RT, McIntosh SM, Seabolt VR, Daniel WA. Iron status of adolescent female athletes. *J Adolescent Health Care*. 1985;6:349-352.

112. Parr RB, Bachman LA, Moss RA. Iron deficiency in female athletes. *Phys Sportsmed*. 1984;12:81-86.

113. Plowman SA, McSwegin PC. The effects of iron supplementation on female cross-country runners. *J Sports Med*. 1981;21:407-416.

114. Schena F, Pattini A, Mantovanelli S. Iron status in athletes involved in endurance and in prevalently anaerobic sports. In: Kies C, Driskell JA, eds. *Sports Nutrition: Minerals and Electrolytes*. Philadelphia, Penn: CRC Press; 1995:65-79.

115. Bank WJ. Myoglobinuria in marathon runners: possible relationship to carbohydrate and lipid metabolism. *Ann N Y Acad Sci.* 1977;301:942-950.
116. Ben BT, Motley CP. Myoglobinemia and endurance exercise: a study on 25 participants in a triathlon competition. *Am J Sports Med.* 1984;12:113-118.
117. Miller BJ, Pate RR, Burgess W. Foot impact force and intravascular hemolysis during distance running. *Int J Sports Med.* 1988;9:56-60.
118. Nickerson HJ, Holubets MC, Weiler BR, Haas RG, Schwartz S, Ellefson ME. Causes of iron deficiency in adolescent athletes. *J Pediatr.* 1989;114:657-663.
119. Viteri FE, Torun B. Anemia and physical work capacity. *Clin Hematol.* 1974;3:609-626.
120. Finch CA, Miller LR, Inamdar A, Person R, Seiler K, Mackler B. Iron deficiency in the rat: physiological and biochemical studies of muscle dysfunction. *J Clin Invest.* 1976;58:447-453.
121. McLane JA, Fell RD, McKay RH, Winder WW, Brown EB, Holloszy JO. Physiological and biochemical effects of iron deficiency on rat skeletal muscle function. *Am J Physiol.* 1981;241:C47-C54.
122. Zhu YI, Haas JD. Iron depletion without anemia and physical performance in young women. *Am J Clin Nutr.* 1997;66:334-341.
123. Martinez-Torres C, Cubeddu L, Dillmann E, et al. Effect of exposure to low temperature on normal and iron-deficient subjects. *J Physiol.* 1984;246:R380-R383.
124. Beard JL, Borel MJ, Derr J. Impaired thermoregulation and thyroid function in iron-deficiency anemia. *Am J Clin Nutr.* 1990;52:13-19.
125. Beard J, Tobin B, Green W. Evidence for thyroid hormone deficiency in iron-deficient anemic rats. *J Nutr.* 1989;119:772-778.
126. Lozoff B. Behavioral alterations in iron deficiency. *Advances Pediatr.* 1988;35:331-359.
127. Yip R, Dallman PR. Iron. In: Ziegler EE, Filer LJ Jr, eds. *Present Knowledge in Nutrition.* 7th ed. Washington, DC: ILSI Press; 1996:277-292.
128. Solvell L. Oral iron therapy—side effects. In: Hallberg L, ed. *Iron Deficiency: Pathogenesis, Clinical Aspects, Therapy.* London, England: Academic Press; 1970:573-583.
129. Nielsen P, Nachtigall D. Iron supplementation in athletes. *Sports Med.* 1998;26:207-216.
130. Cunnane SC. *Zinc: Clinical and Biochemical Significance.* Boca Raton, Fla: CRC Press; 1988.
131. Deuster PA, Day BA, Singh A, Douglass L, Moser-Veillon PB. Zinc status of highly trained women runners and untrained women. *Am J Clin Nutr.* 1989;49:1295-1301.
132. Lukaski HC, Siders WA, Hoverson BS, Gallagher SK. Iron, copper, magnesium and zinc status as predictors of swimming performance. *Int J Sports Med.* 1996;17:534-540.
133. Lukaski HC, Hoverson BS, Gallagher SK, Bolonchuk WW. Physical training and copper, iron, and zinc status of swimmers. *Am J Clin Nutr.* 1990;51:1093-1099.
134. Wada L, King J. Effect of low zinc intakes on basal metabolic rate, thyroid hormones and protein utilization in adult men. *J Nutr.* 1986;48:1045-1053.
135. O'Dell BL. Copper. In: Brown ML, ed. *Sports Nutrition.* 6th ed. Washington, DC: International Life Sciences Institute-Nutrition Foundation; 1990:261-273.
136. Tessier F, Margaritis I, Richard M-J, Moynot C, Marconnet P. Selenium and training effects on the glutathione system and aerobic performance. *Med Sci Sports Exerc.* 1995;27:390-396.
137. Phipps KR. Fluoirde. In: Ziegler EE, Filer LJ Jr, eds. *Present Knowledge in Nutrition.* 7th ed. Washington, DC: ILSI Press; 1996:329-333.
138. Phipps KP. Fluoride and bone health. *J Public Health Dent.* 1995;55:53-56.
139. Nielsen FH. Chromium. In: Shils ME, Olson JA, Shike M, eds. *Modern Nutrition in Health and Disease.* 8th ed. Philadelphia, Penn: Lea & Febiger; 1994:264-268.
140. Hallmark MA, Reynolds TH, Desouza CA, Dotson CO, Anderson AA, Rogers MA. Effect of chromium and resistive training on muscle strength and body composition. *Med Sci Sports Exerc.* 1996;28:139-144.

141. Lukaski HC, Bolonchuk WW, Siders WA, Miline DB. Chromium supplementation and resistance training: effects on body composition, strength, and trace element status of men. *Am J Clin Nutr*. 1996;63:954-965.

142. Volpe SL, Larpadisorn K. Effects of chromium picolinate supplementation on glucose tolerance and body composition in overweight women [abstract]. *Med Sci Sports Exerc*. 1997;29:S-277.

143. Anderson RA, Kozlovsky AS. Chromium intake, absorption and excretion of subjects consuming self-selected diets. *Am J Clin Nutr*. 1985;41:1177-1183.

144. Anderson RA, Polansky MM, Bryden NA. Strenuous running: acute effects on chromium, copper, zinc, and selected clinical variables in urine and serum of male runners. *Biol Trace Element Res*. 1984;6:327-336.

145. Anderson RA, Bryden NA, Polansky MM, Deuster PA. Exercise effects on chromium excretion of trained and untrained men consuming a constant diet. *J Appl Physiol*. 1988;64:249-252.

146. Nielsen FH. Other trace elements. In: Ziegler EE, Filer LJ Jr, eds. *Present Knowledge in Nutrition*. 7th ed. Washington, DC: ILSI Press; 1996:353-377.

147. Meacham SL, Taper LJ, Volpe SL. The effect of boron supplementation on blood and urinary calcium, magnesium, phosphorus, and urinary boron in female athletes. *Am J Clin Nutr*. 1995;61:341-345.

148. Volpe SL, Taper LJ, Meacham SL. The effect of boron supplementation on bone mineral density and hormonal status in college female athletes. *Medicine Exercise Nutrition Health*. 1993;2:323-330.

149. Volpe SL, Taper LJ, Meacham SL. The relationship between boron and magnesium status, and bone mineral density: a review. *Magnes Res*. 1993;6:291-296.

150. Ferrando AA, Green NR. The effect of boron supplementation on lean body mass, plasma testosterone levels, and strength in male bodybuilders. *Int J Sport Nutr*. 1993;3:140-149.

151. Bucci L. Dietary supplements as ergogenic aids. In: Wolinsky I, ed. *Nutrition in Exercise and Sport*. 3rd ed. Boca Raton, Fla: CRC Press LLC; 1998;315-368.

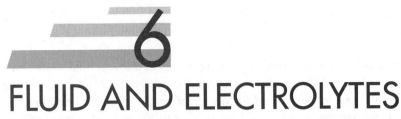

6

FLUID AND ELECTROLYTES

Robert Murray, PhD

It is now widely accepted that consuming adequate fluid before, during, and following physical activity is one of the most important nutritional practices for optimizing performance and protecting health and well-being. Even a slight amount of dehydration can adversely affect the body's ability to cope with physical activity, particularly when that activity is carried out in a warm environment. A comprehensive understanding of the physiological consequences of dehydration can be found in the scientific literature (for selected reviews, see references 1-4) and, perhaps of more relevance, of the physiological and performance benefits of maintaining normal hydration status (5-7). This wealth of research has formed the foundation for practical recommendations regarding fluid replacement during physical activity (6,8-11).

This chapter focuses on the practical consequences, from decades of research, on the physiological and performance-related value of ingesting adequate amounts of fluid during physical activity. This research provides the opportunity to make specific recommendations for fluid-replacement practices.

DAILY FLUID AND ELECTROLYTE BALANCE

Control of Fluid Balance

At rest in thermoneutral conditions, body fluid balance is maintained at ± 0.2% of total body weight (12), a very narrow tolerance befitting the critical importance of hydration status on physiological function, even in nonexercise conditions. Under such circumstances the daily intake of fluid is closely balanced with the volume of fluid that is lost in urine, feces, and sweat; through respiration; and via insensible water loss through the skin. Such a tight regulatory balance requires the constant integration of input from hypothalamic osmoreceptors and vascular baroreceptors so that fluid intake closely matches fluid loss.

Not surprisingly, body fluid balance is regulated by mechanisms that influence water and sodium excretion and affect the sensation of thirst. Sweat loss is accompanied by a decline in plasma volume and an increase in plasma osmolality (due to an increase in plasma sodium and chloride concentrations). These changes are sensed by vascular pressure receptors and hypothalamic osmoreceptors, resulting in an increase in vasopressin (antidiuretic hormone) release from the pituitary gland and in renin release from the kidneys. These hormones (including the angiotensin II and aldosterone that result from an increase in plasma renin activity) serve to increase water and sodium retention by the kidneys and provoke an increase in thirst (13). Whenever fluid intake exceeds fluid losses, plasma volume and osmolality return to normal levels, and water balance is restored by the kidneys (ie, excess fluid is excreted) (14). However, for physically active people, body fluid balance is often compromised because the human thirst mechanism is an imprecise gauge of fluid needs, and it is difficult to ingest enough fluid to offset the large volume of fluid that is lost during physical activity.

Fluid Needs

Daily fluid needs are difficult to predict across a population because of the enormous differences in fluid loss due to physical activity. Many textbooks (15) identify 2 L per day as the fluid requirement for sedentary adults. This minimal need for fluid (2 L = 8 cups per day) can be met from a variety of sources including milk, soft drinks, fruit juices, sports drinks, water, fruit, soup, etc. In physically active individuals daily fluid needs far surpass 2 L per day, rising to over 10 L per day in some athletes and workers (16). These large fluid requirements occur because the volume of sweat lost during physical activity can be prodigious, at times greater than 3 L per hour in highly fit, well acclimated athletes (3). This rapid loss of body fluid is often not accompanied by an equivalent volume of ingested fluid and significant dehydration results.

Fluid is periodically lost from the body by way of the kidneys (urine), gastrointestinal tract (feces), and eccrine sweat glands, and is constantly lost from the respiratory tract and the skin (2,12,15). The total volume of fluid lost from the body on a daily basis is determined by the environmental conditions, the size (and surface area) of the individual, the individual's metabolic rate, and the volume of excreted fluids. Insensible water loss via the skin is relatively constant (see *Table 6.1*), but insensible loss via the respiratory tract is affected by the ambient temperature, relative humidity, and ventilatory volume. Inhaled air is humidified during its passage through the respiratory tract; as a result, exhaled air has a relative humidity of 100% (vapor pressure = 47 mm Hg). Inhaling warm, humid air slightly reduces insensible water loss because the inhaled air already contains substantial water vapor. As indicated in *Table 6.1*, athletes and workers experience a greater insensible water loss via the respiratory tract merely because of the overall increase in breathing that accompanies exercise. The air inhaled during cold weather activity contains relatively little water vapor, so as it is warmed and humidified during its transit through the respiratory tract, an additional water loss occurs. For this reason it is important to keep in mind that even during cold weather activity, fluid losses via the sweat glands and respiratory tract can be quite high.

Urine losses in athletes and workers tend to be lower than in sedentary individuals, a trend that is exacerbated by warm weather as the body strives to conserve fluid. Physical activity results in a reduction in urine production as the kidneys attempt to conserve water and sodium to offset losses due to sweating.

Even in the absence of physical activity, daily fluid losses average a minimum of about 2 to 3 L (see *Table 6.1*). When athletes train and compete in warm environments, their daily fluid needs can be large (16). For example, an athlete who trains 2 hours each day can easily lose an additional 4 L of body fluid, resulting in a daily fluid requirement in excess of 6 to 7 L. Many people are active more than 2 hours each day, further increasing their fluid needs. Such losses can strain the capacity of the fluid regulatory system such that thirst becomes an inadequate stimulus for fluid intake and dehydration results.

TABLE 6.1 Typical Daily Fluid Losses (in mL) for a 70-kg Athlete

	Normal Weather (68°F)	Warm Weather (85°F)	Exercise in Warm Weather (85°F)
Insensible loss			
Skin	350	350	350
Respiratory tract	350	250	650
Urine	1,400	1,200	500
Feces	100	100	100
Sweat	100	1,400	5,000
TOTAL	2,300	3,300	6,600

Adapted from: Guyton AC. *Textbook of Medical Physiology*, 8th ed. Philadelphia, Penn: WB Saunders Co; 1991:150-151.

Note: Daily fluid loss varies widely among athletes and can exceed 10 L per day under some circumstances.

Control of Electrolyte Balance

The concentrations of electrolytes across cell membranes must be tightly regulated to assure proper function of cells throughout the body. In the case of cardiac muscle, for example, electrolyte imbalances can have fatal consequences. For this reason the kidney is well equipped to maintain electrolyte balance by conserving or excreting minerals such as sodium, chloride, potassium, calcium, and magnesium. Aside from the existence of an "appetite" for sodium chloride (17), there is little evidence to suggest that the intake of other minerals is governed by similar responses. Provided that dietary energy intake is adequate, mineral intake is usually in excess of mineral needs, assuring positive mineral balance.

Electrolyte Needs

Electrolyte loss accompanies fluid loss in urine and sweat. Athletes and workers who lose large amounts of sweat on a daily basis can also lose large amounts of electrolytes, particularly sodium and chloride. Potassium is also lost in sweat (17), although the concentration of potassium in sweat (usually < 10 mmol/L) is far less than that of sodium (20 to 100+ mmol/L). The fact that sweat sodium concentration varies widely among individuals means that some people will be prone to large sodium deficits whereas others will not. Increased risk of heat-related problems and muscle cramps has been linked to sodium chloride losses in sweat (18).

The amount of sodium chloride lost in sweat is not trivial. Consider, for example, a football player who practices for 5 hours a day, during which time he loses 8 L of sweat (1.6 L per hour). If his sweat contains an average of 50 mmol Na^+/L, total sodium loss will be 9,200 mg sodium (23 g of NaCl). This sodium loss, which does not include the 100 to 200 mmol of sodium that is typically lost in urine, makes it apparent that many physically active people require a large sodium chloride intake to replace losses in sweat.

Human sweat contains small amounts of dozens of substances, many of which are minerals. Even when sweat losses are large, it is unlikely that minerals such as magnesium, iron, and calcium will be lost in sufficient quantities in sweat to provoke a mineral imbalance in most people. However, there may be some individuals for whom such losses could constitute an additional dietary challenge, as might, in theory at least, be the case with sweat calcium losses in physically active females (see Chapter 5, Vitamins and Minerals for Active People). Additional research will be needed to determine if the current required dietary intake values should be adjusted upwards in these individuals.

ACSM RECOMMENDATIONS

In recognition of recent research on how fluid intake influences physiological and performance responses, the American College of Sports Medicine (ACSM) published a position stand in January 1996 titled *Exercise and Fluid Replacement* (9). This position stand provides clear and practical guidelines regarding fluid, carbohydrate, and electrolyte replenishment for athletes. In preparing the recommendations a panel of experts in fluid homeostasis, carbohydrate feeding, mineral balance, and related fields completed a comprehensive review of the scientific literature in an effort to be certain that each practical recommendation was well substantiated by research. As a result, the ACSM position stand will benefit public health for years to come. In general, the ACSM guidelines emphasize the importance of a fluid replacement plan designed to prevent even slight dehydration during physical activity.

Fluid and Electrolyte Replacement *before* Exercise

Being well hydrated before physical activity helps assure optimal physiological and performance responses. Clearly, athletes who enter competition in a dehydrated state are at a competitive disadvantage (4). For example, in a study by Armstrong et al (19), subjects performed a 5,000-meter (~ 19 minutes) and 10,000-meter (~ 40 minutes) run in either a normally hydrated or dehydrated condition. When dehydrated by ~2% of body weight (by a diuretic given prior to exercise), their running speeds decreased significantly (by 6% to 7%) in both events. To make matters worse, exercise in the heat exacerbates the performance-impairing effects of dehydration (20).

To help assure adequate hydration, the ACSM position stand states that:

"It is recommended that individuals consume a nutritionally balanced diet and drink adequate fluids during the 24-hour period before an event, especially during the period that includes the meal prior to exercise, to promote proper hydration before exercise or competition."(9)

When people live and are physically active in warm environments, voluntary fluid intake is often insufficient to meet fluid needs, as verified by a study conducted on soccer players in Puerto Rico (21). The athletes were studied during 2 weeks of training. When the players were allowed to drink fluids throughout the day as they wished (average intake = 2.7 L per day), their total body water at the end of 1 week was about 1.1 L lower than when they were mandated to drink 4.6 L of fluid per day. In other words, their voluntary fluid consumption did not match their fluid losses, causing them to enter training and competition already dehydrated.

Prior to physical activity:

"It is recommended that individuals drink about 500 mL (about 17 oz) of fluid about 2 hours before exercise to promote adequate hydration and allow time for excretion of excess ingested water." (9)

In fact, laboratory subjects who ingest fluid in the hour before exercise exhibit lower core temperatures and heart rates during exercise than when no fluid is ingested (21,22).

From a practical standpoint noting the color and volume of urine is an important practical tool in helping physically active people assess their hydration status. Darkly colored urine of relatively small volume is an indication of dehydration, a signal to ingest more fluid prior to activity. Monitoring urine output is a common recommendation in occupational settings such as the mining industry in which the workers are constantly exposed to conditions of high heat and humidity.

It has been hypothesized that ingesting a glycerol solution before physical activity in the heat may confer cardiovascular and thermoregulatory advantages. In fact, ingesting glycerol solutions prior to exercise does result in a reduction in urine production and in the temporary retention of fluid (23). Glycerol-induced hyperhydration is accompanied by weight gain that is proportional to the amount of water retained (usually about 0.5 to 1 kg). Fluid retention occurs because after glycerol molecules are absorbed and distributed throughout the body water (with the exception of the aqueous-humor and the cerebral-spinal fluid compartments), their presence provokes a transient increase in osmolality, prompting a temporary fall in urine production. As glycerol molecules are removed from the body water in the subsequent hours, plasma osmolality drops, urine production increases, and the excess water is excreted.

There are a number of reasons why it is unwise to recommend glycerol-induced hydration to athletes.

1. Athletes pay a metabolic cost for carrying extra body weight.
2. There is no compelling evidence that glycerol-induced hyperhydration results in a physiological benefit (24).
3. The side effects of ingesting glycerol can range from mild sensations of bloating and lightheadedness to more severe symptoms of headaches, dizziness, and nausea (25).

Fluid and Electrolyte Replacement *during* Exercise

Recent research has shown that cardiovascular, thermoregulatory, and performance responses are optimized by replacing sweat loss during exercise (see *Table 6.2*) (7,26). These findings are reflected in the recommendation:

> "During exercise, athletes should start drinking early and at regular intervals in an attempt to consume fluids at a rate sufficient to replace all the water lost through sweating, or consume the maximal amount that can be tolerated." (9)

TABLE 6.2   Beneficial Responses to Adequate Fluid Intake during Exercise

Characteristic	Response
Heart rate	Lower
Stroke volume	Higher
Cardiac output	Higher
Skin blood flow	Higher
Core temperature	Lower
Perceived exertion	Lower
Performance	Better

Adapted from: Montain SJ, Coyle EF. The influence of graded dehydration on hyperthermia and cardiovascular drift during exercise. *J Appl Physiol.* 1992;73(4):1340-1350 and Walsh RM, Noakes TD, Hawley JA, Dennis SC. Impaired high-intensity cycling performance time at low levels of dehydration. *Int J Sports Med.* 1994;15:392-398.

This recommendation clearly states that the goal of fluid intake during exercise is to prevent *any* amount of dehydration, but recognizes that such an intake may be difficult under some circumstances. In most instances voluntary fluid intake alone will be insufficient to fully replace sweat loss during physical activity, in part because sweat losses can vary widely among individuals. For example, while light physical activity in a cool, dry environment may result in a sweat loss of only 250 mL per hour, exercise in a warm, humid environment can provoke a sweat loss in excess of 2 L per hour, with some athletes capable of sweating at greater than 3 L per hour (3). For that reason it is essential that athletes and workers follow a prescribed regimen to guide the frequency and volume of their fluid intake. Under ideal circumstances this requires that each individual's sweat rate is known (easily assessed by recording pre- and postactivity body weights and correcting for fluid intake and urine loss; see *Figure 6.1*) and that specific individual recommendations are made regarding fluid intake during activity (see *Figure 6.2; Box 6.1*). Beginning activity with a comfortable volume of fluid already in the stomach, followed by additional fluid intake at 10- to 30-minute intervals (depending upon sweat rate), will help assure rapid gastric emptying by maintaining a large gastric volume, an important driver of gastric emptying (27).

FIGURE 6.1   Determining Sweat Rate

Drinking fluid during exercise to keep pace with sweat loss goes a long way towards helping athletes and workers feel good and work hard. Because sweat rates can vary widely, it is important that athletes and workers are aware of how much sweat they lose during physical activity. Knowing how much fluid is typically lost during an hour of activity provides a goal for fluid replacement. Here are some simple steps to take to determine hourly sweat rate. In the example below, Kelly K. should drink about 1 L (32 oz) of fluid during each hour of activity to remain well hydrated.

A	B	C	D	E	F	G	H	I	J
		Body Weight					Sweat Loss		Sweat Rate
Name	Date	Before Exercise	After Exercise	ΔBW (C–D)	Drink Volume	Urine Volume*	(E+F–G)	Exercise Time	(H/I)
Kelly K.	9/15	61.7 kg	60.3 kg	1,400 g	420 mL	90 mL	1730 mL	90 min	19 mL/min
		(lb/2.2)	(lb/2.2)	(kg x 1,000)	(oz x 30)	(oz x 30)	(oz x 30)	1.5 h	1,153 mL/h
		kg	kg	g	mL	mL	mL	min	mL/min
		(lb/2.2)	(lb/2.2)	(kg x 1,000)	(oz x 30)	(oz x 30)	(oz x 30)	h	mL/h
		kg	kg	g	mL	mL	mL	min	mL/min
		(lb/2.2)	(lb/2.2)	(kg x 1,000)	(oz x 30)	(oz x 30)	(oz x 30)	h	mL/h

*Weight of urine should be subtracted *if urine was excreted prior to postexcercise body weight.*

Reproduced with permission from the Gatorade Sports Science Institute

FIGURE 6.2   Recommendations for Fluid Intake during Stages of Activity

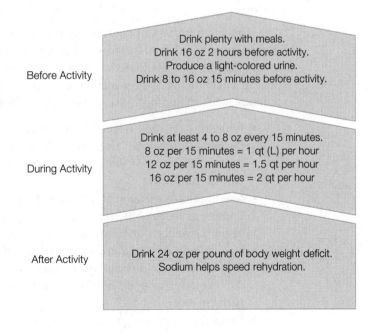

Before Activity
Drink plenty with meals.
Drink 16 oz 2 hours before activity.
Produce a light-colored urine.
Drink 8 to 16 oz 15 minutes before activity.

During Activity
Drink at least 4 to 8 oz every 15 minutes.
8 oz per 15 minutes = 1 qt (L) per hour
12 oz per 15 minutes = 1.5 qt per hour
16 oz per 15 minutes = 2 qt per hour

After Activity
Drink 24 oz per pound of body weight deficit.
Sodium helps speed rehydration.

BOX 6.1   Practical Tips and Recommendations for Encouraging Drinking before, during, and following Physical Activity

1. Take fluid with you. Wear a bottle belt or fluid pack and/or take along a cooler full of drinks. (Freeze fluid bottles overnight to allow the drink to stay cold longer.)
2. Know the warning signs of dehydration (unusual fatigue, lightheadedness, headache, dark urine, dry mouth).
3. Know where to find fluid (water fountains, stores, etc) and always carry money to buy drinks.
4. Drink by schedule—not by thirst.
5. Prehydrate to produce a light-colored urine.
6. Plan for fluid intake during competition. Practice drinking during training.
7. Start activity with a belly full of fluid and keep a comfortably full stomach during activity.
8. Know your sweat rate by weighing before and after activity.
9. Drink 24 oz for every pound of weight loss after activity. (One medium mouthful of fluid equals about 1 oz.)
10. Replace fluid and sodium losses fully to achieve complete rehydration.
11. Put more in your stomach than on your head. Pouring water over your head does nothing to lower body temperature.

"It is recommended that ingested fluids be cooler than ambient temperature [between 15° and 22°C (59° and 72°F)] and flavored to enhance palatability and promote fluid replacement. Fluids should be readily available and served in containers that allow adequate volumes to be ingested with ease and with minimal interruption of exercise." (9)

Not surprisingly, humans prefer beverages that are flavored and sweetened (28). This is an important consideration in preventing dehydration because any step that can be taken to increase voluntary fluid intake will help reduce the risk of health problems associated with dehydration and heat stress. In addition to having palatable beverages available for athletes to drink, a number of other practical steps should be taken. These include the following:

- Educating coaches, trainers, supervisors, parents, and athletes about the benefits of proper hydration. Periodic lectures, locker room posters, take-home flyers, and educational brochures can all be a part of this effort.
- Making fluids easily available at all times. When possible, fluid stations or squeeze bottles should always be nearby and there should be no restrictions on how often people can drink.
- Establishing an organized regimen for fluid replacement. Making individual recommendations regarding fluid intake helps reinforce the message that good drinking habits are important to health and performance.
- Recording body weights before and after physical activity as a way to assess the effectiveness of fluid intake and as a reminder of the importance of drinking adequately (29).

"Addition of proper amounts of carbohydrates and/or electrolytes to a fluid replacement solution is recommended for exercise events of duration greater than 1 hour since it does not significantly impair water delivery to the body and may enhance performance." (9)

Carbohydrate is an important component of a fluid-replacement beverage because it improves palatability by conferring sweetness, provides a source of fuel for active muscles, and stimulates fluid absorption from the intestine (16). The performance benefits of carbohydrate feeding during physical activity are covered in more detail in other chapters. Although it is clear that carbohydrate feeding benefits performance (2,10,16,30), more carbohydrate in a beverage is not necessarily better. Recent research has demonstrated that ingesting drinks containing more than 14 g of carbohydrate per 8 oz serving will decrease the rate of gastric emptying (30) and fluid absorption (31).

"Inclusion of sodium (0.5 to 0.7 g/L of water) in the rehydration solution ingested during exercise lasting longer than 1 hour is recommended since it may be advantageous in enhancing palatability, promoting fluid retention, and possibly preventing hyponatremia in certain individuals who drink excessive quantities of fluid. There is little physiological basis for the presence of sodium in an oral rehydration solution for enhancing intestinal water absorption as long as sodium is sufficiently available from the previous meal." (9)

Sweat contains more sodium and chloride than other minerals and, although sweat electrolyte values are normally substantially lower than plasma values (plasma = 138 to 142 mmol/L; sweat = 25 to 100 mmol/L), physical activity in excess of 2 hours a day can result in considerable salt loss. Normally, sodium deficits are uncommon among athletes and military personnel (32) in large part because a normal diet often provides more than enough salt to replace that which is lost in sweat. However, sodium losses can present problems, as illustrated by Bergeron (33) in a case study of a nationally ranked tennis player who suffered from frequent heat cramps. A high sweat rate (2.5 L per hour) coupled with a higher-than-normal sweat sodium concentration (90 mmol per hour) predisposed him to muscle cramps. The cramps were eliminated when he increased his daily dietary intake of sodium chloride from 5 to 10 g per day to 15 to 20 g per day and increased his fluid intake to assure adequate hydration.

It is also important to understand that ingesting sodium chloride in a beverage consumed during physical activity not only helps ensure adequate fluid intake (34) but also stimulates more complete rehydration following activity (35). Both of these responses reflect the critical role that sodium plays in maintaining the osmotic drive to drink and in providing an osmotic stimulus to retain fluid in the extracellular space.

As indicated in the ACSM position stand, the sodium content of a fluid-replacement beverage does not directly affect the rate of fluid absorption, as demonstrated by research (36). This is because the amount of sodium that can be included in a beverage is small compared to the amount of sodium that can be provided from the bloodstream. Whenever fluid is ingested, plasma sodium diffuses into the gut, driven by an osmotic gradient that strongly favors sodium influx. In brief, sodium chloride is an important constituent of a properly formulated sports drink because it improves beverage palatability, helps maintain the osmotic drive for drinking, reduces the amount of sodium that the blood has to supply to the intestine prior to fluid absorption, helps maintain plasma volume during exercise, and serves as the primary osmotic impetus for restoring extracellular fluid volume following exercise (34,35,37).

A good example of the effect that beverage composition has on voluntary fluid intake is demonstrated by the work of Wilk and Bar-Or (38). Adolescent boys (ages 9 to 12) completed 3 hours of intermittent exercise in the heat, during which time they could drink one of three beverages ad libitum. The boys completed this protocol on three occasions. The beverages tested included water, a sports drink, and a flavored, artificially sweetened replica of the sports drink. The boys drank almost twice as much sports drink as they did water; consumption of the placebo fell in between. Flavoring and sweetness increased voluntary fluid intake (better drinking with placebo versus water), and the presence of sodium chloride in the sports drink further increased consumption (ie, the subjects drank more sports drink than placebo).

These results are consistent with the physiology of the thirst mechanism. In humans the sensation of thirst is a function of changes in plasma sodium concentration (and plasma osmolality) and of changes in blood volume (17). Drinking plain water quickly removes the osmotic drive to drink (dilutes the sodium concentration of the blood) and reduces the volume-dependent drive (by partially restoring blood volume), causing the satiation of thirst. Unfortunately, the resulting decrease in fluid intake occurs prematurely before adequate fluid has been ingested. The osmotic drive for drinking can be maintained by the presence of low levels of sodium chloride in a beverage and greater fluid intake results (35).

Fluid and Electrolyte Replacement *after* Exercise

On those occasions when a fluid deficit (ie, dehydration) exists after physical activity, it is important to be able to rehydrate quickly. An afternoon of working in the yard, two-a-day football practices, a day-long sports tournament, and 8 hours of manual labor are all examples of activities in which dehydration (more precisely referred to in this instance as *hypohydration*) is likely. Fluid intake after physical activity is a critical factor in helping people recover quickly—both physically and mentally. Maughan et al (35) concluded that ingesting plain water is ineffective at restoring euhydration because water absorption causes plasma osmolality to fall, suppressing thirst and increasing urine output. When sodium is provided in fluids or foods, the osmotic drive to drink is maintained (34,35,39), and urine production is decreased. In a very real sense plain water is a good thirst quencher but not an effective rehydrator.

Maughan et al (35) also emphasized the importance of ingesting fluid *in excess* of the deficit in body weight to account for obligatory urine losses. In other words the advice normally given athletes—*"drink a pint of fluid for every pound of body weight deficit"*—must be amended to *"drink at least a pint of fluid for every pound of body weight deficit."* More precise recommendations for how much fluid athletes should ingest to assure rapid and complete rehydration will evolve from future research; existing data indicate that ingestion of 150% or more of weight loss may be required to achieve normal hydration within 6 hours following exercise (38).

Finally, when rapid rehydration is the goal, consumption of alcoholic and caffeinated beverages is contraindicated because of the diuretic properties of each. However, education efforts should reflect the fact that athletes and workers will choose to consume such beverages. For those who do drink coffee, colas, beer, and similar beverages, the best advice is to do so in moderation, especially prior to physical activity.

REFERENCES

1. Murray R. Nutrition for the marathon and other endurance sports: environmental stress and dehydration. *Med Sci Sports Exerc.* 1992;24:S319-S323.
2. Sawka MN. Body fluid responses and dehydration during exercise and heat stress. In: Pandolf KB, Sawka MN, Gonzalez RR, eds. *Human Performance Physiology and Environmental Medicine at Terrestrial Extremes.* Indianapolis, Ind: Benchmark Press; 1988:227-266.
3. Sawka MN, Pandolf KB. Effects of body water loss on physiological function and exercise performance. In: Gisolfi CV, Lamb DR, eds. *Perspectives in Exercise Science and Sports Medicine: Fluid Homeostasis During Exercise.* Indianapolis, Ind: Benchmark Press; 1990:1-38.
4. Sawka MN. Physiological consequences of dehydration: exercise performance and thermoregulation. *Med Sci Sports Exerc.* 1992;24(6):657-670.
5. Below PR, Coyle EF. Fluid and carbohydrate ingestion individually benefit intense exercise lasting one hour. *Med Sci Sports Exerc.* 1995;27(2):200-210.
6. Coyle EF, Montain SJ. Benefits of fluid replacement with carbohydrate during exercise. *Med Sci Sports Exerc.* 1992;24:S324-S330.
7. Montain SJ, Coyle EF. The influence of graded dehydration on hyperthermia and cardiovascular drift during exercise. *J Appl Physiol.* 1992;73(4):1340-1350.
8. American College of Sports Medicine. Position stand on the prevention of thermal injuries during distance running. *Med Sci Sports Exerc.* 1985;17:ix-xiv.
9. American College of Sports Medicine. Position stand on exercise and fluid replacement. *Med Sci Sports Exerc.* 1996;28:i-vii.
10. Coyle EF, Montain SJ. Carbohydrate and fluid ingestion during exercise: are there trade-offs? *Med Sci Sports Exerc.* 1992;24(6):671-678.
11. Gisolfi CV, Duchman SD. Guidelines for optimal replacement beverages for different athletic events. *Med Sci Sports Exerc.* 1992;24(6):679-687.
12. Greenleaf JE. Problem: thirst, drinking behavior, and involuntary dehydration. *Med Sci Sports Exerc.* 1992;24:645-656.
13. Wade CE, Freund BJ. Hormonal control of blood flow during and following exercise. In: Gisolfi CV, Lamb DR, eds. *Perspectives in Exercise Science and Sports Medicine: Fluid Homeostasis During Exercise.* Indianapolis, Ind: Benchmark Press; 1990:3:207-246.
14. Booth DA. Influences on human fluid consumption. In: Ramsay DJ, Booth DA, eds. *Thirst: Physiological and Psychological Aspects.* London: Springer-Verlag; 1991:56.
15. Guyton AC. *Textbook of Medical Physiology.* 8th ed. Philadelphia, Penn: WB Saunders Co; 1991:150-151.
16. Maughan RJ, Shirreffs SM, Galloway DR, Leiper JB. Dehydration and fluid replacement in sport and exercise. *Sports Exerc Inj.* 1995;1:148-153.
17. Hubbard RW, Szlyk PC, Armstrong LE. Influence of thirst and fluid palatability on fluid ingestion during exercise. In: Gisolfi CV, Lamb DR, eds. *Perspectives in Exercise Science and Sports Medicine: Fluid Homeostasis During Exercise.* Indianapolis, Ind: Benchmark Press; 1990:3:39-96.

18. Bauman A. The epidemiology of heat stroke and associated thermoregulatory disorders. In: Sutton JR, Thompson MW, Torode ME, eds. *Exercise and Thermoregulation*. Sydney, Australia: The University of Sydney; 1995:203-208.

19. Armstrong LE, Costill DL, Fink WJ. Influence of diuretic-induced dehydration on competitive running performance. *Med Sci Sports Exerc*. 1985;17:456-461.

20. Sawka MN, Francesconi RP, Young AJ, Pandolf KB. Influence of hydration level and body fluids on exercise performance in the heat. *JAMA*. 1984;252:1165-1169.

21. Rico-Sanz J, Frontera WA, Rivera MA, Rivera-Brown A, Mole PA, Meredith CN. Effects of hyperhydration on total body water, temperature regulation and performance of elite young soccer players in a warm climate. *Int J Sports Med*. 1995;17:85-91.

22. Greenleaf JE, Castle BL. Exercise temperature regulation in man during hypohydration and hyperthermia. *J Appl Physiol*. 1971;30:847-853.

23. Riedesel ML, Allen DY, Peake GT, Al-Qattan K. Hyperhydration with glycerol solutions. *J Appl Physiol*. 1987;63:2262-2268.

24. Latzka WA, Sawka MN, Montain SJ, et al. Hyperhydration: tolerance and cardiovascular effects during uncompensable heat-exercise stress. *J Appl Physiol*. 1998;84:1858-1864.

25. Murray R, Eddy DE, Paul GL, Seifert JG, Halaby GA. Physiological responses to glycerol ingestion during exercise. *J Appl Physiol*. 1991;71(1):144-149.

26. Walsh RM, Noakes TD, Hawley JA, Dennis SC. Impaired high-intensity cycling performance time at low levels of dehydration. *Int J Sports Med*. 1994;15:392-398.

27. Maughan RJ. Gastric emptying during exercise. *Sports Sci Exch*. 1993;6(5):1-6.

28. Greenleaf JE. Environmental issues that influence intake of replacement beverages. In: Marriott BM, ed. *Fluid Replacement and Heat Stress*. Washington, DC: National Academy Press; 1991;XV:1-30.

29. Broad E. Fluid requirements of team sport players. *Sports Coach*. 1996;Summer:20-23.

30. Horswill CA. Effective fluid replacement. *Int J Sports Nutr*. 1988;8:175-195.

31. Ryan AJ, Lambert GP, Shi X, Chang RT, Summers RW, Gisolfi CV. Effect of hypohydration on gastric emptying and intestinal absorption during exercise. *J Appl Physiol*. 1998;84:1581-1588.

32. Armstrong LE, Costill DL, Fink WJ. Changes in body water and electrolytes during heat acclimation: effects of dietary sodium. *Aviat Space Environ Med*. 1987;58:143-148.

33. Bergeron MF. Heat cramps during tennis: a case report. *Int J Sports Nutr*. 1996;6:62-68.

34. Nose H, Mack GW, Shi X, Nadel ER. Role of osmolality and plasma volume during rehydration in humans. *J Appl Physiol*. 1988;65:325-331.

35. Maughan RJ, Shirreffs SM, Leiper JB. Rehydration and recovery after exercise. *Sport Sci Exch*. 1996;9(62):1-5.

36. Gisolfi CV, Summers RW, Schedl HP, Bleiler TL. Effect of sodium concentration in a carbohydrate-electrolyte solution on intestinal absorption. *Med Sci Sports Exerc*. 1995;27:1414-1420.

37. Shirreffs SM, Taylor AJ, Leiper JB, Maughan RJ. Post-exercise rehydration in man: effects of volume consumed and drink sodium content. *Med Sci Sports Exerc*. 1996;28:1260-1271.

38. Wilk B, Bar-Or O. Effect of drink flavor and NaCl on voluntary drinking and hydration in boys exercising in the heat. *J Appl Physiol*. 1996;80:1112-1117.

39. Gonzalez-Alonso J, Heaps CL, Coyle EF. Rehydration after exercise with common beverages and water. *Int J Sports Med*. 1992;13:399-406.

7

ERGOGENIC AIDS

Rob Skinner, RD, CSCS; Ellen Coleman, MA, MPH, RD; and Christine A. Rosenbloom, PhD, RD

Nutritional ergogenic aids are dietary supplements that supposedly enhance performance above levels anticipated under normal conditions. The term "ergogenic" means work-producing. Athletes hope that ergogenic aids will give them a competitive edge and help them win. Since sporting competitions are sometimes won by a difference of $1/100^{th}$ of a second, it is not surprising that athletes want to try the newest ergogenic aid.

By definition, a supplement is something added to the diet to make up for a nutritional deficiency. Athletes, however, consume dietary supplements to improve athletic performance and health. The quest for performance-enhancing supplements is not new. Athletes of ancient days would eat the heart or liver of an animal, such as a lion or deer, to increase their swiftness, courage, or strength (1).

While it is no surprise that competitive athletes use supplements, supplement use is not limited to the elite level. A recent survey by the National Strength and Conditioning Association (NSCA) (2) at its annual convention reported that 71% of coaches encouraged supplement use among their athletes. When asked which athletes were helped by supplementation, 92% of coaches believed that the performance of professional athletes was increased, 91% believed that the performance of collegiate athletes was increased, and 65% believed that the performance of high school athletes was increased (2).

Dietary supplements are a multibillion dollar industry that targets a wide range of populations, including athletes. Between the years 1990 and 1996, supplement sales almost doubled from $3.3 billion to $6.5 billion (3). The Dietary Supplement and Health Education Act of 1994 (DSHEA) bolstered sales by classifying dietary supplements in their own category and not as food additives or drugs. Under DSHEA, dietary supplements are defined as vitamins, minerals, amino acids, herbs, and other botanicals.

Supplement companies do not have to prove a supplement's safety, effectiveness, or potency before placing a product on the market. Manufacturers of supplements are not supposed to make unsubstantiated health claims about their products but easily get around this stipulation with the following disclaimer: "This statement has not been evaluated by the Food Drug and Administration (FDA). This product is not intended to diagnose, treat, cure or prevent disease." This disclaimer is usually in very small print on the back panel of the product. *Box 7.1* highlights the information that must appear on the labels of dietary supplements.

These products generally have very little scientific evidence supporting the validity of claims. Often the studies that are reported as proof that a product

---

BOX 7.1   Information Appearing on Dietary Supplement Labels (3)

As of March 1999, information required on the labels of dietary supplements includes:

1. Statement of identity (eg, "ginseng")
2. Net quantity of contents (eg, "60 capsules")
3. Structure-function claim and the statement, "This statement has not been evaluated by the Food and Drug Administration. This product is not intended to diagnose, treat, cure or prevent any disease."
4. Directions for use (eg, "Take one capsule daily.")
5. Supplement Facts panel (list of serving size, amount, and active ingredients)
6. Other ingredients in descending order of predominance and by common name or proprietary blend
7. Name and place of business of manufacturer, packer, or distributor. This is the address to write to for more product information.

---

works have not been published in peer-reviewed journals or the facts of a published study are extrapolated and misrepresented to support claims. If studies are conducted on a product, many are of poor experimental design or use animal models or human populations different from the populations buying the products.

Interest in supplements has never been greater. According to the advertisements in many fitness magazines, Internet web sites, and television infomercials, nutrition supplements can increase speed, enhance endurance, hasten recovery, improve muscle mass, and reduce body fat. Some advertisements even claim their wonder product does all of the above.

The use of the word "natural" on a supplement label may lead athletes to believe that the supplement is "legal" and "safe." However, several athletes have been disqualified from competitions for taking "natural" products that contained banned or restricted substances such as ephedrine. The belief that "natural" equals "safe" is also common and can be a dangerous misconception as evidenced by the adverse side effects associated with ephedrine-containing products.

Governing organizations such as the National Collegiate Athletic Association (NCAA) and the International Olympic Committee (IOC) have published lists of banned and restricted substances which will disqualify the athlete from competition if he or she tests positive for the substance. The NCAA has reported that not knowing a product is on the banned substance list is not an acceptable excuse for a positive drug test. No appeal on the grounds of ignorance has ever overturned a doping disqualification (4).

New supplements appear almost monthly. This chapter will review some of the most popular supplements, their ergogenic claims, research to support or dispute these claims, and prudent recommendation for persons working with athletes. Although not an all-inclusive report of currently marketed supplements, this chapter provides current information about a topic that is clouded with half-truths and speculation. Herbal products, with the exception of ephedra, will not be covered in this chapter. The sports nutritionist seeking information on other herbal products will find suggested resources in *Box 7.2.*

BOX 7.2   Sources of Information on Herbal Products

Books/Mongraphs

Blumenthal M, Riggins CW. *Popular Herbs in the U.S. Market*. Austin, Tex: The American Botanical Council; 1997.

PDR for Herbal Medicine. 1st ed. Montvale, NJ: Medical Economics Co; 1998.

Schulz V, Hansel R, Tyler VE. *Rational Phytotherapy: A Physician's Guide to Herbal Medicine*. Berlin, Germany: Springer; 1997.

Foster S, Tyler VE. *Tyler's Honest Herbal*. Binghamton, NY: The Haworth Herbal Press; 1999.

Tyler VE, Robbers JE. *Tyler's Herbs of Choice*. Binghamton, NY: The Haworth Herbal Press; 1999.

Periodicals

Journal of Herbal Pharmacotherapy. Lucinda G. Miller, Pharm D, Editor

Journal of Nutraceuticals, Functional, and Medical Foods. Nancy Maressa Childs, PhD, Editor

SCAN's Pulse. Michele Macedonio, MS, RD, Editor

SCAN's Guide to Nutrition and Fitness Resources (published annually)

AMINO ACIDS (ARGININE, LYSINE, ORNITHINE)

Claims

- Increases muscle mass
- Decreases body fat
- Increases growth hormone secretion

Theoretical Basis as an Ergogenic Aid

Arginine and ornithine are two nonessential amino acids, while lysine is an essential amino acid that must be derived from the diet. It has been theorized that oral consumption of one or a combination of these amino acids will raise the circulating level of human growth hormone (hGH) and insulin. The performance advantage to increased levels of hGH and insulin is related to their anabolic properties. It has been speculated that increased hGH and insulin promote accretion of muscle mass and the decrease of body fat.

What Does the Research Show?

A study by Fogelholm et al (5) using a double-blind crossover design examined the ingestion of 2 g of arginine, lysine, and ornithine taken twice per day. Eleven competitive weightlifters were given amino acid or placebo with hGH and insulin levels measured every 24 hours. Spikes in hGH were no different in placebo or supplemented groups, and insulin levels were not elevated postsupplementation. The researchers concluded that the ergogenic value of low-dose amino acids is questionable.

Since hGH levels tend to decrease with age, Corpas et al (6) studied the effects of oral arginine and lysine ingestion on hGH in older men (69 ± 5 yr). Two groups of eight healthy men were given 3 g of arginine and lysine twice per day for 14 days. Levels of hGH were measured in blood samples taken every 20 minutes from 2 AM to 8 AM. The results indicated that neither hGH, growth hormone-releasing hormone, or serum insulin growth factor were significantly altered. The data indicated that oral administration of arginine and lysine is not a practical means of enhancing hGH secretion in older men.

Suminski et al (7) examined amino acid ingestion and resistance training on plasma growth hormone concentration in young men. Sixteen males completed four separate trials. Each subject was randomly assigned to exercise and placebo, amino acid and exercise, amino acids alone, and placebo alone. The amino acid supplement of 1,500 mg of arginine and lysine was consumed immediately before exercise. Concentrations of hGH were elevated at 30, 60, and 90 minutes during exercise, but no differences were noted between the exercise groups. At basal levels the acute secretion of hGH was increased after amino acid ingestion.

Prudent Recommendations

At present, research indicates that the supplementation of arginine, lysine, and ornithine does not have any effect on hGH levels or body composition. Combining the supplements with exercise does not increase hGH levels above what occurs during exercise itself.

The rapid proliferation of free amino acid supplements has made it possible to consume large amounts of single amino acids. This is not possible with protein foods or protein supplements since both contain a variety of amino acids. With the exception of the eosinophilia-myalgia syndrome (due to contaminated tryptophan), significant problems with the ingestion of single amino acids have not been reported. However, large intakes of some single amino acids may interfere with absorption, cause gastrointestinal distress, and lead to metabolic imbalances. It seems prudent to avoid a large intake of any single amino acid until its safety is determined.

ANDROSTENEDIONE

Claims

- Is a natural and legal anabolic steroid
- Increases muscle mass

Theoretical Basis as an Ergogenic Aid

Androstenedione is a precursor in one of the pathways to testosterone synthesis. *Figure 7.1* illustrates where androstenedione occurs in the biochemical pathway. Its proximity (one biochemical step away) from the desired end product is its biggest selling point. Although androstenedione is technically a steroid, presently it is unknown if oral doses of this supplement can significantly raise testosterone levels. The production of testosterone is only one of several paths that androstenedione can take. Most of these reactions are enzyme dependent and rely on complex feedback mechanisms that are not fully elucidated at this time.

FIGURE 7.1   Androstendione Pathway

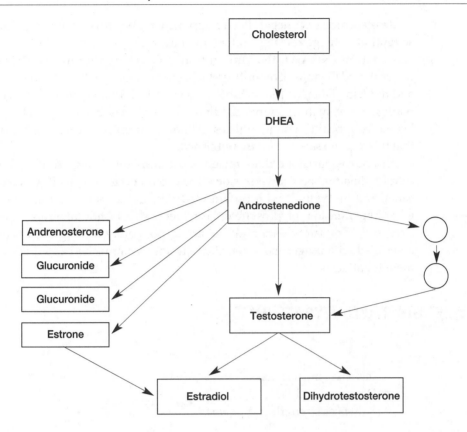

What Does the Research Show?

Androstenedione was synthesized in 1932. A study conducted in 1935 on castrated dogs revealed a mild anabolic effect (8). Androstenedione was virtually forgotten until 1962 when supplements of androstenedione and dehydroepiandrosterone (DHEA) were given to women (n=4) to see if they raised testosterone levels (9). Doses of 100 mg of both androstenedione and DHEA resulted in a transient increase in the women's testosterone levels, which lasted for several hours. Measurements of strength or athletic performance were not taken in the study.

King et al (10) evaluated the effects of androstenedione supplementation (300 mg/day) in untrained men during 8 weeks of resistance training. Serum testosterone and estrogen levels, muscle size and strength, serum lipids, and markers of liver function were measured before and during the study in the supplement (n=10) and placebo (n=10) groups. There were no differences in serum testosterone, muscle size and strength, or body composition between the androstenedione and placebo group. However, the androstenedione group had significant decreases in high-density lipoprotein cholesterol (HDL-C) and significant increases in serum estrogen levels, which may have adverse health consequences during long-term supplementation.

Prudent Recommendations

Androstenedione is a legal dietary supplement, but it is a banned substance by several athletic governing bodies, including the National Collegiate Athletic Association (NCAA), the United States Olympic Committee (USOC), the International Olympic Committee (IOC), the National Football Association (NFL), and the Association of Tennis Professionals (ATP). Several other sports-governing bodies are evaluating androstenedione use and may ban it also. This does not lessen its appeal to young athletes. Although supplement manufacturers claim that it is safe, no safety data are published.

If androstenedione does raise testosterone levels like an illegal anabolic steroid, then the same adverse side effects could occur. Pregnant women, adolescents, and individuals with certain medical conditions (eg, coronary heart disease, hypertension, or prostate enlargement) should not take this supplement. Due to lack of safety data and the strong possibility of long-term health risks associated with usage, androstenedione is not recommended as a dietary supplement for athletes.

BETA-HYDROXY-BETA-METHYLBUTYRATE (HMB)

Claims

- Increases muscle mass
- Decreases body fat
- Enhances strength and power

Theoretical Basis as an Ergogenic Aid

HMB, short for beta-hydroxy-beta-methylbutyrate, is a downstream metabolite of the branched-chain amino acid leucine. Nissen et al (11,12) suggest that HMB, rather than leucine, is responsible for the well-known anticatabolic actions of leucine. HMB may partially prevent exercise-induced proteolysis and/or muscle damage, thereby promoting greater gains in muscle mass and strength during a resistance-training program.

Nissen et al (11,12) hypothesize that HMB supplies a source of beta-hydroxy-beta-methylglutaryl CoA (HMG Co-A) for cholesterol synthesis by the muscle cell. They propose that muscle cells cannot use blood cholesterol effectively and need to manufacture it internally. In stressful conditions the muscle cells require greater cholesterol production for the synthesis of new cell membranes or to regenerate damaged membranes of existing cells. Thus, HMB may be important during periods of stress, such as the stress of resistance exercise, to promote increased muscle cell integrity and function. Further data are needed to support this theory and the exact mechanism behind HMB's proposed effectiveness depends on future research (11,12).

What Does the Research Show?

The claims of reduced muscle proteolysis and increased muscle size and strength are supported by only two studies (published together) by Nissen et al at Iowa State University (13). In the first study, 41 untrained male subjects (ages 19-29, average weight of 82.7 kg) were randomly divided into one of three groups receiving varying amounts of HMB—0 g (placebo), 1.5 g, or 3.0 g per day. The subjects also ingested one of two different amounts of protein: either a normal level of 117 g per day (1.4 g/kg) or a high level of 175 g per day (2.1 g/kg). The subjects lifted weights for an hour and a half, three times a week for 3 weeks.

While not statistically significant, the HMB-supplemented subjects tended to gain lean body mass in a dose-responsive manner—0.4 kg for the placebo group, 0.8 kg for the 1.5 g HMB group, and 1.2 kg for the 3.0 g HMB group. The level of protein intake did not influence body weight change or the amount of weight lifted for any of the exercises. However, the HMB-supplemented subjects lifted more weight than the placebo group during all 3 weeks. The combined HMB groups performed significantly more abdominal exercises (a 50% increase) compared to the placebo group (a 14% increase). Total strength (upper and lower body) increased significantly in both the 1.5 g HMB group (13%) and the 3.0 g HMB group (18.4%), compared to the placebo group (8%). HMB improved lower body strength and abdominal strength more than upper body strength (13).

HMB supplementation was also associated with decreased biochemical indicators of muscle damage. Urinary 3-methylhistidine (3-MH) decreased by 20% and serum levels of muscle creatine phosphokinase (CPK) and lactate dehydrogenase (LDH) fell by 20% to 60% (13).

A second study was conducted to determine whether HMB supplementation would promote changes in body composition and strength over a longer time period. The 32 male trained subjects (ages 19-22, average weight of 99.9 kg) were randomly divided into two groups receiving either no HMB (placebo) or 3.0 g of HMB per day. The subjects lifted weights for 2 to 3 hours daily, 6 days a week for 7 weeks. By day 14 and through day 39, the HM-supplemented subjects gained significantly more fat-free mass than the placebo group. On the last day of the study, fat-free mass was not significantly different between the groups. However, HMB supplementation significantly increased bench press strength by almost threefold (13).

Prudent Recommendations

Athletes who weight train should not consider HMB a magic bullet. The two studies were conducted by the same laboratory group that developed HMB. While these research results are interesting, they must still be considered preliminary.

The following points should be considered before utilizing HMB supplements:

- The results have not been reproduced by other researchers in other labs.
- The subjects in the first study by Nissen et al were untrained, so the results cannot be applied to trained individuals or elite athletes.

- Three weeks of HMB supplementation in untrained subjects did not significantly increase muscle mass compared to a placebo.
- Seven weeks of HMB supplementation in trained subjects did not increase muscle mass compared to a placebo.
- HMB is expensive—a 10-day supply costs about $35.

BRANCHED-CHAIN AMINO ACIDS (BCAA)

Claims

- Prevents fatigue
- Increases aerobic endurance

Theoretical Basis as an Ergogenic Aid

The central fatigue hypothesis suggests that the increase of the neurotransmitter serotonin (5-HT) during prolonged exercise contributes to fatigue and inhibits the ability to sustain work output. An increase in serotonin synthesis occurs when the brain receives elevated levels of blood-borne tryptophan, an amino acid precursor to serotonin. Increased 5-HT levels are associated with a feeling of fatigue and sleepiness.

Tryptophan (TRP) is normally bound to serum albumin, while unbound or free tryptophan (f-TRP) is transported across the blood-brain barrier. BCAA compete with and limit f-TRP entry into the brain. However, plasma BCAA levels decrease during endurance exercise because they are oxidized for energy by the muscles. The increase in plasma-free fatty acids during exercise also increases plasma f-TRP by displacing tryptophan from albumin. These high levels of plasma f-TRP combined with low levels of BCAA (a high free tryptophan/BCAA ratio) increase brain serotonin and cause fatigue during prolonged endurance exercise.

In theory, BCAA supplementation would compete with plasma f-TRP to cross the blood-brain barrier, decrease the f-TRP/BCAA ratio, and reduce central fatigue. Also, carbohydrate supplementation may lower plasma f-TRP by suppressing the rise in free fatty acids which compete with tryptophan for binding sites on albumin.

What Does the Research Show?

Madsen et al (14) examined the performance-enhancing effects of glucose, glucose plus BCAA, or a placebo on nine well-trained cyclists performing a 100-kilometer time trial. The subjects were encouraged to finish the 100-kilometer trial as quickly as possible while consuming a glucose, glucose plus BCAA, or a placebo mixture on three separate occasions. The results indicated that there was no difference in performance times in the three treatments.

Davis et al (15) evaluated the ingestion of a 6% carbohydrate-electrolyte drink, a 12% carbohydrate-electrolyte drink, and water placebo on prolonged cycling to fatigue at 70% of VO_2max. When subjects drank the water placebo, plasma f-TRP increased seven-fold. When subjects drank either the 6% or 12% carbohydrate-electrolyte drink, the increase in plasma f-TRP was greatly reduced and fatigue was delayed by approximately 1 hour.

Prudent Recommendations

Although there appears to be a logical theoretical basis to support BCAA as an ergogenic aid for endurance exercise, the available scientific data are limited and equivocal. Furthermore, the large amounts of BCAA required to make physiologically relevant changes in the plasma f-TRP/BCAA ratio can increase plasma ammonia, which may be toxic to the brain and impair muscle metabolism. Consuming large doses of BCAA during exercise can also slow water absorption from the gut and cause gastrointestinal disturbances (16).

Since BCAA supplements may not be safe or effective, and since it is easy to obtain sufficient quantities from food, BCAA supplements are not recommended at the present time (16).

Carbohydrate feedings, on the other hand, are associated with dramatic reductions in the plasma-free tryptophan/BCAA ratio. It is not possible to determine whether the benefits of carbohydrate feedings are due to decreased central fatigue in the brain or decreased peripheral fatigue in the exercising muscles. However, unlike BCAA supplementation, carbohydrate feedings during exercise can be recommended because their safety, performance, and cost benefits are well-established (16).

BORON

Claims

- Is a natural testosterone booster
- Increases muscle mass/weight gain
- Decreases fat mass

Theoretical Basis as an Ergogenic Aid

In 1987 Nielsen et al (17) evaluated the effect of supplemental boron, aluminum, and magnesium on major mineral metabolism in postmenopausal women. The results indicated that boron supplementation of 3 mg per day increased serum testosterone from 0.3 to 0.6 ng/dL in these subjects. Many supplement companies were quick to point out that increased testosterone levels are associated with increased muscle mass and decreased fat mass. The market was soon flooded with "testosterone booster" supplements containing boron.

What Does the Research Show?

Supplement companies used the Nielson data to launch boron-containing products claiming to be "natural" alternatives to anabolic steroids. However, these supplement companies failed to mention that the study was conducted on 12 postmenopausal women (ages ranging from 48 to 82 years), that estrodiol levels were also increased, and that body composition was never measured. Also, the level of normal male testosterone is approximately 10 times that observed in the Nielson study (17).

Green and Ferrando (18) looked at a more appropriate subject group to examine the ergogenic effects of boron in a double-blind study on 10 male bodybuilders. The subjects consumed 2.5 mg of boron per day or placebo and continued to train for a 7-week period. There was no increase in serum testosterone levels, one repetition max (squat and bench presses), or lean body mass. The researchers concluded that boron supplementation did not have an anabolic affect.

Prudent Recommendations

Boron is a nonessential trace mineral that is found in raisins, prunes, nuts, applesauce, and grape juice. There is no established Recommended Dietary Allowance (RDA) for boron, although some research indicates that humans need about 0.5 to 1.0 mg per day. Ten milligrams of boron per day appears to be safe, but more than 50 mg per day may be toxic. Toxicity symptoms include loss of appetite and gastrointestinal distress. While some research suggests that boron may play a modest role in bone mineral status, boron does not show promise as an ergogenic aid (19).

CAFFEINE

Claims

- Increases energy
- Increases fat loss
- Increases endurance

Theoretical Basis as an Ergogenic Aid

Caffeine has been used for hundreds of years. Although it is non-nutritive, caffeine is prevalent in the average diet. *Table 7.1* identifies the caffeine content of common foods and drugs. Many people equate caffeine with coffee, but chemically coffee consists of hundreds of constituents. Caffeine is metabolized in the liver to three dimethyxanthines (paraxanthine, theophylline, and theobromine).

TABLE 7.1 Caffeine Content of Common Foods and Drugs

Substance	Dose	Caffeine (mg)
NoDoz, Vivarin	1 tablet	200
Excedrin	2 tablets	130
Coffee, brewed	8 oz	135
Coffee, instant	8 oz	95
Snapple tea	16 oz	48
Lipton tea	8 oz	35-40
Mountain Dew	12 oz	55
Surge	12 oz	51
Coca-Cola	12 oz	45
Pepsi-Cola	12 oz	37
Java water	1/2 liter	125
Ben & Jerry's No Fat Coffee Fudge Frozen Yogurt	1 cup	85

Source: Schardt D, Schmidt S. Caffeine: the inside scoop. *Nutrition Action Health Letter*. 1996;23:1,4-7.

Three major theories have been proposed for the ergogenic effects of caffeine.

1. As a central nervous system stimulant, caffeine decreases the perception of fatigue.
2. Caffeine increases the force of muscle contractions by favorably influencing ion transport.
3. Caffeine increases fat utilization and so spares muscle glycogen (20).

Since caffeine enters the central nervous system and skeletal muscle, it is not possible to separate caffeine's central effects from its peripheral effects. It is also possible that different mechanisms are responsible for performance improvement in different exercise situations (20).

What Does the Research Show?

The interest in caffeine as an ergogenic aid was initiated by work from Costill's (21) laboratory over 30 years ago. In a 1978 study (21), nine competitive cyclists consumed 330 mg of caffeine (5 mg/kg) 1 hour prior to cycling at 80% of VO_2max and were able to ride 19% longer (90 minutes compared to 75 minutes) prior to reaching exhaustion. A second study in 1979 demonstrated that consuming 250 mg of caffeine was associated with a 20% increase in the amount of work that could be performed in 2 hours (22). These two studies suggest that the utilization of fat for energy increased by about 30% in the caffeine trials. A third study in 1980 found that consuming 5 mg of caffeine/kg reduced muscle glycogen usage by 42% and increased muscle triglyceride usage by 150% during 30 minutes of cycling at 70% of VO_2max (23).

Following these studies, there was limited well-controlled research on caffeine and exercise performance and the results were inconsistent. However, in the past 10 years an impressive body of research has established that caffeine can improve endurance performance (20).

In 1991 Graham and Spriet (24) evaluated the performance effects of caffeine in a study of competitive distance runners who were given 9 mg caffeine/kg 1 hour prior to cycling and running to exhaustion at intensities of about 85% VO$_2$max. The average increase in endurance for the running test was 44%; for the cycling test it was 51%. However, the urine caffeine levels in 4 of the 12 caffeine trials resulted in levels near or above the IOC threshold (24).

Graham and Spriet (25) conducted another study to examine different doses of caffeine on well-trained subjects. The eight subjects avoided caffeine for 48 hours and consumed 3 mg, 6 mg, or 9 mg of caffeine/kg or placebo 1 hour before exercise at 85% VO$_2$max. Endurance was increased in the 3- and 6-mg/kg doses but was not improved in the 9-mg/kg dose. Plasma epinephrine levels were not increased with the 3 mg dose but were elevated with the higher doses. Also, only the 9 mg dose showed an elevation in glycerol and free fatty acids. These data show that even the lowest dose of 3 mg/kg had an ergogenic effect without increasing epinephrine levels (25).

Prudent Recommendations

Graham and Spriet (20) suggest that the ingestion of 3 to 13 mg of caffeine/kg can improve endurance performance by 20% to 50% in elite and recreationally trained athletes who run or cycle at 80% to 90% of VO$_2$max. They indicate that caffeine dosages of 3 to 6 mg/kg an hour before exercise may produce an ergogenic effect without raising urinary caffeine levels above the IOC doping threshold (20).

Although higher doses of 9 to 13 mg of caffeine/kg may also improve performance, they are more likely to cause side effects and raise urinary caffeine levels above the IOC (12 mcg/dL) and NCAA (15 mcg/dL) doping threshold (20).

Although caffeine is relatively safe, side effects of high caffeine consumption include nausea, muscle tremors, palpitations, and headache. Athletes who are sensitive to caffeine can experience these symptoms at low doses.

Athletes should be aware that the reported ergogenic effect of some over-the-counter supplements might be a result of the caffeine content. Kola nut, mate, and guarana all contain caffeine.

CHROMIUM PICOLINATE

Claims

- Increases muscle mass
- Is a safe alternative to anabolic steroids
- Decreases body fat
- Increases insulin sensitivity

Theoretical Basis as an Ergogenic Aid

Chromium is part of the glucose tolerance factor, an essential cofactor that potentiates the actions of insulin in carbohydrate, lipid, and protein metabolism. Chromium augments the effects of insulin at target tissues and promotes glucose transport by "sensitizing" the body's tissues to insulin. Since insulin also regulates protein synthesis, chromium enhances protein synthesis by promoting amino acid uptake (19).

Picolinic acid is a natural derivative of the amino acid tryptophan and is thought to facilitate chromium absorption. The supposed "enhanced bioavailability" of chromium picolinate forms the basis for claims that it increases muscle mass and decreases body fat. In theory chromium picolinate (CrPl) increases insulin's anabolic properties, allowing more amino acids and glucose to enter cells and promote muscle growth.

What Does the Research Show?

The fat-burning and muscle-building claims for chromium picolinate are based on two studies cited in a review article by Evans (26). His subjects received 200 mcg of CrPl daily during 5 to 6 weeks of weightlifting. The chromium group in both studies had a small increase in lean body mass (1.6 to 2.6 kg) and either no change or decrease in percent body fat (3.6%) compared to the placebo group.

These two studies have been widely criticized. They never underwent peer review; body composition was measured with skinfolds (which is less sensitive to small changes in body composition than hydrostatic weighing); chromium intake prior to supplementation was not assessed; and diet and exercise were not controlled.

Clancy et al (27) examined CrPl supplementation on body composition, strength, and urinary chromium loss in football players. The subjects consumed 200 mcg of CrPl or placebo for a 9-week period during Spring training. The researchers found no significant changes between the treatment and control groups except that urinary chromium loss was five times higher in the CrPl group compared to placebo.

Research by the United States Department of Agriculture (USDA) also does not support the marketing claims made for CrPl (28,29). Hallmark et al (28) evaluated the effects of CrPl supplementation and weight training on muscle strength, body composition, and chromium excretion. Subjects received either 200 mcg of CrPl or a placebo for 12 weeks. The training consisted of weightlifting 3 days per week. The weight training program significantly increased the muscular strength of both groups. The subjects on CrPl had urinary chromium losses (attributed to the supplement) that were nine times greater than the placebo group. No significant changes in strength or body composition were observed between the CrPl and control groups.

Lukaski et al (29) examined the effects of chromium supplementation on body composition, muscle strength, and trace-element status. The subjects received either 200 mcg of chromium chloride, 200 mcg of CrPl, or a placebo for 8 weeks. The training consisted of weightlifting 5 days per week. Chromium supplementation increased serum chromium concentration and urinary chromium excretion. No differences were noted between the chemical forms of chromium. Transferrin saturation decreased more with CrPl supplementation (24%) than with chromium chloride (10%) or placebo (13%). No significant differences were observed among groups in strength or body composition.

Prudent Recommendations

Since exercise increases urinary chromium excretion, athletes should consider the adequacy of their chromium intake. Oral supplementation at the National Research Council-estimated safe and adequate dietary intake level (50 to 200 mcg) appears to be quite safe. However, the amount of chromium obtained from a varied diet should be sufficient to meet the needs of most athletes, since small amounts of chromium are found in almost all foods. Chromium is found in large amounts in whole grains, nuts, molasses, asparagus, brewer's yeast, cheese, mushrooms, and beer (19).

In November 1996, the Federal Trade Commission (FTC) ordered three of the largest distributors of CrPl to cease making unsubstantiated weight loss and health claims about their product (30). The FTC's complaint included charges that supplement companies were unable to support numerous claims (eg, reduced body fat, increased muscle mass, and increased energy) made for the supplement. The FTC also maintained that the companies falsely claimed that chromium picolinate's benefits are proven by scientific studies.

CREATINE

Claims

- Increases energy for high-power activities
- Increases muscle mass

Theoretical Basis as an Ergogenic Aid

Creatine (Cr), or methylguanidine-acetic acid, is an amine comprised of three amino acids (glycine, arginine, and methionine). Creatine phosphate (CrP) and adenosine triphosphate (ATP) supply most of the energy for short-term, maximal exercise (31).

The average creatine content of skeletal muscle is 125 mmol/kg dry muscle and ranges from about 90 to 160 mmol/kg dry muscle. Approximately 60% of muscle creatine is in the form of CrP. The creatine moiety of CrP may be obtained from dietary creatine (found primarily in meat products) or synthesized from the amino acids glycine and arginine. Muscle creatine is replenished at the rate of about 2 g per day, following its irreversible degradation to creatinine (31). *Figures 7.2* and *7.3* illustrate the fate of normal and supplemental creatine intake on liver synthesis of exogenous creatine, muscle stores of creatine, and renal excretion of creatine.

CrP availability is important for performance during brief, high-power exercise because the depletion of CrP prevents ATP from being resynthesized at the rate required. The theory of Cr as an ergogenic aid lies in the ability of CrP to rephosphorylate adenosine diphosphate (ADP) to regenerate ATP during anaerobic metabolism. Creatine supplementation is used in an effort to increase speed and power derived from the ATP-CrP energy system (31).

FIGURE 7.2   Fate of Normal Creatine Intake

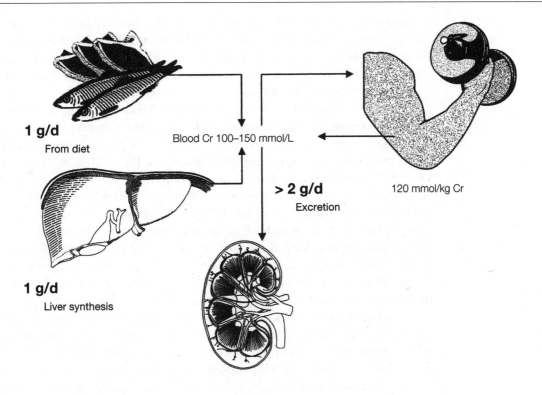

1 g/d
From diet

Blood Cr 100–150 mmol/L

120 mmol/kg Cr

> 2 g/d
Excretion

1 g/d
Liver synthesis

FIGURE 7.3   Fate of Supplemental Dietary Creatine Intake

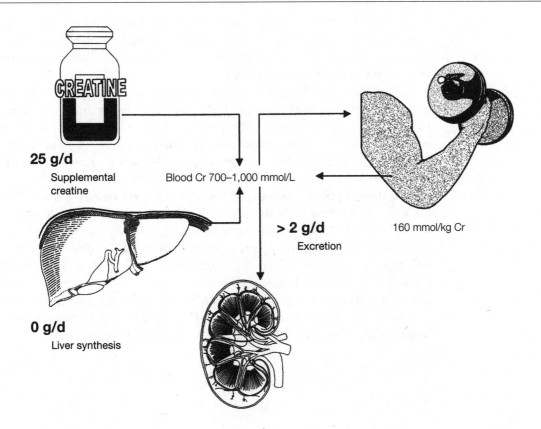

CREATINE

25 g/d
Supplemental
creatine

Blood Cr 700–1,000 mmol/L

160 mmol/kg Cr

> 2 g/d
Excretion

0 g/d
Liver synthesis

What Does the Research Show?

Greenhaff (31) has noted that ingesting 20 to 25 g per day of creatine monohydrate (four to five doses of 5 g) for 5 to 7 days can produce a 20% increase in muscle creatine levels, of which about 20% is CrP. After this loading dose, a maintenance dose of 2 to 5 g per day should maintain elevated creatine levels.

Numerous studies have been conducted examining the effect of Cr supplementation on athletic performance. Volek et al (32) recently investigated the effect of creatine supplementation on muscular performance during repeated sets of high-intensity resistance exercise. The creatine and placebo group performed bench press and jump squat exercise protocols on three different occasions (T1, T2, and T3) separated by 6 days. Before T1, both groups received no supplementation. From T1 to T2, both groups took a placebo. From T2 to T3, the creatine group consumed 25 g (five doses of 5 g) of creatine per day and the placebo group remained on the placebo. Creatine supplementation significantly increased peak power output during all five sets of jump squats and significantly improved the number of repetitions performed during all five sets of bench presses. The investigators concluded that resistance-training athletes might benefit from creatine supplementation by enabling the athlete to train harder.

Additional research has supported the ergogenic effect of creatine for different types of high-power exercise. Creatine supplementation has been associated with increases in strength during resistance exercise in sedentary females (33) and division IA football players (34), maximal power output increases during sprints on a treadmill (35), enhancement of both single and repeated short sprint performance (36), and increased cycling to exhaustion during repeated high-intensity intermittent exercise (37).

However, not all of the research on creatine has found positive results. In some studies creatine supplementation has exhibited no or minimal ergogenic effects on strength and sprint performance. Creatine also does not appear to be effective for endurance exercise (38).

Engelhardt et al (39) examined the effects of creatine supplementation on the performance of regional class triathletes. After receiving 20 g of creatine or a placebo for 5 days, the athletes were tested on endurance performance (30-minute cycle) and intervals (15 seconds of cycling with 45 seconds rest). The results indicated that creatine supplementation significantly increased power performance by 18% but did not influence endurance performance.

Creatine supplementation also seems to increase fat-free mass (FFM). The question still remains: Is the increase in FFM due to increased protein synthesis or to fluid retention? Most studies have indicated an increase in total body mass of 0.7 to 1.6 kg following short-term supplementation (38). Kreider et al (34) examined total body weight compared to total body water in division IA football players over a 28-day period of supplementation versus a control group. The creatine group increased total body mass by an average of 2.42 kg with no significant increase in total body water. More research is needed to determine the effects of creatine supplementation on protein synthesis and fluid retention.

Prudent Recommendations

Many anecdotal reports have claimed that creatine supplementation has been involved in increased incidences of muscle cramps, muscle pulls, tendon pulls, muscular injuries, and delayed recovery from injury. However, none of the studies evaluating highly trained athletes during heavy training periods has reported these side effects (38).

While there is also concern that creatine supplementation may place added stress on the kidneys or liver, this has not been reported in healthy individuals at the doses studied. Currently, the only documented side effect of creatine is increased total body weight (38).

There is no long-term safety data on creatine. The NCAA Committee on Competitive Safeguards and Medical Aspects of Sports has urged that research be done to determine whether long-term use is safe and whether certain individuals might be predisposed to negative side effects.

The current dosage recommendations are to complete a loading phase of 20 to 25 g per day for 5 to 7 days, then a maintenance phase of 5 g per day. While there has been no documentation for the need to cycle on and off creatine, the wash out period for muscular creatine levels to return to normal appears to be about 4 weeks (40).

CONJUGATED LINOLEIC ACID (CLA)

Claims

- Increases lean mass
- Decreases fat mass
- Is a powerful antioxidant

Theoretical Basis as an Ergogenic Aid

CLAs are naturally occurring fatty acids found predominately in beef, lamb, and dairy products. CLA is a true isomer of linoleic acid, an essential fatty acid, with double bonds occurring at carbons 10 and 12 or carbons 9 and 11. Researchers hypothesize that because CLA can be incorporated into cell membranes, it may affect cellular hormonal responses that may inhibit catabolic hormones, thereby creating or maintaining an anabolic state (41).

What Does the Research Show?

Most research using CLA has been conducted in animal models. Miller et al (42) fed CLA to chicks, rats, and mice before injecting them with an endotoxin to induce weight loss and reduce protein synthesis. Following endotoxin injection, the animals that received CLA maintained their body weight or regained body weight more rapidly than the animals not fed CLA. The CLA feeding also promoted increased nitrogen retention and increased albumin levels in these animals. These results suggest that CLA has a protein-sparing effect on muscle (43).

A recent abstract reports that novice male bodybuilders who consumed 7.2 g of CLA per day and exercised for 6 weeks, gained more muscle mass (as measured by skinfolds and bioelectrical impedance) than bodybuilders who received a placebo (44). The researchers concluded that CLA acts as a mild anabolic agent.

Data from another unpublished study discussed in *Environmental Nutrition* (45) reported that Norwegian subjects who took 1.8 g of CLA for 3 months had a 20% reduction in their body fat compared to a placebo group.

Mice fed CLA exhibited 57% and 60% less body fat accumulation and a 5% and 14% increase in lean muscle mass relative to controls (46). The researchers concluded that CLA's effect on body composition appears to be due to reduced fat deposition and increased lipolysis in adipocytes, possibly coupled with enhanced fatty acid oxidation. This study provides a possible mechanism of action for CLA's influence on body fat.

Prudent Recommendations

No adverse reactions to CLA supplementation have been reported. However, the majority of the research has been conducted on animals. The use of CLA as an ergogenic aid warrants further well-controlled research on humans.

DEHYDROEPIANDROSTERONE (DHEA)

Claims

- Increases energy and libido
- Decreases body fat
- Improves mood
- Counteracts stress-releasing hormones

Theoretical Basis as an Ergogenic Aid

DHEA has been called the "youth hormone" and the "mother of all steroids" in popular magazines. DHEA is available over-the-counter but was a prescription drug until the passage of DSHEA of 1994.

DHEA and its precursor dehydroepiandrosterone-3-sulfate (DHEAS) are the most widely circulating steroid hormones in adult males and females. DHEA was isolated as an androgenic steroid in 1934 and DHEAS was isolated from urine in 1944. Research has shown that circulating levels of DHEAS reach maximal levels between 20 to 30 years of age and decrease about 20% for every decade of life (47).

Researchers speculate that some diseases associated with age, such as obesity, diabetes, certain cancers, and heart disease, may be linked to the age-associated decline of DHEA and DHEAS. Although the physiological roles of DHEA and DHEAS are poorly understood, it is recognized that DHEA is a metabolic precursor to testosterone and estradiol. As a precursor to androgenic steroids, promoters claim DHEA supplementation will increase testosterone production, improve sex drive, increase lean body mass, and slow the aging process.

What Does the Research Show?

The antiobesity affect of DHEA supplementation in lower mammals seems to be well documented, but the mechanism of action is as yet undetermined. One theory is that a decline in DHEA levels correlates with an increase in insulin resistance. Clore (48) examined the effect of DHEA supplementation on insulin sensitivity and body composition. In a randomized, double-blind placebo-controlled study, 10 nonobese volunteers were administered 1,600 mg per day of DHEA or placebo for 28 days. The results indicated no significant differences in insulin sensitivity or changes in body fat (48). The age of the subjects was not reported and may be a limitation of the study.

Morales et al (49) examined the hypothesis that the age-related decline in DHEA and DHEAS promotes a shift from an anabolic state in young adults to a catabolic state in older adults. They gave 50 mg of DHEA replacement therapy to 13 men and 17 women 40 to 70 years of age for 6 months. DHEA levels increased in both genders to levels of young adults within 2 weeks in the supplemented group. Serum levels of androgens (androstenedione, testosterone, and dihydrotestosterone) were increased in women with only a small rise in androstenedione in men.

Insulin sensitivity and body fat were unaltered in both groups. There was, however, an increased perception of physical and psychological well-being with no reported change in libido. The researchers did notice an increase in insulin-like-growth-factor-I (IGF-I), a hormone that declines during catabolic states. The increase in IGF-I and the perception of well-being and apparent absence of side effects suggest that DHEA shows promise as a therapy for older adults (49).

Morales et al (50) recently examined a higher dose of DHEA for a longer period on age-advanced men and women. Nine men and 10 women, 50 to 65 years of age, volunteered for a double-blind crossover study that consisted of oral administration of 100 mg of DHEA for 6 months. Sixteen subjects completed the 12-month study. The researchers examined plasma hormone levels, body fat (using dual energy x-ray absorptiometry), and muscular strength (50). The results indicated that DHEA and DHEAS concentrations increased in both men and women.

Serum levels of androstenedione, testosterone, and dihydrotestosterone increased only in the older women to levels of younger women. As in the previous study, IGF-I levels increased in both men and women. Body fat, knee muscle strength, and lumbar back strength increased in men but not women. The researchers concluded that the benefit of DHEA administration may be gender-specific in favor of men. However, estrogen replacement therapy may have been a confounding factor in the female subjects (50).

Prudent Recommendations

Although DHEA is being sold as a safe alternative to illegal anabolic hormones, it is, in fact, an androgenic steroid. Adverse reactions associated with DHEA use can include acne, liver enlargement, unwanted hair growth, irritability, prostate hypertrophy, and masculinizing effects in females. Due to the potential effect on testosterone levels, the USOC, NCAA, and NFL have banned the use of DHEA.

Indiscriminate use of DHEA by young adult athletes is of particular concern, since the hormone's long-term safety has not been established. As with other hormones, adverse effects due to DHEA administration may not appear for years. Individuals who have a family history of breast or prostate cancer should not take DHEA.

Athletes should completely disregard claims that wild yam (Dioscoria) supplements provide the "building blocks" for DHEA. While Dioscoria does contain a plant sterol ring called diosgenin, which is a processor for the semisynthetic production of DHEA and other steroid hormones, this conversion takes place only in the laboratory. The claim that Mexican yam supplements increase the body's production of DHEA (or testosterone) is a complete scam (51).

EPHEDRA/MA HUANG

Claims

- Improves athletic performance
- Promotes weight loss

Theoretical Basis as an Ergogenic Aid

Ephedra, or Ma Huang, is an herb that has been used in Chinese medicine for nearly 5,000 years. Historically, ephedra was used as a nasal decongestant, a central nervous system stimulant, and a treatment for bronchial asthma (51). Its active ingredients are ephedrine and pseudoephedrine. These two ingredients are commonly found in decongestants and cold medications. Ephedra is considered a sympathomimetic agent—it mimics hormones such as epinephrine and norepinephrine that stimulate the central nervous system (52).

In theory, ephedra could enhance athletic performance by increasing cardiac output, enlarging bronchial airways, enhancing muscle contractility, and (possibly) increasing blood glucose during exercise (52).

What Does the Research Show?

White et al (53) recently examined the effect of Ma Huang on heart rate and blood pressure responses in normotensive adults. Twelve volunteers were examined in two phases. In phase one, participants underwent ambulatory blood pressure monitoring every 15 minutes between 7 AM and 8 PM. In phase two, blood pressure was monitored for the same time, but participants ingested 375 mg of Ma Huang with a light breakfast and with their evening meal.

Results revealed that four of the participants experienced a nonsignificant rise in systolic blood pressure 3 hours after ingesting Ma Huang. Six participants had a significant increase in heart rate (from about 72 to 81 beats per minute) 3 hours after ingesting Ma Huang. The rise in systolic blood pressure and increase in heart rate were not accompanied by clinical symptoms. The authors concluded that while ingestion of Ma Haung in normotensive adults is fairly safe in the short term, combining this powerful stimulant with other stimulants such as caffeine could magnify heart rate and blood pressure responses (53).

A recent study by Ramsey et al (54) examined the combination of ephedrine and caffeine on the body composition of rhesus monkeys. Twelve monkeys were separated into lean and obese groups. The monkeys were tested during a 7-week control period, an 8-week drug treatment phase, and a 7-week placebo phase. The monkeys received 6 mg of ephedrine and 50 mg of caffeine three times per day. Food intake was monitored during all phases of the study and energy expenditure was calculated from oxygen consumption. The results indicated that the ephedrine plus caffeine treatment decreased fat mass in both lean and obese rhesus monkeys. In the lean monkeys, this was primarily due to an increase in resting energy expenditure. The loss of fat mass in the obese monkeys was attributed to increased resting energy expenditure and decreased food intake (54).

Prudent Recommendations

There is no substantial evidence that ephedra improves athletic performance. Although some research indicates that ephedra may help promote weight loss, there are safety concerns. According to the FDA, since 1993 at least 17 people have died and 800 made ill by dietary supplements containing ephedrine. Adverse reactions to ephedrine include high blood pressure, heart rate irregularities, insomnia, nervousness, tremors, headaches, seizures, heart attacks, strokes, and death (55).

The FDA recommends a maximum daily ephedrine dose of 24 mg, that supplements contain no more than 8 mg of ephedrine or related alkaloids per serving, and that ephedrine be used for no longer than 1 week. The FDA also recommends that ephedrine-containing products carry a warning label indicating that taking more than the recommended dose may cause heart attack, stroke, seizure, or death. Combining ephedrine-containing products with caffeine greatly increases the adverse effects (55).

There are also doping concerns. Athletes and active people may not realize that ephedrine or other stimulants are in herbal products because an unfamiliar name for the stimulant is used. At the very least, the unwitting use of such herbal products by an elite athlete may result in a doping suspension. Ephedrine is banned by the IOC and NCAA.

GLUCOSAMINE/CHONDROITIN SULFATE

Claims

- Cures osteoarthritis
- Protects against joint destruction
- Heals tendons, ligaments, and cartilage

Theoretical Basis as an Ergogenic Aid

Glucosamine, an amino sugar synthesized by the body, plays a major role in the maintenance and repair of cartilage. It is thought that glucosamine stimulates cartilage cells to synthesize the glycosaminoglycans and proteoglycans that are the building blocks of cartilage. Glucosamine has also been reported to have anti-inflammatory properties by inhibiting the activity of proteolytic enzymes that contribute to cartilage breakdown. Chondroitin is also naturally present in cartilage and composed of repeating units of glucosamine with attached sugar molecules (56).

In theory the dietary supplements glucosamine and chondroitin sulfate work together to rebuild damaged cartilage and halt the progression of osteoarthritis. The interest in glucosamine and chondroitin has been stimulated by books, *The Arthritis Cure* and *Maximizing the Arthritis Cure*, by Jason Theodosakis, MD.

What Does the Research Show?

Interest in glucosamine's potential as an arthritis treatment was initiated in the early 1980s when a number of controlled human studies were conducted in Europe and Asia. Although these studies were small and short-term, many patients reported relief from pain and ease of movement after taking 1.5 g of glucosamine in divided doses daily (57).

A study to compare the validity of using glucosamine as a substitute for ibuprofen (a nonsteriodal anti-inflammatory drug) was conducted on 40 patients with unilateral osteoarthritis of the knee. Patients were given either 1.5 g of glucosamine sulfate or 1.2 g of ibuprofin over a period of 8 weeks. During the first 2 weeks the ibuprofen group reported less pain, but the effects began to taper off in the following 6 weeks. The glucosamine sulfate group reported progressive improvement throughout the study. The authors reported that the differences in the two treatments were not statistically significant and that longer studies were warranted (58).

Further research is required to determine if glucosamine can provide long-term symptomatic benefits. There is also the important and unanswered question of whether glucosamine can stop or retard the process of cartilage deterioration and stimulate cartilage growth (56).

The research studies on glucosamine indicate that the supplement is most effective for early or less severe arthritis and less helpful for severe or late arthritis. Apparently, glucosamine cannot influence the repair of cartilage when there is insufficient (or no) cartilage on joints (56). There is no evidence that glucosamine interferes with the action of anti-inflammatory or analgesic medications. Preliminary animal research suggests that glucosamine may even protect against the long-term, catabolic effects induced by some anti-inflammatory drugs (57).

Prudent Recommendations

Most of the published research on these compounds is short-term. Arthritis is a chronic disease with periods of remission. Long-term, double-blind controlled studies are required to determine the benefits and safety of glucosamine and chondroitin sulfate. They certainly cannot be considered the "cure" for arthritis (59). The Arthritis Foundation encourages people who want to use these supplements to become fully educated about their potential positive and negative effects. In addition, the Arthritis Foundation encourages people to consult with their physician on how to incorporate these supplements into their treatment plan (59).

Above all, the Arthritis Foundation recommends that proven therapies and arthritis-management techniques not be abandoned in favor of supplements. Treatments that are proven to reduce arthritis pain and help disease management include weight control, exercise, appropriate medication(s), joint protection, the use of heat or cold, and (if necessary) surgery (59).

The Arthritis Foundation also notes that some animal studies indicate that glucosamine increases blood sugar levels. Thus, people with diabetes who take glucosamine (an amino sugar) should plan to have their blood sugar levels measured more often. Chondroitin is molecularly quite similar to the blood thinner heparin. Caution is warranted before taking chondroitin when an individual is already taking blood-thinning medications or a daily aspirin (59).

GLUTAMINE

Claims

- Increases immune function
- Prevents overtraining syndrome

Theoretical Basis as an Ergogenic Aid

Glutamine is the most abundant amino acid in human plasma and muscle. Skeletal muscle synthesizes, stores, and releases glutamine at a high rate. Glutamine is a precursor to the synthesis of proteins, a nitrogen donor for the synthesis of nucleotides, a nitrogen transporter between various tissues, and a substrate for the production of urea. Glutamine also serves as the major fuel source for gut enterocytes and the cells of the immune system (60).

Glutamine appears to be conditionally essential during times of metabolic stress and critical illness. Skeletal and plasma glutamine levels are lowered by infection, surgery, trauma, acidosis, and burns. Prolonged endurance exercise, such as the marathon, may also reduce plasma glutamine concentration. Furthermore, plasma glutamine concentrations have been found to be significantly decreased in overtrained athletes compared to control athletes not regarded as being overtrained (19).

Since glutamine is critical for optimal functioning of the immune system, a decreased plasma glutamine concentration may impair immune function and increase the risk of infection. In theory glutamine supplementation may enhance immune function, decrease the risk of infection, and help to prevent the overtraining syndrome.

What Does the Research Show?

The benefits of glutamine supplementation for hospital patients during periods of major physiological stress are well established. Oral or parenteral glutamine supplementation after major trauma or surgery has helped to maintain muscular glutamine concentration, improve nitrogen balance, increase protein synthesis, decrease 3-methylhistidine excretion (a marker of muscle catabolism), prevent intestinal atrophy, improve weight gain, and decrease length of stay (60).

However, the benefits of glutamine supplementation for athletes during periods of heavy training are not well established. Castell et al (61) investigated the effects of feeding glutamine to middle-distance, marathon, and ultra-marathon runners, and to elite rowers during training and competition. The researchers provided a drink containing either glutamine (72 subjects) or a placebo (79 subjects) to athletes immediately after heavy exercise and 2 hours after exhaustive exercise. The athletes completed questionnaires about the incidence of infections during the 7 days following the exercise. The percentage of athletes reporting no infections was significantly higher in the glutamine-supplemented group (81%) than in the placebo group (49%). The incidence of infection was lowest in middle-distance runners and highest in runners after a full or ultra-marathon and in elite rowers after intensive training.

In a later study, however, Castell et al (62) reported that glutamine supplementation did not appear to have an effect on immune function (as assessed by lymphocyte distribution) following completion of the Brussels marathon.

Rohde et al (63) examined glutamine supplementation and repeated exercise on immune cells in a randomized crossover, placebo-controlled study. Eight subjects cycled for 30, 45, and 60 minutes at 75% of VO_2max and rested for 2 hours between exercise sessions. Although plasma glutamine levels were maintained in the glutamine-supplemented group and depressed in the placebo group, the number of lymphocytes and phytohemagglutinin-stimulated lymphocytes declined 2 hours after each bout of exercise in both groups. Thus, the postexercise immune changes did not appear to be caused by decreased plasma glutamine concentrations (63).

Prudent Recommendations

Plasma glutamine concentration may fall after periods of intense training that result in muscle glycogen depletion. However, an adequate daily intake of carbohydrate and energy may help to prevent muscle glycogen depletion and overtraining, as well as help to maintain normal glutamine status. While some preliminary research suggests that glutamine supplementation may reduce the incidence of respiratory infections in athletes, further research is required to provide supporting data (19).

GLYCEROL

Claims

- Enhances aerobic power
- Enhances endurance performance
- Improves thermoregulation

Theoretical Basis as an Ergogenic Aid

Glycerol is a clear, syrupy, sweet liquid that is rapidly absorbed into the body and evenly distributed throughout body fluids. It acts as a sponge, attracting and holding water. Glycerol may increase the volume of fluid between and within cells, thus maintaining plasma volume and reducing the increase in body temperature associated with exercise. An alternative theory is that glycerol affects antidiuretic hormone (ADH) and stimulates the kidneys to reabsorb more water and excrete less water (64).

Glycerol hyperhydration may have an ergogenic effect by reducing heat stress. In theory glycerol hyperhydration prior to endurance exercise would improve performance by increasing plasma volume, decreasing heart rate, and reducing core temperature (64).

What Does the Research Show?

In one of the first glycerol studies, Lyons et al (65) found that glycerol hyperhydration was more effective than water hyperhydration in reducing the thermal stress of moderate exercise in the heat. The subjects consumed either 1 g of glycerol per kilogram along with 21.4 mL of water per kilogram (glycerol trial) or 21.4 mL of water per kilogram (water trial). Two and a half hours after fluid ingestion, the subjects exercised on a treadmill at 60% of VO$_2$max in dry heat (42°C) for 2 hours. The urine volume prior to exercise was decreased in the glycerol trial compared to the water trial, indicating a glycerol-induced hyperhydration. During exercise in the heat, the glycerol trial caused an elevated sweat rate and lowered body temperature compared to the water trial.

In a later, double-blind, crossover study, Montner et al (66) evaluated the effect of glycerol hyperhydration and carbohydrate oral replacement solution (ORS) on thermoregulation and endurance performance. In the first part of the study, the subjects consumed either 1.2 g of glycerol per kilogram along with 26 mL of water per kilogram (glycerol trial) or 26 mL of water per kilogram (water trial) before exercise. The subjects cycled on 2 separate days at 65% of VO$_2$max in a neutral laboratory environment. Glycerol hyperhydration was associated with a significantly longer endurance time (93.8 minutes) and lower heart rate (2.8 beats per minute) compared to water hyperhydration (77.4 minutes).

In the second part of the study, both water and glycerol hyperhydration regimens were followed by ORS every 20 minutes during exercise (3 mL per kilogram of a 5% dextrose solution). Glycerol hyperhydration with ORS was associated with a significantly longer endurance time (123.4 minutes) and lower heart rate (4.4 beats per minute) compared to water hyperhydration with ORS (99.3 minutes). The study indicated that pre-exercise glycerol hyperhydration lowered heart rate and improved endurance even when combined with ORS. The authors speculated that an increased stroke volume and expanded plasma volume were responsible for the benefits associated with glycerol hyperhydration.

Not all studies have found a benefit from glycerol hyperhydration. Latzka et al (67,68) from the U.S. Army Research Institute of Environmental Medicine evaluated the effect of euhydration, water hyperhydration, and glycerol hyperhydration on sweat rate and core temperature during exercise. Their first study applied compensable exercise-induced heat stress—a condition under which the body's thermoregulatory system can maintain a steady-state core temperature (67). The second study utilized uncompensable exercise-induced heat stress, in which the subjects experienced a steady rise in core temperature until exhaustion (68). To produce this effect, the subjects wore full chemical protective suits while exercising. Both studies used the same subjects: 8 fit, heat-acclimated males, exercising on a treadmill in a controlled environment at 35°C.

One hour before exercise in both studies, the subjects consumed either 1.2 g of glycerol/kg per lean body mass along with 29.1 mL of water/kg per lean body mass (glycerol trial) or 29.1 mL of water/kg per lean body mass (water trial). Compared with euhydration, hyperhydration did not alter core temperature, skin temperature, sweat rate, or heart rate. Further, no difference was noted between the glycerol trial and the water trial for these physiological responses, suggesting that glycerol hyperhydration was no more effective than water hyperhydration or euhydration. Thus, while glycerol supplementation did promote hyperhydration, it did not confer any cardiovascular or thermoregulatory benefits for the athletes (67,68).

Prudent Recommendations

The research supporting the effectiveness of glycerol as an ergogenic aid is equivocal. While glycerol ingestion may benefit athletes who participate in endurance sports under hot, humid conditions, the amount of fluid recommended to be taken with glycerol may leave the athlete feeling heavy and bloated (64).

Glycerol supplementation may produce side effects in the form of bloating, nausea, vomiting, headaches, and dizziness. Glycerol should not be used by anyone who has diabetes, high blood pressure, or kidney disorders due to serious health concerns (69).

L-CARNITINE

Claims

- Increases use of fatty acids as fuel
- Decreases body fat
- Increases endurance

Theoretical Basis as an Ergogenic Aid

L-carnitine is synthesized in the body from the amino acids lysine and methionine and is found in animal foods (particularly meat and dairy products) and, to a much lesser extent, plant foods. It is a short-chained carboxylic acid and contains nitrogen. About 90% of the body's supply of carnitine is located in muscle tissues (70). In theory, supplementation of L-carnitine would increase fatty acid oxidation by facilitating the transport of long-chain fatty acids into the mitochondria. L-carnitine may also facilitate the oxidation of pyruvate, which would enhance glucose utilization and reduce lactic acid production during exercise (19).

What Does the Research Show?

The results of studies on L-carnitine supplementation do not support an ergogenic effect (19). Trappe et al (71) evaluated the effect of L-carnitine supplementation on swimmers to determine whether L-carnitine would improve performance by reducing lactic acid accumulation. The subjects were 20 male college varsity swimmers who had been training for 16 weeks prior to the study.

The subjects completed five repeat 100-yard swims, with a 2-minute recovery between intervals, before and after 1 week of L-carnitine supplementation. The supplement group received a 236 mL citrus drink containing 4 g of L-carnitine in the morning and afternoon. The placebo group received the same amount of the citrus drink without L-carnitine. There were no differences between the supplement group and the placebo group with regard to lactic acid, blood pH, or swim velocity in the final swim interval, indicating that L-carnitine did not improve performance (71).

Greig et al (72) examined L-carnitine supplementation and its effect on maximum and submaximum exercise capacity. In two separate trials, two groups of untrained subjects received either 2 g of L-carnitine a day or a placebo for 2 weeks. Exercise capacity was assessed using continuous progressive cycle ergometry. There was a small improvement in submaximal performance at 50% of VO$_2$max in the L-carnitine trial. However, heart rate was not significantly lower at any exercise intensity during the maximal exercise test in the L-carnitine trial. The researchers concluded that L-carnitine supplementation was of little or no benefit to exercise performance.

Prudent Recommendations

The studies on L-carnitine supplementation have largely produced results showing no ergogenic benefits, though further research is warranted. While L-carnitine appears to be a safe supplement, there is a concern that L-carnitine supplements may be adulterated and contain D-carnitine. D-carnitine may be toxic, as it can deplete L-carnitine and lead to a carnitine deficiency (19).

MEDIUM-CHAIN TRIGLYCERIDES (MCTs)

Claims

- Increases energy
- Prolongs endurance
- Spares muscle glycogen
- Decreases body fat

Theoretical Basis as an Ergogenic Aid

Medium-chain triglycerides (MCTs) are 6-12 carbon compounds that yield 8 kcal/g. MCTs are water soluble and readily absorbed into the hepatic system via the portal vein. They have been used in clinical applications for many years to treat fat malabsorption, defects in lipid absorption due to major intestinal resection, and defective lipid transport (73).

It is generally accepted that an increased oxidation of free fatty acids decreases muscle glycogen utilization. Since MCTs are oxidized as quickly as glucose, they could theoretically enhance performance by sparing muscle glycogen during exercise (73). Based on this theory, manufacturers claim that MCTs increase energy, enhance endurance, decrease body fat, and increase lean tissue (19).

What Does the Research Show?

Jeukendrup et al (74) evaluated the oxidation rate of oral MCT feedings in eight well-trained athletes during four different 3-hour bouts of exercise at 50% of maximal work rate. The subjects consumed either carbohydrate (CHO), MCTs, a combination of CHO + MCTs, or placebo. During the second hour of exercise, 72% of the MCTs ingested in the CHO + MCTs trial were oxidized. By comparison only 33% of the MCTs ingested in the MCTs trial were oxidized during the same time period. Thus, the MCTs were oxidized at a higher rate when combined with CHO. Furthermore, the amount of MCTs that could be tolerated by the gastrointestinal tract was small (30 g), which further limited the contribution of MCTs to the total energy expenditure.

In a later study, Jeukendrup et al (75) investigated whether increasing the amount of MCTs from 30 to 85 g would enhance fat oxidation and improve performance during 60% of maximal work rate for 2 hours. The subjects consumed either CHO, MCTs, a combination of CHO + MCTs, or a placebo. The CHO and CHO + MCT feedings had no effect on performance or fat metabolism. When the subjects received only MCTs, performance was decreased compared to the placebo trial. The negative effect of the MCTs was attributed to gastrointestinal (GI) distress.

Van Zyl et al (76) evaluated the effect of MCT + CHO feedings on fat oxidation and performance during 2-hour exercise bouts at 60% of maximal work rate plus a 40-kilometer time trial. Endurance-trained cyclists consumed a CHO + MCT formulation containing 86 g of MCT. The MCT feeding was associated with a small increase in fat oxidation and improved time trial performance, suggesting a glycogen-sparing effect. The subjects did not report any GI distress.

Prudent Recommendations

Although one study (76) indicates that CHO + MCT feedings may improve endurance performance lasting 2 hours or more, more research is needed to replicate these findings. The majority of research does not support an ergogenic effect for MCTs. Even if MCTs do improve performance, the fact that large amounts cause GI distress limits their potential usefulness as an ergogenic aid.

An obvious concern with fat supplementation, even MCTs, is the possibility of an increased risk for cardiovascular disease. Investigators have found that supplementing a normal diet with MCTs had an LDL cholesterol-raising effect similar to that observed with palm oil (77).

OMEGA-3 FATTY ACIDS

Claims

- Increases endurance
- Increases muscle mass

Theoretical Basis as an Ergogenic Aid

Omega-3 fatty acids are 18 carbon fatty acids that cannot be made by the body and are therefore essential nutrients. Linolenic acid is the primary omega-3 fatty acid. The body can manufacture two other omega-3 fatty acids from linolenic acid —eicosapentaenoic acid (EPA) and docosahexaenoic acid (DHA). The primary dietary sources of omega-3 fatty acids are fish (eg, mackerel, tuna, salmon, anchovy, herring, trout, sardines), oils (eg, canola, soybean, walnut, wheat germ), and nuts and seeds (eg, butternuts, walnuts, soybeans).

One theory is that omega-3 fatty acids may be incorporated into the membrane of red blood cells (RBC), making the RBC less viscous and less resistant to flow. Another theory is that omega-3 fatty acids increase the synthesis of the eicosanoids prostaglandin E1 and prostaglandin I2, which promote vasodilation of the blood vessels and may stimulate the release of human growth hormone. The less viscous blood and vasodilation would, in theory, enhance blood flow and benefit the endurance athlete by facilitating the delivery of blood and oxygen to the muscles during exercise. The increased secretion of growth hormone would, in theory, benefit the strength athlete by promoting muscle growth and hastening recovery from intense bouts of resistance training (19).

What Does the Research Show?

The research regarding omega-3 fatty acids and performance is limited. A study conducted in 1990 by Brilla and Landerholm (78) examined the effects of fish oil supplementation and exercise on serum lipids and aerobic fitness. The subjects, 32 previously sedentary males, were divided into the following groups: control, supplement, supplement + exercise, and exercise. The supplemented subjects received 4 g of fish oil per day. The exercise groups engaged in aerobic exercise for 1 hour per day, 3 days per week. After 10 weeks no significant differences were noted between groups for blood lipid values, percent body fat, or dietary composition. Aerobic exercise, with or without fish oil supplements, increased VO$_2$max. Fish oil supplementation, with or without exercise, did not affect blood lipid values or VO$_2$max (78).

Prudent Recommendations

The ergogenic effect of omega-3 fatty acids is not supported by current literature. Potential hazards of fish oil supplements include increased bleeding tendencies (nosebleeds and easy bruising) and impaired immune function. Fish oil supplements may increase the anticoagulant effect of prescription or over-the-counter anticoagulants such as Coumadin, aspirin, or ibuprofen and may be ill-advised for individuals who take these medications. Also, they may dangerously increase the clotting of the blood when combined with dietary supplements such as vitamin E and ginkgo biloba (79).

Other undesirable effects are a fishy breath odor and gastrointestinal upset. Some preparations lack vitamin E, so there is concern for oxidation. Long-term consumption of some products (eg, cod liver oil) may place people at risk for vitamin A and D toxicity. Also, like MCTs, all fish oil supplements provide additional fat calories (79).

PYRUVATE AND DIHYDROXYACETONE

Claims

- Increases aerobic endurance
- Decreases fat mass
- Increases metabolic rate

Theoretical Basis as an Ergogenic Aid

Pyruvate (P) and dihydroxyacetone (DHA) are 3 carbon compounds produced in glycolysis during normal carbohydrate metabolism. Research data suggest that they improve performance by increasing blood glucose utilization, thus sparing muscle glycogen (80).

What Does the Research Show?

The claim of improved endurance is supported by only two studies by Stanko et al (81) using untrained male subjects. The first study evaluated the effects of 7 days of P and DHA supplementation on arm ergometry exercise to exhaustion at 60% of VO$_2$max (81). The 10 subjects consumed diets that provided 35 calories/kg (55% carbohydrate, 15% protein, and 30% fat) and either 100 g of polycose (placebo) or 75 g DHA and 25 g P (triose treatment) substituted for a portion of the carbohydrate. Arm endurance was significantly improved by 20% (160 minutes) for the triose-supplemented group compared to the placebo group (133 minutes).

The triose group had greater pre-exercise triceps glycogen stores (130 mmol/kg) compared to the placebo group (88 mmol/kg). It was also noted that arteriovenous glucose was greater before and 60 minutes after exercise began. The authors suggested that P and DHA supplementation increased arm muscle glucose extraction, thereby enhancing endurance capacity.

The second study (82) evaluated the effects of 7 days of a P and DHA supplementation diet on leg cycle exercise to exhaustion at 70% of VO_2max. The eight subjects consumed diets that provided 35 calories/kg (70% carbohydrate, 18% protein, and 12% fat) and either 100 g of polycose (placebo) or 75 g DHA and 25 g P (triose treatment) substituted for a portion of the carbohydrate. Leg endurance was significantly improved by 20% (79 minutes) for the triose-supplemented group compared to the placebo group (66 minutes). Muscle glycogen at rest and exhaustion did not differ between the treatment and placebo groups. The authors noted that P and DHA supplementation, in conjunction with a high-carbohydrate diet, increased leg muscle glucose extraction, thereby enhancing endurance capacity.

Stanko et al (83,84) have also conducted several studies to evaluate the effect of P and DHA supplementation in conjunction with hypocaloric feedings for 21 days regarding weight loss and body composition in obese women in a metabolic ward. In one study (83), 13 subjects consumed either a 500-calorie placebo diet (60% carbohydrate, 40% protein) or a 500-calorie treatment diet (a 28-g mixture of P and DHA was isocalorically substituted for glucose). The triose-treated subjects lost 16% (0.9 kg) more body weight and 18% (0.8 kg) more body fat than the placebo group.

In another study (84), 14 subjects consumed a 1,000-calorie placebo diet (68% carbohydrate, 22% protein, 10% fat) or a 1,000-calorie treatment diet (22 g of P was isocalorically substituted for glucose) for 21 days. The P-supplemented subjects lost 37% (1.6 kg) more body weight and 48% (1.3 kg) more fat than the placebo group.

Prudent Recommendations

The research supporting the claims of increased fat loss and increased endurance is preliminary. The exercise studies appear valid, as an appropriate experimental design (randomized, crossover, placebo-controlled, double-blind) was utilized; however, Sukala (85,86) has noted that the following points regarding these studies should be considered before pyruvate supplements are recommended to improve performance.

- The results have not been reproduced by other researchers in other labs.
- The subjects were untrained, so the results cannot be applied to trained individuals or elite athletes.
- The triose-supplemented subjects experienced side effects in the form of intestinal gas, flatus, and diarrhea.
- Performance benefits were observed with 75 g DHA and 25 g P, but commercial pyruvate preparations contain only 500 mg to 1 g of pyruvate and may not contain DHA.

- The Dietary Supplement and Health Education Act of 1994 allows products to be marketed without proof of safety, efficacy, or potency, so there is no guarantee of consistent dosage.

The weight loss studies suggest that substitution of P and DHA for glucose in a hypocaloric diet will increase weight and fat loss. However, Sukala (85,86) has noted that the following points should be considered before pyruvate supplements are recommended for weight loss.

- Can the results be reproduced?
- The subjects were obese and completely sedentary, so the results cannot be applied to lean, active population.
- The population at large does not live on a metabolic ward and subsist on a hypocaloric diet providing 500 to 1,000 calories.
- The differences in body weight loss and fat loss were statistically significant, but such a small change (about 1.0 to 1.5 kg) is physiologically insignificant and difficult to measure accurately.
- Weight loss was observed with a 28-g triose mixture and with 22-g pyruvate, but commercial pyruvate preparations contain minuscule doses and the potency of the preparation is questionable.

VANADIUM (VANADYL SULFATE)

Claims

- Increases lean mass
- Decreases fat mass and increases vascularity
- Increases muscle fullness and produces a "pumped up" feeling
- Promotes anabolic effects similar to insulin
- Increases glycogen synthesis and storage

Theoretical Basis as an Ergogenic Aid

Vanadium is a trace mineral present in nature and the human body. Research with animals suggests that vanadium is important in enzymatic reactions (including carbohydrate and lipid metabolism) and cellular function in the human body (19). Although vanadium is not considered an essential nutrient, the normal human diet provides 12 to 28 µg per day.

Vanadium exists in several forms, but vanadate and vanadyl are the most common with vanadyl sulfate (VS) being the most common form sold as a dietary supplement. Vanadium compounds have been reported to have insulin-mimicking effects on protein and glucose metabolism (87). In theory vanadium would benefit the strength athlete by inducing an anabolic effect on muscle similar to insulin (19). The mechanism by which vanadium enhances insulin action remains unclear.

What Does the Research Show?

The research on vanadium compounds largely revolves around the treatment of diabetes. Sakurai et al (88) looked at the effect of VS injections on rats with streptozotocin (STZ)-induced type 1 diabetes. The results indicated that VS normalized the blood glucose levels of rats with STZ-induced type 1 diabetes. Rats with STZ-induced type 1 diabetes that were supplemented with VS also have shown reduction in the frequency of secondary conditions, like cataracts, when compared to nonsupplemented rats (89). These results suggest that VS seems to have an insulin-mimetic action in rat muscle.

Human studies on persons with type 2 diabetes have revealed results similar to the animal studies. Cohen et al (90) examined blood glucose control in six type 2 diabetic subjects during a 7-week period. In the first 2 weeks the subjects received a placebo, followed by 3 weeks of supplementation with 100 mg VS, followed by another 2 weeks of placebo. There was no change in blood glucose control during the first 2 weeks (placebo). During the 3-week treatment phase with VS, there was a significant increase in blood glucose control. After the last 2-week placebo period, the beneficial effects of VS supplementation seemed to be sustained. Researchers concluded that the decreased fasting blood glucose and glycated hemoglobin values were a result of improved hepatic and peripheral insulin sensitivity.

Fawcett et al (91) examined body composition and performance in weight-training athletes in a 12-week double-blind, placebo-controlled trial. The subjects (30 males and 10 females between the ages of 19 and 39) were given either a placebo or VS supplement of 0.5 mg/kg per day. This was the dosage recommended by the manufacturer to maximize muscle strength and mass. Body composition was measured by DXA (dual x-ray absorptiometry). Performance was measured by 1 rep max and 10 repetitions on both the bench press and leg extensions. The VS supplement did not have an anabolic effect on muscle mass. Although the 1 rep max for the leg extension did increase modestly in the treatment group at the fourth week, the authors indicated that the VS group started at a lower baseline than the control group. The VS supplement seemed to be well tolerated, but 20% of the supplemented individuals complained of a subjective feeling of tiredness after exercise.

Prudent Recommendations

Vanadyl sulfate use is normally well tolerated, but there have been reports of transient diarrhea, abdominal cramps, and nausea in type 2 diabetic subjects (92). There is also a concern about the cumulative effect of supplementing with VS over time. Research has shown an accumulation of vanadium in the testes and spleen of rats (93). Although VS does show promise as a treatment for diabetes, it shows little promise as an ergogenic aid.

WHEY PROTEIN

Claims

- High biological value
- Greater nitrogen retention
- Greater muscular gains

Theoretical Basis as an Ergogenic Aid

Whey protein is a by-product of the manufacture of cheese. It has been a disposal problem for the dairy industry and is a typical ingredient in low-cost commodity protein powders (94).

Recent marketing claims of the high biological value of whey, as well as the profit to be made from this waste product, have led to the spray drying of whey protein for use in commercial protein powders. In theory whey protein increases nitrogen retention, thus promoting a positive nitrogen balance.

What Does the Research Show?

Advertisements for the benefits of whey protein are aimed at active individuals and athletes. However, the data on whey protein formulas (WPF) are largely derived from studies on animals and low-birth-weight infants.

One particular study has been used to promote the benefits of whey protein and is featured by advertisers in most print ads (95). These ads have indicated that WPF were proven to increase weight gain compared to other dietary treatments. However, the advertisers fail to mention that the experimental subjects were starved rats given WPF or a free amino acid mixture. The starved rats that were fed the WPF regained their lost weight faster than the starved rats that were fed the free amino acid mixture (95). Increased nitrogen retention has also been seen in thermally injured animals that received either a WPF or free amino acid mixture (96).

Whey protein has also been studied in low-birth-weight infants. Both casein and whey proteins have been shown to adequately nourish very-low-birth-weight infants, but the whey protein may aid in preventing metabolic acidosis (97).

An interesting and promising benefit of whey protein is its apparent ability to increase glutathione levels. Glutathione, an antioxidant, may have an important role in immune function. Bounous et al (98) fed mice a whey or casein diet and measured glutathione levels. The whey protein diet increased glutathione levels in the mice compared to the casein diet. This may have occurred due to the high cysteine content of whey protein, as cysteine is part of the tripeptide that makes up glutathione.

In a later study, Bounous et al (99) investigated the effect of whey protein on glutathione levels and body weight in HIV-seropositive individuals. The subjects were given adequate calories and the majority of protein was provided by intact whey protein. The results showed an increase in both body weight and glutathione levels (99).

Prudent Recommendations

Although whey protein may enhance immune function by increasing glutathione levels, it does not appear to increase muscle mass in athletes. Athletes who want to gain muscle mass should continue to follow those strategies that have been demonstrated to increase lean tissue. In short, the athlete should consume sufficient calories and protein and engage in a resistance-training program.

WORKING WITH ATHLETES

Discussing supplements with athletes is not easy. In many cases the health professional is concerned about safety and cost, while the athlete is concerned with immediate athletic success. If the product is ineffective but safe, the health professional should consider working with the athlete to find a way to use the product on a trial basis. This helps to improve the health professional's credibility with the athlete (100).

Butterfield (101) recommends four tactics when discussing supplement use with athletes:

1. Gain an understanding of the athlete's motives and beliefs. Determine what sources influence the athlete (eg, coaches, popular sports magazines, celebrity endorsements) and realize that athletes usually care about short-term benefits, while health professionals care about long-term risks.
2. Assess the athlete's knowledge. Discussing sound nutrition practices and supplements demonstrates concern in helping athletes to reach their goals—with or without supplements.
3. Evaluate the overall diet. By definition, a supplement is a substance to augment the diet. Supplements alone will not enable athletes to reach their goals; rather, supplements must be used as part of a sound nutrition and training program.
4. Promote healthful dietary practices as the cornerstone to improved athletic performance. Give the athlete positive feedback for the sound nutrition practices she or he already follows. Educate athletes about healthy dietary practices—from choosing healthier fast foods to optimizing fluid intake.

Note: Some of the material contained in this chapter was previously published in *SCAN's Pulse* (Skinner R. Medium chain triglycerides and conjugated linoleic acid. 1999;18:10-13) and *SCAN's Guide to Nutrition and Fitness Resources* (Sarubin A, Skinner R. Ergogenic aids: reported facts and claims. Winter;1998:14-22). Used with permission.

REFERENCES

1. Applegate EA, Grivetti LE. Search for the competitive edge: a history of dietary fads and supplements. *J Nutr.* 1997;127:S869-S873.
2. National Strength and Conditioning Association. Use of dietary supplements in sports training. *Bulletin.* 1998;19:1.

3. Kurtzweil P. An FDA guide to dietary supplements. *FDA Consumer Magazine.* September-October 1998. http://www.fda.gov/fdac/features/1998/598_guid.html. Accessed December 13, 1998.

4. Hawes K. Athletes buying trouble with dietary supplements. *NCAA News: News & Features.* http://www.ncaa.org/news/19980511/active/3519n03.html. Accessed January 6, 1999.

5. Fogelholm GM, Naveri HK, Kiilavuori KT, Harkonen MH. Low-dose amino acid supplementation: no effects on serum human growth hormone and insulin in male weightlifters. *Int J Sport Nutr.* 1993;3:290-297.

6. Corpas E, Blackman MR, Roberson R, Scholfield D, Harman SM. Oral arginine-lysine does not increase growth hormone or insulin-like growth factor-I in old men. *J Gerontol.* 1993;48:128-133.

7. Suminski RR, Robertson RJ, Goss FL, et al. Acute effect of amino acid ingestion and resistance exercise on plasma growth hormone concentration in young men. *Int J Sport Nutr.* 1997;7:48-60.

8. Kochakian CD, Murlin JR. The relationship of synthetic male hormone androstene-dione to the protein and energy metabolism of castrated dogs and the protein metabolism of a normal dog. *Am J Physiol.* 1936;117:642-657.

9. Mahesh VB, Geenblatt RB. The in-vivo conversion of dehydroepiandrosterone and androstenedione to testosterone in humans. *Acta Endocrinol.* 1962;41:400-406.

10. King DS, Sharp RL, Vukovich MD, et al. Androstenedione on serum testosterone and adaptations to resistance training in young men. *JAMA.* 1999;281:2020-2028.

11. Nissen SL, Abumrad NN. Nutritional role of the leucine metabolite beta-hydroxy-beta methylbutyrate (HMB). *J Nutr Biochem.* 1997;8:300-311.

12. Nissen S, Fuller J Jr, Rathmacher J, Baier S. HMB (Beta-hydroxy beta-methylbu-tyrate) supplementation and exercise. *SCAN's Pulse.* 1998;17:1-3.

13. Nissen SL, Sharp R, Ray M, et al. Effect of leucine metabolite beta-hydroxy-beta-methylbutyrate on muscle metabolism during resistance-exercise training. *J Appl Physiol.* 1996;81:2095-2104.

14. Madsen K, Maclean DA, Kiens B, Christensen D. Effects of glucose, glucose plus branched-chain amino acids, or placebo on bike performance over 100 km. *J Appl Physiol.* 1996;18:2644-2650.

15. Davis JM, Bailey SP, Woods JA, Galiano FJ, Hamilton M, Bartoli WP. Effects of car-bohydrate feedings on plasma free tryptophan and branched-chain amino acids during prolonged cycling. *Eur J Appl Physiol.* 1992;65:513-519.

16. Davis JM. Carbohydrates, branched-chain amino acids, and endurance: the central fatigue hypothesis. *Int J Sport Nutr.* 1995;5(suppl):S29-S38.

17. Nielsen FH, Hunt CD, Mullen LM, Hunt JR. Effect of dietary boron on mineral, estrogen, and testosterone metabolism in postmenopausal women. *FASEB J.* 1987;1:394-397.

18. Green NR, Ferrando AA. Plasma boron and the effects of boron supplementation in males. *Environ Health Perspect.* 1994;102:73-77.

19. Williams MH. *Nutrition for Health, Fitness and Sport.* 5th ed. Dubuque, Ia: WCB-McGraw Hill; 1999.

20. Graham TE, Spriet LL. Caffeine and exercise performance. *Sport Sci Exch.* 1996;9(1).

21. Costill DL, Dalsky GP, Fink WJ. Effects of caffeine ingestion on metabolism and exercise performance. *Med Sci Sport.* 1978;10:155-158.

22. Ivy JL, Costill DL, Fink WJ, Lower RW. Influence of caffeine and carbohydrate feed-ings on endurance performance. *Med Sci Sport.* 1979;11:6-11.

23. Essig D, Costill DL, VanHandel PJ. Effects of caffeine ingestion on utilization of muscle glycogen and lipid during leg ergometer cycling. *Int J Sports Med.* 1980;1:86-90.

24. Graham TE, Spriet LL. Performance and metabolic responses to a high caffeine dose during prolonged exercise. *J Appl Physiol.* 1991;71:2292-2298.

25. Graham TE, Spriet LL. Metabolic, catecholamine, and exercise performance responses to various doses of caffeine. *J Appl Physiol.* 1995;78:8750-8787.

26. Evans GW. The effect of chromium picolinate on insulin-controlled parameters in humans. *Int J Biosocial Med Res.* 1989;11:163-180.

27. Clancy SP, Clarkson PM, DeCheke ME, et al. Effects of chromium picolinate supplementation on body composition, strength, and urinary chromium loss in football players. *Int J Sport Nutr.* 1994;4:142-153.

28. Hallmark MA, Reynolds TH, DeSouza CA, Dotson DO, Anderson RA, Rogers MA. Effects of chromium and resistive training on muscle strength and body composition. *Med Sci Sports Exerc.* 1996;28:139-144.

29. Lukaski HC, Bolonchuk WW, Siders WA, Milne DB. Chromium supplementation and resistance training: effects on body composition, strength, and trace element status of men. *Am J Clin Nutr.* 1996;63:954-965.

30. Federal Trade Commission. Companies advertising popular dietary supplement chromium picolinate can't substantiate weight loss and health claims, says FTC. November 7, 1996. http://www.ftc.gov. Accessed April 26, 1998.

31. Greenhaff PL. Creatine and its application as an ergogenic aid. *Int J Sports Nutr.* 1995;5(suppl):S100-S110.

32. Volek JS, Kraemer WJ, Bush JA, et al. Creatine supplementation enhances muscular performance during high-intensity resistance exercise. *J Am Diet Assoc.* 1997;97:765-770.

33. Vandenberghe K, Goris M, Van Hecke P, Van Leemputte M, Vangerven L, Hespel P. Long-term creatine intake is beneficial to muscle performance during resistance training. *J Appl Physiol.* 1997;83:2055-2066.

34. Kreider RB, Ferreira M, Wilson M, et al. Effects of creatine supplementation on body composition, strength, and sprint performance. *Med Sci Sports Exerc.* 1998;30:73-82.

35. Bosco C, Tihanyi J, Pucspk J, et al. Effect of oral creatine supplementation on jumping and running performance. *Int J Sports Med.* 1997;18:369-372.

36. Dawson B, Cutler M, Moody A, Lawrence S, Goodman C, Randall N. Effects of oral creatine loading on single and repeated maximal short sprints. *Aust J Sci Med Sport.* 1995;27:56-61.

37. Prevost MC, Nelson AG, Morris GS. Creatine supplementation enhances intermittent work performance. *Res Q Exerc Sport.* 1997;68:233-240.

38. Kreider RB. Creatine supplementation: analysis of ergogenic value, medical safety, and concerns. *J Exerc Physiol.* 1998;1:1-12.

39. Engelhardt M, Neumann G, Berbalk A, Reuter I. Creatine supplementation in endurance sports. *Med Sci Sports Exerc.* 1997;30:1123-1129.

40. Febbraio MA, Flanagan TR, Snow RJ, Zhao S, Carey MF. Effect of creatine supplementation on intramuscular TCr, metabolism and performance during intermittent, supramaximal exercise in humans. *Acta Physiol Scand.* 1995;155:387-395.

41. Burke ER. Nutritional ergogenic aids. In: Berning JR, Steen SN, eds. *Nutrition for Sport and Exercise.* 2nd ed. Gaithersburg, Md: Aspen Publishers; 1998:119-142.

42. Miller CC, Park Y, Pariza MW, Cook ME. Feeding conjugated linoleic acid to animals partially overcomes catabolic responses due to endotoxin injection. *Biochemical and Biophysical Communications.* 1994;198:1107-1112.

43. Furst P. New parenteral substrates in clinical nutrition Part II. *Eur J Clin Nutr.* 1994;48:681-691.

44. Lowery LM, Appiceili PA, Lemon PWL. Conjugated linoleic acid enhances muscle size and strength gains in novice bodybuilders [abstract]. *Med Sci Sports Exerc.* 1998;30:S182.

45. Ask EN. Conjugated linoleic acid supplements: cure-all or craze? *Environmental Nutr.* 1998;21:7.

46. Park Y, Albright KJ, Liu W, Storkson JM, Cook ME, Pariza MW. Effect of conjugated linoleic acid on body composition in mice. *Lipids.* 1997;32:853-858.

47. Labrie F, Belanger A, Simard J, Luu-the V, Labrie C. DHEA and peripheral androgen and estrogen formation: intracrinology. *Ann N Y Acad Sci.* 1995:774;16-28.

48. Clore J. Dehydroepiandrosterone and body fat. *Obes Res.* 1995:3;613-616.

49. Morales AJ, Nolan JJ, Nelson JC, Yen SS. Effects of replacement doses of dehydroepiandrosterone in men and women of advancing age. *J Clin Endocrinol Metab.* 1994:78;1360-1367.

50. Morales AJ, Haubrich RH, Hwang JY, Asakura H, Yen SS. The effect of six months treatment with 100 mg daily dose of dehydroepiandrosterone (DHEA) on circulating sex steroids, body composition and muscle strength in age-advanced men and women. *Clin Edocrinol.* 1998;49:421-432.

51. Foster S, Tyler VE. *Tyler's Honest Herbal.* 4th ed. Binghampton, NY: Haworth Herbal Press; 1999.

52. Williams MH. *The Ergogenics Edge.* Champaign, Ill: Human Kinetics; 1998.

53. White LM, Gardner SF, Gurley BJ, Marx MA, Wang PL, Estes M. Pharmacokinetics and cardiovascular effects of Ma Haung (ephedra sinica) in normotensive adults. *J Clin Pharmacol.* 1997;37:116-122.

54. Ramsey JJ, Colman RJ, Swick AG, Kemnitz JW. Energy expenditure, body composition, and glucose metabolism in lean and obese rhesus monkeys treated with ephedrine and caffeine. *Am J Clin Nutr.* 1998;68:42-51.

55. Food and Drug Administration Center for Food Safety and Applied Nutrition. FDA proposes safety measures for ephedrine dietary supplements. June 2, 1997. http://vm.cfsan.gov/~lrd/hhsephed.html. Accessed August 23, 1998.

56. Is there an arthritis cure? *Tufts University Health & Nutrition Letter.* April 1997;15:1.

57. Bucci LR. Glycosaminoglycans. In: Bucci LR, ed. *Nutrition Applied to Injury Rehabilitation and Sports Medicine.* Boca Raton, FL: CRC Press; 1994:177-203.

58. Vaz AL. Double-blind clinical evaluation of the relative efficacy of ibuprofen and glucosamine sulfate in the management of osteoarthritis of the knee in outpatients. *Curr Med Res Opin.* 1982;8:145-149.

59. The Arthritis Foundation. Glucosamine sulfate and chondroitin sulfate. http://www.arthritis.org/resource/statements/glucosamine.asp.html. Accessed June 14, 1998.

60. Lacey JM, Wilmore DW. Is glutamine a conditionally essential amino acid? *Nutr Rev.* 1990;48:297-309.

61. Castell LM, Poortmans JR, Newsholme EA. Does glutamine have a role in reducing infections in athletes? *Eur J Appl Physiol.* 1996;73:488-490.

62. Castell LM, Poortmans JR, Leclercq R, Brasseur M, Duchateau J, Newsholme EA. Some aspects of the acute phase response after a marathon race, and the effects of glutamine supplementation. *Eur J Appl Physiol.* 1997;75:47-53.

63. Rohde T, MacLean DA, Pedersen BK. Effect of glutamine supplementation on changes in the immune system induced by repeated exercise. *Med Sci Sports Exerc.* 1998;30:856-862.

64. Wagner DR. Hyperhydrating with glycerol: implications for athletic performance. *J Am Diet Assoc.* 1999;99:207-212.

65. Lyons TP, Reidesel ML, Meuli LE, Chick TW. Effects of glycerol-induced hyperhydration prior to exercise in the heat on sweating and core temperature. *Med Sci Sports Exerc.* 1990;22:477-483.

66. Montner P, Stark DM, Reidesel ML, et al. Pre-exercise glycerol hydration improves cycling endurance time. *Int J Sport Med.* 1996;17:27-33.

67. Latzka WA, Sawka MN, Montain SJ, et al. Hyperhydration: thermoregulatory effects during compensable exercise-heat stress. *J Appl Physiol.* 1997;83:860-866.

68. Latzka WA, Sawka MN, Montain SJ, et al. Hyperhydration: tolerance and cardiovascular effects during uncompensable heat-exercise stress. *J Appl Physiol.* 1998;84:1858-1864.

69. Murray R, Eddy DE, Paul GL, Seifert JG, Halaby GA. Physiological responses to glycerol ingestion during exercise. *J Appl Physiol*. 1991;71:144-149.

70. Broquist HP. Carnitine. In: Shils ME, Olson JA, Shike M, eds. *Modern Nutrition in Health and Disease*. 8th ed. Philadelphia, Penn: Lea & Febiger; 1994:459-465.

71. Trappe SW, Costill DL, Goodpaster B, Vukovich MD, Fink WJ. The effects of L-carnitine supplementation on performance during interval swimming. *Int J Sport Med*. 1994;15:181-185.

72. Grieg C, Finch KM, Jones DA, Cooper M, Sargeant AJ, Forte CA. The effect of oral supplementation with L-carnitine on maximum and submaximum exercise capacity. *Eur J Appl Physiol*. 1987;56:457-460.

73. Berning JR. The role of medium chain-triglycerides in exercise. *Int J Sport Nutr*. 1996;6:121-133.

74. Jeukendrup AE, Saris WHM, Schrauwen P, Brouns R, Wagenmakers AJM. Metabolic availability of medium-chain triglycerides coingested with carbohydrates during prolonged exercise. *J Appl Physiol*. 1995;79:736-762.

75. Jeukendrup AE, Thielen JHC, Wagenmakers AJM, Brouns F, Saris AE. Effect of medium-chain triglycerol and carbohydrate ingestion during exercise on substrate utilization and subsequent cycling performance. *Am J Clin Nutr*. 1998;67:397-404.

76. Van Zyl CG, Lambert EV, Hawley JA, Noakes TD, Dennis SC. Effects of medium-chain triglyceride ingestion on fuel metabolism and cycling performance. *J Appl Physiol*. 1996;80:2217-2225.

77. Carter NB, Heller HJ, Denke MA. Comparison of the effects of medium-chain triacyglyerols, palm oil, and high oleic acid sunflower oil on lipid and lipoprotein concentrations in humans. *Am J Cin Nutr*. 1997;65:41-45.

78. Brilla LR, Landerholm TE. Effect of fish oil supplementation and exercise on serum lipids and aerobic fitness. *J Sports Med Phys Fitness*. 1990;30:173-180.

79. Stone NJ. Fish consumption, fish oil, lipids, and coronary heart disease. *Circulation*. 1996;94:2337-2346.

80. Ivy J. Effect of pyruvate and dihydroxyacetone on metabolism and aerobic endurance capacity. *Med Sci Sports Exer*. 1998;30:837-843.

81. Stanko RT, Robertson RJ, Galbreath RW, Reilly JJ, Greenwalt KD, Goss FL. Enhancement of arm exercise endurance capacity with dihydroxyacetone and pyruvate. *J Appl Phys*. 1990;68:199-124.

82. Stanko RT, Robertson RJ, Spina RJ, Reilly JJ, Greenwalt KD, Goss FL. Enhanced leg exercise endurance with a high-carbohydrate diet and dihydroxyacetone and pyruvate. *J Appl Phys*. 1990;69:1651-1656.

83. Stanko R, Tietze D, Arch J. Body composition, energy utilization, and nitrogen metabolism with a severely restricted diet supplemented with dihydroxyacetone and pyruvate. *Am J Clin Nutr*. 1992;55:771-776.

84. Stanko R, Tietze D, Arch J. Body composition, energy utilization, and nitrogen metabolism with a 4.25 MJ/d low-energy diet supplemented with pyruvate. *Am J Clin Nutr*. 1992;56:630-635.

85. Sukala W. Pyruvate research: preliminary at best. *SCAN'S Pulse*. 1998;17:6-8.

86. Sukala W. Pyruvate: beyond the marketing hype. *Int J Sport Nutr*. 1998;8:241-249.

87. Crans D, Mahroof-Tahir M, Keramidas A. Vanadium chemistry and biochemistry of relevance for use of vanadium compounds as antidiabetic agents. *Molecular and Cellular Biochemistry*. 1995;153:17-24.

88. Sakurai H, Tsuchiya K, Nukatsuka M, Sofue M, Kawada J. Insulin-like effect of vanadyl ion on streptozotocin-induced diabetic rats. *J Endocrinol*. 1990;126:451-459.

89. Ramadadham S, Mongold J, Brownsey R, Cros G, McNeill J. Oral vanadyl sulfate in treatment of diabetes mellitus in rats. *Am J Physiol*. 1989;257:H904-H911.

90. Cohen N, Halberstam M, Shlimovich P, Chang C, Shamoon H, Rossetti L. Oral vanadyl sulfate improves hepatic and peripheral insulin sensitivity in patients with non-insulin-dependent diabetes mellitus. *J Clin Inves*. 1995;95:2501-2509.

91. Fawcett J, Farquhar S, Walker R, Thou T, Lowe G, Goulding A. The effect of oral vanadyl sulfate on body composition and performance in weight-training athletes. *Int J Sport Nutr*. 1996;6:382-390.

92. Boden G, Chen X, Ruiz J, Van Rossum G, Turco S. Effects of vanadyl sulfate on carbohydrate and lipid metabolism in patients with non-insulin-dependent diabetes mellitus. *Metabolism*. 1996;45:1130-1135.

93. Hamel F, Duckworth W. The relationship between insulin and vanadium metabolism in insulin target tissues. *Mol Cell Biochem*. 1995;153:95-102.

94. Smithers GW, Ballard FJ, Copeland AD, et al. New opportunities from the isolation and utilization of whey proteins. *J Dairy Sci*. 1996;79:1445-1459.

95. Poullain MG, Cezard JP, Roger L, Mendy F. Effect of whey proteins, their oligopeptide hydrolystas and free amino acid mixtures on growth and nitrogen retention in fed and starved rats. *JPEN J Parenter Enteral Nutr*. 1989;13:382-386.

96. Trocki O, Moxhizuki H, Dominioni L, Alexander JW. Intact protein versus free amino acids in the nutritional support of thermally injured animals. *JPEN J Parenter Enteral Nutr*. 1986;10:139-144.

97. Shenai JP, Dame MC, Churella HR, Reynolds JW, Babson SG. Nutritional balance studies in very low birth weight infants: role of whey formula. *J Gastroenterol Nutr*. 1986;5:428-433.

98. Bounous G, Batist G, Gold P. Immunoenhancing property of dietary whey protein in mice: role of glutathione. *Clin Invest Med*. 1989;12:154-161.

99. Bounous G, Baruchel S, Falutz J, et al. Whey proteins as a food supplement in HIV-seropositive individuals. *Clin Invest Med*. 1992;16:204-209.

100. Rosenbloom C, Storlie J. A nutritionist's guide to evaluating ergogenic aids. *SCAN's Pulse*. 1998;17:1-5.

101. Butterfield G. Ergogenic aids: evaluating sports nutrition products. *Int J Sport Nutr*. 1996;6:191-197.

SECTION 2 ASSESSMENT OF THE BODY'S RESPONSE TO PHYSICAL ACTIVITY

Assessment of nutritional status is a standard practice for sports nutrition professionals. Increasingly, athletes are requesting information on nutritional deficiency, body composition, and general physical fitness. Because of the availability of many techniques and formulas, the nutrition practitioner may find it difficult to select the most appropriate one for the individual being evaluated. This section provides an overview of medical, nutrition, physical fitness, and dietary assessment and offers guidance on the potential limitations and inherent advantages of assessment methods and techniques. Because computer-generated nutrition information has become a mainstay of many assessments, guidelines for selecting computer programs for diet, fitness, and body composition assessment are presented. This section closes with a thought-provoking discussion on documenting sports nutrition outcomes. While documenting outcomes is widely accepted in other health arenas, sports nutrition professionals need to be challenged to design and conduct outcome research that will provide the data needed to support the value of our services.

SECTION 2 CONTENTS

HEALTH SCREENING AND MEDICAL EVALUATION

Katherine A. Beals, PhD, RD and Melinda M. Manore, PhD, RD

Prior to beginning a fitness program, it is recommended that individuals undergo a health screening and, when appropriate, a complete medical evaluation. Health screening identifies medical risks and their nutritional relationships. Such identification of potential risks is the first step in planning an appropriate and safe exercise program and nutrition regimen. A complete medical assessment should include measurements that lead to a better understanding of general health, physical fitness, and nutritional status.

HEALTH SCREENING AND RISK STRATIFICATION

To optimize safety during exercise participation and to develop a sound and effective exercise prescription, an initial health screening is recommended (1). The purposes of a preparticipation health screening include the following (1):

- Identification and exclusion of individuals with medical contraindications to exercise
- Identification of individuals with disease symptoms and risk factors for disease development who should receive medical evaluation before starting an exercise program
- Identification of persons with clinically significant disease considerations who should participate in a medically supervised exercise program
- Identification of individuals with other special needs

The health screening procedure or tool utilized should be valid, cost-effective, and time-efficient (2). The procedure can range from a self-administered questionnaire to more sophisticated diagnostic tests (1). Two practical tools for health screening include the Physical Activity Readiness Questionnaire (PAR-Q) (3) and the American Heart Association (AHA)/American College of Sports Medicine (ACSM) Health/Fitness Facility Preparticipation Screening Questionnaire (2). The PAR-Q focuses primarily on symptoms that might suggest cardiovascular disease, although it is also useful in identifying musculoskeletal problems that should be evaluated before participation because they may require modification in the exercise program (2). The AHA/ACSM questionnaire is slightly more complex than the PAR-Q and uses history, symptoms, and risk factors (including age) to direct prospective exercise participants to either participate in an exercise program or contact their physician (or appropriate health care provider) prior to exercise participation (2).

Using information from the health screening and the guidelines and categories established by the ACSM, dietetics professionals can stratify clients according to health and/or risk status prior to beginning their exercise program. The ACSM risk categories or "strata" are outlined in *Table 8.1*. Additionally, the ACSM has published recommendations (see *Table 8.2*) for determining when a diagnostic medical examination and exercise test are appropriate and when physician coverage of exercise testing is recommended (1).

TABLE 8.1   Initial Risk Stratification

Apparently Healthy	Individuals who are asymptomatic and apparently healthy with no more than one of the following coronary risk factors:
	• Age (men >45 years; women >55 years or premature menopause without estrogen replacement therapy)
	• Family history of myocardial infarction (MI) or sudden death before 55 years of age in father or other male first-degree relative or before 65 years of age in mother or other female first-degree relative
	• Current cigarette smoking
	• Hypertension (blood pressure ≥140/90 mm Hg, confirmed by measurements on at least two separate occasions, or taking antihypertensive medication)
	• Hypercholesterolemia (total serum cholesterol >200 mg/dL or 5.2 mmol/L, or HDL <35 mg/dL or 0.9 mmol/L)
	• Diabetes mellitus (Persons with type 1 diabetes mellitus who are >30 years or who have had type 1 for >15 years and persons with type 2 diabetes mellitus who are >35 years should be classified as patients with known disease.)
	• Sedentary lifestyle/physical inactivity (25% of the population, as defined by the combination of sedentary jobs involving sitting for a large part of the day and no regular exercise or active recreation pursuits)
Increased Risk	Individuals who have signs or symptoms suggestive of possible cardiopulmonary (see *Box 8.1*) or metabolic disease and/or two or more coronary risk factors
Known Disease	Individuals with known cardiac, pulmonary, or metabolic disease

Source: American College of Sports Medicine. *Guidelines for Exercise Testing and Prescription.* Media, Penn: Williams and Wilkens; 1995. Reprinted with permission.

TABLE 8.2   ACSM Recommendations for (A) Medical Examination and Exercise Testing prior to Participation and (B) Physician Supervision of Exercise Tests

A. Medical examination and exercise test prior to participation recommended:

	Apparently Healthy		Increased Risk*		Known Disease[a]
	Younger[b]	Older	No Symptoms	Symptoms	
Moderate exercise[c]	No[d]	No	No	Yes	Yes
Vigorous exercise[e]	No	Yes[f]	Yes	Yes	Yes

B. Physician supervision of exercise test recommended:

	Apparently Healthy		Increased Risk*		Known Disease
	Younger[b]	Older	No Symptoms	Symptoms	
Submaximal testing	No[d]	No	No	Yes	Yes
Maximal testing	No	Yes[f]	Yes	Yes	Yes

*Persons with two or more risk factors or one or more signs or symptoms

[a] Persons with known cardiac, pulmonary, or metabolic disease

[b] Younger implies ≤40 years for men and ≤50 years for women.

[c] Moderate exercise is defined by intensity of 40% to 60% VO$_2$max. If intensity is uncertain, moderate exercise may alternately be defined as an intensity well within the individual's current capacity, one which can be comfortably sustained for a prolonged period of time (ie, 60 minutes) which has a gradual initiation and progression and is generally noncompetitive.

[d] A "no" response means that an item is deemed "not necessary." The "no" response does not mean that the item should not be done.

[e] Vigorous exercise is defined by an exercise intensity >60% VO$_2$max. If intensity is uncertain, vigorous exercise may alternately be defined as exercise intense enough to represent a substantial cardiorespiratory challenge or if it results in fatigue within 20 minutes.

[f] A "yes" response means that an item is recommended. For physician supervision this suggests that a physician is in close proximity and readily available should there be an emergent need.

Source: American College of Sports Medicine. *Guidelines for Exercise Testing and Prescription.* Media, Penn: Williams and Wilkens; 1995. Reprinted with permission.

MEDICAL EVALUATION

The extent to which medical evaluation is necessary prior to exercise participation largely depends on the assessment of risk as determined by the health screen and risk stratification (1). The medical evaluation may include any or all of the following: medical history, nutrition history, and physical exam, including an evaluation of general systems, blood pressure, blood lipids, and pulmonary function.

Medical History

The medical history should include both remote and recent past medical events and be sufficiently comprehensive to give the health professional a good understanding of the individual's risk of developing an illness. (See the sample medical history questionnaire in the Tools section.) The medical history should address the following areas (1):

- Medical diagnoses—cardiovascular disease including myocardial infarction, angioplasty, cardiac surgery, coronary artery disease, angina, and hypertension; pulmonary disease including asthma, emphysema, and bronchitis; cerebrovascular disease, including stroke; diabetes; peripheral vascular disease; anemia; phlebitis or emboli; cancer; pregnancy; osteoporosis; emotional disorders; eating disorders

- Previous physical examination findings—murmurs, clicks, other abnormal heart sounds, other unusual cardiac findings, abnormal blood lipids and lipoproteins, high blood pressure, or edema
- History of symptoms—discomfort (pressure, tingling, pain, heaviness, burning, numbness) in the chest, jaw, neck, or arms; lightheadedness, dizziness, or fainting; shortness of breath; rapid heart beats or palpitations, especially if associated with physical activity, eating a large meal, emotional upset, or exposure to cold (See *Box 8.1.*)
- Recent illnesses, hospitalizations, or surgical procedures
- Orthopedic problems—including arthritis, joint swelling, and any condition that would make ambulation or use of certain test modalities difficult
- Medication use and drug allergies
- Other habits—including caffeine, alcohol, tobacco, or recreational drug use
- Menstrual history—including age of menarche, typical cycle length, and any episodes of menstrual dysfunction (ie, amenorrhea, oligomenorrhea, annovulation, shortened luteal phase, etc)
- Exercise history—information on habitual level of activity including type, frequency, duration, and intensity of exercise
- Work history—with an emphasis on current or expected physical demands noting upper and lower extremity requirements
- Family history—of cardiac, pulmonary, or metabolic disease, stroke, or sudden death

---

BOX 8.1   Major Symptoms or Signs Suggestive of Cardiopulmonary Disease*

- Pain, discomfort (or other anginal equivalent) in the chest, neck, jaw, arms, or other areas that may be ischemic in nature
- Shortness of breath at rest or with mild exertion
- Dizziness or syncope
- Orthopnea or paroxysmal nocturnal dyspnea
- Ankle edema
- Palpitations or tachycardia
- Intermittent claudication
- Known heart murmur
- Unusual fatigue or shortness of breath with usual activities

---

* The symptoms must be interpreted in the clinical context in which they appear, since they are not all specific for cardiopulmonary or metabolic disease.

Source: American College of Sports Medicine. *Guidelines for Exercise Testing and Prescription.* Media, Penn: Williams and Wilkens; 1995. Reprinted with permission.

Diet History

In addition to a medical history, an in-depth assessment of the client's diet should be obtained. The diet history usually involves a one-on-one interview with the client to obtain current and past diet and activity information. This information can then be used to estimate energy intake and nutrient requirements

For the physically active individual, diet history data can be gathered through the medical (patient) chart, interview, or both. It is especially important that information be obtained on the type, duration, and intensity of activity the individual is, or will be, engaged in. This information will assist the health professional in assessing any dietary or nutrient issues relevant to a given activity. The following diet history interview format has been adapted for use with physically active individuals (4):

- Weight—current weight, usual weight, weight goal for sport, recent weight loss or gain, percent body fat, goal body fat, and frequency of dieting for weight loss
- Appetite/intake—appetite changes and factors affecting appetite/intake such as training routine, activity level, anorexia, stress, allergies, medications, chewing/swallowing problems (bulimia, oral health), and gastrointestinal problems (gastritis, laxative abuse, constipation)
- Eating patterns—typical patterns (weekdays/weekends); primary eating place (dorm, home, cafeteria, training table); primary food shopper at home; dietary restrictions (understanding of and compliance with these restrictions); frequency of eating out; effect of training, precompetition, competition, and travel on typical eating patterns; ethnicity of diet
- Food preferences/dietary practices—food likes and dislikes; any food restrictions due to dietary practices or beliefs (ie, vegetarianism, religious dietary practices, food allergies, food intolerances (eg, lactose intolerance)
- Estimation of typical energy and nutrient intake—standards include the 1989 Recommended Dietary Allowances (5), recommended macronutrient intakes for athletes (see section 1); the Dietary Reference Intakes (DRIs) (6,7), *Dietary Guidelines for Americans* (8), and the American Heart Association guidelines (9). Food intake information may be obtained from a 24-hour recall, food frequency questionnaire, and/or food diary.
- Psychosocial data—economic status, occupation, educational level, living/cooking arrangements, and mental status
- Medication and/or supplement use—current use of medications and supplements, including amounts and reason for use. Drug-nutrient or nutrient-nutrient interactions may necessitate special dietary consideration (10,11). Effect of medication on physical performance and eating habits.
- Other—age; gender; types of physical activity and amount (minutes per day, miles per week) engaged in during competition, training, and nontraining periods; fitness level (VO$_2$max; strength tests; and flexibility)

PHYSICAL EXAMINATION

The physical examination should be conducted by a properly licensed physician, nurse practitioner, or physician's assistant. Vital signs (ie, temperature, pulse rate and regularity, blood pressure, respiration), head-to-toe inspection, resting 12-lead electrocardiogram (ECG), stress test, heart sounds, anthropometric measurements, laboratory (biochemical) data, tests of neurological function (including reflexes), and physical fitness evaluation are all components of this examination (1,12). (A more in-depth description of physical fitness assessment, anthropometric assessment, and interpretation of biochemical data is provided in Chapter 10, Physical Fitness Assessment, and Chapter 11, Assessment of Body Size and Composition.)

The frequency with which an individual should have a physical examination depends on the individual's medical history, age, and physical condition. *Table 8.3* provides an outline of the recommended frequency of medical examinations provided by the National Conference on Preventive Medicine (12).

TABLE 8.3   Recommended Frequency of Medical Examinations

Age (years)	Frequency of Medical Examinations
0-1	At least four times
2, 5, 8, 15, 18, 25	At each age listed
35 to 65	Every 5 years
Over 65	Every 2 years

PREPARTICIPATION EXAMINATIONS FOR ATHLETES

Prior to participating in an organized sport at the high school or college level, athletes customarily undergo a physical examination. The specific objectives of the preparticipation sports examination (PSE) include (13-15):

- Determine the general health of the athlete.
- Detect any conditions that may limit participation or predispose the athlete to injury.
- Determine the athlete's physical fitness.
- Assess the athlete's physical maturity.
- Institute treatment that will help the athlete reach optimal performance.
- Counsel the athlete about health and personal issues.
- Meet legal and insurance requirements.

The PSE should be conducted 4 to 6 weeks prior to beginning the competitive season. This allows time to evaluate and treat problems identified during the physical examination and rehabilitate any residual injuries prior to the start of the season (14,15). The NCAA requires only one PSE at the athlete's initial entrance into a college athletic program (16). Other organizations recommend a comprehensive PSE any time the athlete enters a new "level" of participation (17). Most athletic programs require that athletes complete a yearly health history to identify any problems that may have developed since the initial PSE (15).

The PSE is generally conducted via one or a combination of the following methods: by the athlete's private physician in the office, by a physician as part of a mass "assembly line" examination, or by multiple examiners as part of a "station" examination. Which method or combination of methods to use depends on the specific objectives of the examination as well as the time and resources available (15). Graffe et al (15) and Hergenroeder (14) provide a detailed description of these methods and the indications for their use.

The components of the PSE are similar to those for the health screening and medical evaluation of the adult exercise participant outlined earlier in this chapter. The PSE should include an in-depth medical and diet history, with an additional focus on previously sustained sports-related injuries. For female athletes an in-depth menstrual history and assessment of current menstrual status are a necessity (13). In addition, all female athletes should be screened for disordered eating and/or pathogenic weight control behaviors (13). Although most schools do not have the resources to provide female athletes with bone mineral density screening, an in-depth history of stress fractures (13) should be obtained. A sample medical history questionnaire can be found in the Tools section.

The PSE physical examination should also include an evaluation of general body systems and an in-depth musculoskeletal examination including an overall assessment, evaluation of areas at increased risk of injury for the athlete's specific sport, and examination of sites of previous injury (13). An assessment of growth and maturity is strongly recommended for the adolescent athlete (14). Detailed explanations of the components of the PSE physical examination for various athletic populations have been published elsewhere (13-15,17).

REFERENCES

1. American College of Sports Medicine. *Guidelines for Exercise Testing and Prescription.* Media, Penn: Williams and Wilkens; 1995.
2. ACSM and AHA Joint Position Statement: recommendations for cardiovascular screening, staffing, and emergency policies at health/fitness facilities. *Med Sci Sports Exerc.* 1998;30:1009-1017.
3. Thomas S, Reading J, Shephard RJ. Revision of the Physical Activity Readiness Questionnarie (PAR-Q). *Can J Sport Sci.* 1992;17:338-345.
4. Chicago Dietetic Association, South Suburban Dietetic Association. *Manual of Clinical Dietetics.* 5th ed. Chicago, Ill: The American Dietetic Association; 1996.
5. Food and Nutrition Board. *Recommended Dietary Allowances.* 10th ed. Washington, DC: National Academy Press; 1989.
6. Institute of Medicine, Food and Nutrition Board. *Dietary Reference Intakes for Calcium, Phosphorous, Magnesium, Vitamin D, and Fluoride.* Washington, DC: National Academy Press; 1997.
7. Institute of Medicine, Food and Nutrition Board. *Dietary Reference Intakes for Thiamin, Riboflavin, Niacin, Vitamin B-6, Folate, Vitamin B-12, Pantothenic Acid, Biotin, and Choline.* Washington, DC: National Academy Press; 1998.
8. *Nutrition and Your Health: Dietary Guidelines for Americans.* 4th ed. Washington, DC: US Dept of Agriculture, US Dept of Health and Human Services; 1995. Home and Garden Bulletin No. 232.

9. American Heart Association. *Dietary Guidelines for Healthy American Adults*. Dallas, Tex: American Heart Association; 1996. AHA publication 21-0030.

10. Allen AM. *Food-Medication Interactions*. 7th ed. Pottstown, Penn: Food Medication Interactions; 1991.

11. Mahan LK, Escott-Stump S. *Krause's Food, Nutrition and Diet Therapy*. 9th ed. Philadelphia, Penn: W B Saunders Co; 1996.

12. Howley ET, Franks BD. *Health Fitness Instructors Handbook*. 2nd ed. Champaign, Ill: Human Kinetics; 1992.

13. Johnson MD. Tailoring the preparticipation exam to female athletes. *Phys Sportsmed*. 1992;20:61-72.

14. Hergenroeder AC. The preparticipation sports examination. *Ped Clin of N Am*. 1997;44:1525-1540.

15. Grafe MW, Paul GR, Foster TE. The preparticipation sports examination for high school and college athletes. *Clin Sports Med*. 1997;16(4):569-591.

16. National Collegiate Athletic Association 1995-1996. *Sports Medicine Handbook*. Overland Park, Kan: National Collegiate Association; 1995.

17. American Medical Association Board of Trustees, Group on Science and Technology. Athletic preparticipation examinations for adolescents. *Arch Pediatr Adolesc Med*. 1994;148:93-98.

9

DIETARY ASSESSMENT

Katherine A. Beals, PhD, RD and Melinda M. Manore, PhD, RD

Assessment of dietary intake is one of the most frequently used procedures in dietetics practice and human nutrition research. In both of these settings, the goal is to achieve the most accurate description of an individual's or group's typical food and nutrient intake. Therefore, the dietary assessment method utilized must be not only valid and reliable, but appropriate for the individual or population being studied.

Dietary assessment involves not only collecting the food intake information but also analyzing and evaluating the data. Selecting the appropriate dietary intake tool can go a long way toward increasing the accuracy of the overall assessment. Factors to consider when selecting a dietary intake tool include the objectives of the assessment, the individual or group being assessed, the dietary information of interest (ie, energy, specific nutrients, food groups, dietary patterns, etc), the time frame involved, the costs versus resources, and the interviewer's qualifications and experience (1).

Collection of the food intake data is only one part of dietary assessment. Once the diet data have been collected, they must be analyzed for nutrient content and subsequently evaluated, which typically entails comparing the data to nutrient standards or goals. Today, dietary intake data are most often analyzed for nutrient content using computerized nutrient-analysis programs (2,3). To avoid introducing additional error into the diet assessment technique, care should be taken in the selection and use of these computer programs. The evaluation and selection of diet-analysis computer programs are covered in Chapter 12, Computer Programs for Nutrition, Diet, Fitness, and Body Composition Assessment.

Although a variety of dietary standards or references are available for evaluating nutrient intake, those most commonly used are the latest RDAs (4) (see Tools section), the 1995 *Dietary Guidelines for Americans* (5), and the 1996 American Heart Association guidelines (6). The newly established Dietary Reference Intakes (DRIs) provide another set of dietary standards by which nutrient intakes may be evaluated (7-10) (see Tools section). Research on the nutrient needs of athletes has also produced dietary recommendations by sport and nutrition organizations. For example, the United States Olympic Committee (USOC) has published a set of *Guidelines on Dietary Supplementation* (see Chapter 18, Elite and Olympic Athletes) which can be readily tailored to meet the needs of a particular client (11).

METHODS FOR COLLECTING DIETARY INTAKE DATA

Table 9.1 summarizes the currently available methods for obtaining dietary intake information along with the strengths and weaknesses of each. These methods can be broadly classified as either retrospective, prospective, or some combination of the two.

TABLE 9.1 Diet Assessment Methods

METHOD AND DESCRIPTION	STRENGTHS	WEAKNESSES/LIMITATIONS
24-Hour Recall		
• Interviewer prompts respondent to recall and describe all foods and beverages consumed over the past 24 hours, usually starting with the meal immediately preceding the interview. • Food models and measuring cups and spoons are used to get a rough estimate of portion sizes. • May be done face-to-face or via telephone	• Easy to administer • Respondent burden is low. • Time required to administer is short. • Bias introduced by record keeping is avoided. • Inexpensive • Useful in clinical situations • More objective than dietary history • Does not alter usual diets • Good reliability between interviewers • Serial 24-hour recalls can provide estimates of usual intakes on individuals. • Data obtained can be repeated with reasonable accuracy.	• Does not provide adequate quantitative data on nutrient intakes • Individual diets vary daily so that a single day's intake may not be representative of habitual intake. • An experienced interviewer is required. • Relies heavily on memory • Desire to please the interviewer may result in inaccurate intakes. • Data may not accurately reflect nutrient intakes for populations because of variations in food consumption from day to day. • May be a tendency to over-report intake at low levels and under-report intake of high levels, leading to a "flat slope syndrome" with reports of group intakes.
Food Frequency Questionnaire		
• Respondent records or describes usual intakes as a list of different foods and the frequency of consumption per day, week, or month, over a period of several months or a year. • The number and type of food items vary depending on the purpose of the assessment.	• Easy to standardize • Does not require highly trained interviewers, and some types may be self-administered • Inexpensive • Easy and quick to administer • No observer bias • Good at describing food intake patterns for diet and meal planning • Can be used for large population studies • Useful when purpose is to study associations of a specific food or small number of foods and disease (eg, alcohol and birth defects) • Specific information about nutrient intakes may be obtained if food sources of nutrients are limited to a few sources. • Can be analyzed rapidly for nutritients or food groups using a computer • Foods can be ranked in relation to intakes of certain food items or groups of foods. • Does not alter usual diets	• Does not provide adequate data to determine quantitative nutrient intake • Incomplete responses may be given. • Response rates may be lower if questionnaire is self-administered. • Lists compiled for the general population are not useful for obtaining information on groups with different eating patterns (eg, vegetarians or those on special ethnic or therapeutic diets). • Estimation of total consumption is difficult to obtain because not all foods can be included in the lists; thus, underestimation can occur. • Respondent burden rises as number of items queried increases. • Analysis is difficult without the use of computers. • Reliability is lower for individual foods than for groups of foods. • Foods differ in extent to which they are over- or under-reported (errors are not random).

continued

TABLE 9.1 Diet Assessment Methods (continued)

METHOD AND DESCRIPTION	STRENGTHS	WEAKNESSES/LIMITATIONS
Food Frequency Questionnaire (continued)		
		• Amount and frequency with which a food is consumed influence errors in estimation; staples and large quantities are better estimated than accessories or items eaten less frequently. • Each questionnaire requires validation. • Translation of food groups to nutrient intakes requires many assumptions.
Semiquantitative Food Frequency Questionnaire		
• Similar to a food frequency questionnaire. • Portion sizes are specified as standardized portion size or choice (of a range of sizes). • Foods are chosen to encompass the most frequently consumed foods as well as the most common sources of nutrients. • The major sources of nutrients for a given population should be included for the questionnaire to be valid.	• Inexpensive and rapid to administer • May be self-administered • Usual diets are not altered. • Precoding and direct data entry to computer available to speed analysis on some versions • Can rank or categorize individuals by rank of nutrient intakes rather than measuring group means • Correlations between this and other methods are satisfactory for food items and targeted nutrients when groups are the focus of analysis. • Sufficiently simple to obtain dietary information on large epidemiological studies that would not otherwise be possible with other methods • Can provide useful information on intake of a wide variety of nutrients • Respondent burden varies.	• Good for the general population but not necessarily for specific groups. • Culture-specific-ie, assessment of intake in a culturally distinct group requires the creation and validation of another instrument. • Not validated for individual dietary assessments • Questionnaires available for adults cannot be used for children. • Must be constantly updated • Specific nutrient intakes, rather than all nutrient intakes or food constituents, are measured. • Not yet validated for those who eat modified or unusual diets • Ability to monitor short-term changes in food intake (weeks or months) is unknown. • Correlations for individual nutrient intakes obtained with semiquantitative food frequency questionnaires are poor when compared to diet histories and food records in household measures. • May be reliable but invalid in some cases • May reflect "core diets" of a week's duration • Default codes with estimated variables may influence the results unduly.
Burke-type Dietary History		
• Respondent orally reports all foods and beverages consumed on a usual day, then the interview progresses to questions about the frequency and amount of consumption of the foods. • Often the respondent provides additional documentation of several days' intakes in the form of food diaries. • Food models, crosschecks on food consumption, careful probing, and other techniques are frequently used.	• Provides a more complete and detailed description of both qualitative and quantitative aspects of food intake than do food records, 24-hour recalls, or food frequency questionnaires • Eliminates individual day-to-day variations • Takes into consideration seasonal variations in diet • Good for longitudinal studies • Does not alter usual diets • Provides good description of usual intake	• Highly trained interviewers required to administer dietary histories. • Highly dependent on subject's memory • Difficult to standardize because of considerable variability among and within interviewers • Diet histories overestimate intakes compared with food records collected over the same period because of bigger portion sizes and greater frequencies reported; also does not account for missed meals or snacks.

continued

TABLE 9.1   Diet Assessment Methods (continued)

METHOD AND DESCRIPTION	STRENGTHS	WEAKNESSES/LIMITATIONS
Burke-type Dietary History (continued)		
	• Provides some data on previous diet before beginning prospective studies	• Costs of analyses are high because records must be checked, coded, and entered appropriately. • Time frame actually used by subject for reporting intake history is uncertain, probably no longer than a few weeks. • Validity must be established in each study.
Food Diary		
• Respondent records all foods and beverages consumed in a food diary, including estimated portion sizes, at the time of consumption for several days or only at specified times.	• What is eaten is recorded (or should be recorded) at the time of consumption; thus, errors of recall are less than with retrospective methods. • Does not rely heavily on memory • Respondent can be instructed in advance to reduce recording errors.	• Food intake may be altered during reporting periods. • Respondent burden is great. • Individual must be literate and physically able to write. • Respondent may not record intakes on assigned days, compromising representativeness. • Difficult to estimate portion sizes • Underreporting is common. • Number of sampled days must be sufficient to provide usual intakes. • Records must be checked and coded in a standardized way. • Measured food intakes are more valid than records. • Costs of coding and analysis are high. • Requires competency in recording food items and quantities • Number of days surveyed depends on the nutrient being studied. • The very act of recording may change what is eaten.
Weighed Food Diary		
• Similar to a food record except the individual weighs on a small scale all food and drink consumed rather than simply estimating portion sizes. All food is recorded at the time it is eaten.	• Increased accuracy of portion sizes over food diaries (where errors are substantial-up to 40% for foods and 25% for nutrients)	• Expensive and time-consuming • May restrict choice of food • Subjects must be highly motivated. • Requires reliable equipment (eg, calibrated, operable scales) • Other disadvantages similar to those of a food diary
Telephone Record		
• Instead of personal, face-to-face interviews, telephones are used to report food intakes as soon as they have occurred.	• Some anonymity is maintained. • Validity is good. • Respondent burden is low. • Respondent acceptance is good. • Effect of forgetting is minimum. • Outreach is greater. • May be easier to carry out after face-to-face interview and instruction	• Assumption is made that portion sizes reported are actually eaten. • Validation studies are incomplete.

TABLE 9.1   Diet Assessment Methods (continued)

METHOD AND DESCRIPTION	STRENGTHS	WEAKNESSES/LIMITATIONS
Photographic or Videotape Records		
• Individual photographs or videotapes of all foods to be eaten at a standard distance	• Validity is good.	• Problems with estimating portion sizes and identifying some foods from photographs. • Food waste may not be taken into account, leading to overestimation. • Obtrusive • Respondent burden is high.
Electronic Records (Food Recording Electronic Device or FRED)		
• Respondent records food intake on a specially programmed electronic recording device (hand-held computer or small tape recorder).	• Preliminary validations are good. • Deceased respondent burden • Eliminates time for coding and data entry, and associated errors occurring at those stages	• Requires considerable instruction and training • Special food groups must be constructed for population to be studied. • Portion size estimates often imprecise
Duplicate Portion Collection and Analysis		
• A duplicate portion of the foods and beverages consumed by an individual is collected. Foods are then chemically analyzed to obtain a direct nutrient analysis.	• Highly accurate in metabolic research • Duplicate portion permits direct chemical analysis. • Helpful for validating other methods for constituents on which food composition data are incomplete • Good for individuals consuming unusual foods • Can be used with patients who cannot write	• Intakes may be altered. • High respondent burden • Expensive, time-consuming, and messy • Differences between duplicate portions and weighed records are large (7% for energy, larger for other nutrients).
Measured Intakes and Outputs		
• Applicable to confined individuals, usually in institutions • All foods entering and leaving the room are measured. The differences between them are assumed to be equivalent to what the respondents ate.	• Low respondent burden • Assessment can be accomplished without the individual knowing about it. • Good for individuals incapable of writing or remembering	• Others in the room may have eaten the food. • Individual may hide or throw away food (eg, clients with anorexia nervosa). • Staff may forget to deliver or collect the food.
Direct Observation by Video Recording		
• Video camera are used to monitor the individual's food intake over a certain period. • Videotapes may then be reviewed and intakes recorded accordingly.	• Low respondent burden • Measures usual and habitual food intake • Highly accurate • Details may be observed. • Individual may or may not know he or she is being observed.	• High initial cost • Not good for large studies • May have technical problems (eg, angle of camera, low-quality picture detail) • Intakes may be altered if individual is aware of observation.
Direct Observation by Trained Observers		
• In controlled or highly supervised environments, intakes may be directly watched by trained observers who use any of the methods mentioned above. Sometimes this observation is covert.	• Low respondent burden • Overt or covert observation is possible. • Precise measurements may be obtained.	• Obtrusive • Expensive and time-consuming for observer • Not ideal for large studies • Intakes may be altered, especially if person is aware of observation. • Details may be overlooked.

Adapted from: Dwyer JT. Dietary assessment. In: Shils ME, Olson JA, Shike M, eds. *Modern Nutrition in Health and Disease.* 9th ed. Philadelphia, Penn: Lea & Febiger; 1998:937-957. Used by permission.

Retrospective Methods

Retrospective methods involve looking back at, or "recalling," dietary intake over a specified time period. Consequently, these methods rely heavily on memory and, thus, are limited by the individual's ability to remember dietary intake in the near or more distant past. Nonetheless, with a skilled interviewer and respondent motivation and commitment, the data generated can approximate or even equal that derived from prospective methods (1). The most commonly used retrospective methods include the 24-hour recall and food frequency questionnaire (FFQ).

24-hour recall. The 24-hour recall is the easiest and fastest method available for assessing food and nutrient intake. This method requires that a client recall in detail all the foods and beverages consumed during the previous 24 hours. Knowing the preparation methods, the brand names of foods and beverages, and any vitamin-mineral supplements is critical to an effective evaluation. In addition to the limitations listed in *Table 9.1,* a major limitation of the 24-hour recall is the tendency for some clients to minimize food choices they perceive to be less healthful or acceptable and to overstate those they perceive to be more healthful or acceptable (1,12)

The success of the 24-hour recall will depend in large part on the client's memory, motivation to respond accurately, and ability to convey precise information. The accuracy of a 24-hour recall can be improved by a skilled interviewer's use of "probing" questions, measuring devices, and food models to help the client remember the types and amounts of foods consumed. Indeed, the persistence and skill of the interviewer are critical factors in obtaining accurate information from a 24-hour recall (1).

A single 24-hour recall is most appropriately used for estimating the nutrient intake of a group or population, as opposed to assessing the usual food and nutrient intake of an individual (1,13). If the 24-hour recall is to be used for estimating individual food intakes, the US Committee on Food Consumption Patterns recommends that a minimum of four 24-hour recalls be collected over a 1-year period (14).

Food frequency questionnaire (FFQ). A FFQ is designed to provide descriptive information about an individual's usual dietary pattern. The information collected can then be used to assess food patterns and preferences that may not be evident from a food recall or diet record (15). For best results the FFQ should be brief, requiring less than 30 minutes for administration and completion (14). As with the 24-hour recall, a major limitation of the FFQ is that it relies heavily on memory and, thus, may not be appropriate for use with very young children or with individuals who have poor memories (1,16). Additionally, while FFQs are good for describing dietary patterns of populations, they are seriously limited in their ability to provide quantitative information about specific nutrient intakes of individuals (1,17,18). However, if only a single nutrient is of interest, it may be possible to estimate intake of that particular nutrient with a comprehensive FFQ.

Lists are now available for approximately 100 foods that, by virtue of their composition, portion size, and the frequency with which they are eaten, contribute the most to intakes of that nutrient in national surveys of representative samples of Americans (19). In addition, some researchers have developed a picture approach to the FFQ. In this method a color picture or black-and-white line drawing of the food is shown. The subjects then identify the foods they eat and sort them into categories based on frequency of consumption (eg, "daily," "once per week," "never," etc). Portion sizes can also be reviewed since the pictures indicate standard portion sizes (20).

The FFQ can be designed to provide either qualitative or semiquantitative information on a client's typical food intake (14,16,18). Questionnaires that provide qualitative data (ie, list only typical foods consumed) are most useful for obtaining general, descriptive information about an individual's dietary patterns or for comparing consumption of certain foods before and after nutrition intervention (13,14). Semiquantitative FFQs not only list typical foods consumed, but also attempt to quantify the usual intake of these foods. This type of questionnaire allows the assessment of specific nutrient intakes in addition to dietary patterns. Selective FFQs can also be created to inquire about specific nutrient concerns such as fat (21,22), carbohydrate (23), and cholesterol (24,25).

Because the aim of the FFQ is to assess the frequency with which certain food items or food groups are consumed during a specified period, it is important that the questionnaire be designed and tested specifically for the population and nutrient being measured. A variety of FFQs have been designed and validated for various populations (18,19,26,27). For example, Moses and Manore (23) have developed and tested an FFQ to monitor carbohydrate intake in athletes. Similarly, Rockett et al (26) have recently tested and validated a youth and adolescent FFQ and Coates and Monteilh (27) have published a FFQ for minority populations.

Prospective Methods

Prospective methods of collecting dietary intake data involve recording food intake at the time the food is eaten or shortly thereafter. The most commonly used prospective methods are food records or diaries. Other techniques that are applicable in certain situations are: collection of duplicate portions of all food eaten; observations of intakes and food wastes; and photographic, videotaped, and electronic microcomputer records of consumption (28). Because prospective methods are less dependent upon memory, they tend to be more accurate than the retrospective methods. Nonetheless, they have limitations. The very act of recording intake tends to influence food choices and nutrient intakes or may otherwise lead the respondent to alter intake during the recording period (1,14,29).

Food records. A food record is a list of all foods consumed, including a description of food preparation methods and brand names used, over a specified time period (typically 3 to 7 days). To predict nutrient content accurately, it is best if the foods consumed are weighed or measured. However, it is most common for consumed foods to be recorded by common portion sizes expressed in common household measuring units. Depending on the reasons for recording food intake, more in-depth information on eating habits, such as time, place, feelings, and behaviors associated with eating, can also be included on a food record. When the records are completed, the nutrient contribution from each food is determined and average nutrient intake for the time period being monitored can be calculated.

Determining the number of days that food intake should be recorded to give an accurate and reliable estimate of typical dietary intake has been addressed by a number of researchers (30-35). Schlundt (33) determined that, for most purposes, diet records collected for 3 to 4 days will provide accurate estimates of nutrient intake; however, both reliability and accuracy tend to increase with each additional day up to day 7 (32,33). For most nutrients, there is little advantage to measuring intakes beyond 2 or 3 weeks (33,34). The disadvantage to longer periods of recording food consumption is that the increased respondent burden decreases accuracy (1). For shorter records (3 to 4 days), at least 1 weekend day should be included (13,32).

The accuracy of a food record relies heavily on the client's cooperation and skill in recording foods consumed. Under-reporting of food intake remains a significant problem that can severely compromise the accuracy of the dietary analysis (16,17). Research indicates that certain individuals are more prone to under-reporting energy intake, including women and those who are older, overweight, or trying to lose weight (16,36). Knowing who is likely to under-report food intake will allow the dietetics professional to take extra precautions when selecting and administering the food intake protocol and analyzing the record. The accuracy of the food record may be increased if the client is given adequate incentive and proper instructions. Specific guidelines for keeping records should be included in the instruction sheet given to the client and also be reviewed verbally. (A sample 3-day food record and instructions is provided in the Tools section.)

Combination methods. Another perhaps more comprehensive approach to obtaining a representative estimate of an individual's or group's food intake is to combine two or more dietary intake methods. Using a combination of dietary assessment methods not only provides a more complete picture of an individual's typical dietary habits and nutrient intake, but also may increase the accuracy of the assessment as the shortcomings of one method may be counterbalanced by the strengths of another (1). For example, the National Health and Nutrition Examination Surveys used a combination of a 24-hour recall and FFQ. Similarly, the Nationwide Food Consumption Surveys of 1977-1978 and 1987-1988 conducted by the USDA used a combination of a 24-hour food recall and a 2-day food record (37).

VALIDITY OF DIETARY INTAKE METHODS

The validity of dietary intake methods, particularly 24-hour recalls and food records, has been difficult to determine, at least without the use of direct observation which is time-consuming, costly, and largely unrealistic. However, with the development of various biochemical markers, most notably doubly-labeled water, it is now possible to assess the validity of different dietary intake methods (38,39). Doubly-labeled water allows for the estimation of energy expenditure in free living humans. Under conditions of weight maintenance, energy intake is equal to energy expenditure. Thus, if energy expenditure is measured, the validity of reports of energy intake can be assessed (38). Similarly, protein (nitrogen) intake can be checked against crude nitrogen balance (40).

ANALYSIS OF FOOD INTAKE INFORMATION

Currently, computerized diet analysis is the most popular and widely used method for analyzing dietary intake information. When properly applied this method is considered the most efficient, accurate, and timely means available for analyzing the nutrient content of consumed foods (3). Recorded foods are entered into a computerized nutrient-analysis program and a computer printout containing information regarding daily energy and macro- and micronutrient intake is subsequently generated. Most dietary analysis programs calculate total calories as well as grams and percentages of carbohydrates, protein, fat, and selected vitamins and minerals. Some programs also give information regarding the type of fat and sugar consumed, the polyunsaturated/saturated fat ratio, or the cholesterol-saturated fat index of the diet. In addition, most programs will compare the calculated vitamin and mineral intakes to the appropriate RDA (or DRI) based on age and gender, and many will compare current food intake to the Food Guide Pyramid (41). Some programs even offer specific recommendations for improving nutrient intake. See Chapter 12, Computer Programs for Nutrition, Diet, Fitness, and Body Composition Assessment, for more information on computerized dietary analysis.

EVALUATION/INTERPRETATION OF DIETARY ANALYSIS

Once dietary intake information has been collected and analyzed, it must be evaluated. This generally entails comparing nutrient intakes to accepted standards in order to make the information more meaningful to the client and to help set the groundwork for formulating dietary goals.

Several methods are used for dietary evaluation. A simple and quick method is to compare dietary intake to the Food Guide Pyramid and determine if any major food groups are completely omitted from the individual's diet or are consumed infrequently. Because no single food can provide all the nutrients needed, the diet must also be checked for variety within each food group. In general, a monotonous diet will increase the risk of poor nutritional status. In addition, because foods within each group vary in their fat and sodium content, the frequency of consumption of foods high in fat and/or sodium within each group should also be checked. Finally, if an individual consistently consumes foods high in simple sugars and/or fats (eg, rich desserts, high-fat spreads, highly processed foods), fat and energy intake can be high, even though he or she is eating a variety of other foods (42). It is generally assumed that if adequate energy (kcal) and a variety of foods are consumed from each group, the nutrients provided by these food groups will be adequately represented in the diet.

REFERENCES

1. Dwyer JT. Dietary assessment. In Shils ME, Olson JA, Shike M, eds. *Modern Nutrition in Health and Disease.* 9th ed. Philadelphia, Penn: Lea & Febiger; 1998:937-957.

2. Byrd-Bredbenner C. Computer nutrient analysis software packages: considerations selection. *Nutrition Today.* Sept/Oct 1988;13-21.

3. Lee RD, Nieman DC, Rainwater M. Comparison of eight microcomputer dietary analysis programs with the USDA nutrient data base for standard reference. *J Am Diet Assoc.* 1995:95:858-867.

4. Food and Nutrition Board. *Recommended Dietary Allowances.* 10th ed. Washington, DC: National Academy Press; 1989.

5. *Nutrition and Your Health: Dietary Guidelines for Americans.* 4th ed. Washington, DC: US Depts of Agriculture and Health and Human Services; 1995. Home and Garden Bulletin No. 232.

6. American Heart Association. *Dietary Guidelines for Healthy American Adults.* Dallas, Tex: American Heart Association; 1996. AHA publication 21-0030.

7. Institute of Medicine, Food and Nutrition Board. *Dietary Reference Intakes for Calcium, Phosphorous, Magnesium, Vitamin D, and Fluoride.* Washington, DC: National Academy Press; 1997.

8. Institute of Medicine, Food and Nutrition Board. *Dietary Reference Intakes for Thiamin, Riboflavin, Niacin, Vitamin B-6, Folate, Vitamin B-12, Pantothenic Acid, Biotin, and Choline.* Washington, DC: National Academy Press; 1998.

9. Yates AA, Schlicker SA, Suitor CW. Dietary Reference Intakes: The new basis for recommendations for calcium and related nutrients, B vitamins, and choline. *J Am Diet Assoc.* 1998;98:699-706.

10. Translating the science behind the DRIs. *J Am Diet Assoc.* 1998;98:756.

11. United States Olympic Committee. *Guidelines on Dietary Supplements.* 1998. http://www.usoc.org.html. Accessed May 23, 1999.

12. Karvetti R, Knuts L. Validity of the 24-hour dietary recall. *J Am Diet Assoc.* 1985;85:1437-1444.

13. Todd KS, Hudes M, Calloway DH. Food intake measurement: problems and approaches. *Am J Clin Nutr.* 1983;37:139-146.

14. Gibson RS. *Principles of Nutritional Assessment.* New York, NY: Oxford University Press; 1990.

15. Zulkifli SN, Yu SM. The food frequency method for dietary assessment. *J Am Diet Assoc.* 1992;92:681-685.

16. Dwyer JT, Coleman KA. Insights into dietary recall from a longitudinal study: accuracy over four decades. *Am J Clin Nutr.* 1997:65(suppl):1153S-1158S.

17. Briefel RR, Flegal KM, Winn DM, Loria CM, Johnson CL, Sempos CT. Assessing the nation's diet: limitations of the food frequency questionnaire. *J Am Diet Assoc.* 1992;92:959-962.

18. Willett WC. Future directions in the development of food-frequency questionnaires. *Am J Clin Nutr.* 1994;59(suppl):171S-178S.

19. Block G, Hartman AM, Dresser CM, Carroll MD, Gannon J, Gardner L. A data-based approach to diet questionnaire design and testing. *Am J Epidemiol.* 1986;124:453-469.

20. Kumanyika SK, Tell GS, Shemanski L, Martel J, Chinchilli VM. Dietary assessment using a picture-sort approach. *Am J Clin Nutr.* 1997;65(suppl):1123S-1129S.

21. Block G, Clifford C, Naughton MD, Henderson M, McAdams M. A brief dietary screen for high fat intake. *J Nutr Ed.* 1989;21:199-207.

22. Coates RJ, Serdula MK, Byers T, et al. A brief, telephone-administered food frequency questionnaire can be useful for surveillance of dietary fat intakes. *J Nutr.* 1995;125:1473-1483.

23. Moses K, Manore MM. Development and testing of a carbohydrate monitoring tool for athletes. *J Am Diet Assoc*. 1991;91:962-965.

24. Ammerman AS, Haines PS, DeVellis RF, et al. A brief dietary assessment to guide cholesterol reduction in low-income individuals: design and validation. *J Am Diet Assoc*. 1991;91:1385-1390.

25. Lee J, Kolonel LN, Hankin JH. Cholesterol intake as measured by unquantified and quantified food frequency interviews: implications for epidemiological research. *Int J Epidemiol*. 1985;14:249-253.

26. Rockett HRH, Breitenbach M, Frazier LA, et al. Validation of a youth/adolescent food frequency questionnaire. *Prev Med*. 1997;26:808-816.

27. Coates RJ, Monteilh CP. Assessments of food-frequency questionnaires in minority populations. *Am J Clin Nutr*. 1997;65(suppl):1108S-1115S.

28. Thompson FE. Dietary assessment resource manual. *J Nutr*. 1994;124(suppl):2245S-2317S.

29. Bingham SA. Limitations of the various methods for collecting dietary intake data. *Ann Nutr Metab*. 1991;35:117-127.

30. Basiotis PP, Welsh SO, Cronin FJ, Kelsay JL, Mertz W. Number of days of food intake records required to estimate individual and group nutrient intakes with defined confidence. *J Nutr*. 1987;117:1638-1641.

31. Heaney RP, Davies KM, Recker RR, Packard PT. Long-term consistency of nutrient intakes in humans. *J Nutr*. 1990;120:869-875.

32. Jackson B, Dujovne CA, DeCoursey S, Beyer P, Brown EF, Hassanein K. Methods to assess relative reliability of diet records: minimum records for monitoring lipid and calorie intake. *J Am Diet Assoc*. 1986;86:1531-1535.

33. Schlundt EG. Accuracy and reliability of nutrient intake estimates. *J Nutr*. 1988;118:1432-1435.

34. Sempos CT, Johnson NE, Smith EL, Gilligan C. Effects of intraindividual and interindividual variation in repeated dietary records. *Am J Epidemiol*. 1985;121:120-130.

35. Conner SL, Gustafson JR, Artaud-Wild SM, Classick-Kohn CJ, Conner WE. The cholesterol-saturated fat index for coronary prevention: background, use, and a comprehensive table of foods. *J Am Diet Assoc*. 1989;89:807-816.

36. Briefel RR, Sempos CT, McDowell MA, Chien S, Alaimo K. Dietary methods research in the third National Health and Nutrition Examination Survey: underreporting of energy intake. *Am J Clin Nutr*. 1997;65(suppl):1203S-1209S.

37. Pao EM, Sykes KE, Cypel YS. *USDA Methodological Research for Large-scale Dietary Intake Surveys, 1975-1988*. Washington, DC: US Government Printing Office; 1989. Home Economics Research Report No. 49.

38. Bandini LG, Cyr H, Must A, Dietz WH. Validity of reported energy intake in preadolescent girls. *Am J Clin Nutr*. 1997:65(suppl):1138S-1141S.

39. Kaaks RJ. Biochemical markers as additional measurements in studies of the accuracy of dietary questionnaire measurements: conceptual issues. *Am J Clin Nutr*. 1997:65(suppl):1232S-1239S.

40. Bingham SH, Day NE. Using biochemical markers to assess the validity of prospective dietary assessment methods and the effect of energy adjustment. *Am J Clin Nutr*. 1997;65(suppl):1130S-1137S.

41. *Food Guide Pyramid: A Guide to Daily Food Choices*. Washington, DC: US Dept of Agriculture, Human Nutrition Information Service; 1992. Home and Garden Bulletin No. 252.

42. McCrory MA, Fuss PJ, McCallum JE, et al. Dietary variety within food groups: association with energy intake and body fatness in men and women. *Am J Clin Nutr*. 1999;69:440-447.

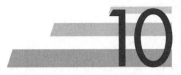

PHYSICAL FITNESS ASSESSMENT

Katherine A. Beals, PhD, RD and Melinda M. Manore, PhD, RD

The term "physical fitness" has numerous connotations and, thus, may be defined in a number of ways. Until recently, definitions have focused largely on proficiencies and/or elements relating to athletic performance but not necessarily health. However, because of increasing evidence supporting a positive relationship between physical activity and health, more "health-related" definitions of physical fitness are more prevalent (1-3). The primary concept that underlies health-related fitness is that improvement in any of the fitness components is associated with a lower risk for chronic diseases and functional disabilities (4-6). The components of health-related fitness typically include body composition, cardiorespiratory endurance, muscular strength and endurance, and flexibility.

The measurement of physical fitness is an important component of any preventive or rehabilitative exercise program and serves several purposes (4):

- Provides a basis for developing an exercise prescription
- Allows for collection of baseline and follow-up data for evaluation of progress
- Motivates participants by establishing reasonable and attainable fitness goals
- Educates participants about the concepts of physical fitness and health
- Allows for stratification of participants based on risk for disease (ie, risk stratification)

A sound, well-conducted physical fitness test should be valid, reliable, relatively inexpensive, and easy to administer. Additionally, the test should yield results that can be directly and appropriately compared to normative data (4).

FITNESS ASSESSMENT COMPONENTS

A comprehensive fitness assessment should include at least one test to measure each of the components of fitness (ie, body composition, cardiorespiratory endurance, muscular strength and endurance, and flexibility). The organization of the testing session can be very important, especially if multiple tests are being administered (4). If all of the components are assessed during a single session, body composition measures should be taken first, followed (in order) by tests of cardiorespiratory endurance, muscular strength and endurance, and flexibility. Testing cardiorespiratory endurance after assessing muscular strength and endurance, which elevates heart rate, may lead to an underestimation of an individual's cardiorespiratory endurance, especially if submaximal tests are used (4).

Similarly, assessing body composition after cardiorespiratory endurance and/or muscular strength and endurance may lead to an overestimation of body fat due to loss of water via sweating. If the testing protocol involves assessing resting measures (eg, heart rate, blood pressure, and blood lipids), such measures should be taken before any fitness testing begins (4).

BODY COMPOSITION

Body composition refers to the relative percentages of body weight comprised of fat mass (FM) and fat-free mass (FFM). It is well established that excess body fat can be harmful to health; however, many misconceptions exist regarding the assessment and interpretation of body composition data (4). This section will briefly describe the most commonly used techniques for assessing body composition. For a more detailed account of body composition assessment, refer to Chapter 11, Assessment of Body Size and Composition and the *ACSM Resource Manual for Guidelines for Exercise Testing and Prescription* (7).

Hydrostatic Weighing

Hydrostatic or "underwater" weighing (UUW) is one of the most common laboratory methods for estimating body composition (FM and FFM) and remains the criterion measurement technique or "gold standard" (8,9). This technique is based on Archimedes' principle, which states that a submerged object will be "buoyed up" by a counterforce equal to the volume of the water it displaces. This buoyant force causes the object to weigh less underwater than it does on land. The difference between land weight and underwater weight is used to calculate body volume and, subsequently, body density. Bone and muscle tissues are more dense than water, whereas FM is less dense; thus, an individual with more FFM for the same total body weight will weigh more in water, have a higher body density, and a lower percentage of body fat. While hydrostatic weighing is currently considered the "gold standard," several sources of error are inherent in the procedure and must be considered. First, an estimate of lung residual volume is required to calculate body density. Second, the great variability in bone density among individuals is not accounted for by this method. Finally, hydrostatic weighing requires expensive, complex equipment and the procedure is somewhat complicated and time-consuming (4,10). Moreover, this method requires that the individual be completely submerged for an extended period of time, which may be extremely difficult and anxiety-provoking for many individuals.

Plethysmography

Another method that uses the concept of density as the ratio of body weight to body volume is air displacement plethysmography, also known as the Bod Pod (Life Measurement Instruments, Concord, Calif). In this method the individual simply sits inside a sealed chamber and breathes normally. Body volume is then derived from the difference between the empty chamber air volume and the air volume with the individual inside (10). The Bod Pod has several advantages over

UUW: It is portable and relatively easy to operate; measurement time is short; and it may be better able to accommodate special populations such as young children, obese individuals, the elderly, or disabled persons (9).

Dual-energy X-ray Absorptiometry (DXA)

Originally developed to assess bone mineral content (bone density), DXA is now an accepted method for estimating body composition and may one day replace UUW as the "gold standard" or criterion measure. The technique is based on measuring the attenuation of two energies of x-rays through the body. As the x-ray beams pass through the subject, the density of all parts of the body is determined. Because fat is less dense than bone or nonbone lean tissue, the percentage of total body weight composed of fat can be calculated (9,11). DXA has several advantages over other techniques used to determine body composition. Perhaps its greatest advantage is that it provides both regional and whole-body estimates of bone, fat, and lean tissue from a single whole-body scan. Thus, visceral versus subcutaneous fat can be determined, providing a better indication of disease risk (9,11). Moreover, because DXA is based on a three-component model of composition (ie, bone, fat, and lean soft tissue), it may provide a more accurate estimate of body composition in individuals with both below- and above-average bone mineral contents and, thus, avoid some of the limitations seen in the two-component models described above (9,11). Nonetheless, the method is not widely available, is very expensive, and requires a highly skilled technician to administer the scan and interpret the data output.

Anthropometry

Anthropometry includes measures such as height, weight, limb and torso circumferences, and skinfold thickness. Anthropometric measurements can be used in equations to either directly predict percent fat or indirectly predict whole-body density that can then be used to estimate percent fat (9,12). Measuring skinfolds is one of the most commonly used anthropometric methods for estimating body fat percentage. This method is based on the assumption that the thickness of the subcutaneous adipose tissue is proportional to the total amount of body fat mass, and the sites selected for measurement represent the average thickness of the subcutaneous adipose tissue. The accuracy and reliability of percentage of fat estimated from skinfolds depend on the technician's skill, type of skinfold caliper used, and the prediction equation employed to estimate body fatness (9). If done correctly, body composition determined from skinfold measurements correlates well (r ≥0.80) with body composition as assessed by hydrostatic weighing (4).

Body mass index (BMI) is used to assess weight relative to height and provides an acceptable approximation of total body fat in population-based studies. In addition, BMI demonstrates a strong positive correlation with both morbidity and mortality; thus, it provides a direct indication of health status and disease risk (13). Calculating BMI is simple, quick, and inexpensive (BMI = weight in kg ÷ height in m^2). The major limitations of BMI are that it does not provide information regarding regional body fat distribution, it is difficult to explain to clients, and it is difficult to project changes in actual weight loss to BMI changes (4). In addition, BMI has been shown to overestimate body fat in persons who are very muscular (eg, many athletes) and underestimate body fat in persons who have lost muscle mass (eg, the elderly) (13).

Recent data indicate that the pattern of body fat distribution is an important predictor of the health risks of obesity (14-17). Specifically, individuals with high amounts of fat in the abdominal region, especially visceral abdominal fat, are at increased risk for premature death and a number of chronic diseases including hypertension, type 2 diabetes, hyperlipidemia, and coronary artery disease (14-17). The waist-to-hip ratio (WHR) is a simple method for determining an individual's body fat pattern or the relative ratio of abdominal to gluteal-femoral body fat (18). Ratios of >0.90 for men and >0.80 for women place the individual at significantly increased risk of disease (18).

It has recently been suggested that a combination of BMI, waist circumference, and risk factors for disease be used to assess whether a person is overweight and evaluate the need for weight loss (13). According to the recently published *Clinical Guidelines on the Identification, Evaluation, and Treatment of Overweight in Adults* (13), overweight is defined as a BMI of 25 to 29.9 kg/m^2 and obesity is defined as a BMI greater than 30 kg/m^2. Similarly, a waist circumference >40" in men and >35" in women signifies an increased risk for obesity-related diseases in those with a BMI of 25 to 34.8 kg/m^2 (13).

Bioelectrical Impedence Analysis (BIA)

BIA is a simple, quick, and noninvasive method for estimating FFM or total body water that involves passing a small electric current through the body and measuring the resistance encountered. The technique is based on the assumption that tissues that are high in water content (eg, muscle) will conduct electrical currents with less resistance or "impedence" than those with little water (eg, adipose). The BIA method has the advantage that is does not require a high degree of technical skill to administer. Nonetheless, body composition estimates from BIA are generally less accurate and require more assumptions than those obtained from accurate skinfold measurements (4,19). A major limitation of BIA is that it is greatly affected by state of hydration. Moreover, BIA has been shown to consistently overestimate percent body fat in very lean individuals and underestimate percent body fat in obese individuals (9,19).

Near-infrared Interactance

Near-infrared interactance was originally developed for commercial use to measure the fat content of meat and grains (9) and has become a commonly used method for estimating body fat percentage in health clubs and at fitness fairs. It is based on the principle of light absorption and reflection using near-infrared spectroscopy to provide information about the chemical composition of the body (4). In general, the instrument can be used to estimate fatness over the biceps area of the body but does not provide accurate estimates of whole-body composition (9).

CARDIORESPIRATORY ENDURANCE

Cardiorespiratory endurance is defined as the ability to perform large muscle, dynamic, moderate- to high-intensity exercise for prolonged periods and is considered one of the most important components of physical fitness (4,20). Every fitness test should include an assessment of cardiorespiratory fitness at rest and during exercise.

Resting Evaluation

A resting evaluation of cardiorespiratory function should be taken prior to exercise testing and should include the following (20):

- Heart rate
- Supine, sitting, and standing blood pressure
- 12-lead electrocardiogram (ECG)

Heart rate. The resting heart rate (RHR) is the heart rate measured when an individual is resting but not sleeping. It can be measured in a seated or supine position via auscultation (using a stethoscope), radial or carotid palpitation, or ECG recordings (20). Regardless of the method used, the client should rest 5 to 10 minutes in either the supine or seated position prior to taking the measurement. The average RHR for men and women is 60 to 80 beats per minute (bpm). RHRs as low as 28 to 48 bpm have been reported for highly conditioned endurance athletes, while poorly trained, sedentary individuals may have an RHR of ≥100 bpm (20). Care should be taken in using RHR as a measure of cardiorespiratory fitness because it is a highly variable measure that fluctuates easily due to such factors as environmental temperatures, anxiety, stress, caffeine, time of day, and body position. A low RHR may indicate a pathologically diseased heart (21).

Another valuable heart rate measure in the assessment of cardiorespiratory fitness is maximum heart rate (MHR). MHR is the highest heart rate that an individual can achieve and can be determined directly via a graded exercise test (ie, when a client is brought to total exhaustion) or indirectly by subtracting age in years from 220 (ie, MHR = 220 – age [in years]). The direct measurement of MHR is preferred because individuals of the same sex and age have heart rates that vary greatly (22,23). Because this formula provides only an estimate of MHR, caution is advised when using it to develop a fitness program. For example, a 45-year-old individual may have a true heart rate of 145 to 205 bpm, rather than the estimated 175 bpm. However, two-thirds of the population at this age would have MHRs of 165 to 185 bpm. Although heart rate will increase in direct proportion to the intensity of exercise, MHR changes little with training.

To monitor heart rate before, during, and after exercise, count the number of heartbeats (starting with zero) in 10 seconds and multiply by 6.

Blood pressure. Blood pressure (BP) is a measure of the force or pressure exerted by the blood on the arteries. The highest pressure or systolic BP reflects the pressure in the arteries during systole of the heart when myocardial contraction forces a large volume of blood into the arteries; diastolic BP reflects the lowest pressure in the arteries during the cardiac cycle. Blood pressure should be taken in the supine, sitting, or standing position prior to exercise testing. More detailed information on procedures for obtaining proper blood pressure measurement is found elsewhere (20). Optimal blood pressure with respect to cardiovascular risk is a systolic pressure <130 mm Hg and diastolic pressure <85 mm Hg. A systolic blood pressure in the range of 130 to 159 and/or a diastolic blood pressure in the range of 85 to 109 is indicative of mild to moderate hypertension. Severe hypertension is indicated if diastolic blood pressure exceeds 110 mm Hg and systolic blood pressure exceeds 180 mm Hg (24). In addition to high blood pressure readings, unusually low readings should also be evaluated for clinical significance (4). More detailed information on blood pressure is found in Chapter 23, Hypertension, Diet, and Exercise.

12-lead ECG. The ECG is a composite record of the electrical events of the heart during the cardiac cycle. As the heart depolarizes and repolarizes during contraction, an electrical impulse spreads to the tissues surrounding the heart. Electrodes placed on opposite sides of the heart transmit the electrical potential to an ECG recorder. In addition to obtaining baseline data, the resting ECG is used to detect such contraindications to exercise testing as evidence of previous myocardial infarction, ischemic ST segment changes, conduction defects, and left ventricular hypertrophy (20). The reading and interpretation of ECGs require a high degree of skill and should be undertaken only by a qualified exercise test technologist or physician (20).

Exercise Evaluation

The graded exercise test (GXT) is a frequently used technique to determine cardiorespiratory fitness and to assess a client's exercise capacity prior to starting an exercise program. A GXT is also commonly used in the detection, treatment, and rehabilitation of cardiovascular disease. A variety of GXT protocols (maximal and submaximal) and modalities (bike, treadmill, bench-step, walk/run) have been developed for assessing cardiorespiratory fitness. The choice of the most appropriate protocol and/or modality depends on several factors. These include the client's age, fitness level, known health problems, risk factors for heart disease, and fitness goals, as well as the availability of equipment and qualifications/skill level of the health professional administering the test (10). For an in-depth review of cardiorespiratory fitness and testing modalities, consult *ACSM's Guidelines for Exercise Testing and Prescription,* 5th edition (4) and *ACSM's Resource Manual for Guidelines for Exercise Testing and Prescription* (7).

The concept of maximal oxygen uptake. The traditionally accepted criterion measure of cardiorespiratory fitness is maximal oxygen uptake (VO_2max) (4). In healthy individuals oxygen consumption increases as work load increases until a plateau is reached. This threshold is referred to as VO_2max. Thus, VO_2max is the greatest rate of oxygen consumption attained during exercise and is usually expressed in liters per minute (absolute) or milliliters per kilogram of body weight per minute (relative to body weight). Measurement of VO_2max involves direct analysis of expired air samples collected while the subject performs exercise of progressing intensity (25).

Maximal aerobic capacity is often assessed in athletes to predict performance, with direct measurement of VO_2max preferred over an estimation. In general, the higher the VO_2max value obtained, the greater the client's potential for sustaining high-intensity aerobic work (23). However, other factors besides VO_2max contribute to an individual's exercise performance including motivation, state of training, and nutritional status (26).

Percentage of VO_2max utilized during exercise is the amount of oxygen consumed relative to max VO_2 and is useful for determining how stressful the exercise is with respect to one's maximum capacity. Percentage of VO_2max is calculated by dividing the oxygen consumption during exercise by the VO_2max and multiplying by 100:

$$\% \ VO_2max = \frac{(VO_2 \ during \ exercise)}{VO_2max} \times 100$$

While VO_2max appears to be genetically influenced, training has been shown to produce an increase in VO_2max in the range of 10% to 30% and can improve the ability to utilize a higher percentage of VO_2max without lactic acid accumulation (22,26,27).

Exercise Testing Protocols

Mode of testing. Commonly used modes of exercise testing include treadmill walking or running and stationary cycling. Arm crank ergometry is useful for paraplegics and patients who have limited use of the lower extremities. Bench or step tests, while not as well-founded or precise as treadmill or cycle ergometer, are frequently used in the health/fitness industry where time, equipment, and qualified personnel may be limited. In addition, a variety of running and walking field tests have been developed for mass fitness testing. Two of the most widely used running tests are the Cooper 12-minute run and the 1.5-mile run test for time (4). The most common walking test is the Rockport One-mile Fitness Walking Test. For more information on the administration and interpretation of these tests, see *ACSM's Resource Manual for Guidelines for Exercise Testing and Prescription* (7).

Maximal versus submaximal exercise test. VO_2max can be directly measured during maximal exercise testing by direct analysis of expired gases or estimated from a submaximal exercise test (28). The decision to select a maximal or submaximal exercise test depends on the reasons for the test, the type of subject to be tested, and the availability of the appropriate equipment and personnel (28). Direct measurement of expired gases during maximal-effort exercise yields the most accurate determination of VO_2max; however, it is costly (in terms of equipment), requires specially trained personnel, and tends to be time-consuming (4). Thus, direct measurement of VO_2max is generally reserved for the research or clinical setting, while the vast majority of health/fitness facilities utilize submaximal tests to estimate VO_2max and assess cardiorespiratory fitness.

The basic aim of submaximal exercise testing is to determine the relationship between a subject's heart rate response and his or her VO_2 during progressive exercise, and then to use that relationship to predict VO_2max (4). To accurately determine this relationship, heart rate and VO_2 need to be measured at two or more submaximal exercise intensities.

Any of the GXT protocols can be used for submaximal or maximal testing (ie, bike ergometer, treadmill, bench)—the only difference is the criteria for stopping the test. Either test should be terminated if any of the abnormal responses listed in *Box 10.1* occur. In the absence of abnormal responses, the submaximal test is usually terminated when the person reaches a predetermined heart rate (typically 85% of predicted maximum heart rate reserve), and the maximal test is terminated when the person reaches a stage of voluntary exhaustion (10).

BOX 10.1   Contraindications to Exercise Testing

Absolute Contraindications

- A recent significant change in the resting ECG suggesting infarction or other acute cardiac event
- Recent complicated myocardial infarction (unless patient is stable and pain-free)
- Unstable angina
- Uncontrolled ventricular arrhythmia
- Uncontrolled atrial arrhythmia that compromises cardiac function
- Third degree atrial-ventricular heart block without pacemaker
- Acute congestive heart failure
- Severe aortic stenosis
- Suspected or known dissecting aneurysm
- Active or suspected myocarditis or pericarditis
- Thrombophlebitis or intracardiac thrombi
- Recent systemic or pulmonary embolus
- Acute infections
- Significant emotional distress (psychosis)

Relative Contraindications

- Resting diastolic blood pressure >115 mm Hg or resting systolic blood pressure >200 mm Hg
- Moderate valvular heart disease
- Known electrolyte abnormalities (hypokalemia, hypomagnesemia)
- Fixed-rate pacemaker (rarely used)
- Frequent or complex ventricular ectopy
- Ventricular aneurysm
- Uncontrolled metabolic disease (eg, diabetes, thryotoxicosis, or myxedema)
- Chronic infectious disease (eg, mononucleosis, hepatitis, AIDS)
- Neuromuscular, musculoskeletal, or rheumatoid disorders that are exacerbated by exercise
- Advanced or complicated pregnancy

Source: American College of Sports Medicine. *Guidelines for Exercise Testing and Prescription.* 5th ed. Media, Penn: Williams and Wilkins; 1996. Reprinted with permission.

Use of Subjective Ratings Scales

A valuable parameter for determining exercise intensity and monitoring individual tolerance to an exercise load is a subjective measure of effort level known formally as the "rating of perceived exertion" (RPE) (4,29). RPE is frequently used when conducting a GXT and has been shown to be significantly and positively correlated with measured exercise heart rates and calculated oxygen consumption (4). The original RPE scale developed by Borg (30) was based on a scale of 6 to 20 (roughly based on resting to maximal heart rate (ie, 60 to 200 bpm) (10). A revised and simplified scale of 0 to 10 has been developed which is easier for most individuals to understand or interpret and, thus, provides the tester with more valid information to further direct the GXT (31). While both scales account for the linear increase in VO$_2$ and heart rate during exercise, the revised scale also considers the nonlinear responses of variables such as blood lactic acid accumulation and ventilation (see *Table 10.1*). It has been found that a cardiorespiratory training effect and the threshold for blood lactate accumulation are achieved at a rating of "somewhat hard" or "hard," which corresponds to a rating of 13 to 16 on the original scale or 6 to 8 on the revised scale (4,29).

TABLE 10.1 Original and Revised Scales for Ratings of Perceived Exertion (RPE)

Original Scale		Revised Scale	
6		0	Nothing at all
7	Very, very light	0.5	Very, very weak
8		1	Very weak
9	Very light	2	Weak
10		3	Moderate
11	Fairly light	4	Somewhat strong
12		5	Strong
13	Somewhat hard	6	
14		7	Very strong
15	Hard	8	
16		9	
17	Very hard	10	Very, very strong
18			Maximal
19	Very, very hard		
20			

Source: American College of Sports Medicine. *Guidelines for Exercise Testing and Prescription.* 5th ed. Media, Penn: Williams and Wilkins; 1996. Reprinted with permission.

GXT Guidelines, Measures, and Termination Criteria

Healthy young individuals (men ≤40 years of age and women ≤50 years of age) can usually begin a moderate or vigorous exercise program without a GXT (4). Older individuals (men >40 years and women >50 years) can begin a moderate exercise program without a GXT; however, they should undergo a complete medical evaluation including a GXT prior to starting a vigorous exercise program (4). In addition, all individuals, regardless of age, who demonstrate signs or symptoms suggestive of cardiopulmonary disease and/or have known cardiac, pulmonary, or metabolic disease should have a complete medical exam and clinical GXT (with a physician present) prior to exercise participation (4). The American College of Sports Medicine (ACSM) guidelines for exercise testing are listed in *Table 8.2* in Chapter 8, Health Screening and Medical Evaluation.

As previously described, a resting (pre-exercise) heart rate (HR) and BP should be obtained during the period immediately preceeding the GXT. Additionally, HR, BP, and RPE should be obtained at regular intervals during the GXT (typically every 3 minutes or at least once during each stage of the test). During the recovery period (ie, approximately 3 to 5 minutes of low-intensity exercise), HR and BP measures should be taken at 1- to 2- minute intervals (4,10).

The criteria for test termination depend on the testing protocol used. That is, a maximal test is terminated when oxygen uptake plateaus and does not increase with a further increase in workload or the subject reaches volitional exhaustion (20); while submaximal testing often uses a predetermined criteria for termination, typically 85% of predicted maximal heart rate reserve (max HRR) (ie, [max HRR – RHR] x .85). Occasionally, however, the test should be terminated prior to the aforementioned end-points. The indications for terminating a GXT are outlined in *Box 10.1*. For more specific termination criteria, consult *ACSM's Guidelines for Exercise Testing and Prescription* (4).

When the graded exercise test is completed, the following information should be included in the laboratory report: .

- Pre-exercise heart rate and blood pressure
- Maximum exercise level achieved and the energy cost of the maximum workload
- Heart rate and blood pressure at each stage of the test
- Heart rate and blood pressure during recovery
- ECG abnormalities noted on the pre-exercise recording, at any test stage, and during recovery
- Any symptoms that occurred during the testing period, and the test stage at which they appeared
- Reason for termination of the test (eg, target achieved, symptoms, volitional exhaustion, ECG findings)
- Test interpretations, including risks and the likelihood of disease, and any relevant findings and their significance

This information can then be used in client education and exercise prescription.

Additional Cardiorespiratory-related Measures

Power. By definition, power is work produced per unit of time and can be expressed as force (f) times distance (d) divided by time (t):

$$p = \frac{f \times d}{t}$$

Power, therefore, is a combination of both speed and strength, and refers to the rate at which one performs work (32).

Some simple anaerobic tests for power consist of running up a flight of stairs or timing a 50-yard dash with a 15-yard running start (32). Tests (such as the Wingate Anaerobic Test) have been developed to measure peak power, mean power, and rate of fatigue by using a predetermined force to produce a supramaximal effort (32).

Anaerobic threshold. The anaerobic threshold occurs when the ventilatory response during graded exercise is no longer linear (25). The physiological mechanism behind anaerobic threshold is not fully understood. It usually occurs close to the work rate at which blood lactic acid concentrations start to accumulate. Regular exercisers may perceive anaerobic threshold as the exercise intensity at which breathing and talking become somewhat difficult. In most individuals the onset of blood lactic acid accumulation is a marker for determining the upper end of the intensity range for "aerobic" exercise programs (10). Fitness programs emphasizing aerobic exercise will want exercise intensity to be below the anaerobic threshold to prevent the rapid accumulation of lactic acid, which usually causes discomfort and necessitates an earlier termination of the exercise.

Lactate threshold. The lactate threshold occurs when the relatively constant blood lactate level observed during graded exercise suddenly increases. Endurance training programs can increase the lactate threshold, thereby delaying fatigue (10).

Metabolic equivalents (METS). METS are often used to measure the workload at various stages of a graded exercise test. One MET is equal to the resting oxygen consumption of the "average human" and equals 3.5 mL/kg/min or approximately 1 kcal/kg per hour of oxygen consumed. The following formula can be used to determine the MET level for a particular exercise (4):

$$\text{METs} = \frac{\text{oxygen required for exercise}}{\text{oxygen required at rest (3.5 mL/kg/min)}}$$

Healthy, sedentary people can usually exercise up to 10 to 12 METS, while well-conditioned athletes often exercise above 15 METS (32). See the Tools section for more information on METs.

MUSCULAR STRENGTH AND ENDURANCE

Muscular strength and endurance are important components of both physical fitness and overall health. Development and maintenance of muscular strength and endurance help to preserve functional capacity and attenuate the loss of FFM and bone density that often accompanies advancing age (33). In addition, since skeletal muscle is more metabolically active than fat tissue, development of muscle mass via strength training will cause a corresponding increase in resting metabolic rate, which is an important factor in the prevention and management of obesity (33). Finally, improvements in muscular strength and endurance can improve personal appearance and self-esteem (4).

Muscular strength can be defined as the maximum amount of force that can be exerted by a muscle, while muscular endurance is the ability of a muscle to exert a force repeatedly over a period of time (10). Because of the interrelationship between muscular strength and endurance, an increase in one of these components usually results in some degree of improvement in the other. The assessment of muscular strength and endurance is reviewed in-depth elsewhere (10,33,34) and will be addressed only briefly here.

Muscular strength. Static or isometric muscle strength can be conveniently measured using a variety of devices including cable tensiometers and handgrip dynamometers (4,33). Unfortunately, measures of static strength are specific both to the muscle group and joint angle involved in testing and, therefore, their utility in assessing overall muscular strength is limited. Dynamic strength measures provide a more comprehensive test of muscular strength and involve movement of the body or an external load. The most common measures of dynamic strength involve various 1-repetition maximum (1-RM) weightlifting tests, defined as the heaviest weight that can be lifted only once. Isokinetic strength testing involves the assessment of muscle tension generated throughout a range of joint motion at a constant angular velocity. Equipment that allows control of the speed of joint rotation (degrees/second) as well as physical adjustability to test movement around various joints (eg, knee, hip, shoulder, elbow) is available from several commercial sources; however, it is extremely expensive compared to other strength-testing modalities (4,33).

Muscular endurance. Simple field tests such as the 60-second sit-up test or the maximum number of push-ups that can be performed without rest may be used to evaluate the endurance of the abdominal muscle groups and upper body muscles, respectively (4,33). Methods of administration and age- and gender-specific percentile norms for these tests have been published (35). Resistance training and isokinetic equipment can also be adapted to measure muscular endurance by selecting an appropriate submaximal level of resistance and measuring the number of repetitions or duration of static contraction before fatigue (4). For example, the YMCA bench-press test involves performing standardized repetitions at a rate of 30 per second using an 80-lb (men) or 30-lb (women) weight (35).

FLEXIBILITY

Flexibility is the maximum ability to move a joint through a range of motion. A number of specific variables influence flexibility including distensibility of the joint capsule, muscle temperature, muscle viscosity, and others. Additionally, compliance ("tightness") of various other tissues, such as ligaments and tendons, affects the range of motion (ROM) (4,36). Having functional ROM at all joints of the musculoskeletal system is desirable to ensure efficient body movement. In addition, increasing evidence suggests that improving flexibility can enhance muscular performance and, perhaps, aid in the prevention and treatment of musculoskeletal injuries (27). The assessment of flexibility has been reviewed in detail by Protas (36) and Corbin (37). In general, assessment of flexibility is not complicated and can be done with minimal equipment (tape and measuring stick) and cost. The most common flexibility test used for mass screening is the "sit-and-reach" (trunk flexion) test (4).

EXERCISE PRESCRIPTION

The fundamental objective of exercise prescription is the successful integration of exercise principles with behavioral techniques to promote long-term program compliance and the attainment of personal fitness goals. A comprehensive exercise prescription should include the appropriate mode(s), intensity, duration, frequency, and progression of physical activity (4). These five components apply regardless of the client's age, functional capacity, or risk factors for disease; however, each should be adjusted to meet the individual's needs, goals, motivation, and initial fitness level. Prior to giving the client an exercise prescription, the health professional should obtain information on his or her medical history, current health, and fitness (38). Even though a GXT is not required for all individuals prior to beginning an exercise program, the exercise prescription should be developed with careful consideration of the individual's health status including risk factor profile and medications currently being taken (38).

Aerobic activity should be a major part of the exercise prescription because of its association with cardiovascular fitness (ie, VO_2max and prevention of cardiovascular disease) (2,5,39,40). The most common aerobic activities are walking, jogging, cycling, swimming, stepping, rowing, aerobic dancing, or some combination of these. Clearly, this wide range of activities provides ample individual variability in terms of skill level and enjoyment factors that are paramount to exercise program compliance and desired outcomes (4). The ACSM provides the following exercise recommendations for improving cardiorespiratory fitness (27):

- Frequency of training: 3 to 5 days per week
- Intensity of training: 55%/65% to 90% of maximum HR or 40%/50% to 85% of maximum oxygen uptake reserve (VO_2 reserve) of maximum HRR. The lower intensity values (ie, 40% to 49% of VO_2 or HRR and 55% to 64% of maximum HR) are most applicable to individuals who are very unfit.
- Duration of training: 20 to 60 minutes of continuous or intermittent (minimum of 10-minute bouts accumulated throughout the day) aerobic activity. Duration is highly dependent on the intensity of the activity; thus, lower-intensity exercise should be conducted over a longer period of time ($\geq$30 minutes), while higher-intensity exercise can be conducted over a slightly shorter time period (>20 minutes).

These recommendations, particularly those regarding the intensity of exercise, are necessary for individuals wishing to improve their VO_2max. However, it should be stressed that research has shown that exercise of lower intensity may promote significant health benefits and decrease one's risk of chronic disease (5,6,41). Moreover, because of the potential hazards and adherence problems associated with high-intensity activity, moderate-intensity activity of longer duration and greater frequency is probably more appropriate for adults not training for athletic competition (27).

Resistance training should also be an integral part of any adult fitness program. The resistance training prescription should include exercises for all major muscle groups, be progressive in nature, and be of sufficient intensity to enhance muscular strength and endurance and maintain FFM and bone density (27,42).

One set (8 to 12 repetitions) of 8 to 10 exercises that condition the major muscle groups performed 2 to 3 days per week is the general recommendation. However, multiple set regimens and/or varying numbers of repetitions performed with more frequency may provide greater and/or more specific (ie, muscular strength versus muscular endurance) benefits (27,42).

Flexibility exercises sufficient to develop and maintain optimal range of motion should also be incorporated into the overall fitness program (27). A well-rounded stretching program should include exercises for all the major muscle/tendon groups. At least four repetitions per muscle/tendon group should be performed at a minimum of 2 to 3 days per week (27).

An effective physical activity program should include methods for keeping clients motivated and preventing relapse to their more sedentary, and potentially unhealthy, habits. Strategies aimed at making exercise more enjoyable should be emphasized and periodic follow-ups for fitness assessment, positive reinforcement, and permanent lifestyle change should be encouraged (32).

REFERENCES

1. *Surgeon General's Report on Physical Activity and Health.* Washington, DC: US Dept of Agriculture Health and Human Services; 1988. DHHS (PHS) publication 88-50210.
2. Pate RR, Pratt M, Blair SN, Haskell WL, Marcera CA, Bouchard C. Physical activity and public health: a recommendation from the Centers for Disease Control and Prevention and the American College of Sports Medicine. *JAMA.* 1995;273:402-407.
3. National Institutes of Health Consensus Development Conference. *Physical Activity and Cardiovascular Health.* Rockville, Md; 1996.
4. American College of Sports Medicine. *Guidelines for Exercise Testing and Prescription.* 5th ed. Media, Penn: Williams and Wilkins; 1995.
5. Blair SN, Kohl HW III, Barlow CE, Paffenbarger RS Jr, Gibbons LW, Marcera CA. Changes in physical fitness and all-cause mortality. *JAMA.* 1995;273:1093-1098.
6. Bouchard C, Shephard RJ, Stephens T, eds. *Physical Activity, Fitness, and Health: International Proceedings and Consensus Statement.* Champaign, Ill: Human Kinetics; 1994.
7. Roitman JL, ed. *Resource Manual for Guidelines for Exercise Testing and Prescription.* 3rd ed. Baltimore, Md: Williams and Wilkins; 1988.
8. Going SB. Densitomitry. In: Roche AF, Heymsfield SB, Lohman TG, eds. *Human Body Composition.* Champaign, Ill: Human Kinetics Publishers Inc; 1996:1-24.
9. Lohman TG, Houtkooper L, Going SB. Body fat measurement goes high-tech: not all are created equal. *ACSM's Health and Fitness Journal.* 1997;1:30-35.
10. Howley ET, Franks BD. *Health Fitness Instructor's Handbook.* Champaign, Ill: Human Kinetics; 1997.
11. Lohman TG. Dual energy X-ray absorptiometry. In: Roche AF, Heymsfield SB, Lohman TG, eds. *Human Body Composition.* Champaign, Ill: Human Kinetics; 1996:63-78.
12. Gibson RS. *Principles of Nutritional Assessment.* New York: Oxford University Press; 1990.
13. National Institutes of Health and National Heart, Lung, and Blood Institute. *Clinical Guidelines on the Identification, Evaluation, and Treatment of Overweight and Obesity in Adults.* Bethesda, Md; 1998.
14. Bjorntorp P. Abdominal fat distribution and disease: an overview of epidemiological data. *Ann Med.* 1992;24:15-28.

15. Kissebah AH, Vydelingum N, Murray R, et al. Relation of body fat distribution to metabolic complications of obesity. *J Clin Edocrin Metab*. 1982;54:254-260.

16. Van Itallie TB. Topography of body fat: relationship to risk of cardiovascular and other diseases. In: Lohman TG, Roche AF, Martorell R, eds. *Anthropometric Standardization Reference Manual*. Champaign, Ill: Human Kinetics; 1988.

17. Walton C, Lees B, Crook D, Worthington M, Godsland IF, Stevenson JC. Body fat distribution, rather than overall adiposity, influences serum lipids and lipoproteins in healthy men independently of age. *Am J Med*. 1995;99:459-464.

18. Bray GA. Pathophysiology of obesity. *Am J Clin Nutr*. 1992;55:488S-494S.

19. Baumgartner RN. Electrical impedance and total body electrical conductivity. In: Roche AF, Heymsfield SB, Lohman TG, eds. *Human Body Composition*. Champaign, Ill: Human Kinetics; 1996:79-108.

20. Heyward V. *Advanced Fitness Assessment and Exercise Prescription*. 2nd ed. Champaign, Ill: Human Kinetics; 1991.

21. McArdle WD, Katch FL, Katch VL. *Exercise Physiology, Energy, Nutrition, and Human Performance*. 4th ed. Baltimore, Md: Williams and Wilkins; 1996.

22. Pollock ML, Wilmore JH. *Exercise in Health and Disease: Evaluation and Prescription for Prevention and Rehabilitation*. 2nd ed. Philadelphia, Penn: W B Saunders Co; 1990.

23. Astrand PO, Rodahl K. *Textbook of Work Physiology*. 3rd ed. New York, NY: McGraw-Hill; 1986.

24. National Institutes of Health and National Heart, Lung, and Blood Institute. *The Fifth Report of the Joint Committee on Detection, Evaluation, and Treatment of High Blood Pressure*. Bethesda, Md: National Institutes of Health; 1995.

25. Franklin BA. Normal cardiorespiratory responses to acute aerobic exercise. In: Roitman JL, ed. *Resource Manual for Guidelines for Exercise Testing and Prescription*. 3rd ed. Baltimore, Md: Williams and Wilkins; 1998:137-145.

26. Franklin BA, Roitman JL. Cardiorespiratory adaptations to exercise. In: Roitman JL, ed. *Resource Manual for Guidelines for Exercise Testing and Prescription*. 3rd ed. Baltimore, Md: Williams and Wilkins; 1998:156-163.

27. American College of Sports Medicine. Position stand: the recommended quantity and quality of exercise for developing and maintaining cardiorespiratory and muscular fitness, and flexibility in healthy adults. *Med Sci Sports Exerc*. 1998;30:975-991.

28. McConnell TR. Cardiorespiratory assessment of apparently health populations. In: Roitman JL, ed. *Resource Manual for Guidelines for Exercise Testing and Prescription*. 3rd ed. Baltimore, Md: Williams and Wilkins; 1998:347-351.

29. Carton RL, Rhodes EC. A critical review of the literature on ratings scales for perceived exertion. *Sports Med*. 1985;2:198-222.

30. Borg G. Perceived exertion as an indicator of somatic stress. *Scand J Rehabil Med*. 1970;2:92-98.

31. Borg G. Psychophysical bases of perceived exertion. *Med Sci Sports Exerc*. 1982;14:377-381.

32. Nieman DC. *Fitness and Your Health*. Palo Alto, Calif: Bull Publishing Co; 1993.

33. Graves JE, Pollock ML, Bryant CX. Assessment of muscular strength and endurance. In: Roitman JL, ed. *Resource Manual for Guidelines for Exercise Testing and Prescription*. 3rd ed. Baltimore, Md: Williams and Wilkins; 1998:363-367.

34. Skinner JS, Oja P. Laboratory and field tests for assessing health-related fitness. In: Bouchard C, Shephard RJ, Stephens T, eds. *Physical Activity, Fitness, and Health: International Proceedings and Consensus Statement*. Champaign, Ill: Human Kinetics; 1994:160-179.

35. Golding LA, Myers CR, Sinning WE, eds. *Y's Way to Physical Fitness*. 3rd ed. Champaign, Ill: Human Kinetics; 1989.

36. Protas EJ. Flexibility and range of motion. In: Roitman JL, ed. *Resource Manual for Guidelines for Exercise Testing and Prescription*. 3rd ed. Baltimore, Md: Williams and Wilkins; 1998:368-377.

37. Corbin C. Flexibility. *Clin Sports Med.* 1984;3:101-117.
38. Gordon NF. Pre-participation health appraisal in the non-medical setting. In: Roitman JL, ed. *Resource Manual for Guidelines for Exercise Testing and Prescription.* 3rd ed. Baltimore, Md: Williams and Wilkins; 1998:341-346.
39. Holly RG, Shaffrath JD. Cardiorespiratory endurance. In: Roitman JL, ed. *Resource Manual for Guidelines for Exercise Testing and Prescription.* 3rd ed. Baltimore, Md: Williams and Wilkins; 1998:437-447.
40. Lee CD, Blair SN, Jackson AS. Cardiorespiratory fitness, body composition, and all-cause cardiovascular mortality in men. *Am J Clin Nutr.* 1996;68:373-380.
41. Shephard RJ. How much physical activity is needed for good health? *Int J Sports Med.* 1999;20:23-27.
42. Bryant CX, Peterson JA, Graves JE. Muscular strength and endurance. In: Roitman JL, ed. *Resource Manual for Guidelines for Exercise Testing and Prescription.* 3rd ed. Baltimore, Md: Williams and Wilkins; 1998:448-455.

ASSESSMENT OF BODY SIZE AND COMPOSITION

Christopher M. Modlesky, MA and Richard D. Lewis, PhD, RD

The body is an elaborate structure consisting of many components that change with growth, development, and aging. Monitoring these changes assists health professionals in their assessment of nutritional status, physical fitness, and physical performance. Specifically, measurement of body size allows for tracking the changes in the physical dimensions of the body, while measurement of body composition allows for following changes in its gross chemical composition (ie, fat and fat-free mass). Excess body weight, especially in the form of body fat often reflects high caloric intake and reduced levels of physical activity, and can contribute to poor physical performance. Adiposity is also believed to contribute to disease risk, since it is positively associated with cardiovascular disease, diabetes mellitus, and other chronic diseases (1). Extremely low body weight and low body fat reflect diseased states associated with under-nutrition, such as anorexia nervosa. The purpose of this chapter is to review the application and measurement of body size and body composition.

ASSESSMENT OF BODY SIZE

There are advantages and disadvantages associated with being a particular body size, which are evident in different sports. Taller people tend to be successful in sports where reaching a level high above the ground is required, such as basketball and volleyball. Shorter people may have an advantage in sports that require rotation of the body around an axis, such as tumbling in gymnastics. Within a sport a particular position may dictate a size advantage. In football a large body weight is advantageous to offensive linemen, giving them the size and power to move players in their path. Conversely, wide receivers tend to be much lighter, allowing them to run at great speeds.

Size, specifically body weight, has also been negatively associated with health. Because of the inverse relationship between body weight and longevity, and the strong societal and cultural pressure for a thinner, leaner body, the search for an ideal or desirable body weight has followed.

Height-Weight Tables

Defining an ideal body weight for a population might seem simple; however, such a task is likely impossible. Insurance companies and other organizations have attempted to present ideal body weights through the development of height-weight tables that provide gross weight range estimates for given heights associated with the greatest longevity and the lowest mortality rate (2). They are used to compare the body weight of an individual to a reference population or a standard believed to be ideal. Using the standard or ideal, individuals who are over- or underweight can be identified. Studies conducted by insurance companies and the American Cancer Society (3) have concluded that, in general, non-smokers with body weights 80% to 89% of average tend to live longer than individuals with average or above-average body weight (4). While this observation has been supported by reports from the Framingham Heart Study (5) and other large-scale studies, height-weight tables have undergone scrutiny, particularly during recent years.

Two of the most commonly used height-weight tables were developed by the Metropolitan Life Insurance Company in 1959 (6) and 1983 (7). The 1959 and 1983 tables were developed using the weight ranges of individuals with the lowest mortality rates in the Build and Blood Pressure Study 1959 and the Build Study 1979 (7,8), respectively. Although widely used, the Metropolitan tables have been criticized for a variety of reasons (8,9), including:

- They were developed using a sample that was not representative of the total population, consisting primarily of upper- and middle-class white males without the chronic diseases prevalent in the obese.
- If a person held a life insurance policy with more than one insurance company included in the study, that person was represented more than once in the sample.
- Twenty percent of the heights and weights used to develop the 1959 Metropolitan tables and 10% of those used to develop the 1983 tables were self-reported, and individuals who were actually measured wore shoes and clothes.
- Frame size, which is used in the tables to determine an individual's appropriate weight range, was not actually measured in the samples.

In addition to the problems shared by the 1959 and 1983 tables, the 1983 table gave weight ranges 2% to 13% higher than the older table, with the greatest discrepancy at the shorter heights. For instance, using the 1959 table a weight range of 99 to 107 lb is suggested for a small-framed woman 61 in tall, whereas the 1983 table suggests a weight range of 106 to 118 lb. Conversely, suggested weight ranges for a small-framed woman 72 in tall are very similar (138 to 148 lb versus 138 to 151 lb).

In 1973 a modification of the 1959 Metropolitan table was presented at the Fogarty International Center Conference on Obesity held at the National Institutes of Health (NIH), and in 1985 NIH released a modification of the 1983 Metropolitan tables. Both modifications excluded frame size and recalculated the data from Metropolitan tables to express height without shoes and weight without clothes.

In 1990 the US Department of Agriculture (USDA) released a height-weight table representing healthy weight ranges for adults (10). The USDA table was different from others because it gave one weight range for both men and women. Furthermore, it gave higher weight ranges for people 35 years of age and older, which prompted criticism by some obesity experts (11). Although some reports suggest that with increasing age weights associated with a lower risk of mortality are higher (12), the latest table released by the USDA in 1995 eliminated the higher weight recommendations for those 35 years of age and older (13) (see the Tools section).

Because of the uncertainty surrounding the height-weight tables, it is difficult to recommend the use of one particular table. Even if one set of weight ranges more accurately predicts optimal health than the other ranges, they all suffer from the inability to assess body composition and body fat distribution (9). Therefore, in some instances healthy individuals who are highly muscular might be considered overweight and at risk for disease, whereas individuals with high amounts of body fat but body weights in the desirable range would be considered at low risk for mortality. Despite the many flaws associated with height-weight tables, they are often used in conjunction with other markers of disease risk, such as diet, blood lipid profile, and anthropometric measurements, to identify those at risk for chronic disease.

Body Mass Index

Body mass index (BMI) is another measure of body size based on height and weight used to assess disease risk. In people with a BMI >20 kg/m^2, morbidity for many health conditions increases as BMI increases (14). Similar to height-weight tables, there are several versions of BMI that are commonly used. The most widely accepted BMI is the Quetelet Index in which weight (kg) is divided by height^2 (m^2). BMI can also be calculated as follows:

$$BMI = [weight (lb)/height (in)^2] \times 704.5$$

or by using *Tables 11.1A* and *11.1B*. Some advantages to using BMI rather than height-weight tables are:

- It is moderately correlated with percent body fat (r = 0.58) (15).
- It is a single value that can be readily used for comparisons among men, women, children, and individuals of different heights.
- It is associated with conditions detrimental to health.

TABLE 11.1A   Body Mass Index (BMI) at Specific Heights and Weights

Height (inches)	Body Weight (lb)																	
58	91	96	100	105	110	115	119	124	129	134	138	143	148	153	158	162	167	172
59	94	99	104	109	114	119	124	128	133	138	143	148	153	158	163	168	173	178
60	97	102	107	112	118	123	128	133	138	143	148	153	158	163	168	174	179	184
61	100	106	111	116	122	127	132	137	143	148	153	158	164	169	174	180	185	190
62	104	109	115	120	126	131	136	142	147	153	158	164	169	175	180	186	191	196
63	107	113	118	124	130	135	141	146	152	158	163	169	175	180	186	191	197	203
64	110	116	122	128	134	140	145	151	157	163	169	174	180	186	192	197	204	209
65	114	120	126	132	138	144	150	156	162	168	174	180	186	192	198	204	210	216
66	118	124	130	136	142	148	155	161	167	173	179	186	192	198	204	210	216	223
67	121	127	134	140	146	153	159	166	172	178	185	191	198	204	211	217	223	230
68	125	131	138	144	151	158	164	171	177	184	190	197	203	210	216	223	230	236
69	128	135	142	146	155	162	169	176	182	189	196	203	209	216	223	230	236	243
70	132	139	146	153	160	167	174	181	188	195	202	209	216	222	229	236	243	250
71	136	143	150	157	165	172	179	186	193	200	208	215	222	229	236	243	250	257
72	140	147	154	162	169	177	184	191	199	206	213	221	228	235	242	250	258	265
73	144	151	159	166	174	182	189	197	204	212	219	227	235	242	250	257	265	272
74	148	155	163	171	179	186	194	202	210	218	225	233	241	249	256	264	272	280
75	152	160	168	176	184	192	200	208	216	224	232	240	248	256	264	272	279	287
76	156	164	172	180	189	197	205	213	221	230	238	246	254	263	271	279	287	295
BMI (kg/m^2)	19	20	21	22	23	24	25	26	27	28	29	30	31	32	33	34	35	36

TABLE 11.1B   Body Mass Index (BMI) at Specific Heights and Weights

Height (inches)	Body Weight (lb)																	
58	177	181	186	191	196	201	205	210	215	220	224	229	234	239	244	248	253	258
59	183	188	193	198	203	208	212	217	222	227	232	237	242	247	252	257	262	267
60	189	194	199	204	209	215	220	225	230	235	240	245	250	255	261	266	271	276
61	195	201	206	211	217	222	227	232	238	243	248	254	259	264	269	275	280	285
62	202	207	213	218	224	229	235	240	246	251	256	262	267	273	278	284	289	295
63	208	214	220	225	231	237	242	248	254	259	265	270	278	282	287	293	299	304
64	215	221	227	232	238	244	250	256	262	267	273	279	285	291	296	302	308	314
65	222	228	234	240	246	252	258	264	270	276	282	288	294	300	306	312	318	324
66	229	235	241	247	253	260	266	272	278	284	291	297	303	309	315	322	328	334
67	236	242	249	255	261	268	274	280	287	293	299	306	312	319	325	331	338	344
BMI (kg/m^2)	37	38	39	40	41	42	43	44	45	46	47	48	49	50	51	52	53	54

continued

TABLE 11.1B   Body Mass Index (BMI) at Specific Heights and Weights (continued)

Height (inches)	Body Weight (lb)																	
68	243	249	256	262	269	276	282	289	295	302	308	315	322	328	335	341	348	354
69	250	257	263	270	277	284	291	297	304	311	318	324	331	338	345	351	358	365
70	257	264	271	278	285	292	299	306	313	320	327	334	341	348	355	362	369	376
71	265	272	279	286	293	301	308	315	322	329	338	343	351	358	365	372	379	386
72	272	279	287	294	302	309	316	324	331	338	346	353	361	368	375	383	390	397
73	280	288	295	302	310	318	325	333	340	348	355	363	371	378	386	393	401	408
74	287	295	303	311	319	326	334	342	350	358	365	373	381	389	396	404	412	420
75	295	303	311	319	327	335	343	351	359	367	375	383	391	399	407	415	423	431
76	304	312	320	328	336	344	353	361	369	377	385	394	402	410	418	426	435	443
BMI (kg/m²)	37	38	39	40	41	42	43	44	45	46	47	48	49	50	51	52	53	54

Several BMI ranges have been proposed to represent healthy body weights for the general population. Using data from the National Health and Nutrition Examination Survey (NHANES II), the National Center for Health Statistics defined overweight as the sex-specific 85th percentile of the BMI distribution of men and women 20 to 29 years of age (16). The BMI ranges that resulted are 20.7 to 27.8 kg/m² for men and 19.1 to 27.3 kg/m² for women. Other ranges recommended by different agencies are reported in *Table 11.2*.

TABLE 11.2   Body Mass Index (BMI) Ranges Recommended by Different Agencies

Agency	Sex	Age (years)	Recommended BMI (kg/m²)
National Center for Health and Statistics	Male	20-74	20.7-27.8
	Female	20-74	19.1-27.3
US Departments of Agriculture and Health and Human Services	Both	19-34	19-25
		≥35	21-27
National Academy of Sciences	Both	19-24	19-24
		25-34	20-25
		35-44	21-26
		45-54	22-27
		55-64	23-28
		≥65	24-29
World Health Organization	Both	Adult	20-25
Minister of National Health and Welfare Canada (Canadian)	Both	20–65	20-27

Adapted from: Sichieri R, Everhart JE, Hubbard VS. Relative weight classifications in the assessment of underweight and overweight in the United States. *Int J Obes.* 1992;16:303-312.

Similar to the enigma associated with height-weight tables, it is unclear which BMI ranges are most representative of optimal health. Furthermore, some studies suggest recommended BMI ranges should increase with age (12,17) and are affected by ethnicity (18,19). A study by Sichieri et al (17) examined the ability of the different BMI recommendations to detect morbidity and mortality. It concluded that the BMI ranges proposed by the National Academy of Sciences (NAS) performed the best in determining population-attributable risk for hospitalization and death. Interestingly, the recommended ranges proposed by NAS increase 1 kg/m^2 for every decade after 24 years of age. Likewise, some studies suggest the BMI-related increase in disease risk is 1 to 3 kg/m^2 higher in African-Americans than in whites (18,19).

As with height-weight tables, BMI is insensitive to varying degrees of fat mass, fat-free mass, and fat distribution (20), which may lead to inappropriate weight recommendations. For example, a very large, physically fit athlete standing 76 in (1.93 m) tall and weighing 250 lb (113.6 kg) with a very lean body (<10% fat) would have a BMI of 30.5 kg/m^2. Such a value would be considered overweight or obese by any BMI recommendations currently available. On the other hand, a sedentary woman with a poor diet and a high percent body fat standing 65 in (1.65 m) tall and weighing 140 lb (63.4 kg) would have an optimal BMI by any standard (23.4 kg/m^2). Similar to height-weight tables, BMI has limitations and should be used in conjunction with other markers when assessing health risk and making weight loss or weight gain recommendations.

Waist-to-Hip Ratio and Waist Circumference

Fat distribution has been identified as an important marker of disease risk (21,22), with those exhibiting a larger proportion of fat in the upper half of the body (android obesity or apple shape) being at greater risk for health complications than individuals having a larger proportion of fat in the lower half (gynoid obesity or pear shape). More specifically, deep abdominal (visceral) fat is a strong independent predictor of disease (21,22). Diseases associated with android obesity include hypertension, hypercholesterolemia, diabetes, cardiovascular disease, gallbladder disease, and death (23,24), with women also being at greater risk for oligomenorrhea (25) and breast cancer (26).

One of the easiest and most common assessments of body fat distribution and obesity type is waist-to-hip ratio (WHR). A higher WHR reflects android obesity and is associated with greater disease risk. Risk increases steeply when WHR is above 0.95 in men and 0.8 in women (27). Waist circumference is another simple measure used to assess deep abdominal fat and disease risk. The girth of the abdomen is highly correlated (r = 0.77 to 0.87) with deep abdominal fat measured using computed tomography, an expensive technique that provides precise measurement of deep and subcutaneous adipose tissue (21,22). Since waist circumference has been found to provide a better measure of deep abdominal fat than waist-to-hip ratio (21,22), its use is preferred when assessing risk of disease (14,22).

Federal Obesity Clinical Guidelines

While height-weight tables, BMI, and waist circumference each give some insight into disease risk, a combined approach can provide more definitive information. Accordingly, the National Heart, Lung, and Blood Institute (NHLBI) of the National Institutes of Health released guidelines on the identification, evaluation, and treatment of overweight and obesity in adults (14). They were developed based on an extensive review of the literature by a 24-member expert panel. Assessment of overweight and obesity involves three important measures: BMI; waist circumference; and risk factors for diseases and conditions associated with obesity. The guidelines identify overweight as a BMI of 25 to 29.9 kg/m^2 and obesity as a BMI of 30 kg/m^2 and greater. All clients ≥18 years of age with a BMI ≥25 kg/m^2 are considered at risk. Treament is recommended in overweight or obese clients with two or more risk factors (see *Table 11.3*) or a waist circumference greater than 40 in (102 cm) in men and greater than 35 in (88 cm) in women. Because waist circumference cutpoints lose their predictive power in clients with a BMI ≥35 kg/m^2, the guidelines are appropriate only for those with a BMI of 25 to 34.9 kg/m^2.

TABLE 11.3   Risk Factors to Consider before Recommending Obesity Treatment

Disease Conditions

- Established coronary disease
- Other atherosclerotic diseases (peripheral arterial disease, abdominal aortic aneurysm, symptomatic carotid artery disease)
- Type 2 diabetes mellitus
- Sleep apnea

Other Obesity-related Diseases

- Gynecological abnormalities
- Osteoarthritis
- Gallstones and their complications
- Stress incontinence

Cardiovascular Risk Factors

- Cigarette smoking
- Hypertension (systolic BP ≥ 140 mm Hg or diastolic BP ≥ 90 mm Hg, or patient is taking antihypertensive agents)
- High-risk LDL-cholesterol (≥160 mg/dL)
- Low HDL-cholesterol (<35 mg/dL)
- Impaired fasting glucose (110 to 125 mg/dL)
- Family history of premature CHD (definite myocardial infarction or sudden death at or before 55 years of age in father or other male first-degree relative, or at or before 65 years of age in mother or other female first-degree relative)
- Age (≥ 45 years and women ≥ 55 years or postmenopausal)

Other Risk Factors

- Physical inactivity
- High serum triglycerides (>200 mg/dL)

Adapted from: National Heart, Lung, and Blood Institute. *Clinical Guidelines on the Identification, Evaluation, and Treatment of Overweight and Obesity in Adults: The Evidence Report.* Washington, DC: National Institutes of Health. US Dept Health and Human Services; June 1998.

BODY SIZE MEASUREMENT TECHNIQUES

Standing Height

Standing height is one of the most fundamental physical measures used to quantify body size. In addition to being used in combination with body weight to screen for disease risk, it is used to detect growth deficiencies in children and skeletal diseases, such as osteoporosis, that lead to a significant reduction in standing height in the elderly.

Equipment. A stadiometer (a vertical measurement board or rod with a horizontal head piece) is often used (see *Figure 11.1*), following this procedure (28):

1. The client is measured while standing on a flat horizontal surface that is at a right angle to the stadiometer.
2. The client should wear as little clothing as possible to facilitate optimal body position, and should be barefoot or wearing thin socks.
3. The head, upper back (or shoulder blades), buttocks, and heels should be positioned against the vertical board or rod of the stadiometer. If a reasonable natural stance cannot be maintained while these body parts are touching the vertical board, the person can be positioned so that only the buttocks and heels or head are touching the board.
4. Weight should be distributed evenly on both feet with heels together, arms to the side, palms facing the thighs, legs straight, and the head in the Frankfort Horizontal Plane ("looking straight ahead").
5. Before measurement, a deep breath should be taken and held until the headpiece is pressed against the head (enough to compress the hair) and measurement is attained.
6. Measurement should be made to the nearest 0.5 cm or 0.125 in while viewing the measure at eye level to the headboard.

Measuring height using a tape measure against the wall is not recommended, but if done, a wall that is free of a base board and is not in contact with a carpeted floor should be chosen (28).

Recumbent Length

Recumbent length is measured in those unable to stand without assistance, such as infants or bedridden individuals.

Equipment. A recumbent length table (see *Figure 11.2*) is often used, following this procedure (28):

1. The client lies supine on the recumbent length table.
2. The body is positioned so that the top of the head touches the vertical headboard attached to the table and the center line of the body matches up with the center line of the table.
3. One measurer stands behind the end of the table with the vertical board and holds the head of the person being measured in the Frankfort Plane, perpendicular to the plane of the table.

FIGURE 11.1 Measurement of Standing Height Using a Stadiometer

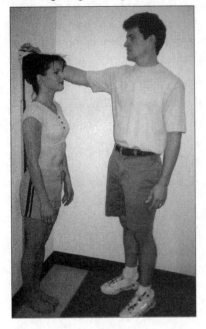

FIGURE 11.2 Measurement of Recumbent Length

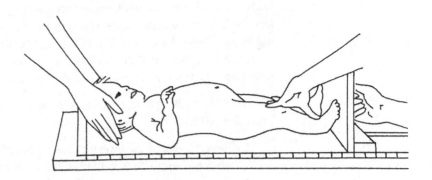

4. The shoulders and hips are at right angles to the long axis of the body, while the shoulders and buttocks are flat against the table.
5. A second measurer places one hand on the knees of the client to ensure the legs are flat against the table and uses the other hand to press the movable board against the heels of the feet.
6. Length is recorded to the nearest 0.5 cm or 0.125 in.

Body Weight

Body weight is another fundamental physical measure used to quantify body size. Periodic measurement of body weight is important because extremes are associated with nutritional, metabolic, and cardiovascular disorders. It is also used to calculate energy expenditure and body composition.

Equipment. A beam scale with movable weights is often used, following this procedure (28):

1. The scale should be on a hard, flat, horizontal surface.
2. Before measurement, the scale should be calibrated to zero.
3. It is important to calibrate the scale monthly or quarterly, and whenever the scale is moved. Measurement accuracy can be verified using standard weights.
4. Ideally, weight should be measured before consumption of the first meal and after the bladder has been emptied.
5. When measured, the client should be nude or wearing as little clothing as possible.
6. The client should stand still over the center of the scale platform with weight evenly distributed between both feet.
7. Weight is determined to the nearest 0.5 lb or 0.2 kg using the movable beam. Body weight in lb divided by 2.2 yields weight in kg (1 kg = 2.2 lb).

If the person being measured cannot stand without assistance, a beam chair scale or a bed scale can be used. When measuring an infant, a leveled pan scale with a pan at least 100 cm in length is recommended (28).

Body Circumference

Body circumference measurements are used to estimate muscularity (29), fat patterning (30), nutritional status, changes in the physical dimensions of a child during growth, and changes in adults during weight-loss programs. When combined with skinfold thickness, circumference measurements can also estimate adipose tissue and the underlying muscle and bone (30).

Equipment. A flexible but inelastic tape measure is often used, following this procedure (30):

1. The zero end of the tape measure is held in the left hand while the other end of the tape is held in the right hand.
2. The areas being measured should be free of clothing or covered by as little clothing as possible.
3. All circumference measurements, other than the head and neck, should be taken with the plane of the tape around the body part perpendicular to the long axis of the segment being measured.
4. When measuring the head the tape should compress the hair and the soft tissue of the scalp. For all circumference measurements other than the head, the tape should be snug but not tight enough to compress the soft tissue.
5. Measurements should be recorded to the nearest 0.5 cm or 0.125 in.

Circumference measurements of the head, neck, mid-upper arm, wrist, chest, waist, abdomen, hips, buttocks, and thigh are found in *Figures 11.3 to 11.13.*

FIGURE 11.3   Head circumference is taken just above the eyebrows and posteriorly so that maximum circumference is measured.

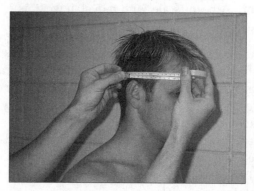

FIGURE 11.4   Neck circumference taken just below the laryngeal prominence (Adam's Apple) with the head in the Frankfort Horizontal Plane (looking straight ahead)

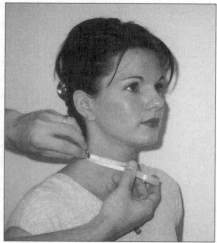

FIGURE 11.5 Midarm circumference of the upper arm taken midway between the acromion process of the scapula and the olecranon process of the ulna

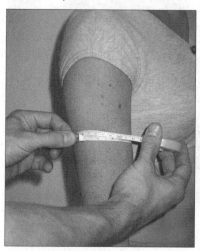

FIGURE 11.6 Wrist circumference is measured just distal to the styloid processes of the radius and ulna.

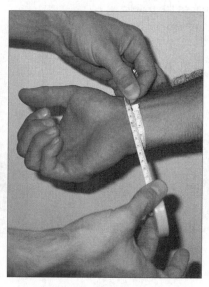

FIGURE 11.7 Chest circumference taken horizontally at the 4th costosternal joints (at the level of the 6th ribs), after normal expiration

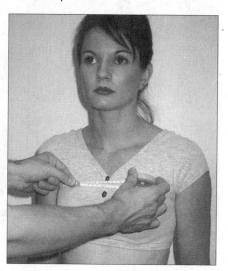

FIGURE 11.8 Waist circumference taken at the smallest circumference of the torso. Abdomen circumference, rather than waist circumference, is used to calculate waist-to-hip ratio.

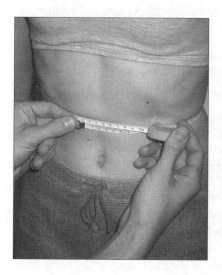

FIGURE 11.9 Abdomen circumference taken at the maximal circumference of the abdomen. This measurement, not waist circumference, is used to calculate waist-to-hip ratio.

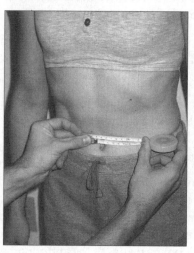

FIGURE 11.10 Hip (buttocks) circumference taken over the maximal circumference of the buttocks

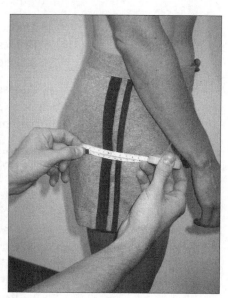

FIGURE 11.11   Proximal thigh circumference taken horizontally, just distal to the gluteal fold

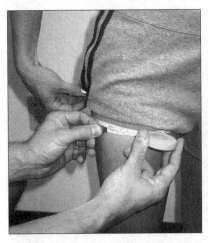

FIGURE 11.12   Midthigh circumference taken midway between the inguinal crease and the proximal border of the patella

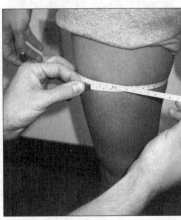

FIGURE 11.13   Distal thigh circumference taken just proximal to the femoral epicondyles

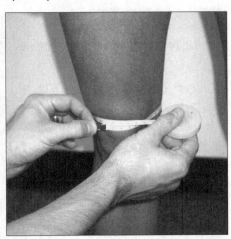

Body Breadth

Body breadth measurements are useful in the determination of body type and frame size (31). Somatotyping is one body typing technique in which body breadths, along with circumference measures, are used to categorize individuals into three distinct categories:

1. Endomorph: relative fatness and leanness
2. Mesomorph: relative musculoskeletal development per unit of height
3. Ectomorph: relative linearity

Assessing frame size can help determine desirable weight for a given height and can help determine appropriate lean weight gains in athletes and the malnourished.

Procedure.   A standard anthropometer, sliding caliper, or spreading caliper may be used, following this procedure (31):

1. The client being measured should wear as little clothing as possible to facilitate identification of measurement sites.
2. Using the tips of the fingers, identify the bony landmarks of the area to be measured.
3. Using both hands, hold the anthropometer or caliper so that the tips of the index fingers are adjacent to the projecting blades.
4. Position the blades of the anthropometer or sliding caliper at the bony landmarks.
5. Apply enough pressure to the blades so that the underlying skin, fat, and muscle contribute minimally to the measurement.
6. Measurements are made to the nearest 0.1 cm or 0.125 in.

To minimize experimenter bias, measurements should be made sequentially, such that all sites are measured once and then the sequence is repeated until a minimum of three measurements are made at each site. The average measurement at each site is recorded.

Proper measurement of the elbow and ankle breadth is demonstrated in *Figures 11.14* and *11.15*. Elbow breadth, regarded as the best marker of frame size, can also be measured using a Frameter (9) (see *Figure 11.16*). Frame size can be categorized using *Table 11.4*, which was developed based on NHANES I and NHANES II data sets (32).

FIGURE 11.14 Standard anthropometer used for measuring elbow breadth. Measurement is taken at the epicondyles of the humerus.

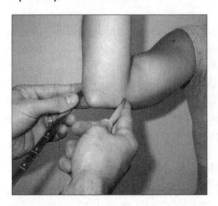

FIGURE 11.15 Measurement of ankle breadth using a spreading caliper taken at the maximum distance between the most medial extension of the medial malleolus and the most lateral extension of the lateral malleolus in the same horizontal plane.

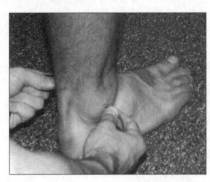

FIGURE 11.16 Elbow Breadth Measured Using a Frameter

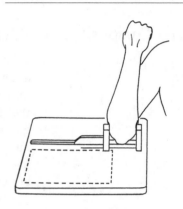

TABLE 11.4 Frame Size by Elbow Breadth (cm) of US Male and Female Adults*

Age (years)	Frame Size		
Males	Small	Medium	Large
18-24	≤6.6	>6.6 and <7.7	≥7.7
25-34	≤6.7	>6.7 and <7.9	≥7.9
35-44	≤6.7	>6.7 and <8.0	≥8.0
45-54	≤6.7	>6.7 and <8.1	≥8.1
55-64	≤6.7	>6.7 and <8.1	≥8.1
65-74	≤6.7	>6.7 and <8.1	≥8.1
Females			
18-24	≤5.6	>5.6 and <6.5	≥6.5
25-34	≤5.7	>5.7 and <6.8	≥6.8
35-44	≤5.7	>5.7 and <7.1	≥7.1
45-54	≤5.7	>5.7 and <7.2	≥7.2
55-64	≤5.8	>5.8 and <7.2	≥7.2
65-74	≤5.8	>5.8 and <7.2	≥7.2

*Derived from NHANES I and II combined data sets

Adapted from: Frisancho R. New standards of weight and body composition by frame size and height for assessment of nutritional status of adults and the elderly. *Am J Clin Nutr.* 1984;40:806-819.

ASSESSMENT OF BODY COMPOSITION

While height-weight charts and BMI are used to determine appropriate weights and to assess disease risk, they have poor sensitivity for classifying body composition (9,20). Body composition, the relative amount of fat and other gross chemical constituents within the body, is affected by age, gender, race, genetics, diet, activity, and environmental factors (20). Higher degrees of total body fatness are believed to be related to increased disease risk (33).

Body Composition and Disease Risk

While many of the adverse conditions associated with obesity are linked to excess amounts of total body fatness (33), the actual contribution has yet to be determined. The reason for such a lack of understanding of such a compelling issue is that large, prospective, epidemiological randomized studies that use the most accurate techniques to assess body composition have yet to be conducted (20). Further, causal associations with chronic diseases likely take years to detect, making it unclear whether changes in body composition precede or follow the onset of disease (20).

Because of the uncertainty surrounding the role of total body fatness in disease risk, the development of standards has been difficult. According to Lohman (34), the mean percent body fat is 15% in men and 25% in women. Body fat values of 10% to 22% in men and 20% to 32% in women are generally considered satisfactory (34). However, the data supporting these values have not been clearly defined, such as for BMI and waist circumference cutpoints described in the Federal Obesity Clinical Guidelines. Until more research examining the relationship between body composition and disease risk is conducted, the use of percent body fat as a marker of health risk is limited.

Body Composition and Performance

Body composition is related to athletic success, especially in sports that require translocation of the body horizontally (ie, running) or vertically (ie, jumping) (35). In these instances, excess body fat is deleterious because it adds to the load (ie, body mass) without contributing to the body's force-producing capacity. Furthermore, a greater metabolic cost is incurred, limiting prolonged performance (36-38). Specific body composition recommendations for athletes have yet to be determined; however, several studies have reported mean body fat percentages for different athletic groups (39-68). A summation of some of these reports is found in *Table 11.5* (69). These body fat percentages should not be viewed as recommended values of percent body fat, but as percentages that have been observed in elite athletes.

TABLE 11.5 Summary of Body Composition Characteristics of Athletes (Means ± SD)

Sport/specialty	Gender	N	Age (years)	Height (cm)	Weight (kg)	% Body Fat	Source
Ballet	F	34	21.9 ± 4.3	168.0 ± 6.8	54.4 ± 6.0	16.9 ± 4.7	Calabrese et al (39)
Baseball and Softball							
• Baseball	M	—	27.4	183.1	88.0	12.6	Wilmore (40)
• Softball	F	14	22.6 ± 4.1	167.1 ± 6.1	59.6 ± 5.8	19.1 ± 5.0	Withers et al (41)
Basketball	F	49	19.3 ± 1.4	176.5 ± 8.8	66.8 ± 6.7	19.2 ± 4.6	Walsh et al (42)
	M	10	20.9 ± 1.3	194.3 ± 10.2	87.5 ± 7.2	10.5 ± 3.8	Siders et al (43)
Bicycling	M	11	22.2 ± 3.6	176.4 ± 7.1	68.5 ± 6.4	10.5 ± 2.4	Withers et al (44)
Field Events							
• Decathlon	M	3	22.5 ± 2.2	186.3 ± 1.4	84.1 ± 9.2	8.4 ± 5.1	Withers et al (44)
• Pentathlon	F	9	21.5 ± 3.1	175.4 ± 3.0	65.4 ± 5.7	11.0 ± 3.3	Krahenbuhl et al (45)
• Throwing	F	9	18.8 ± 3.0	173.9 ± 6.9	80.8 ± 21.1	27.0 ± 8.4	Wilmore et al (46)
• Discus	M	7	28.3 ± 5.0	186.1 ± 2.6	104.7 ± 13.2	16.4 ± 4.3	Fahey et al (47)
• Shot	M	5	27.0 ± 3.9	188.2 ± 3.6	112.5 ± 7.3	16.5 ± 4.3	Fahey et al (47)
• Jumping	F	13	17.4 ± 0.9	173.6 ± 8.0	57.1 ± 6.0	12.9 ± 2.5	Thorland et al (48)
	M	16	17.6 ± 0.8	181.7 ± 6.1	69.2 ± 7.2	8.5 ± 2.1	Thorland et al (48)
Field Hockey	F	13	19.8 ± 1.4	159.8 ± 5.5	58.1 ± 6.6	21.3 ± 7.2	Sinning and Wilson (49)
Football							
• Defensive backs	M	26	24.5 ± 3.2	182.5 ± 4.5	84.8 ± 5.2	9.6 ± 4.2	Wilmore et al (50)
• Offensive backs and wide receivers	M	40	24.7 ± 3.0	183.8 ± 4.1	90.7 ± 8.4	9.4 ± 4.0	
• Line backers	M	28	24.2 ± 2.4	188.6 ± 2.9	102.2 ± 6.3	14.0 ± 4.6	
• Offensive line	M	38	24.7 ± 3.2	193.0 ± 3.5	112.6 ± 6.8	15.6 ± 3.8	
• Defensive line	M	32	25.7 ± 3.4	192.4 ± 6.5	117.1 ± 10.3	18.2 ± 5.4	
• Quarterbacks	M	16	24.1 ± 2.7	185.0 ± 5.4	90.1 ± 11.3	14.4 ± 6.5	
Gymnastics	F	26	19.7	158 ± 1.1	54.1 ± 1.2	17.0 ± 0.5	Kirchner et al (51)
	M	19	—	168.7 ± 6.7	65.8 ± 4.3	6.5 ± 2.4	Sinning et al (52)
Lacrosse	F	17	24.4 ± 4.5	166.3 ± 7.5	60.6 ± 7.3	19.3 ± 5.7	Withers et al (41)
	M	26	26.7 ± 4.2	177.6 ± 5.5	74.0 ± 8.6	12.3 ± 4.3	Withers et al (44)
Orienteering	M	7	25.9 ± 8.5	176.2 ± 6.8	64.7 ± 5.0	10.7 ± 2.9	Withers et al (44)
Racket Sports							
• Badminton	F	6	23.0 ± 5.3	167.7 ± 2.5	61.5 ± 2.6	21.0 ± 2.1	Withers et al (41)
	M	7	24.5 ± 3.6	180.0 ± 5.2	71.2 ± 5.6	12.8 ± 3.1	Withers et al (44)
• Tennis	F	7	21.3 ± 0.9	164.7 ± 4.2	59.6 ± 4.6	22.4 ± 2.0	Sinning and Wilson (49)
	M	9	—	179.1 ± 4.5	73.8 ± 7.3	11.3 ± 5.2	Sinning et al (52)
• Squash	M	9	22.6 ± 6.8	177.5 ± 4.1	71.9 ± 8.3	11.2 ± 3.7	Withers et al (44)
Skating							
• Ice hockey	M	27	24.9 ± 3.6	182.9 ± 6.1	85.6 ± 7.1	9.2 ± 4.6	Agre et al (53)

continued

TABLE 11.5   Summary of Body Composition Characteristics of Athletes (Means ± SD) (continued)

Sport/specialty	Gender	N	Age (years)	Height (cm)	Weight (kg)	% Body Fat	Source
• Speed skating	F	9	19.7 ± 3.0	165.0 ± 6.0	61.2 ± 6.9	16.5 ± 4.1	Pollock et al (54)
	M	6	22.2 ± 4.1	178.0 ± 7.1	73.3 ± 7.1	7.4 ± 2.5	Pollock et al (54)
Skiing (Nordic)	F	5	23.5 ± 4.7	164.5 ± 3.3	56.9 ± 1.1	16.1 ± 1.6	Sinning et al (55)
	M	11	22.8 ± 1.9	179.0 ± 5.0	71.8 ± 5.4	7.2 ± 1.9	Sinning et al (55)
Soccer	F	11	22.1 ± 4.1	164.9 ± 5.6	61.2 ± 8.6	22.0 ± 6.8	Withers et al (41)
	M	19	—	176.8 ± 6.6	72.4 ± 8.9	9.5 ± 4.9	Sinning et al (52)
Swimming	F	9	13.5 ± 0.9	164.5 ± 7.4	53.3 ± 5.3	17.2 ± 3.6	Meleski et al (56)
	F	13	16.4 ± 0.9	168.8 ± 7.1	57.9 ± 5.5	15.6 ± 4.0	
	F	19	19.2 ± 0.8	169.6 ± 4.7	56.0 ± 3.1	16.1 ± 3.7	
	M	27	—	178.3 ± 6.4	71.0 ± 5.9	8.8 ± 3.2	Sinning et al (52)
Track Events							
• Distance runners	F	15	27	161.0 ± 4.0	47.2 ± 4.0	14.3 ± 3.3	Graves et al (57)
	M	20	—	177.0 ± 6.0	63.1 ± 4.8	4.7 ± 3.1	Pollock et al (58)
• Sprinters and hurdlers	F	8	15.9 ± 2.7	166.5 ± 9.3	54.0 ± 8.4	10.9 ± 3.6	Wilmore et al (46)
	M	5	28.4 ± 0.1	179.9 ± 0.7	66.8 ± 0.9	8.3 ± 5.2	Withers et al (44)
• Walkers	F	4	24.9 ± 6.3	163.4 ± 3.9	51.7 ± 4.8	18.1 ± 4.4	Withers et al (41)
	M	3	20.3 ± 2.0	178.4 ± 2.1	66.1 ± 1.8	7.3 ± 1.3	Withers et al (44)
• Masters runners/walkers	M	11	40-49	180.7	63.1	4.7	Pollock et al (59)
	M	5	50-59	174.2	67.2	10.9	
	M	6	60-69	175.4	67.1	11.3	
	M	3	70.8	175.6	66.7	13.6	
Triathlon	F	16	24.2 ± 4.3	162.1 ± 6.3	55.2 ± 4.6	16.5 ± 1.4	Leake et al (60)
	M	14	36.0 ± 9.9	176.4 ± 8.6	73.3 ± 8.6	12.5 ± 5.9	Loftin et al (61)
Volleyball	F	14	21.6 ± 0.8	178.3 ± 4.2	70.5 ± 5.5	17.9 ± 3.6	Puhl et al (62)
	M	11	20.9 ± 3.7	185.3 ± 10.2	78.3 ± 12.0	9.8 ± 2.9	Withers et al (44)
Weightlifting and Bodybuilding							
• Olympic lift	M	10	30.1 ± 8.1	179.3 ± 6.1	91.3 ± 8.9	9.9 ± 1.9	Spitler et al (63)
• Power lift	F	10	25.2 ± 6.0	164.6 ± 3.7	68.6 ± 3.6	21.5 ± 1.3	Johnson et al (64)
	M	13	24.8 ± 1.6	173.5 ± 2.8	80.8 ± 3.2	9.1 ± 1.2	Katch et al (65)
• Bodybuilders	F	10	30.4 ± 8.2	165.2 ± 5.6	56.5 ± 0.9	13.5 ± 1.5	Johnson et al (64)
	M	18	27.8 ± 1.8	177.1 ± 1.1	82.4 ± 1.0	9.3 ± 0.8	Katch et al (65)
Wrestling							
• Adult	M	37	19.6 ± 1.34	174.6 ± 7.0	74.8 ± 12.2	8.8 ± 4.1	Sinning (66)
• Adolescent	M	409	16.2 ± 1.0	171.0 ± 7.1	63.2 ± 10.0	11.0 ± 4.0	Housh et al (67)
• Sumo	M	23	27.3 ± 1.1	178.8 ± 1.1	115.1 ± 4.2	27.3 ± 1.1	Kanehisa et al. (68)

Adapted from: Sinning WE. Body composition in athletes. In: Roche AF, Heymsfield SB, Lohman TG, eds. *Human Body Composition*. Champaign, Ill: Human Kinetics; 1996:257-273. Data rounded to 0.1. Reported SEMs converted to SD on the basis of sample size.

Because each athlete probably has a fat percentage and body weight at which he or she performs best, the values reported in *Table 11.5* may be too low for one athlete but suitable for another. A more appropriate use of body composition measurements is to identify the levels of fat and fat-free mass at which a particular athlete performs best. Body composition can also be used to monitor the health of an athlete and to track compositional changes following weight loss or gain during training. Often, when an athlete is trying to lose weight during a training period that incorporates resistance training, body weight may not change but an increase in fat-free mass and a decrease in fat mass are likely. Unless body composition is assessed, these positive changes may go unnoticed.

While body composition differs from one athlete to another, some athletes believe that extremely low levels of body fat are necessary for success in their sport. On the contrary, very low body fat levels can have deleterious effects on health and physical performance. Minimum levels have not been clearly defined for most sports, but body fat percentages below 5% in men and 12% in women are not recommended (70). In 1996 the American College of Sports Medicine (ACSM) released a position stand on weight loss in wrestlers (71). It recommended that males 16 years of age and younger with a body fat below 7% and those over 16 years of age with a body fat below 5% receive medical clearance before they compete. Body fat levels below 12% to 14% are not recommended in female wrestlers. Several skinfold equations considered appropriate for estimating percent body fat in male wrestlers (71) are reported by Thorland et al (72); however, the equations have not been validated using current criterion methods.

When considering minimum percent body fat values, bear in mind that error is associated with all methods of assessment. Under the best conditions, most methods have an error of 3% to 4% body mass (33,73). Therefore, a body fat percentage may actually be lower than reported. For example, a body fat of 13% may actually be 9% to 10 % or even lower, which is a dangerously low level in females. Because of the error associated with all body composition assessment techniques, it is more appropriate to recommend a percent body fat range rather than a specific percent body fat value (70).

BODY COMPOSITION MEASUREMENT TECHNIQUES

In its simplest form, body composition is based on a two-component model in which the body is divided into fat and fat-free mass. Fat mass includes nonessential and essential portions. Nonessential fat has been described as all fat stored within adipose tissue, while essential fat encompasses all other fat stores, including fat within the bone marrow, spinal cord, brain, and certain organs (74). The fat-free mass includes all substances that are not fat, primarily water, protein, and mineral. Muscle, skin, bone, connective tissue, and organs are the primary fat-free tissues.

Hydrodensitometry (Underwater Weighing)

The densitometric technique for body composition assessment relies upon the two-component model. Assuming the density of fat mass (~0.9 g/cm^3), fat-free mass (~1.1 g/cm^3), and the total body are known, the contribution of each component to the total can be calculated. Researchers and clinicians can determine body density by dividing body weight by body volume, which is typically measured using underwater weighing (water displacement). Based on these assumptions and the measurement of total body density, percent body fat can be calculated using equations developed by Siri (75) or Brozek (76) found in *Table 11.6*. Percent body fat equations based on three- and four-component models, also reported in *Table 11.6*, are discussed later in this chapter (see Criterion Methods of Body Composition).

TABLE 11.6 Percent Body Fat Equations Based on Two-, Three-, and Four-component Models

Model	Body Measurement(s)	Equation
Two-component[1]	density	% body fat = 495/D$_b$ − 450
Two-component[2]	density	% body fat = 457/D$_b$ − 414.2
Two-component	water	% body fat = $\left(\dfrac{\text{weight (kg)} - (\text{water (kg)}/.73)}{\text{weight (kg)}} \right) \times 100$
Three-component[3]	density and water	% body fat = (2.1176/D$_b$ − 0.78w − 1.351) × 100
Four-component[4]	density, water, and mineral	% body fat = (2.747/D$_b$ − 0.714w + 1.146m − 2.0503) × 100

D$_b$ = body density (g/cm^3)

w = water (kg)/weight (kg)

m = mineral (kg)/weight (kg)

[1]Siri WE. Body composition from fluid spaces and density: analysis of methods. In: Brozek J, Henschel A, eds. *Techniques for Measuring Body Composition.* Washington, DC: National Academy of Sciences; 1961:223-244.

[2]Brozek J, Grande F, Anderson JT, Keys A. Densitometric analysis of body composition: revision of some quantitative assumptions. *Annals of the New York Academy of Sciences.* 1963;110:113-140.

[3]Modlesky CM, Cureton KJ, Lewis RD, Prior BM, Sloniger MA, Rowe DA. Density of the fat-free mass and estimates of body composition in male weight trainers. *J Appl Physiol.* 1996;80(6):2085-2096.

[4]Lohman TG. Applicability of body composition techniques and constants for children and youths. In: Pandolf K, ed. *Exercise and Sports Science Reviews.* 14th ed. New York: Macmillian; 1986:325-357.

Until recently, underwater weighing was considered one of the gold standard techniques of body composition assessment against which all other methods were compared. Although measurements of body composition have become more sophisticated with multiple body components being examined (ie, water, mineral, protein, and fat), underwater weighing alone is still a good method of assessment. The technique is based on Archimedes' principle that a body immersed in a fluid is acted on by a buoyancy force equal to the volume of the fluid displaced (77). Because fat is less dense than fat-free tissue, a greater proportion of body fat will cause a person to be more buoyant (float) and weigh less in the water. Conversely, a greater proportion of fat-free tissue will cause the person to be less buoyant (sink) and weigh more in the water. This contrast is demonstrated in *Figure 11.17*. The clients are the same height and weight, but the client on the left has a higher body density and a lower percent body fat.

FIGURE 11.17 Underwater weighing of two men with the same height and weight but different degrees of density and fatness. The man on the left has a greater body density and lower percent body fat.

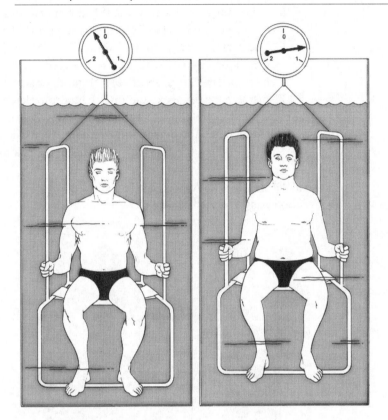

Equipment

1. Underwater weighing tank, pool, or hot tub 4- to 5-ft deep
2. 9 kg Chatillion autopsy scale with 10 g increments (A 15-kg scale with 25-g increments may be necessary for very obese subjects.)
3. Overhead beam or diving board from which the scale can hang
4. Chair (32 in wide with a back height of 24 in) made from 3/4 to 1 in plastic pipe with holes drilled in the pipe to avoid air entrapment
5. Weights to give the chair a minimum weight in the water of 3 kg (4 to 6 kg with the obese)
6. Thermometer to record the temperature of the water during measurement

Procedure (78)

1. The chair hangs from the scale into the tank.
2. The water in the tank should be filtered, chlorinated, 89° to 95°F (~32° to 35°C), and range from shoulder to chin height when the client is sitting in the chair.
3. When placed in the water, the chair minus the client should weigh at least 3 kg. A higher weight (4 to 6 kg) may be required for obese people. These weights can be obtained by adding weights to the chair.

4. The person should report to the clinic following a 2- to 3-hour fast of food and drink. Foods that can cause an excess amount of intestinal gas should be avoided.

5. Following a bowel movement and urinary void (if necessary), the person is weighed on land while wearing only a bathing suit.

6. The person is instructed to sit in the chair that is suspended from the Chatillion autopsy scale and submerged in the water. The feet should be positioned on the front bar of the chair which serves as a foot rest.

7. Just as a maximal exhalation is being completed, full submersion under the water is accomplished by slowly leaning forward. Upon submersion, the person must remain still in the chair with feet on the foot rest and hands on the side rails of the chair (see *Figure 11.18*).

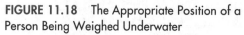

FIGURE 11.18   The Appropriate Position of a Person Being Weighed Underwater

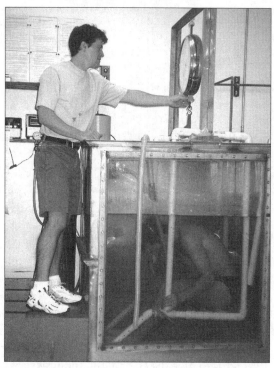

8. While underwater, the measurer should keep one hand on the scale to steady it and observe the weight of the person underwater to the nearest 10 g.

9. The test should be repeated 4 to 10 times until consistent readings are obtained.

10. During each trial, temperature of the water should be recorded.

11. The density of the water during measurement can be determined using *Table 11.7* (79).

TABLE 11.7   Water Density at Different Temperatures

Water Temperature (Celcius)	Water Density (g/cm³)
28	0.9962371
29	0.9959486
30	0.9956511
31	0.9953450
32	0.9950302
33	0.9947071
34	0.9943756
35	0.9940359

Adapted from: Lide DR ed. *Handbook of Physical Chemistry.* 76th ed. Boca Raton, Fla: CRC Press; 1998.

12. Because some air remains in the lungs following forced exhalation, the residual lung volume of air (RLV) must be measured or estimated (measurement is preferred). The RLV can be measured using nitrogen washout, oxygen dilution, or helium dilution techniques before, after, or during the underwater weighing procedure. Measurement during the procedure is preferred. Residual lung volume can be estimated using the following equations:

$$RLV_{males} = (0.017 \times age) + (0.06858 \times ht) - 3.447$$

$$RLV_{females} = (0.009 \times age) + (0.08128 \times ht) - 3.9$$

*age = age in years and ht = height in inches

13. Body density (D_b) is calculated using the following equation:

$$D_b = \frac{W_a}{\dfrac{(W_a - W_a)}{D_w} - (RLV + 100)}$$

*100 mL is an estimate of gastrointestinal volume
during underwater weighing
W_a = weight in air
W_w = weight in water
D_w is density of the water at the time of measurement

14. Percent body fat is calculated using the Siri (75) or Brozek (76) equation (see *Table 11.6*), which yield almost identical estimates of percent body fat.

The advantage of using underwater weighing to determine body fatness is that it has good accuracy and is an established technique. The accuracy of percent body fat from underwater weighing is approximately ± 4% in the general population (75) and ± 2.7% in the population from which the Siri and Brozek equations were developed (young white males) (80). Thus, in the general population, a 20%

estimate of fat from underwater weighing typically varies between 16% and 24%. While these equations yield reasonably accurate measurements, especially in young white males, the density of the fat-free mass can stray markedly in population groups other than young white males and result in larger error. For instance, children have been found to have a much lower density of the fat-free tissue than assumed (~1.086 g/cm^3 versus 1.1 g/cm^3), resulting in significant overestimation of percent body fat when the Siri or Brozek equations are used (81). In this instance, an equation developed specifically for children (81) would be more appropriate. Other equations have been proposed for African Americans (82), women (33), and individuals with extreme muscularity (83); however, more testing is needed to verify their validity.

Air Displacement Plethysmography (Bod Pod)

Another technique for determining body composition from body density is air displacement plethysmography. The Bod Pod Body Composition System (see *Figure 11.19*), a recently developed air displacement plethysmograph, appears to have overcome many of the problems experienced with its predecessors. The Bod Pod determines body volume from air displacement and percent body fat is calculated using the Siri and Brozek equations (see *Table 11.6*). The few studies that have examined the applicability of the Bod Pod suggest it provides estimates of body volume (84) and percent body fat (85,86) similar to underwater weighing. However, more research is needed to determine the validity of the Bod Pod for assessment of body composition in specific population groups, such as the elderly and children.

The advantages of using the Bod Pod for body composition assessment are

FIGURE 11.19   The Bod Pod Body Composition System assesses body fatness using air displacement plethysmography.

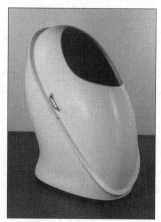

the lack of stress placed upon the client (no submersion in water or pinching required) and the minimal time required. Disadvantages of the Bod Pod are the high expense of the system, the large space required to house the chamber and other system components, and the limited research supporting its validity.

Skinfold Thickness

Skinfold thickness measurement is one of the most commonly used field methods for assessing body composition. The method is based on the assumptions that subcutaneous fat represents a certain proportion of the total body fat, and total subcutaneous fat can be accurately determined by measuring skinfold thickness at a few specific sites on the body.

FIGURE 11.20   Harpenden and Lange Skinfold Caliper Used for Assessing Skinfold Thickness

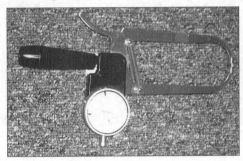
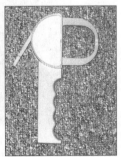

Procedure. Skinfold calipers that apply a constant pressure of 10 g/mm² are often used. Harpenden and Lange calipers are preferred (*Figure 11.20*). The following procedure is used (87).

1. Using anatomical landmarks and a tape measure when necessary, carefully identify the site to be measured.
2. The site should be felt prior to measurement.
3. Those with little experience may mark the site with a black felt pen.
4. Measurement sites for the 3 skinfold technique are the chest (*Figure 11.21*), abdomen (*Figure 11.22*), and thigh (*Figure 11.23*) in men, and the triceps (*Figure 11.24*), suprailium (*Figure 11.25*), and thigh in women.

FIGURE 11.21   Chest skinfold taken with the long axis of the fold directed to the nipple

FIGURE 11.22   Abdomen skinfold taken immediately lateral of the umbilicus

FIGURE 11.23   Midthigh skinfold taken midway between the inguinal crease and the proximal border of the patella

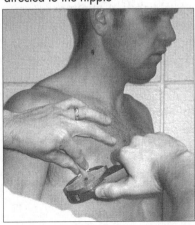
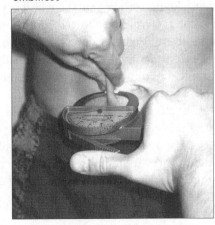
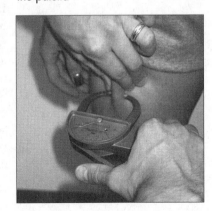

FIGURE 11.24   Triceps skinfold taken on the midline posterior surface of the arm over the triceps muscle, at the midpoint between the acromion process of the scapula and the olecranon process of the ulna

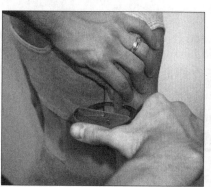

FIGURE 11.25   Suprailiac skinfold taken on the midaxillary line just superior to the iliac crest

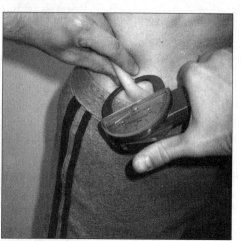

5. The skinfold is grabbed and elevated by the thumb and index finger of the left hand. The amount of tissue being grabbed must be able to form a fold with sides being approximately parallel.

6. Hold skinfold calipers in the right hand, with the heads perpendicular to the site being measured and the dial facing up. After opening the caliper arms with pressure, the caliper heads are applied to the fold and pressure is gradually released. The heads should be applied where the sides of the fold are parallel, approximately midway between the body site where the skinfold originates and the crest of the skinfold.

7. Read the dial to the nearest 1 mm approximately 4 seconds after the heads have been applied to the site. Waiting longer to observe the measurement causes smaller readings because fluids are forced from the tissues at the site.

8. After the measurement is read the calipers should be opened and then removed from the site.

9. A minimum of two measurements should be taken for each site. If the first two measurements vary by more than 1 mm, additional measurements should be taken until consistency is established. A minimum of 15 seconds should be allowed between measurements.

10. In the obese, it may be necessary to grab the skinfold with two hands while a partner measures the skinfold thickness. If the fold is too thick to apply the calipers, an alternative body composition method may be necessary.

11. Sites should not be measured when the skin is moist to avoid grabbing excess skin and elevating skinfold measures, or directly after exercise because body fluid shifts may increase the skinfold size.

12. When all sites are measured, adult percent body fat is determined using *Tables 11.8* and *11.9* (88), derived using skinfold equations developed by Jackson et al (89,90).

TABLE 11.8   Percent Fat Estimate for Men: Sum of Chest, Abdomen, and Thigh Skinfolds

Sum of Skinfolds (mm)	Age to Last Year								
	Under 22	23-27	28-32	33-37	38-42	43-47	48-52	53-57	Over 57
8-10	1.3	1.8	2.3	2.9	3.4	3.9	4.5	5.0	5.5
11-13	2.2	2.8	3.3	3.9	4.4	4.9	5.5	6.0	6.5
14-16	3.2	3.8	4.3	4.8	5.4	5.9	6.4	7.0	7.5
17-19	4.2	4.7	5.3	5.8	6.3	6.9	7.4	8.0	8.5
20-22	5.1	5.7	6.2	6.8	7.3	7.9	8.4	8.9	9.5
23-25	6.1	6.6	7.2	7.7	8.3	8.8	9.4	9.9	10.5
26-28	7.0	7.6	8.1	8.7	9.2	9.8	10.3	10.9	11.4
29-31	8.0	8.5	9.1	9.6	10.2	10.7	11.3	11.8	12.4
32-34	8.9	9.4	10.0	10.5	11.1	11.6	12.2	12.8	13.3
35-37	9.8	10.4	10.9	11.5	12.0	12.6	13.1	13.7	14.3
38-40	10.7	11.3	11.8	12.4	12.9	13.5	14.1	14.6	15.2
41-43	11.6	12.2	12.7	13.3	13.8	14.4	15.0	15.5	16.1
44-46	12.5	13.1	13.6	14.2	14.7	15.3	15.9	16.4	17.0
47-49	13.4	13.9	14.5	15.1	15.6	16.2	16.8	17.3	17.9
50-52	14.3	14.8	15.4	15.9	16.5	17.1	17.6	18.2	18.8
53-55	15.1	15.7	16.2	16.8	17.4	17.9	18.5	19.1	19.7
56-58	16.0	16.5	17.1	17.7	18.2	18.8	19.4	20.0	20.5
59-61	16.9	17.4	17.9	18.5	19.1	19.7	20.2	20.8	21.4
62-64	17.6	18.2	18.8	19.4	19.9	20.5	21.1	21.7	22.2
65-67	18.5	19.0	19.6	20.2	20.8	21.3	21.9	22.5	23.1
68-70	19.3	19.9	20.4	21.0	21.6	22.2	22.7	23.3	23.9
71-73	20.1	20.7	21.2	21.8	22.4	23.0	23.6	24.1	24.7
74-76	20.9	21.5	22.0	22.6	23.2	23.8	24.4	25.0	25.5
77-79	21.7	22.2	22.8	23.4	24.0	24.6	25.2	25.8	26.3
80-82	22.4	23.0	23.6	24.2	24.8	25.4	25.9	26.5	27.1
83-85	23.2	23.8	24.4	25.0	25.5	26.1	26.7	27.3	27.9
86-88	24.0	24.5	25.1	25.7	26.3	26.9	27.5	28.1	28.7
89-91	24.7	25.3	25.9	26.5	27.1	27.6	28.2	28.8	29.4
92-94	25.4	26.0	26.6	27.2	27.8	28.4	29.0	29.6	30.2
92-97	26.1	26.7	27.3	27.9	28.5	29.1	29.7	30.3	30.9
98-100	26.9	27.4	28.0	28.6	29.2	29.8	30.4	31.0	31.6
101-103	27.5	28.1	28.7	29.3	29.9	30.5	31.1	31.7	32.3
104-106	28.2	28.8	29.4	30.0	30.6	31.2	31.8	32.4	33.0
107-109	28.9	29.5	30.1	30.7	31.3	31.9	32.5	33.1	33.7
110-112	29.6	30.2	30.8	31.4	32.0	32.6	33.2	33.8	34.4
113-115	30.2	30.8	31.4	32.0	32.6	33.2	33.8	34.5	35.1
116-118	30.9	31.5	32.1	32.7	33.3	33.9	34.5	35.1	35.7
119-121	31.5	32.1	32.7	33.3	33.9	34.5	35.1	35.7	36.4
122-124	32.1	32.7	33.3	33.9	34.5	35.1	35.8	36.4	37.0
125-127	32.7	33.3	33.9	34.5	35.1	35.8	36.4	37.0	37.6

Adapted with permission from: Jackson AS, Pollock ML. Practical assessment of body composition. *Phys Sports Med.* 1985;13(5):76-90.

TABLE 11.9   Percent Fat Estimate for Women: Sum of Triceps, Suprailium, and Thigh Skinfolds

Sum of Skinfolds (mm)	Age to Last Year								
	Under 22	23-27	28-32	33-37	38-42	43-47	48-52	53-57	Over 57
23-25	9.7	9.9	10.2	10.4	10.7	10.9	11.2	11.4	11.7
26-28	11.0	11.2	11.5	11.7	12.0	12.3	12.5	12.7	13.0
29-31	12.3	12.5	12.8	13.0	13.3	13.5	13.8	14.0	14.3
32-34	13.6	13.8	14.0	14.3	14.5	14.8	15.0	15.3	15.5
35-37	14.8	15.0	15.3	15.5	15.8	16.0	16.3	16.5	16.8
38-40	16.0	16.3	16.5	16.7	17.0	17.2	17.5	17.7	18.0
41-43	17.2	17.4	17.7	17.9	18.2	18.4	18.7	18.9	19.2
44-46	18.3	18.6	18.8	19.1	19.3	19.6	19.8	20.1	20.3
47-49	19.5	19.7	20.0	20.2	20.5	20.7	21.0	21.2	21.5
50-52	20.6	20.8	21.1	21.3	21.6	21.8	22.1	22.3	22.6
53-55	21.7	21.9	22.1	22.4	22.6	22.9	23.1	23.4	23.6
56-58	22.7	23.0	23.2	23.4	23.7	23.9	24.2	24.4	24.7
59-61	23.7	24.0	24.2	24.5	24.7	25.0	25.2	25.5	25.7
62-64	24.7	25.0	25.2	25.5	25.7	26.0	26.7	26.4	26.7
65-67	25.7	25.9	26.2	26.4	26.7	26.9	27.2	27.4	27.7
68-70	26.6	26.9	27.1	27.4	27.6	27.9	28.1	28.4	28.6
71-73	27.5	27.8	28.0	28.3	28.5	28.8	29.0	29.3	29.5
74-76	28.4	28.7	28.9	29.2	29.4	29.7	29.9	30.2	30.4
77-79	29.3	29.5	29.8	30.0	30.3	30.5	30.8	31.0	31.3
80-82	30.1	30.4	30.6	30.9	31.1	31.4	31.6	31.9	32.1
83-85	30.9	31.2	31.4	31.7	31.9	32.2	32.4	32.7	32.9
86-88	31.7	32.0	32.2	32.5	32.7	32.9	33.2	33.4	33.7
89-91	32.5	32.7	33.0	33.2	33.5	33.7	33.9	34.2	34.4
92-94	33.2	33.4	33.7	33.9	34.2	34.4	34.7	34.9	35.2
95-97	33.9	34.1	34.4	34.6	34.9	35.1	35.4	35.6	35.9
98-100	34.6	34.8	35.1	35.3	35.5	35.8	36.0	36.3	36.5
101-103	35.3	35.4	35.7	35.9	36.2	36.4	36.7	36.9	37.2
104-106	35.8	36.1	36.3	36.6	36.8	37.1	37.3	37.5	37.8
107-109	36.4	36.7	36.9	37.1	37.4	37.6	37.9	38.1	38.4
110-112	37.0	37.2	37.5	37.7	38.0	38.2	38.5	38.7	38.9
113-115	37.5	37.8	38.0	38.2	38.5	38.7	39.0	39.2	39.5
116-118	38.0	38.3	38.5	38.8	39.0	39.3	39.5	39.7	40.0
119-121	38.5	38.7	39.0	39.2	39.5	39.7	40.0	40.2	40.5
122-124	39.0	39.2	39.4	39.7	39.9	40.2	40.4	40.7	40.9
125-127	39.4	39.6	39.9	40.1	40.4	40.6	40.9	41.1	41.4
128-130	39.8	40.0	40.3	40.5	40.8	41.0	41.3	41.5	41.8

Adapted with permission from: Jackson AS, Pollock ML. Practical assessment of body composition. *Phys Sports Med.* 1985;13(5):76-90.

Some advantages of using skinfolds to assess body composition include low expense, little space required to store the equipment, quick measurement, and reasonably accurate estimates of percent body fat. When population-specific equations are used, the accuracy of skinfold estimates of percent body fat is generally 3% to 4% body weight (80). One disadvantage of the skinfold technique is that subcutaneous fat may not represent a predictable proportion of the total body fat among and within different population groups. Furthermore, very few studies have examined the applicability of different skinfold equations using a multicomponent model as the criterion. In a recent study the validity of skinfold equations developed specifically for boys and girls (*Table 11.10*) (91) was questioned (92). Percent body fat estimates from the equations were approximately 3.5% body mass lower than estimates from a four-component model (a criterion method) in children 8 to 12 years of age (92).

TABLE 11.10   Percent Body Fat Estimates Using Skinfold Measurements

Boys (all ages)	Girls (all ages)
percent fat = 0.735 (SF) + 1.0	percent fat = 0.610 (SF) + 5.0

SF = triceps plus calf skinfolds

Adapted from: Slaughter MH, Lohman TG, Boileau RA, et al. Skinfold equations for estimation of body fatness in children and youth. *Human Biol.* 1988;60(5):709-723.

Hydrometry

Another technique that was considered a gold standard in body composition assessment is hydrometry. This technique also involves a two-component model in which water is assumed to represent ~73% of the body's fat-free component. Thus, a higher measure of body water indicates a higher amount of fat-free tissue. Total body water is measured by the dilution of a known quantity of nonmetabolizable tracer. A lower concentration of tracer after ingestion and equilibration (~3 to 4 hours) reflects a higher amount of body water and vice versa. The error associated with hydrometry is similar to that of underwater weighing.

Procedure. An infrared spectrophotometer or mass spectrophotometer is used, following this procedure (93,94):

1. The client reports to the clinic or laboratory following an overnight fast.
2. A baseline sample of body fluid (blood, urine, or saliva) is collected.
3. The client consumes a known quantity of the tracer, usually tritium or deuterium, that is mixed with water.
4. A 3- to 4-hour equilibration period follows to allow the tracer to distribute itself evenly throughout the body fluids. During this time the client must avoid food, drink, or physical exertion.
5. The equilibration period is followed by collection of a body fluid sample. Both samples are stored frozen.
6. The fluid is thawed and analyzed for tracer concentration using an infrared spectrophotometer or a mass spectrophotometer. A lower tracer concentration reflects a larger quantity of total body water and fat-free mass.

7. The body water measurement is reduced by 4% to correct for tracer binding to substances other than water (93).
8. Percent body fat can be calculated using the appropriate equation in *Table 11.6*.

The advantage of using body water to assess body composition is that it provides a good measure of body fatness in the general population. Body water is primarily used in research settings in combination with other body measures using a multicomponent approach to assessing body composition. The disadvantages of hydrometry are the long hours required to analyze the data and the exposure to body fluids. Furthermore, the water concentration of the fat-free component may vary from one population group to another. For instance, a child has a higher water concentration in the fat-free tissue than an adult. Thus, an equation developed for adults will overestimate percent body fat in children (81).

Bioelectrical Impedance Analysis (BIA)

The use of bioelectrical impedance analysis (BIA) to assess body composition has increased markedly during the past 10 years, especially in hospitals and field settings. The technique is based on the conductive and dielectric properties of different tissues within the body at different frequencies. Tissues that contain large amounts of fluid and electrolytes, such as blood, have high conductivity, whereas fat, bone, and lungs have high resistance or are dielectric (95,96). A small alternating current that is passed through the body (~500 to 800 µA), typically at a frequency of 50 kHz, will flow predominantly through tissue with higher conductivities. Bioelectrical impedance analysis determines the resistance to flow (impedance) of the current as it passes through the body. While it is generally believed that BIA measures body fat, it actually provides estimates of body water from which body fat is calculated using selected equations (96). The standard error of estimate of body water measurement from BIA is typically below 2 L (96).

FIGURE 11.26   Measurement of Body Composition Using Bioelectrical Impedance Analysis

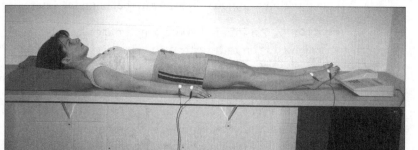

Procedure. A bioelectrical impedance analyzer is used, following this procedure using the Four-Electrode Technique (see *Figure 11.26*) (95,96):

1. Measurement occurs while the client is lying supine on a flat surface that is nonconductive, such as a bed or cot free of metal framing.
2. The head should be flat or supported by a thin pillow.

3. The arms are abducted slightly so they do not touch the trunk.
4. Legs are separated so that the ankles are at least 20 cm apart and the thighs are not touching.
5. The subject must be free of shoes, socks, and metallic jewelry.
6. The client and analyzer should be at least 50 cm from metallic objects and electronic equipment
7. The skin at each site is cleaned with alcohol before application of the electrodes.
8. Placement of electrodes is demonstrated in *Figure 11.27*. Electrodes are attached to the wrist (midway between the styloid processes), hand (at least 5 cm distal to the wrist electrode), ankle (midway between the malleoli), and foot (at least 5 cm distal to the ankle electrode).

FIGURE 11.27   Position of Electrodes when Assessing Body Composition Using Bioelectrical Impedance Analysis

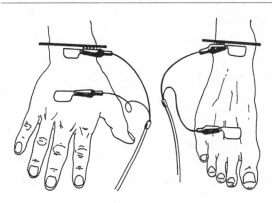

9. The source cable (black) is attached to the electrodes on the hand and foot. The source cable introduces the current to the client.
10. The sensing cable (red) is attached to the electrodes on the wrist and ankle.
11. An excitation current ranging from 500 to 800 µA at a frequency of 50 kHz is transmitted by the electrolytes within body fluids and impeded by the resistive tissues.
12. The electrical impedance of the tissues provides an estimate of total body water, from which fat-free and fat components are determined.

The advantages of using BIA to assess body composition are its convenience, ease of use, precise measurement, and relatively low expense. The disadvantages are its limited accuracy in the severely obese, its inability to accurately assess short-term changes in body composition, and the lack of validation studies using populations other than white European and North American non-Hispanic white subjects (96). Furthermore, the accuracy of body fat assessment may be compromised in very muscular athletes with disproportionately high concentrations of water in the fat-free mass, amputees, and those suffering from unilateral hemiparesis, edema, or tissue atrophy (96). Although body fat estimates from BIA can vary by as much as 10% of body mass due to differences in instrumentation and methodologies, most prediction errors for young adults are 5% or less (96).

It has been recommended that population-specific equations be used to reduce potential error associated with the BIA technique. Nevertheless, very few population-specific equations have been validated against the most recently accepted criterion techniques. Population-specific equations that have been validated using multicomponent models are reported in *Table 11.11* (33,97). More research examining the accuracy of body composition measures from BIA versus measures from multicomponent models are needed, particularly in specific population groups.

TABLE 11.11   Equations to Estimate Body Composition from Bioelectrical Impedance Analysis in Different Groups

Children and Youth (10-19 years of age)[1]

FFM (kg) = [0.61 height^2 ÷ resistance (ohms)] + 0.25 weight + 1.31

Women 18-35 years of age[2]

FFM (kg) = [0.666 height^2 ÷ resistance (ohms)] + 0.164 weight + 0.217 reactance − 8.78

Women 36-70 years of age[2]

FFM (kg) = [0.475 weight^2 ÷ resistance (ohms)] + 0.295 weight + 5.49

Males[2]

FFM (kg) = [0.485 height^2 ÷ resistance (ohms)] + 0.338 weight + 5.32

Height is measured in cm.

Weight is measured in kg.

FFM = fat-free mass

[1]Houtkooper LB, Going SB, Lohman TG, Roche AF, Van Loan M. Bioelectrical impedance estimation of fat-free body mass in children and youth: a cross validation study. *J Appl Physiol.* 1992;72:366-373.

[2]Lohman TG: *Advances in Body Composition Assessment.* Champaign, Ill: Human Kinetics; 1992.

Near Infrared Interactance (NIR)

Near infrared interactance (NIR) is based on the principles of light absorption and reflection. The method was originally developed to determine the amount of protein, water, and fat in agriculture products, which are assumed to have different bands of light absorption (98). The commercially available portable NIR device produced by Futrex uses a light probe with a silicon detector, two near-infrared diodes that emit light at a wavelength of 940 nm, and two near-infrared diodes that emit light at a wavelength of 950 nm. At a measurement site, typically the bicep, the intensity of light or optical density emitted at the different wavelengths is determined. The machine estimates body fat using the optical density at the two different wavelengths, body weight, height, gender, and activity level. The accuracy of NIR has been assessed using underwater weighing as the criterion with conflicting results. While few studies suggest NIR has reasonable accuracy (99), others suggest its use is problematic in children and adolescents (100), women (79), the obese (101,102), and collegiate football players (103). Discrepancies have also been found when different models of the instrument are used (104). Furthermore, the ability of NIR to detect changes in fat and fat-free mass has not been determined. In conclusion, NIR may be a promising method for assessing body composition; however, research to date suggests further development of this technology is necessary before it can be used with confidence.

Dual-energy X-ray Absorptiometry

Dual-energy x-ray absorptiometry (DXA), derived from single and dual photon absorptiometry, is one of the newest body composition technologies available. DXA was originally developed to measure bone mineral density (g/cm^2). The technology is based on the x-ray energy attenuation properties of bone mineral and soft tissue (105). X-ray energy transmitted through the client is attenuated (lost) in proportion to the material's composition and thickness, and thickness of the components within the material. Bone mineral, because it has a much higher density, attenuates an x-ray beam to a greater degree than soft tissue. Soft tissue is broken down further into fat and fat-free tissue based on their different attenuation properties. Measurements are made while the client is lying supine on the DXA table (*Figure 11.28*). Low dose x-rays are passed through the client in the posterior to anterior position. The x-rays pass from head to toe in 0.6- to 1.0-cm increments (106). Most total body scans require between 2.5 to 15.0 minutes depending upon the instrumentation. Up to 30 minutes may be required with larger subjects. When compared to body composition, estimates from a criterion four-component model, the accuracy appears to be as good as or slightly better than densitometry in college-aged athletes and nonathletes (SEE = 2.9%) (107) but is questionable in children (108,109) and the elderly (108,110). Although the scanning region of most DXA instruments is limited to approximately 6 ft in length, athletes can be assessed using a two-scan approach (111).

FIGURE 11.28   Dual-energy x-ray absorptiometry (DXA) is used to assess body composition and bone mineral density (g/cm^2). It is based on the different x-ray attenuation properties of fat mass, fat-free mass, and bone.

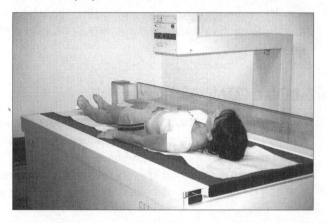

The advantages of using DXA for body composition measurement are:

- It provides three body components (bone mineral, fat-free soft tissue, and fat) versus two components from most other methods (fat and fat-free mass)
- It provides regional estimates of body composition (arms, legs, head, and trunk)
- The procedure is fairly quick, comfortable, and noninvasive.

The major disadvantages of DXA are the cost of the instrument and the space needed to house it.

CRITERION METHODS OF BODY COMPOSITION

Hydrodensitometry, based on a two-component model, was long considered the criterion method of body composition assessment against which all other techniques were judged. However, more elaborate multicomponent models are now considered the criterion of body composition assessment. There are basically two types of multicomponent models:

1. Elaborate models based on in vivo measurement of the elemental constituents within the body, using in vivo neutron activation analysis (IVNAA)
2. Simpler, less expensive chemical models based on the in vivo measurement of water and/or mineral (bone) and body density

Although IVNAA is the most accurate body composition technique, measuring percent body fat within 1% body mass (112), its extreme expense and radiation exposure limit its use and availability. Although not quite as accurate as the IVNAA multicomponent model, the simpler chemical multicomponent models are believed to be acceptable criterion methods, with the four-component chemical model measuring percent body fat within 1.5% body mass (112).

Three- and four-component models are most frequently used in body composition research. Percent fat equations based on the three- and four-component models are presented in *Table 11.6*. Although the four-component model involves measurement of more body components than the three-component model (ie, bone mineral), the added accuracy is minimal (83,113).

Despite the advances with multicomponent models, a paucity of studies has used them to assess the accuracy of body composition techniques that are simpler, less expensive, and more accessible (83,108-110,114,115). Until the simpler techniques are validated against these criterion methods, their accuracy will remain limited.

TIPS FOR MEASURING BODY COMPOSITION

- Clients should not exercise several hours before measurement.
- For many measurement techniques, clients should be adequately hydrated before measurement.
- Measurements that are included in the assessment, such as height and weight, should be performed as precisely and accurately as possible.
- When assessing changes in body composition, the same measurer using the same technique and instrument should perform measurements.
- Error associated with many methods of body composition assessment can be substantially larger when performed by an inexperienced measurer.
- Most methods for estimating body fat have an accuracy of 3% to 4% or greater under the best circumstances.
- Use population-specific equations to determine body fat when appropriate, especially equations that have been validated against a multi-component model.

REFERENCES

1. Bray GA. Complications of obesity. *Ann Intern Med.* 1985;103:1052-1062.
2. Robinett-Weiss N, Hixson ML, Keir B, Sieberg J. The metropolitan height-weight tables: perspectives for use. *J Am Diet Assoc.* 1984;84:1480-1481.
3. Lew EA, Garfinkel L. Variations in mortality by weight among 750,000 men and women. *J Chron Dis.* 1979;32:563-576.
4. Simopoulos AP. The health implications of overweight and obesity. *Nutr Rev.* 1985;43:33-40.
5. Garrison RJ, Feinleib M, Castelli WP, McNamara PM. Cigarette smoking as a confounder of the relationship between relative weight and long-term mortality. *JAMA.* 1983;249:2199-2203.
6. Metropolitan Life Insurance Company: new weight standards for men and women. *Stat Bull.* 1959;40:1-4.
7. 1983 Metropolitan height and weight tables. *Stat Bull.* 1983;64:9.
8. Knapp TR. A methodological critique of the 'ideal weight' concept. *JAMA.* 1983;250:506-510.
9. Frisancho RF. Nutritional anthropometry. *J Am Diet Assoc.* 1988;88(5):553-555.
10. *Nutrition and Your Health: Dietary Guidelines for Americans.* 3rd ed. Washington, DC: US Dept of Agriculture and US Dept of Health and Human Services; 1990. Home and Garden Bulletin No. 232.
11. Marwick C. Obesity experts say less weight still best. *JAMA.* 1993;269:2617-2618.
12. Andres R, Elahi D, Tobin JD, Muller DC, Brant L. Impact of age on weight goals. *Ann Intern Med.* 1985;103:1030-1033.
13. *Report of the Dietary Guidelines Advisory Committee on the Dietary Guidelines for Americans.* Washington, DC: U.S. Dept of Agriculture, Agriculture Research Service, and Dietary Guidelines Advisory Committee; 1995.
14. *Clinical Guidelines on the Identification, Evaluation, and Treatment of Overweight and Obesity in Adults: The Evidence Report.* Washington, DC: National Heart, Lung, and Blood Institute. National Institutes of Health. US Dept of Health and Human Services; June 1998.
15. Revicki DA, Israel RG. Relationship between body mass indices and measures of body adiposity. *Am J Public Health.* 1986;76:992-994.
16. Najjar MF, Rowland M. Anthropometric data and prevalance of overweight. In: *National Center for Health Statistics.* Hyattsville, Md: 1987:238-230.
17. Sichieri R, Everhart JE, Hubbard VS. Relative weight classifications in the assessment of underweight and overweight in the United States. *Int J Obes.* 1992;16:303-312.
18. Wienpahl J, Ragland DR, Sidney S. Body mass index and 15-year mortality in a cohort of black men and women. *J Clin Epidemiol.* 1990;43(9):949-960.
19. Durazo-Arvizu R, Cooper RS, Luke A, Prewitt TE, Liao Y, McGee DL. Relative weight and mortality in US blacks and whites: findings from representative national population samples. *Ann Epidemiol.* 1997;7:383-395.
20. Baumgartner RN, Heymsfield SB, Roche AF. Human body composition and the epidemiology of chronic disease. *Obes Res.* 1995;3:73-95.
21. Despres JP, Prud'homme D, Pouliot MC, Tremblay A, Bouchard C. Estimation of deep abdominal adipose tissue accumulation from simple anthropometric measurements in men. *Am J Clin Nutr.* 1991;54:471-477.
22. Pouliot MC, Despres JP, Lemieux S, et al. Waist circumference and abdominal sagital diameter: best simple anthropometric indexes of abdominal visceral adipose tissue accumulation and related cardiovascular risk in men and women. *Am J Cardiol.* 1994;73:460-468.

23. Larsson B, Svardsudd K, Welin L, Wilhelmsen L, Bjorntorp P, Tibblin G. Abdominal adipose tissue distribution, obesity, and risk of cardiovascular disease and death: 13-year follow-up of participants in the study of men born in 1913. *Br Med J.* 1984;288:1401-1404.

24. Wannamethee G, Shaper AG. Body weight and mortality in middle aged British men: impact of smoking. *Br Med J.* 1989;299:1497-1502.

25. Rimm AA, Hartz AJ, Fischer ME. A weight shape index for assessing risk of disease in 44,820 women. *J Clin Epidemiol.* 1988;41:459-465.

26. Shapira DV, Kumar NB, Lyman GH, Cox CE. Abdominal obesity and breast cancer risk. *Ann Intern Med.* 1990;112:182-186.

27. Ducimetiere RP, Cambien F, Avons P, Jacqueson A. Relationships between adiposity measurements and the incidence of coronary heart disease in a middle-aged male population—The Paris Prospective Study I. In: Vague J, Bjorntorp P, GuyGrand M, Rebuffe-Scrive M, Vague P, eds. *Metabolic Complications of Human Obesities.* Amsterdam: Elsevier; 1985:31-38.

28. Gordon CC, Chumlea WC, Roche AF. Stature, recumbent length, and weight. In: Lohman TG, Roche AF, Martorell R, eds. *Anthropometric Standardization Reference Manual.* Champaign, Ill: Human Kinetics; 1988:3-8.

29. Carter JEL, Heath BH. *Somatotyping—Development and Applications.* Cambridge, England: Cambridge University Press; 1990.

30. Callaway CW, Chumlea WC, Bouchard C, et al. Circumferences. In: Lohman TG, Roche AF, Martorell R, eds. *Anthropometric Standardization Reference Manual.* Champaign, Ill: Human Kinetics; 1988:39-54.

31. Wilmore JH, Frisancho RA, Gordon CC, et al. Body breadth equipment and measurement techniques. In: Lohman TG, Roche AF, Martorell R, eds. *Anthropometric Standardization Reference Manual.* Champaign, Ill: Human Kinetics; 1988:27-38.

32. Frisancho R. New standards of weight and body composition by frame size and height for assessment of nutritional status of adults and the elderly. *Am J Clin Nutr.* 1984;40:806-819.

33. Lohman TG. *Advances in Body Composition Assessment.* Champaign, Ill: Human Kinetics; 1992.

34. Lohman TG. Body composition methodology in sports medicine. *Phys Sports Med.* 1982;10(12):47-558.

35. Beunen G, Malina RM, Ostyn M, Renson R, Simons J, Van Gerven D. Fatness, growth, and motor fitness of Belgian boys 12 through 20 years of age. *Hum Biol.* 1983;55(3):599-613.

36. Cureton KJ, Sparling PB. Distance running performance and metabolic responses to running in men and women with excess weight experimentally equated. *Med Sci Sports Exerc.* 1980;12:288-294.

37. Cureton KJ, Sparling PB, Evans BW, Johnson SM, Kong UD, Purvis JW. Effect of experimental alterations in excess weight on aerobic capacity and distance running performance. *Med Sci Sports Exerc.* 1978;15:218-223.

38. Buskirk ER, Taylor HL. Maximal oxygen intake and its relation to body composition, with special reference to chronic physical activity and obesity. *J Appl Physiol.* 1957;11:72-78.

39. Calabrese LH, Kirkendall DT, Floyd M, et al. Menstrual abnormalities, nutrition patterns, and body composition in female classical ballet dancers. *Phys Sports Med.* 1983;11:86-89.

40. Wilmore JH. Body composition in sport and exercise: directions for future research. *Med Sci Sports Exerc.* 1983;15:21-31.

41. Withers RT, Whittingham NO, Norton KI, La Forgia J, Ellis MW, Crockett A. Relative body fat and anthropometric prediction of body density of female athletes. *Eur J Appl Physiol.* 1987;56:169-180.

42. Walsh FK, Heyward VH, Schau CG. Estimation of body composition of female inter-collegiate basketball players. *Phys Sports Med.* 1984;12:74-79.

43. Siders WA, Bolonchuk WA, Lukaski HC. Effects of participation in a collegiate sport season on body composition. *J Sports Med Phys Fitness.* 1991;31:571-576.

44. Withers RT, Craig NP, Bourbon PC, Norton KI. Relative body fat and anthropometric prediction of body density of male athletes. *Eur J Appl Physiol.* 1987;56:191-200.

45. Krahenbuhl GS, Wells CL, Brown CH, Wood PE. Characteristics of national and world class female pentathletes. *Med Sci Sports Exerc.* 1979;11:20-23.

46. Wilmore JH, Brown CH, Davis JA. Body physique and compostition of the female distance runner. *Ann N Y Acad Sci.* 1977;301:764-776.

47. Fahey TD, Akka L, Ralph R. Body composition and VO$_2$max of exceptional weight trained athletes. *J Appl Physiol.* 1975;39:559-561.

48. Thorland WG, Johnson GO, Fagot TG, Tharp GD, Hammer RW. Body composition and somatotype characteristics of junior olympic athletes. *Med Sci Sports Exerc.* 1981;13:332-338.

49. Sinning WE, Wilson JR. Validity of "generalized" equations for body composition analysis in women athletes. *Res Q Exerc Sport.* 1984;55:153-160.

50. Wilmore JH, Parr RB, Haskell WL. Football pro's strengths and CV weaknesses charted. *Phys Sports Med.* 1976;4:45-54.

51. Kirchner EM, Lewis RD, O'Connor PJ. Bone mineral density and dietary intake of female college gymnasts. *Med Sci Sports Exerc.* 1995;27(4):543-549.

52. Sinning WE, Dolny DG, Little KD, et al. Validity of generalized equations for body composition analysis in male athletes. *Med Sci Sports Exerc.* 1985;17:124-130.

53. Agre JC, Casal DC, Leon AS, McNally MC, Baxter TL, Serfass RC. Professional ice hockey players: physiologic, anthropometric, and musculoskeletal characteristics. *Arch Phys Med Rehab.* 1988;69:188-192.

54. Pollock ML, Pels AE III, Foster C, Holum D. Comparison of male and female speed-skating candidates. In: Landers DM, ed. *Sports and Elite Performance.* Champaign, Ill: Human Kinetics; 1986:143-152.

55. Sinning WE, Cunningham LN, Racaniello AP, Sholes JL. Body composition and somatotype of male and female Nordic skiers. *Res Q Exerc Sport.* 1977;48:741-749.

56. Meleski BW, Shoup RF, Malina RM. Size, physique, and body composition of competitive female swimmers 11 through 20 years of age. *Hum Biol.* 1982;54:609-625.

57. Graves JE, Pollock ML, Sparling PB. Body composition of elite female distance runners. *Res Q Exerc Sport.* 1987;60:239-245.

58. Pollock ML, Gettman LR, Jackson A, Ayers J, Ward A, Linnerud AC. Body composition of elite class distance runners. *Ann N Y Acad Sci.* 1977;301:351-370.

59. Pollock ML, Miller HS Jr, Wilmore J. Physiological characteristics of champion American track athletes 40 to 75 years of age. *J Gerontol.* 1974;29:645-649.

60. Leake CN, Carter JEL. Comparison of body composition and somatotype of trained female triathletes. *J Sport Sci.* 1991;9:125-135.

61. Loftin M, Warren BL, Zingraf S, Brandon JE, Skudle A, Scully B. Peak physiological function and performance of recreational triathletes. *J Sports Med Phys Fitness.* 1988;28:330-335.

62. Puhl J, Case S, Fleck S, Van Handel P. Physical and physiological characteristics of elite volleyball players. *Res Q Exerc Sport.* 1982;53:257-262.

63. Spitler DL, Diaz FJ, Horvath SM, Wright JE. Body composition and maximal aerobic capacity of body builders. *J Sports Med Phys Fitness.* 1980;20:181-188.

64. Johnson GO, Housh TJ, Powell DR, Ansorge CJ. A physiological profile comparison of female body builders and power lifters. *J Sports Med Phys Fitness.* 1990;30:361-364.

65. Katch VL, Katch FI, Moffatt R, Gittleson M. Muscular development and lean body weight in bodybuilders and weightlifters. *Med Sci Sports Exerc.* 1980;12:340-344.

66. Sinning WE. Body composition assessment of college wrestlers. *Med Sci Sports Exerc.* 1974;6:139-145.

67. Housh TJ, Johnson GO, Kenney KB, et al. Validity of anthropometric estimations of body composition in high school wrestlers. *Res Q Exerc Sport.* 1989;60:239-245.

68. Kanehisa H, Kondo M, Ikegawa S, Fukunaga T. Body composition and isokinetic strength of professional Sumo wrestlers. *Eur J Appl Physiol.* 1998;77(4):352-359.

69. Sinning WE. Body composition in athletes. In: Roche AF, Heymsfield SB, Lohman TG, eds. *Human Body Composition.* Champaign, Ill: Human Kinetics; 1996:257-273.

70. Houtkooper LB, Going SB. Body composition: how should it be measured? Does it affect performance? *Sports Sci Exch.* 1994;7(5).

71. ACSM position stand on weight loss in wrestlers. *Med Sci Sports Exerc.* 1996;28(2):ix-xii.

72. Thorland WG, Tipton CM, Lohman TG, et al. Midwest wrestling study: prediction of minimal weight for high school wrestlers. *Med Sci Sports Exerc.* 1991;23(9):1102-1110.

73. Lukaski HC. Methods for the assessment of human body composition: traditional and new. *Am J Clin Nutr.* 1987;46:537-556.

74. Martin AD, Drinkwater DT. Variability in the measures of body fat: assumptions or technique? *Sports Med.* 1991;11:277-288.

75. Siri WE. Body composition from fluid spaces and density: analysis of methods. In: Brozek J, Henschel A, eds. *Techniques for Measuring Body Composition.* Washington, DC: National Academy of Sciences National Research Council; 1961:223-244.

76. Brozek J, Grande F, Anderson JT, Keys A. Densitometric analysis of body composition: revision of some quantitative assumptions. *Ann N Y Acad Sci.* 1963;110:113-140.

77. Behnke AR. Comment of the determination of whole body density and a resume of body composition data. In: Brozek J, Henschel A, eds. *Techniques for Measuring Body Composition.* Washington, DC: National Academy of Sciences National Research Council; 1961:118-133.

78. Going SB. Densitometry. In: Roche AF, Heymsfield SB, Lohman TG, eds. *Human Body Composition.* 3rd ed. Champaign, Ill: Human Kinetics; 1996:3-23.

79. Eaton AW, Israel RG, O'Brien KF, Hortobagyi T, McCammon MR. Comparison of four methods to assess body composition in women. *Eur J Clin Nutr.* 1993;47:353-360.

80. Lohman TG. Skinfolds and body density and their relation to body fatness: a review. *Hum Biol.* 1981;53:181-225.

81. Lohman TG. Applicability of body composition techniques and constants for children and youths. In: Pandolf K, ed. *Exercise and Sports Science Reviews.* 14th ed. New York, NY: Macmillian; 1986:325-357.

82. Schutte JE, Townsend EJ, Hugg J, Shoup RF, Malina RM, Blomqvist CG. Density of lean body mass is greater in blacks than in whites. *J Appl Physiol.* 1984;56:1647-1649.

83. Modlesky CM, Cureton KJ, Lewis RD, Prior BM, Sloniger MA, Rowe DA. Density of the fat-free mass and estimates of body composition in male weight trainers. *J Appl Physiol.* 1996;80(6):2085-2096.

84. Dempster P, Aitkens S. A new air displacement method for the determination of human body composition. *Med Sci Sports Exerc.* 1995;27(12):1692-1697.

85. McCrory MA, Mole PA, Gomez TD, Dewey KG, Bernauer EM. Body composition by air-displacement plethysmography by using predicted and measured thoracic gas volumes. *J Appl Physiol.* 1998;84:1475-1479.

86. Biaggi RR, Volman MW, Nies MA, et al. Comparison of air-displacement plethysmography with hydrostatic weighing and bioelectrical impedance analysis for the assessment of body composition in healthy adults. *Am J Clin Nutr.* 1999;69:898-903.

87. Harrison GC, Buskirk ER, Carter JEL, et al. Skinfold thicknesses and measurement technique. In: Lohman TG, Roche AF, Martorell R, eds. *Anthropometric Standardization Reference Manual.* Champaign, Ill: Human Kinetics; 1988:55-70.

88. Jackson AS, Pollock ML. Practical assessment of body composition. *Phys Sports Med.* 1985;13(5):76-90.

89. Jackson AS, Pollock ML. Generalized equations for predicting body density of men. *Br J Nutr*. 1978;40:497-504.

90. Jackson AS, Pollock ML, Ward A. Generalized equations for predicting body density of women. *Med Sci Sports Exerc*. 1980;12(3):175-182.

91. Slaughter MH, Lohman TG, Boileau RA, et al. Skinfold equations for estimation of body fatness in children and youth. *Hum Biol*. 1988;60(5):709-723.

92. Wells JCK, Fuller NJ, Dewit O, Fewtrell MS, Elia M, Cole TJ. Four-component model of body composition in children: density and hydration of fat-free mass and comparison with simpler models. *Am J Clin Nutr*. 1999;69:904-912.

93. Schoeller DA. Hydrometry. In: Roche AF, Heymsfield SB, Lohman TG, eds. *Human Body Composition*. Champaign, Ill: Human Kinetics; 1996:25-43.

94. Davis JM, Lamb DR, Burgess WA, Bartoli WP. Accumulation of deuterium oxide in body fluids after ingestion of D2O-labeled beverages. *J Appl Physiol*. 1987;63(5):2060-2066.

95. Baumgartner RN. Electrical impedance and total body electrical conductivity. In: Roche AF, Heymsfield SB, Lohman TG, eds. *Human Body Composition*. Champaign, Ill: Human Kinetics; 1996:79-107.

96. NIH Technological Assessment Statement. *Bioelectrical Impedance Analysis in Body Composition Measurement*. December 12-14, 1996:1-35.

97. Houtkooper LB, Going SB, Lohman TG, Roche AF, Van Loan M. Bioelectrical impedance estimation of fat-free body mass in children and youth: a cross-validation study. *J Appl Physiol*. 1992;72:366-373.

98. Lanza E. Determination of moisture, protein, fat, and calories in raw pork and beef by near infrared spectroscopy. *J Food Sci*. 1983;48:471-474.

99. Nielsen DH, Cassady SL, Wacker LM, Wessels AK, Wheelock BJ, Oppliger RA. Validation of Futrex 5000 near-infrared spectrophotometer analyzer for assessment of body composition. *J Orthop Sports Phy Ther*. 1992;16:281-287.

100. Cassady SL, Nielsen DH, Janz KF, Wu Y, Cook JS, Hansen JR. Validity of near infrared body composition analysis in children and adolescents. *Med Sci Sports Exerc*. 1993;25(10):1185-1191.

101. Heyward VH, Cook KL, Hicks VL, Jenkins KA, Quatrochi JA, Wilson WL. Predictive accuracy of three field methods for estimating relative body fatness of nonobese and obese women. *Int J Sport Nutr*. 1992;2:75-86.

102. Wilmore KM, McBride PJ, Wilmore JH. Comparison of bioelectric impedance and near-infrared interactance for body composition assessment in a population of self-perceived overweight adults. *Int J Obes Relat Metab Disord*. 1994;18:375-381.

103. Houmard JA, Israel RG, McCammon MR, O'Brien KF, Omer J, Zamora BS. Validity of a near-infrared device for estimating body composition in a college football team. *J Appl Sport Sci Res*. 1991;5:53-59.

104. Smith DB, Johnson GO, Stout JR, Housh TJ, Housh DJ, Evetovich TK. Validity of near-infrared interactance for estimating relative body fat in female high school gymnasts. *Int J Sports Med*. 1997;18:531-537.

105. Lukaski HC. Soft tissue composition and bone mineral status: evaluation by dual energy x-ray absorptiometry. *J Nutr*. 1993;123:438-443.

106. Lohman TG. Dual-energy x-ray absorptiometry. In: Roche AF, Heymsfield SB, Lohman TG, eds. *Human Body Composition*. Champaign, Ill: Human Kinetics; 1996:63-78.

107. Prior BM, Cureton KJ, Modlesky CM, et al. In vivo validation of whole-body composition estimates from dual-energy x-ray absorptiometry. *J Appl Physiol*. 1997;83(2):623-630.

108. Bergsma-Kadijk JA, Baumeister B, Deurenberg P. Measurement of body fat in young and elderly women: comparison between a four-component model and widely used reference methods. *Br J Nutr*. 1996;75:649-657.

109. Roemmich JN, Clark PA, Weltman A, Rogol AD. Alterations in growth and body composition during puberty. I. Comparing multicomponent body composition models. *J Appl Physiol*. 1997;83(3):927-935.

110. Clasey JL, Hartmen ML, Kanaley J, et al. Body composition by DEXA in older adults: accuracy and influence of scan mode. *Med Sci Sports Exerc*. 1997;29(4):560-567.

111. Modlesky CM, Prior BM, Lewis RD, Cureton KJ. Measurement of body composition in tall individuals using dual-energy x-ray absorptiometry. *Med Sci Sports Exerc*. 1997;29(5):S37.

112. Heymsfield SB, Lichtman S, Baumgartner RN, et al. Body composition of humans: comparison of two improved four-component models that differ in expense, technical complexity, and radiation exposure. *Am J Clin Nutr*. 1990;52:52-58.

113. Withers RT, LaForgia J, Pillans RK, et al. Comparisons of two-, three-, and four-compartment models of body composition analysis in men and women. *J Appl Physiol*. 1998;85(1):238-245.

114. Cote KD, Adams WC. Effect of bone density on body composition estimates in young adult black and white women. *Med Sci Sports Exerc*. 1993;25:290-296.

115. Oritz O, Russell M, Daley TL, et al. Differences in skeletal muscle and bone mineral mass between black and white females and their relevance to estimates of body composition. *Am J Clin Nutr*. 1992;55:8-13.

COMPUTER PROGRAMS FOR NUTRITION, DIET, FITNESS, AND BODY COMPOSITION ASSESSMENT

Marie Dunford, PhD, RD

Much computer wisdom stems from a single proverb: "Garbage in, garbage out." Ease of operation and program features must take a backseat to the most important issues—quality of the database used for calculations and standards used for assessments and recommendations. Incomplete, out-of-date databases or inappropriate norms or formulas represent "garbage in." Misinterpretations or inappropriate recommendations result in "garbage out." Determining the "best" computer program begins with a thorough assessment of the databases and standards used (1).

A final decision will be based on many factors such as price, available hardware, ease of operation, appearance of the computer screen, ability to customize, frequency of updates, quality and quantity of printed client material, graphics, readability of the program manual, statistical capabilities, and file export options (1,2). The *Journal of the American Dietetic Association* regularly publishes software reviews (3-7). Be aware that software programs rapidly evolve and publishing timely evaluations of software is difficult at best (8). Talking to other dietitians and health professionals and viewing "demo" disks are ways to learn more about specific programs.

Computer software has made dietary and fitness analysis easier by compiling information, performing mathematical calculations, and analyzing data. Clients have come to expect computer printouts as part of the evaluation process. The ultimate goal is to use the computer as a tool resulting in less time calculating and more time counseling (9).

Multimedia software, often sold as a CD-ROM, allows the use of more than one media (eg, video, slides, graphics, animation, sound, and text) and can be interactive. Clients may enter their dietary intake. Pictures may be used to show unfamiliar foods and to help clients visualize portion size. The multimedia CD-ROM appears to be an emerging technology for dietary assessment (6,9,10).

COMPUTER PROGRAMS FOR DIETARY ASSESSMENT

Evaluation of Computerized Nutrient Databases

The primary consideration in software evaluation is the quality of the nutrient database (1,2). The nutrient database contains the numerical values that are the foundation of all dietary calculations performed by the computer program and is the basis for estimating nutrient intake. Therefore, an accurate nutrient database is essential. The inherent limitations of all nutrient databases, computerized or not, are well-recognized (1,11,12). Professionals and clients alike should keep the following in mind:

- Many foods listed in a nutrient database have not undergone chemical evaluation for nutrient content; therefore, their nutrient values are estimated.
- Estimated nutrient values may be obtained by calculating values from a similar food, a different form of the same food, a household recipe, or a similar product formulation.
- Many foods in the database have missing values because they were never analyzed for certain nutrients, and there are no similar foods that have been analyzed from which to project nutrient content.
- Methods used for chemically analyzing the nutrient content of foods are of variable sophistication and accuracy.
- Nutrient databases do not consider the variability of nutrient content for foods grown in different areas.
- The bioavailability of any nutrient may be influenced by the food in which it resides and the other foods consumed at the same meal, neither of which can be considered in a nutrient database.

Lee, Nieman, and Rainwater (2) entered a 3-day food record containing 73 food items into each of eight microcomputer dietary analysis programs and analyzed the food record for energy and 36 nutrients. The nutrient database was judged against the 1993 US Department of Agriculture Nutrient Data Base for Standard Reference (USDA NDB). Seven of the eight programs were within 15% of the USDA NDB for energy, protein, total fat, and total carbohydrate. The nutrients that varied more than 15% from the USDA NDB (and differed considerably among programs) were total tocopherols, α tocopherols, dietary fiber, fatty acids, and cholesterol. The nutrients most likely to be missing from the eight program databases were total tocopherols, α tocopherols, manganese, some amino acids, some fatty acids, pantothenic acid, copper, magnesium, and caffeine. The study found that the eight software programs had from 0% to 15.1% missing values. The authors note that these numbers would have been higher if brand-name foods and recipes had been used in the 3-day food record since the USDA NDB does not contain data for brand-name foods other than ready-to-eat cereals and some kinds of candy.

Results of other studies comparing databases have been mixed (13-16). LaComb, Taylor, and Noble (16) compared four microcomputer nutrient analysis programs using 24-hour dietary recalls of homeless children and found no significant differences in energy and nutrient values among the databases. Another study of four computerized databases revealed no statistically significant differences among three of the databases when analyzing 60 24-hour recalls (14). There were significant differences ($p < 0.01$) between one database and the other three, but the reasons for the differences could not be detected. Taylor et al (13) analyzed 24-hour dietary records using three computerized nutrient databases. Results of this study demonstrated that 9 of the 19 nutrient value means differed, although no database consistently reported high or low values. In a study published in 1992, Nieman et al (15) compared six microcomputer nutrient analysis programs with the USDA NDB. All six programs were within 7% of the USDA

NDB for energy, protein, total fat, and total carbohydrate; however, the other nutrients varied by more than 15%. There is a compelling argument for a peer-reviewed, national, nutrient database for use in dietary analysis (17).

When reviewing a computerized dietary assessment program, the health professional should consider a number of database issues:

- Source(s) and currency of data
- Missing and imputed values
- Number and definition of nutrients analyzed
- Type and number of foods in the database
- Portion size
- Standards used

Sources and currency of data. The most commonly cited source of nutrient values is the USDA Handbook 8 series (USDA Nutrient Data Base for Standard Reference), *Nutrient Composition of Foods*. Many databases rely on Home and Garden Bulletin 72, *Nutrient Values of Foods*, which is a subset of USDA Handbook 8. These databases are generally accepted as valid. However, both have the limitation that few brand-name food values are included (only ready-to-eat-cereals and some candy). This limitation has forced software developers to add nutrient values of brand-name food items that have been derived from other sources such as manufacturer's information, journal articles, food composition tables from other countries, and unpublished sources (18).

The USDA Nutrient Data Base for Standard Reference contains about 6,000 items; however, the databases of some computer software programs contain as many as 23,000 items. As the number of food items in the database increases, the number of data sources increases. One computer program lists more than 1,100 data sources. Each data source must be valid and identified. It has become increasingly difficult for dietitians to judge the validity of a program's data sources due to the sheer volume of sources listed (1).

Due to changing consumer demand, food manufacturers are reformulating products, but the reformulated products may retain the same name. Database developers must be diligent about checking current product formulations. Database updates are provided by software companies and should include new products as well as reformulated ones (1).

Missing and imputed values. For a substantial number of foods there are no data available for some nutrients. Thus, the issue of missing values is an important one. Each software developer must determine how to deal with missing values. Some choose to calculate missing values as zeroes. Unless a missing value is flagged, the user cannot distinguish between a food that contains none of a particular nutrient and a food that contains an unknown amount of a particular nutrient. Missing values usually result in an underestimate of nutrient intake. To avoid such errors, many software developers impute values. An imputed value is an educated guess (18). Some professionals believe it is better for nutrient database developers, using published guidelines, to impute values than to leave missing values (19). It is important to note that currently all databases have missing or imputed values.

Number and definition of nutrients analyzed. Potential users must determine the number of analyzed nutrients essential to best serve their populations (1). Some programs offer a small number (12 to 15 nutrients), while other programs contain more than 125 nutrients. Programs analyzing large numbers of nutrients can be cumbersome and may serve to confuse clients. On the other hand, the additional nutrients may be helpful for certain clients and some programs may be customized so that a limited number of nutrients are routinely analyzed.

If a particular nutrient is of concern, care should be taken to determine how that nutrient is defined. For example, is fiber measured as crude or dietary fiber? How precise is the fatty acid analysis? Are the individual fatty acids calculated or do just the major classifications appear? These are essential questions when determining the utility of the database (1).

Type and number of foods in the database. The computer program literature usually includes the number of foods contained in the database. Although the total number of foods is important, the breadth and depth of the food included should also be considered. Evaluation should be based on the number of foods in the database that most completely reflects the diets of the client population. In some work environments a database with a strong list of ethnic and regional foods may be a necessity. Athletes often consume low-fat or nonfat food items, energy bars, sports drinks, and supplements, and these foods should be included in the database. Some users may want to have the capacity to analyze recipes. If this is the case, the database should be evaluated for the availability of ingredients (1).

In some databases the actual number of different foods may be inflated because a single food is listed several times with different portion sizes (1). Thus, a stick of butter, a pat of butter, and a tablespoon of butter may be counted as three different foods. In reality these entries represent one food item with three different portion sizes. Similarly, there may be separate entries for foods that differ little in nutrient value (ie, cakes made from cake mixes and cakes commercially prepared) (18). By itself, the quantity of foods in the database may be misleading.

In most cases foods can be added by the user as a means of enhancing the database. However, this can be an extremely time-consuming task if a substantial number of foods must be added. If foods are added by the user, care must be taken to ensure that accurate values are obtained and accurately entered into the database (1).

Portion size. The accuracy of any nutrient evaluation is dependent on the accuracy of the portion-size estimates. The serving sizes used in the database must be represented by common household or other widely recognized measures. Some entries appear as "one piece" or "one serving." While this may be an appropriate description for some foods, such measures may leave the user and the client guessing, which increases the chance of error (18). The program should allow the user to enter exact volume measurements and to use grams or ounces.

Standards used. Equally important to the quality of the database are the standards used for comparison. Commonly used standards include the Recommended Dietary Allowances (RDA) and Dietary Reference Intakes (DRI), the Food Guide Pyramid, the Percent Daily Value from the food label, the US Dietary Guidelines, the Exchange Lists, and the American Heart Association recommendations. Energy requirements are often determined using height, weight, gender, age, and activity levels. Because energy requirements differ substantially between sports and among athletes, it is important to check if the default standard can be altered by the user. Although there is not an "athletic RDA," some clients may wish to create their own standards based on an understanding of what is required by a specific athletic population (ie, 1.5 g protein/kg of body weight per day, or 70% of calories derived from carbohydrate) (20).

System Requirements

Before purchasing software a decision must be made regarding hardware. Increasing program sophistication has resulted in greater system requirements, especially for memory and hard drive space. The newest generation of computer programs now requires a CD-ROM to store the huge volume of information in the program and databases and to run a wide variety of graphics. Most programs require, at a minimum, a 486/33 MHz CPU and 8 MB RAM. Some may require a specific operating system or a CD-ROM drive. Some programs do not have a Macintosh version.

If new or upgraded hardware is not an option, examine the minimum system requirements and consider only those programs that are compatible with the current hardware. On the other hand, purchasing new software may be the impetus for upgrading or purchasing new hardware. Hardware (including the printer) and software incompatibility is often a source of great frustration.

Speed is an important consideration. Searching a large database at a slow speed results in what seems like an inordinate amount of time for the food to appear on the screen. If data entry is done during a counseling session, this could considerably increase the length of the session.

Program Features

After evaluating the database and identifying programs compatible with current hardware, it is important to evaluate a variety of program features. These include:

- Overall ease of operation
- Data entry
- Verification procedures
- On-line and program documentation help features
- Printed format and design
- Statistical capabilities and file export options
- Cost (1,2)

Demonstration diskettes may be helpful in the evaluation process (21), but the demonstration program may not be representative of the entire database (1).

Data entry. Always a tedious task, data entry deserves close attention. Evaluate the data entry features with efficiency in mind. Entering data is not a good use of the dietitian's time; however, data must be accurately entered to ensure valid results (18). Most programs are menu driven, allowing the user to highlight and select a food which then appears on the screen. Foods are selected from the database by entering a complete or partial name of the food or by accessing food categories and viewing a list of foods. Portion sizes are displayed when a food is selected.

Data verification and correction procedures. Careful data entry can minimize errors, but the need to verify and correct data will always be present. Some programs have built in error-detection functions that flag potential data-entry errors (eg, values that appear to be out of the normal range, such as 100 lb of ground beef as part of a 24-hour diet recall). When errors are not so obvious, the user must detect incorrect entries and edit them. Editing procedures may be cumbersome and are an important consideration. Determine how easily input can be edited as part of the evaluation process (18).

Help features. No matter how experienced, all users rely on help features to some degree. On-line help menus are handy features that briefly explain or clarify the information appearing on the screen and can increase the user's efficiency. Some users prefer written program documentation materials. Manuals should be reviewed for clarity. The degree of technical support offered by software companies varies. Some software companies offer toll-free phone numbers to reach knowledgeable staff and on-site programmers who can answer questions; others offer limited technical support.

Printout format and design. The end product of most computerized nutrient analyses will be a printout. Printout formats and designs will vary, but all formats should be accurate, clear, concise, interpretable, and appropriate for the intended audience. Determine if the amount of information to be printed can be chosen by the user. Programs can generate a large amount of data, some of which might not be useful or may be confusing for the client. Most software programs offer samples of printouts so this feature can easily be reviewed.

Clarity of information is an important issue. Too much information on a page or the presence of too many symbols will serve only to confuse the client trying to read the printout. Make certain that any abbreviations are clearly understood. Charts and graphs, which are common features, often make data interpretation easier and are appropriately used with many client populations. Ranking food in ascending or descending order based on a particular nutrient is a feature of some programs.

Interpretation of data is a key issue. Clients may attach importance to computer-generated information, even though they have been told of its limitations. The potential for misinterpretation is great, especially when a large amount of material is printed out. To reduce the incidence of misinterpretation, printouts should bear a statement of their limitations as well as the name, address, and phone number of the health professional who generated the reports and to whom questions should be directed (18,20).

Preprogrammed text ("boiler plate") should be checked to ensure accuracy. A common feature is a list of recommendations generated by matching the estimated dietary intake against program standards. Carefully review the preprogrammed interpretations. For example, if vitamin C is consumed at 125% of the Recommended Dietary Allowances (RDA), how is this interpreted by the program? Some programs using a strict cutoff point of 100% of the RDA would advise the client to reduce intake of vitamin C. If text does not accompany the printout, consider how the client would receive information about proper interpretation. The dietitian must also determine how to address apparent deficiencies that are in fact a result of missing values in the database.

Finally, check carefully that information visible on the screen can be printed in its entirety. Some programs require long-carriage printers or must alter the format shown on the screen when printing.

Statistical capabilities and file export options. There may be a need to transfer files from the dietary analysis program to another computer program to perform tasks the dietary analysis program cannot do. These tasks could include statistical analysis of data (eg, SAS, SPSSX) or database management. To be able to transfer files, the dietary analysis program must be able to export data as an ASCII file.

Cost. The cost of the software varies and is usually dependent on the sophistication of the program. As part of the cost analysis, one should include the original cost of the program, costs of any updates, the cost of an extended service agreement, and the cost of any hardware (including increased costs for printing) that will be needed to run the program.

COMPUTER PROGRAMS FOR FITNESS AND BODY COMPOSITION

Many dietary assessment programs also include a fitness assessment component. Additionally, programs focused only on fitness and body composition are also available. Fitness assessment may include measures of cardiovascular and respiratory fitness (heart rate, blood pressure, and maximum oxygen uptake) as well as strength, endurance, and flexibility. Body composition may be assessed using height, weight, skinfold measurements, and arm circumference (22). Estimates of total daily energy expenditure and resting metabolic rate are frequently included. The most important evaluation criteria are the formulas and standards used for generating recommendations.

Formulas and Standards

The limitation of using a fitness and body composition program lies in the formulas and standards used for interpretation. Evaluate all formulas used in the program to determine if they are the most appropriate for the client population being served, with consideration given to age, sex, ethnicity, and sport (22). The written documentation should contain an explanation of the norms and criteria used and the known limitations of the methods chosen.

All methods of assessing body composition have measurement error in the range of 2% to 5%. Some assessment methods overestimate body fat; others underestimate it (22). The biggest issue is the rigidity of the standard used to interpret the estimates of body fat. Programs should report desirable body fat as a range since the "ideal" body fat for a particular client or sport is difficult to pinpoint (22,23).

The program may be capable of estimating the approximate calorie expenditure for a single activity or for a 24-hour period. This is typically done by selecting an activity and indicating body weight. A calorie per minute estimate is then multiplied by the number of minutes the activity was performed to determine an estimated calorie expenditure. Such figures may include the resting energy expenditure as part of the total figure.

Program Features

Once the database and standards have been evaluated, program features should be considered. In this respect fitness and body composition programs differ little from dietary assessment programs. Evaluate the ease with which the data can be entered, available help features, clarity of written materials, and cost of the program.

Box 12.1 lists pertinent questions to consider when choosing a computer program.

BOX 12.1   Questions to Ask when Evaluating Computer Programs for Nutrition, Diet, Fitness, and Body Composition

Quality of the Nutrient Database:
- Are the nutrient values in the database valid?
- What are the sources for the nutrient values in the database?
- How are missing values treated?
- How many nutrients are analyzed and how are the nutrients measured?
- Does the database contain the foods representative of the intake of the client population?
- Can foods be added to the database?
- How are portion sizes entered?
- How frequently are updates available?

Standards for Evaluation:
- Are the standards used for nutrient analysis and/or fitness and body composition assessment valid?
- Are the standards used representative of the client population?
- How are the standards interpreted?

System Requirements:
- Is the current hardware (including the printer) compatible with the software?
- If the current system is not compatible, what will be required to make it compatible?

---

continued

BOX 12.1   Questions to Ask when Evaluating Computer Programs for Nutrition, Diet, Fitness, and Body Composition (continued)

Program Features:
- How are data entered?
- How are data edited?
- How are data errors brought to the attention of the user?
- How helpful is on-line help?
- How clear is the written manual?
- Is technical support available?
- Is printed material accurate?
- Is printed material clear to the professional and the client?
- Is printed material open to misinterpretations by the client?
- Is printed material concise?
- Do "boiler plate" recommendations reflect the philosophy of the professional?
- Can data be exported?
- How much does the original program cost?
- What other expenses might be incurred to make and keep the program operational?

REFERENCES

1. Buzzard IM, Price KS, Warren RA. Considerations for selecting nutrient-calculation software: evaluation of the nutrient database. *Am J Clin Nutr*. 1991;54:7-9.
2. Lee RD, Nieman DC, Rainwater M. Comparison of eight microcomputer dietary analysis programs with the USDA Nutrient Data Base for Standard Reference. *J Am Diet Assoc*. 1995;95:858-867.
3. Nieman DC. The food processor for windows [review]. *J Am Diet Assoc*. 1997;97:1337.
4. Nieman DC. Food intake analysis system [review]. *J Am Diet Assoc*. 1997;97:697-698.
5. Lee RD. Nutrition profile 100 [review]. *J Am Diet Assoc*. 1997;97:559.
6. Nieman DC. Nutrition DISCovery Personalized CD-ROM Diet Assessment Program [review]. *J Am Diet Assoc*. 1997;97:338.
7. Lee RD. Nutribase nutrition manager [review]. *J Am Diet Assoc*. 1997;97:219.
8. Byrd-Bredbenner C. How should nutrient databases be evaluated [letter]? *J Am Diet Assoc*. 1996;96:120.
9. Kolasa KM, Miller MG. Developments in nutrition education using computer technology. *J Nutr Ed*. 1996;28:7-14.
10. Kohlmeier L, Mendez M, McDuffie J, Miller M. Computer-assisted self-interviewing: a multimedia approach to dietary assessment. *Am J Clin Nutr*. 1997;65(suppl):1275S-1281S.
11. Schakel SF, Buzzard IM, Gebhardt SE. Procedures for estimating nutrient values for food composition databases. *J Food Compos Anal*. 1997;10:102-114.
12. Schakel SF, Sievert YA, Buzzard IM. Sources of data for developing and maintaining a nutrient database. *J Am Diet Assoc*. 1988;88:1268-1271.
13. Taylor ML, Kozlowski BW, Baer MT. Energy and nutrient values from different computerized data bases. *J Am Diet Assoc*. 1985;85:1136-1138.
14. Eck LH, Klesges RC, Hanson CL, Baranowski T, Henske J. A comparison of four commonly used nutrient database programs. *J Am Diet Assoc*. 1988;88:602-604.

15. Nieman DC, Butterworth DE, Nieman CN, Lee KE, Lee RD. Comparison of six microcomputer dietary analysis systems with the USDA Nutrient Data Base for Standard Reference. *J Am Diet Assoc.* 1992;92:48-56.

16. LaComb RP, Taylor ML, Noble JM. Comparative evaluation of four microcomputer nutrient analysis software packages using 24-hour dietary recalls of homeless children. *J Am Diet Assoc.* 1992;92:1391-1392.

17. Juni R. How should nutrient databases be evaluated [letter] *J Am Diet Assoc.* 1996;96:120-121.

18. Byrd-Bredbenner C. Computer nutrient analysis software packages: considerations for selection. *Nutrition Today.* 1988;Sept/Oct:13-21.

19. Lee RD, Nieman DC. Authors' reply [letter]. *J Am Diet Assoc.* 1996;96:122.

20. Frank GC, Pelican S. Guidelines for selecting a dietary analysis system. *J Am Diet Assoc.* 1986;86:72-75.

21. Ralston CE, Matthews ME. Software selection: can a demonstration computer package help? *J Am Diet Assoc.* 1988;88:72-75.

22. Williams MH. *Nutrition for Health, Fitness and Sport.* 5th ed. Boston, Mass: McGraw-Hill; 1999.

23. Houtkooper L. Fast anthropometric assessment body profile software [review]. *J Nutr Ed.* 1996;28:363-364.

13

DOCUMENTING SPORTS NUTRITION OUTCOMES

Nancy Clark, MS, RD, FADA, FACSM

Clinical nutritionists are familiar with how to document the outcomes of medical nutrition therapy. Counseling protocols have been established to help dietetics professionals and clients work together as partners to achieve desired health goals or outcomes (1). For example, among clients with hypertension a desired outcome is lower blood pressure and among clients with heart disease a desired outcome is lower blood lipids.

Studies suggest a high level of patient satisfaction with this client-centered approach. In a survey of 400 clients at two academic health centers (both inpatient and outpatient), 83% of the patients reported the dietitian's advice helped them know what to eat. The majority of patients made dietary changes, felt better emotionally, and felt more in control of their medical condition. Forty-three percent reported health-related changes (2). These positive benefits help to "prove our worth" and provide data to support the value and cost benefits of medical nutrition therapy.

Because athletes' nutrition needs are generally related to performance enhancement, not medical nutrition therapy, the incentive to develop outcomes for sports nutrition counseling has been low. Yet, the same client-centered, outcome-based approach to nutrition counseling could help define the best practices for sports nutrition education and the best standards of care.

To date, very few published studies document the outcomes of sports nutrition counseling. Frentsos and Baer (3) published an article entitled, "Increased Energy and Nutrient Intake During Training and Competition Improves Elite Triathletes' Endurance Performance," but it is one of just a few studies that document the outcomes of nutrition education.

WHY DOCUMENT OUTCOMES?

"Why bother to document outcomes?" Nobody wants more paperwork. Why bother? We should "bother" because dietetics professionals need to be able to prove the benefits of individual sports nutrition counseling and the benefits of having a sports nutritionist as part of the sports medicine team. How can sports nutritionists claim to meet The American Dietetic Association (ADA) and Sports, Cardiovascular, and Wellness Nutritionist (SCAN) vision for their members to be considered nutrition experts when the worth and value of nutrition services are unproven? Knowing the outcomes of sports nutrition efforts can enhance the value of services, create jobs, and answer the following questions:

- Why should a college or professional sports team hire a sports nutritionist when a coach or athletic trainer is already handling the nutrition concerns?
- How do we know a registered dietitian (RD) could do a better job and enhance athletes' ability to perform better, eat more healthfully, and better invest in their overall well-being?
- Why should a professional team retain a sports nutritionist to work with the athletes when there were no obvious changes visible from the first season's nutrition education program?

The bottom-line question is: "How can jobs be created if the value or the worth of nutrition services for athletes is not known?" Sports nutritionists need to identify how to provide consistent, high-quality sports nutrition services and how to demonstrate the impact this care has on athletes. People will be more interested in hiring sports nutritionists when the ensuing benefits are clearly documented. Examples of such benefits might include:

- Saving a college a year's worth of tuition if a borderline anorexic student with an athletic scholarship is in danger of being asked not to compete. The sports nutritionist, along with others on the eating disorders team, could help the athlete transform the fear of eating into optimal fueling patterns.
- Enhancing the chances of becoming the championship team by teaching the athletes how to delay fatigue and maintain strength and stamina throughout the entire season. The sports nutritionist who can educate professional athletes to properly fuel-up before a game, and refuel after the game (even when the team is traveling), offers incredibly valuable information. As one coach said, "Good nutrition is our secret weapon!"
- Helping a person achieve his or her athletic dreams. For example, individual counseling for an aspiring marathoner by a sports nutritionist can help that novice athlete complete the grueling event.

SPORTS NUTRITIONISTS: AN ENDANGERED SPECIES

In two-thirds of the health clubs in the Boston area, personal trainers and group exercise leaders are the nutrition educators. RDs provide nutrition services in only one-third of the clubs (4). It is likely that this happens because personal trainers/group exercise leaders are the first to establish a caring relationship with the client; they want to help their clients meet health and weight goals. The clients respond by entrusting the exercise leaders with their nutrition questions and weight concerns.

Are personal trainers as good at nutrition education as the RDs? Who knows? RDs have no way to proclaim themselves nutrition experts because they have no data. Clearly, a vehicle for monitoring the results of our work needs to be created. Otherwise, many jobs will be lost to the exercise leaders who are often the first contact with people interested in improving their physical fitness. Registered dietitians could become an endangered species.

CASE STUDY

Outcomes of Individual Counseling in a Private Practice

Like most sports nutritionists, I never got around to documenting outcomes—until 1997. In that year I took the time to assess the needs of the clients whom I counseled and the outcomes of my counseling sessions. I addressed the following questions:

- Who comes to see a sports nutritionist in a private practice?
- What do they want?
- What counseling and/or intervention do they get?
- What are the outcomes of the counseling sessions?
- How can I use those (positive) outcomes to create jobs?

The answers became obvious. Exercisers and athletes interested in nutrition guidance come to see a sports nutritionist for private, personalized counseling. Most are self-referred. They generally are fueling themselves well and/or are committed to eating well for top performance. Their main concerns are:

- How to lose weight and have energy to exercise
- How to resolve eating disorders/disordered eating patterns
- How to have more energy for sports and life
- How to eat the best balance of carbohydrate, protein, and fat
- How to eat well for top athletic performance

These issues may vary slightly according to age group. Concerns with *eating disorders* are more prevalent in the teens to 21-year age group. *How to lose weight gained because of the stress of work and juggling a busy lifestyle* is the biggest issue among clients aged 22 to 35 years. *Weight reduction for health/medical reasons* is the biggest concern among clients over 50 years of age.

Each of my clients received at least 1 hour of personalized nutrition counseling. What benefits did he or she get from the nutrition education sessions? Of the 50% who returned for two or more visits, 80% reported positive outcomes. (The remaining 20% demonstrated lack of readiness to change.) Across the board, the successful clients commented they had more energy, performed better during exercise sessions, felt better about their bodies, and were more at peace with food.

One 44-year-old female executive and triathlete commented, "It's only been a week and I can't begin to tell you how much better I feel. I have lots more energy. I'm drinking less coffee and don't even want to drink wine at night." Three weeks later she commented, "I've never felt better in my whole life—I feel fabulous! I've lost a few pounds. I have more energy than ever before. And every sport I do, I knock minutes off my time."

PUTTING POSITIVE OUTCOMES TO GOOD USE

Positive outcomes derived from sports nutrition counseling can powerfully promote the value of working with a sports nutritionist. The testimonials of satisfied clients singing praises via "word of mouth" can persuade others to seek the same services. But sports nutritionists need more than just testimonials; we need to document in a systematic way the value of what we do.

Documenting outcomes will help create jobs and ensure the future of our profession. The more positive outcomes that can be documented as a result of nutrition education, the more job opportunities that will open up. For example:

- Would you want your niece to enroll in a nutrition program for teens that has a documented 90% success rate in helping the participants reach their desired weight goals and maintain them for at least 2 years?
- Would a professional baseball team want to continue its nutrition education program with an RD who can document that each player, on average, made six nutritional changes that could potentially enhance his health and performance as a result of attending a 45-minute nutrition workshop?

Most likely, the answer to each question is a resounding "Yes!"

SO WHAT IS A SPORTS NUTRITIONIST TO DO?

If you are interested in documenting the outcomes of your sports nutrition education efforts, where do you start? An action plan might look like this:

- Identify what your athletes want and/or what you think they need. For example, an assessment of the nutrition needs of a Division I men's basketball team identified the following concerns (C. Rosenbloom, unpublished data, 1999):
  1. How to maintain weight throughout the season
  2. How to stay well-hydrated throughout practices and games
  3. How to delay fatigue during games
  4. How to enter the postseason with high muscle-glycogen stores
  5. How to select an appropriate pregame meal
  6. How to best replenish muscle glycogen stores during the season
  7. How to make more healthful food choices when eating out
- Develop a defined care plan that meets the needs of the athletes and targets behaviors that can negatively affect their health or athletic performance (such as skipping breakfast). For the basketball team, the nutritionist developed a series of five 10-minute nutrition education sessions that were offered either before or after the strength and conditioning preseason workouts. The topics included fluids, carbohydrates, pregame meals, eating out, and maintaining weight throughout the season.
- Collect outcomes data (via questionnaire or a checklist of dietary changes) to document the effectiveness of the plan and determine if nutrition education helped athletes achieve their desired goals. Coaches and trainers who spend a significant amount of time with the athletes can also record their observations.

Box 13.1 offers one example of a questionnaire that has been used to document the effectiveness of nutrition classes. It was administered to weight-conscious athletes, 4 weeks after the nutrition education sessions. Alternatively, a questionnaire could be administered at the end of the season to document team nutrition outcomes.

In addition to documenting the changes made by an individual athlete, the sports nutritionist who works with teams (either high school, college, amateur, or professional) should document athlete interest in nutrition. For example, a year-end report for a university-based RD might include the following data to validate the sports nutritionist's job:

- The sport of athletes who requested and/or participated in nutrition seminars
- Number of athletes in attendance per seminar
- Questions generated from the presentation
- Follow-up plan presented to the coach
- Statements of appreciation for the sports nutritionist's efforts (written by the athletes, coaches, and/or parents of the athletes) (5)

Using the positive outcomes documented from one sports nutrition education program, you can justify an RD's salary and also promote the value of additional sports nutrition workshops to other teams, schools, and athletic groups. For example, if every member of a football team reported making four to six potentially performance-enhancing dietary changes as a result of a nutrition workshop series, the athletic director might want to expand the nutrition education program to other sports.

WHAT ARE THE LIMITS OF SPORTS NUTRITION?

Sports nutritionists would love to be able to say their advice results in improved athletic performance, winning championships, and gold medals. Clearly, sports success involves more than just nutrition; many other training, coaching, psychological, and injury-related factors are involved. But, success can be attributed to increased strength, increased muscle mass, and decreased body fat (3).

In real life it may be hard, if not impossible, to isolate the effects of nutrition intervention to confirm the value of the sports nutritionist. But perhaps with several well-controlled nutrition outcomes studies, the profession will be able to answer these questions:

- Is proper nutrition a significant performance-enhancer for all athletes?
- Is optimal nutrition necessary for maximum performance?
- Do teams have a better chance of optimizing performance if all members, rather than only a few players, eat and drink appropriately for a game?

Of course, sports nutritionists would like to believe the answer is "yes" to all of those questions, but it is no secret that plenty of athletes perform very well with suboptimal fueling habits. Clearly, our work is cut out for us. Let's get busy collecting outcomes and demonstrating the value of nutrition education for active people.

BOX 13.1   Form for Documenting Outcomes

The following form has been used for weight-conscious athletes (eg, dancers, female basketball players)
to document changes made as a result of a nutrition education program.

Dear Athlete,

*Thanks for completing the following brief questionnaire. We are trying to document the effectiveness of nutrition
education for active people and appreciate your contributions. Feel free to add as many comments as you'd like.*

Please check the dietary changes you have made as a result of the nutrition session.

BREAKFAST:

☐ My breakfast has always been fine; I've made no changes.

☐ I now think more about the importance of breakfast and try to eat a better breakfast.

☐ I now look forward to breakfast and feel less guilty about eating a good breakfast.

☐ I'm eating more at breakfast.

☐ I'm eating a healthier breakfast.

☐ I feel better because I've improved my breakfast.

☐ I have more energy because I'm eating a bigger breakfast.

☐ I think I exercise better because I'm fueling myself better at breakfast.

☐ I am less hungry later in the day because I'm eating a bigger breakfast.

☐ I still struggle with eating a proper breakfast.

As a result of the nutrition class, I've made the following breakfast changes:

_____

_____

_____

_____

SNACKS:

☐ My snacking habits have always been fine; I have made no changes.

☐ I look forward to snacks and feel less guilty about snacking.

☐ I now plan to eat snacks at appropriate times.

☐ I'm eating healthier snacks.

☐ Adding planned pre-exercise snacks has helped me to have more energy.

☐ I have replaced "snacks" with an added meal (such as a second lunch).

☐ I still need help snacking more healthfully.

As a result of the nutrition class, I've made the following changes in my snacking habits:

_____

_____

_____

_____

continued

BOX 13.1   Form for Documenting Outcomes (continued)

FRUITS/VEGETABLES:

☐ I have always eaten plenty of fruits and vegetables and continue to do so.

☐ I am now eating more fruits.

☐ I am now drinking more orange juice.

☐ I am now eating more colorful vegetables.

☐ I feel better about my intake of fruits and vegetables.

☐ I still need help improving my intake of fruits and vegetables.

As a result of the nutrition class, I have made the following changes in my intake of fruits and vegetables:

_____

_____

_____

_____

FLUIDS:

☐ My fluid intake has always been fine; I have made no changes.

☐ I'm making an effort to drink more fluids before and during exercise.

☐ I always bring my own water bottle with me when I exercise.

☐ In general, I am drinking more fluids throughout the day.

☐ I still need to drink more fluids so I'll be better hydrated.

As a result of the nutrition class, I have made the following changes in my fluid intake:

_____

_____

_____

_____

CALCIUM/DAIRY FOODS:

☐ I have always eaten 2 to 4 servings of calcium-rich foods daily.

☐ I now think more about calcium and try to have more milk and yogurt.

☐ I'm now drinking more milk; I generally drink ____8-oz glasses per day.

☐ I'm now eating more yogurt; I generally eat ____8-oz cups per day.

☐ I'm now choosing to drink calcium-fortified orange juice.

☐ I still need help with my calcium intake.

As a result of the nutrition class, I have made these changes in my calcium intake:

_____

_____

_____

_____

continued

BOX 13.1   Form for Documenting Outcomes (continued)

CALORIES/FUEL:

☐ I have always fueled myself well and have made no changes in my fueling patterns.

☐ As a result of the class, I now feel less guilty about eating.

☐ Knowing my calorie needs has helped me fuel myself better during the day.

☐ Knowing my calorie budget has helped me improve the quality of my diet.

☐ I feel better because I am distributing my calories more evenly throughout the day.

☐ I have more energy because of better fueling patterns.

☐ I think I am performing better because of better fueling patterns.

☐ I still struggle with spending my calories during the day; I tend to save them for PM.

As a result of the nutrition class, I have made the following changes in my fueling patterns:

_____

_____

_____

_____

WEIGHT:

☐ Weight is not an issue for me; I have always been at peace with my weight.

☐ I now focus more on proper fueling than on dieting to lose weight.

☐ By eating better since the nutrition class, I have been able to lose weight (____lbs).

☐ I am more at peace with my body.

☐ I still struggle with weight and constantly try to diet.

☐ I think I would benefit from personalized advice to help me reach my weight goals.

As a result of the nutrition class, I have made the following attitudinal changes about my weight:

_____

_____

_____

_____

Thank You!

This form was developed by Nancy Clark, MS, RD.

REFERENCES

1. *Medical Nutrition Therapy Across the Continuum of Care.* Chicago, Ill: The American Dietetic Association; 1996.

2. Schiller MR, Miller M, Moore C, et al. Patients report positive nutrition counseling outcomes. *J Am Diet Assoc.* 1998;98:977-982.

3. Frentsos J, Baer J. Increased energy and nutrient intake during training and competition improves elite triathletes' endurance performance. *Int J Sport Nutr.* 1997;7:61-71.

4. Baron H, Clark N. Who provides nutrition information at health clubs in the Boston area [abstract]? *J Am Diet Assoc.* 1997;97(suppl):A-71.

5. Clark KL. Sports nutrition counseling: documentation of performance. *Top Clin Nutr.* 1999;14:34-40.

SECTION 3 SPORTS NUTRITION GUIDELINES FOR SPECIAL POPULATION GROUPS

The pursuit of fitness is no longer the domain of the young and healthy. People of all ages and abilities are embarking on fitness programs. However, as more and more people with diverse backgrounds and varying levels of fitness and health become involved in physical exercise, it is increasingly important for health professionals to have knowledge of the physiological and health-related issues of special population groups. Knowing how factors such as age, health status, physical ability, eating habits, and exercise environment affect exercise performance and nutrition needs can help the professional design the most effective care plan for a client. Section 3 opens with pointers on how to communicate effectively with athletes about nutrition. This is followed by discussion of nutritional considerations and physiological concerns during various stages of the lifecycle and under a variety of conditions and disease states.

SECTION 3 CONTENTS

14

COMMUNICATING WITH ATHLETES ABOUT NUTRITION

Nancy Clark, MS, RD, FADA, FACSM

Communicating effectively with athletes about nutrition is an essential skill if you want to help them make the positive changes in their eating behaviors that contribute to enhanced health and athletic performance. Each athlete wants to be listened to as a unique individual, be respected for his or her strengths, and be offered appropriate food solutions. The job of the sports nutrition counselor becomes that of facilitator and mentor, with wisdom to ask the right questions and provide the "how to" guidance that will help the client meet his or her personal nutrition, weight, and performance goals.

The keys to successful communication with athletes about nutrition include:

- Knowing (or being willing to learn about) their sport so you can understand the perspective from which they speak
- Learning why they have come to you, so you have a clear understanding of their nutrition and performance goals
- Building a relationship with the client(s) by being empathetic, genuine, and a good listener
- Attending to the athletes' needs and help them explore the problems; offering a respectful, business-like approach
- Being sensitive to athlete-specific issues and multicultural differences
- Assessing their concerns and then teaching the skills that empower the athlete(s) to succeed with optimal fueling (1)

BE PREPARED

Athletes' common request of a sports nutritionist: "Tell me what to eat—and I'll eat it!" But before being able to tell them what to eat, the effective sports nutrition communicator must first assess the athlete's following characteristics:

- Normal nutrition needs to support growth and health
- Nutrition needs during daily training
- Sport-specific needs preceeding, during, and following competition
- Special nutrition needs due to health concerns (hypertension, diabetes, and so on) (2)

For more detailed information on how to assess athletes' nutritional status, refer to Chapter 8, Health Screening and Medical Evaluation; Chapter 9, Dietary Assessment; and Chapter 11, Assessment of Body Size and Composition.

The job of sports nutrition communicators is to identify and understand all the factors that affect food intake including the following:

- The athletes' training schedule:
  — How often do they train per day—once, twice, or more?
  — At what times do they exercise?
  — Does training interfere with regularly scheduled meals?
  — How often are rest days included in the training program?
- Personal food preferences and lifestyle factors:
  — Who provides the athlete's food—The school? The parents? or Is the athlete responsible for his or her own foods acquisition and preparation?
  — Does the athlete have a limited food budget?
  — Is the athlete weight-conscious and trying to maintain a low-calorie diet?
  — Is the athlete a vegetarian?
  — Does the athlete have any special health issues that require a special diet?
- Supplementation practices common to the sport: (See Chapter 7, Ergogenic Aids for more information.)
  — What supplements are commonly taken by athletes in this sport?
  — Does peer-reviewed research support the use of these supplements?
  — Is your client currently taking or interested in taking these supplements?
  — What goals does the athlete hope to achieve by using supplements?
  — Can these goals be met with dietary improvements?
- Weight demands of each sport:
  — Does the sport have weight classes?
    • If so, what are the weight classes?
    • How many days or weeks does the athlete have to attain the desired weight?
    • What is the time span between weigh-in and competition?
    • Will the athlete be able to eat or drink after weigh-in?
  — Does the sport favor heavier athletes?
    • Is the athlete trying to gain weight?
- Nutrition demands surrounding competition:
  — What time is the event?
    • What meals or snacks will the athlete be able to eat preevent?
  — How long does a game or event last?
    • Will the athlete have ready access to fluids during the event?
    • What foods and fluids, if any, will be available at breaks?
  — Will the event include multiple competitions, such as a swim meet?
    • If so, what is the time span between competitions?
    • Who is responsible for providing fluids and foods?

Sports nutrition professionals need to be knowledgable and credible so the athlete will respect their counsel. Being athletic can enhance a sports nutritionist's credibility. For example, a sports nutritionist who has been a competitive gymnast has a wealth of personal experience that can strengthen his or her rapport with other gymnasts. Even a sports nutritionist who had no formal school sports experiences can gain credibility by joining sports groups such as running or bicycling clubs. This offers more professional credibility (and learning opportunities) than simply running or biking solo.

ATHLETES AS EAGER LEARNERS

Most athletes and active people recognize that proper fueling is an important and integral part of a training program, and they commonly have a keen interest in nutrition. They come to a sports nutritionist with an open ear and an earnest interest in finding answers to their nutrition questions and food concerns. Most are ready and willing to make changes but, like many of today's busy people, they face barriers that interfere with optimal fueling (3). It is not uncommon to hear:

- "I have no time to eat well."
- "Eating well is too difficult."
- "Healthy food does not taste good."
- "I'm confused about what to eat."

When communicating with athletes, keep in mind they want practical advice that helps them overcome these barriers and eat well in a variety of sport-specific situations. This includes eating well when they are rushing to practice and need a quick energy boost, eating the pregame meal at a fast-food restaurant, traveling to an event in a different time zone, selecting a sports diet at a sumptuous hotel buffet, trying to lose weight while maintaining energy to exercise, cooking solo and opting for meals that require minimal preparation. *Box 14.1* lists tips on how to offer practical advice.

BOX 14.1 Offer Practical Advice

Athletes welcome not only general advice but also specific "how to" information about various topics:

- Calorie needs
- Optimal distribution of calories throughout the day
- Appropriate amount of grams of protein and fat
- How to easily select the right balance of protein, fat, and carbohydrates
- Fluid needs
- How to stay well-hydrated

The information is best provided both as numbers and examples of appropriate foods and fluids that provide the desired amounts of nutrients. For example, an athlete who is told she needs 60 g of protein can better visualize the concept: 60 g of protein = One 6-oz can of tuna + 3 glasses of skim milk.

---

continued

BOX 14.1   Offer Practical Advice (continued)

When communicating with athletes, be sure to present the information in a simple, doable manner that enables the athletes to put the tips into use. The sports nutritionist can help athletes achieve their desired, positive outcomes by:

- Processing their concerns, understanding the problem from their perspective, and recognizing the barriers they face (such as, "I don't have time to eat well.")
- Asking open-ended questions to help the athletes create the solution ("When do you think you could consume more calories so you can attain your weight-gain goal?")
- Offering specific, practical suggestions ("Here are three ways you can easily boost your calorie intake...")
- Creating a personalized nutrition program *with* the athlete that works *for* the athlete ("Could you drink four more glasses of juice in place of water throughout the day?")

THE RESISTANT ATHLETE

Not all athletes are ready for change. For example, athletes with eating disorders commonly deny any problems with fueling and may reject your suggestions for dietary improvements. If you are asked to communicate with a resistant athlete who seemingly lacks interest in making dietary changes, a good place to start is to communicate the benefits associated with optimal fueling. Three important benefits are:

1. Delaying fatigue
2. Enhancing healing of illness and/or injuries
3. Improving performance

Once the athlete can relate to the benefits, he or she will be more likely to display interest in the topic and may be more willing to experiment with making small dietary changes "one step at a time."

Often the counseling needs to focus on the source of the resistance and then how to overcome the resistance. For example, a swimmer with an eating disorder may hesistate to fuel herself better for fear of "getting fat." By exploring this fear and providing appropriate education, the nutrition counselor can help the athlete transform that fear into appropriate fueling for better sports performance and overall good health.

COMMUNICATION OBSTACLES

Sports nutritionists commonly encounter obstacles that hinder their ability to communicate with athletes. Three common obstacles include:

1. "No thank you"
2. "No time"
3. "No money"

"No thank you"

Each team has a "gatekeeper" who controls the dissemination of nutrition information. When that gatekeeper is the coach who declines your invitation to work together with him or her and his or her team, you will rightfully feel frustrated. Clearly, if you cannot get through the gate, you will be unable to communicate your important message to the athletes.

Two solutions may be:

- Educate the coach about the benefits of nutrition education. (See Chapter 13, Documenting Sports Nutrition Outcomes.) If the coach understands what you have to offer and how you can help the team improve its performance, he or she will be more likely to listen to your request.
- Explore other ways to open the gate. For example, a coach may display little interest in working with a sports nutritionist, but the athletic trainer, who commonly deals with the myriad of nutrition concerns and questions, may enthusiastically welcome a sports nutritionist and persuade the coach to see the benefits of having a nutrition professional handle the food and weight problems.

"No time"

Time is a big obstacle that hinders effective nutrition communication. Most coaches hesitate to donate more than 10 to 15 minutes of practice time to nutrition education. Solutions to this resistance include:

- Propose a series of short (10-minute) nutrition sessions, with each session covering only one topic such as fluids, carbohydrates, protein, calories, alcohol, supplements, or pregame eating. The session would be best given at the start of practice when the athletes are fresh, as opposed to at the end of the practice when they are tired, hungry, and eager to leave. A sports nutritionist should plan to concisely make three key points, answer the athletes' questions, and honor the time schedule.
- Propose a one-time nutrition class to replace the training session. This might be done on the day after a competition when the athletes need and welcome a rest day from exercise.

"No money"

If you are a paid staff member at a college or university, funding for nutrition services may be less of an issue than for an outside consultant. Consultants are commonly confronted with budget constraints that close the door to nutrition education and communication. The solution is to explore funding possibilities.

- If the cost is too high for one team's budget, you can offer to talk to three teams, each chipping in one-third of the fee.

- Perhaps money is available from the health center, sports medicine department, booster club, Parent Teacher Association, or special athletic fund.
- Sometimes an interested parent is willing to pay. For example, the parents of a weight-cycling wrestler are often interested in supporting nutrition education.

COMMUNICATION ENHANCERS

Helpful factors that enhance the sports nutritionist's ability to be an effective communicator include:

- Be a good listener. *Table 14.1* illustrates basic listening skills.
- Create educational sessions with small but clear goals and objectives for each session. For example, a session on fluids might include information on how to identify when an athlete is dehydrated, which fluids are best to drink, when to drink, and how to determine sweat losses and fluid needs.
- Leave adequate time to teach each athlete how to create the winning program (ie, more than 5 minutes right before practice). Mini-classes can sometimes be preferable to presenting a large amount of information in a one-time-only team workshop. This will depend on both the nutrition professional's time schedule and the athlete's availability. If time is available, supermarket tours and cooking classes may also interest the team, in addition to being fun.
- Secure an appropriate counseling space for team seminars—not the gym with a hard floor for sitting during an hour-long workshop.
- Reserve an appropriate counseling space for individuals—not the locker room that lacks privacy.
- Show genuine empathy for and caring and concern about the athlete. Attendance at athletic events can enhance communication by visibly demonstrating interest in the sport and athletes.

TABLE 14.1   Basic Listening Skills (1)

Skill	Description	Function in Interview
Active Listening Skills		
Silence or minimal response	Nod of head; "um-um"	Provides neutral feedback that the message was heard but does not indicate judgment
Reflective responses	Statements which summarize the content or feeling of the client	Encourages elaboration, acts as promoter for discussion, shows understanding and a willingness to help, checks clarity of counselor's understanding, elucidates emotions underlying client's words and actions

continued

TABLE 14.1   Basic Listening Skills (continued)

Skill	Description	Function in Interview
Leading Skills		
Open questions	"What": facts "How": process or feelings "Tell me more." "Could you be more specific?"	Brings out major data and facilitates the helping interaction. Elicits client response in an open-ended yet focused manner. Can be in the form of questions or open statements
Closed questions	Usually begin with "do," "is," or "are," and can be answered with a "yes" or "no" or one or two words	Quickly obtains specific data. Use with caution.
Why questions	Questions which seek the reason, cause, or purpose	Can result in learning more about how the client reasons. Caution: May put the client on the defensive. Use sparingly.
Influencing responses	"That's a good idea." (encourages) "Maybe that's not the real issue." (interprets) "It's self-defeating to think that." (discourages)	Encourages or discourages the client's ideas, thoughts, or course of action to change or reinforce behavior
Advice	Provides suggestions, instructional ideas, homework, and advice on how to act, think, or behave	May provide client with new and useful ideas to try. Use sparingly.
Information	A statement made to instruct the client on appropriate nutrition practices.	Provides clients with more data to enable them to design their own solutions. Note that too much information is overwhelming. Counselors must determine the amount that is really necessary.
Self-referent Skills		
Self-involving responses	The counselor shares a personal response to what the client said or did.	Can be used to provide feedback or praise, or to gently comfort. Gives counselor a way to use his or her own feelings and reaction to the client during counseling.
Self-disclosure	Counselor shares personal experiences from the past or factual information about himself or herself.	Can build a good relationship with the client through similar, shared experiences.

Source: Helm K, Klawitter B. *Nutrition Therapy: Advanced Counseling Skills*. Lake Dallas, Tex: Helm Seminars; 1995. Reprinted by permission.

SUMMARY

Effective communication with athletes follows the same rules as effective communication with all other clients. The main difference is that with athletes it is important to know the specific demands each sport places on the athletes' nutrition needs and eating schedule. If necessary, take time to attend practice sessions and events to better learn about each sport. This will help the sports nutritionist to create a personalized program for each athlete that supports normal nutrition needs, additional nutrition needs resulting from training and competition, and special nutrition needs related to health problems, including weight management (3). The skilled nutrition communicator can help athletes overcome the barriers that impede optimal fueling and make good nutrition and optimal fueling easy, practical, and beneficial.

REFERENCES

1. Helm K. In: King N, Klawitter B, eds. *Nutrition Therapy: Advanced Counseling Skills.* Lake Dallas, Tex: Helm Seminars; 1995.
2. Storlie J. Nutrition assessment of athletes: a model for integrating nutrition and physical performance indicators. *Int J Sport Nutr.* 1991;1:192-204.
3. *1997 Nutrition Trends Survey.* Chicago, Ill: The American Dietetic Association; 1997.

15

ELEMENTARY AND MIDDLE SCHOOL ATHLETES

Suzanne Nelson Steen, DSc, RD

Whether it is training for a soccer game or playing a backyard game of catch, children's health and athletic performance depend largely on adequate nourishment and hydration. This chapter provides guidelines to help ensure that young athletes are fueled and hydrated for exercise, compatible with their needs for growth and development (1-4).

GROWTH AND DEVELOPMENT

Growth Charts

All children should have their weight, height, weight-for-height, and standard-height-for-age evaluated and assessed using National Center for Health Statistics growth charts (5). Routine plotting of weight and height is essential to track normal growth and to identify patterns that are indicative of acute or chronic malnutrition (stunting, failure to thrive) or over-nutrition (obesity).

Measurements should be recorded at regular intervals in order to accurately reflect the growth patterns of the child (6). Usually, normal childhood growth occurs between the 5th and 95th percentile. During the first 2 years of age, some fluctuation in height and weight within the 5th and 95th percentile is expected as both infants and children demonstrate individual spurts in growth. However, children generally maintain their height and weight between the same percentiles (ie, 25th to 50th percentile; also referred to as growth channel) during the preschool and early childhood years. Although individual children differ in their rates of growth, they should follow the same channels. When either height or weight deviates from the child's usual growth percentiles, the etiology of the change should be investigated.

A more precise evaluation of growth is necessary when height and weight fall in markedly different percentiles (ie, height 10th percentile, weight 50th percentile) since the height and weight of a child should be in proportion. Assessment of weight in relation to height enables evaluation of current nutrition status and growth that is specific to the child's body size. At a single point in time, weight-for-height is a more sensitive index of appropriate growth than weight-for-age, since appropriateness of body weight is dependent on total body size, not on age.

In contrast to the weight-for-height assessment, height-for-age comparison is an index of previous nutrition and growth status. A reduction in height velocity is slower to develop in the presence of under-nutrition than a decrease in weight velocity. Therefore, it is an index of *chronic* malnutrition.

Age- and sex-specific standards have been developed to separate the genetic contribution of parental stature from other factors that affect a child's linear growth, such as malnutrition or disease. A child's actual height can be adjusted with a factor derived from the average of each parent's height. This method is recommended for evaluating children whose height-for-age is less than the 5th percentile (7,8).

The actual increments in height and weight during the school age years are small compared with those during infancy and adolescence. Weight increases an average of 2 to 3 kg each year until the child is 9 or 10 years old. Then, rate of weight gain increases, which is an initial sign of approaching puberty. Height increments average 5 to 6 cm per year from age 2 until the pubertal acceleration (6). At puberty, children undergo hormonal changes that mark the beginning of adolescence. Nutrition needs prior to and during this period of rapid growth increase significantly.

Body Composition Assessment

It is now widely recognized that weight, *per se,* is not an appropriate marker of performance capabilities, and that the existing weight of an athlete should not be used to establish goal weights (9). Instead, the athlete's body composition needs to be evaluated, with an estimate of the amount of lean and fat tissue.

However, in children and youth, evaluation of body composition is complicated by several factors that affect the conceptual basis for estimating fat and lean tissue (10-12). First, children have higher body-water content and lower bone-mineral content (10-12) and, therefore, have a lower body density than adults. Equations developed for prepubescent children that use conversion constants derived from adult samples are not appropriate for children because they may overestimate body fatness by 3% to 6% and underestimate lean body weight (11-12).

Another limitation is that the chemical composition of the fat-free mass changes as the child passes through puberty (10-12). Significant changes in the relation of skinfolds to density occur from prepubescence to puberty and from puberty to postpubescence. As a result, estimates of body fatness by skinfolds, body widths, and circumferences may reflect alterations in the composition of the fat-free body components, which include water, mineral, and protein, rather than alterations in actual fat content.

To overcome these limitations, estimates of body fat in children and youth must take a multicomponent approach to assessing body composition rather than the traditional two-compartment model of fat and fat-free densities (10-12). Lohman (13) has proposed equations for estimating percent body fat from body density on the basis of age and gender. These equations were derived by substituting estimated fat-free body densities by age and sex (along with the assumed fat density of 0.90 g/mL) into the Siri equation (a prediction equation used for calculating percentage body fat). These equations are listed in *Table 15.1.*

TABLE 15.1   Body-fat Equations

Age (years)	Males	Females
7–8	% fat = 5.38 Db – 4.97	% fat = 5.43 Db – 5.03
9–10	% fat = 5.30 Db – 4.89	% fat = 5.35 Db – 4.95
11–12	% fat = 5.23 Db – 4.81	% fat = 5.25 Db – 4.84
13–14	% fat = 5.07 Db – 4.64	% fat = 5.12 Db – 4.69
15–16	% fat = 5.03 Db – 4.59	% fat = 5.07 Db – 4.64

Db = body density (determined by underwater weighing)

Adapted with permission from Loman TG. Assessment of body composition in children. *Pediatric Exercise Science. Vol. 1.* 1989:19-30.

Skinfold equations that use a multicomponent approach to assess body composition and account for the chemical immaturity of children have been developed by Slaughter et al (12). The Tanner Scale (14) of pubertal development was used to assess the maturational level of the children. These equations (see *Table 15.2*) are recommended for predicting percent body fat in children and youth 8 to 18 years. Another approach is to simply track changes in skinfold thickness

TABLE 15.2   Skinfold Equations

Skinfold equations are for predicting % body fat in children and youth (8 to 18 years).

For sum of triceps and subscapular <35 mm use:

White male:

Prepubescent   % fat = 1.21 (T+S) – 0.008 (T+S)^2 – 1.7

Pubescent   % fat = 1.21 (T+S) – 0.008 (T+S)^2 – 3.4

Postpubescent   % fat = 1.21 (T+S) – 0.008 (T+S)^2 – 3.5

Black male:

Prepubescent   % fat = 1.21 (T+S) – 0.008 (T+S)^2 – 3.2

Pubescent   % fat = 1.21 (T+S) – 0.008 (T+S)^2 – 5.2

Postpubescent   % fat = 1.21 (T+S) – 0.008 (T+S)^2 – 6.8

All females: % fat = 1.33 (T+S) – 0.013 (T+S)^2 – 2.5

For sum of triceps and subscalpular >35 mm use:

All males   % fat = 0.783 (T+S) + 1.6

All females   % fat = 0.546 (T+S) + 9.7

For triceps and calf use:

All males   % fat = 0.735 (T+C) + 1.0

All females   % fat = 0.610 (T+C) + 5.1

Skinfold Measurement Locations

- Triceps (upper arm): Vertical fold raised midway between right olecranon and acromion processes on posterior of brachium.
- Subscapular (back): Skinfold picked up 1 cm below inferior angle of right scapula inclined downward laterally in natural cleavage.
- Medial calf: Vertical skinfold raised on medial side of right calf just above level of maximal calf girth.

C = calf; S = subscapular; T = triceps

Source: Slaughter MH, et al. *Skinfold Equations for Evaluation of Body Fatness in Children and Youth. Vol. 60.* Detroit, Mich: Wayne State University Press; 1988.

instead of calculating percentage body fat. The sum of specific skinfolds (for example, triceps plus subscapular) may be used.

Body composition tables that show percent body fat values for male and female athletes are not suitable for children because the majority of measurements were taken on athletes 19 years and older. There are currently no standards of comparison for young athletes that are specific for sport and gender. No tables are available that provide an "optimal or ideal weight" for performance (if one does in fact exist) for children or older athletes.

From a practical standpoint, body composition measures can be used by a qualified health professional to monitor changes in fat and lean tissue during training. Growth charts in combination with skinfold measures and sound clinical judgment can be used to determine a range of weights for a particular young athlete. Body composition measures should not be used in the prepubescent athlete to set stringent weight-loss or body-fat guidelines. Doing so may adversely affect normal growth and development. This point needs to be made clear to coaches, parents, and athletes.

NUTRITION ASSESSMENT

School-age children tend to be repetitious in their food choices, causing the foods they include in their diets to remain relatively constant from month to month (15). In addition to evaluating the caloric and nutrient content of the diet, excess consumption of high-calorie/low-nutrient density foods, unusual foods, and consistently omitted food categories should be noted.

Most children recall food items fairly reliably but quantities less accurately. Therefore, the methodology used to assess dietary intake (24-hour recall, food records) should consider the maturity level of the child. Most important is to establish a good rapport with the child to facilitate acceptance of the recommendations that will be made.

The parent(s) need to be interviewed about the child's diet. Ideally, the child and parent(s) should be interviewed separately. Otherwise, children may report what they think the parent wants them to be eating instead of actual intake. Comparing and combining information from both parent and child provides a complete picture of the child's habits and rationale for consumption of certain foods.

Meal Patterns

Meal patterns can be identified by asking the child when he or she typically eats, where he or she eats, and with whom. For example:

- Does the child eat breakfast?
- Does the child have lunch at school or at home?
- What is the frequency of snacking?
- Are dinners spent with family or eaten alone?
- What time of day does the child eat meals in relation to practice?
- When are fluids consumed?

Many children skip breakfast (15). Some studies suggest that children who eat breakfast have a better attitude, school record, and problem-solving abilities compared to children who do not eat breakfast (16,17). In addition, breakfast helps to replenish glycogen stores depleted during an overnight fast, to ensure that the child has adequate energy stores for afternoon training or competition. It is important to encourage children to find foods they like to eat for breakfast. These do not need to be traditional foods. Food composition, not social tradition, is the best strategy. Breakfast should provide between a quarter to a third of the nutrients for the day.

The child's lunch may be provided by the school or brought from home. Because the child's friends often influence food choices, it is important to ask the child with whom he or she typically eats lunch and why he or she chooses certain foods. Studies have shown that the school lunch is usually more nutritious than a lunch brought from home (18). This is because box lunches typically contain less variety and include only favorite foods (18). In addition, they are limited to foods that travel well and do not require heating or refrigeration. Even if a nutritious lunch is packed at home, the parent does not necessarily know what portion is eaten, traded, or thrown away. Timing of meals is also a consideration. Depending on scheduling at the school cafeteria, some children may eat breakfast at 8:30 AM followed by lunch at 11:30 AM. Practice may not be until 2:30 PM. If the time between lunch and practice is more than 2 hours, the child should pack a snack to eat during this time.

Snacks may significantly contribute to the child's nutrient intake and eating style (15). The quality of snacks eaten may determine whether nutrient requirements are being met. Therefore, the frequency of snacking and type of snacks are important considerations. For example:

- Does the child typically snack during the morning, afternoon, and/or evening?
- What are the child's favorite snacks?
- Are snacks prepared at home or purchased from a vending machine?

Ideas for snacks to pack (or choose from a vending machine as available) for school-age children are listed in *Box 15.1*.

BOX 15.1   Snacks to Pack for Children

Crunchy	Chewy	Creamy	Juicy
Pretzels	Raisins	Pudding packs	Juice packs
Popcorn	Dried fruit	Cheese cubes	Jello packs
Mini flavored rice cakes	Bagels	Milk	Applesauce
Animal crackers	Breakfast bars	Yogurt	Canned fruit
Trail mix	Rice Krispie Treats	Peanut butter	Cherry tomatoes
Granola bars	Graham Treats	Banana	Tangerine
Baked chips	Chewy granola bars		Orange
Graham crackers			Grapes
Cereal			
Air Crisps			
Apples			
Baby carrots			
Celery sticks			

Energy Requirements

Energy requirements should consider current dietary intake, rate of growth, age, gender, weight, and energy demands of the sport. Prior to puberty, nutrition needs are modest compared to the adolescent period of rapid growth and high-nutrition demands. However, a large variability in energy intakes may exist for healthy growing children of the same age and sex. For example, a 7-year-old boy and a 10 1/2-year-old girl approaching puberty have significantly different factors determining their energy needs, even though they are in the same Recommended Dietary Allowance (RDA) category (19). The RDA can be used to estimate caloric needs for normal growth and development per kilogram of body weight.

Although data on adult athletes have shown that differences in daily energy requirements depend on the volume of training and the energy cost of their specific sport, no similar data exist for young children. In children, energy needs are different because of lower body mass and lower skill level, and the metabolic cost per kg body mass decreases with age (20). Frost et al (21) have shown that energy "wastefulness" in children's movement is due to a lack of adequate co-contraction of antagonist muscles during walking and running.

To estimate how many calories the child may be expending during activity, specific questions should be asked about the training schedule:

- In what sport(s) is the child involved?
- Does the child participate in competitions, and if so, at what level?
- How often does the child train, and for how long?
- What is the intensity of the activity? This can be estimated by asking the child to describe a typical training session or, more precisely, by having the child/parent keep an exercise log that documents time spent doing various activities.

Caloric expenditures for various activities that are specific for children are presented in *Table 15.3*. These data can be used as a guide to calculate calories expended per kilogram of body weight.

Other factors to consider that may affect the young athlete's food intake are socioeconomic status, the individual responsible for food purchase and preparation, access to sufficient calories, intentional weight loss, body image disturbance, peer pressure, and health problem(s) (22,23).

TABLE 15.3   Caloric Equivalents of Child's Activities in Kcal per 10 Minutes of Activity

Activity	Body Weight (kg)									
	20	25	30	35	40	45	50	55	60	65
Basketball	34	43	51	60	68	77	85	94	102	110
Calisthenics	13	17	20	23	26	30	33	36	40	43
Cycling										
10 km/hour	15	17	20	23	26	29	33	36	39	42
15 km/hour	22	27	32	36	41	46	50	55	60	65
Figure skating	40	50	60	70	80	90	100	110	120	130
Ice hockey										
(on ice time)	52	65	78	91	104	117	130	143	156	168
Running										
8 km/hour	37	45	52	60	66	72	78	84	90	95
10 km/hour	48	55	64	73	79	85	92	100	107	113
Soccer (game)	36	45	54	63	72	81	90	99	108	117
Swimming 30 m/minute										
Breast	19	24	29	34	38	43	48	53	58	62
Front crawl	25	31	37	43	49	56	62	68	74	80
Back	17	21	25	30	34	38	42	47	51	55
Tennis	22	28	33	39	44	50	55	61	66	72
Walking										
4 km/hour	17	19	21	23	26	28	30	32	34	36
6 km/hour	24	26	28	30	32	34	37	40	43	48

Adapted with permission from Bar-Or O. *Pediatric Sports Medcine*. New York, NY: Springer-Verlag; 1983.

Dietary Recommendations

What is the most appropriate diet for the child athlete? Adequate energy and nutrients should be obtained from a diet that emphasizes complex carbohydrates and moderate amounts of protein and fat to support growth and physical activity (24). This can be achieved by planning to include a variety of foods from each of the major food groups as illustrated by the Food Guide Pyramid (25). The key messages of variety, balance, and moderation in food choices should be promoted.

Especially for the young child, the pyramid serves as a visual guide for choosing foods and helping to plan healthful meals. Each day the young athlete should consume at least two to three servings from the milk group, two to three servings from the meat/protein group, four servings from the vegetable group, three servings from the fruit group, and nine servings from the bread/grain group. Foods containing the majority of calories from fat or sugars (at the top of the pyramid) are not eliminated but should be consumed occasionally as an addition to, and not in place of, other nutrient-dense foods. In general, providing servings within these recommended ranges will supply the necessary vitamins, minerals, and calories (2,200 kcal) most active children require. However, depending on the frequency, intensity, and duration of physical activity, the exercising child may need an additional 500 to 1,000 kcal each day. Children should be encouraged to distribute calories throughout the day at regular meal times and snacks. This will ensure the presence of readily available sources of energy to support growth and training activity.

Young athletes can meet their vitamin and mineral needs on diets that include the foods and servings recommended in the Food Guide Pyramid (24). If it is determined that the child's intake is low for certain micronutrients, strategies to increase consumption from foods should be discussed with the parent. Because the young child relies for the most part on the foods that are brought into the house, an evaluation of foods that are purchased by the parents/caretakers is essential.

In addition to purchasing more healthful foods, favorite foods can be made more nutrient-dense or acceptable substitutions can be made with similar foods. For example, fortified cereals can be served rather than sugary ones, and peanut butter cookies can be offered instead of vanilla cream cookies. Many different food choices are available to supply adequate amounts of vitamins and minerals for even the choosiest of eaters. Small changes that are acceptable to the child can be encouraged to increase nutrient density.

Variety in the family menu underscores the importance of eating different foods to provide the range of nutrients necessary for growth and development. Ideally, this variety is most easily achieved in regularly scheduled meals at home, plus nutritious snacks. However, this may not be possible. An important issue facing parents with children in sports is how to provide nutritious meals around hectic practice schedules. Workouts may interfere with home meals, resulting in a greater reliance on convenient fast foods or the child eating alone after the family has finished the evening meal.

It is important for children to learn how to make nutritious food choices at fast-food restaurants since most popular choices are high in fat and salt, and low in vitamins A and C and fiber. Examples of healthier choices are pancakes, baked potato with chili, salad bar, grilled chicken sandwich, plain hamburgers versus super deluxe burgers, and thick-crust vegetable pizza. Beverage suggestions include low-fat milkshakes, low-fat milk, and juices.

Vegetarian Diet

When carefully planned, a diet that derives its protein from vegetable sources can provide adequate protein, carbohydrate, vitamins, and minerals that the young athlete needs to sustain growth and prolonged workouts. Protein intake on a lacto-ovo vegetarian diet or a semivegetarian diet should provide adequate calories and high-quality protein from eggs and dairy products. However, on a strict vegetarian diet, the athlete may have difficulty obtaining calories, protein, and other nutrients such as calcium, vitamin D, zinc, iron, and vitamin B-12 (4). Eliminating foods that contain important vitamins and minerals can be risky unless the parent is well informed and motivated to carefully plan intake so that good health and proper growth are maintained (4).

FLUID NEEDS OF CHILDREN

All athletes need to maintain adequate hydration to replace losses during exercise. However, compared with adults and even adolescents, preadolescent children must be especially careful to drink enough during exercise for several reasons. Although children's physiologic responses to exercise are generally similar to those of adults, there are several age- and maturation-related differences in their response (26-28). As shown in *Table 15.4,* children respond to the combined stresses of exercise and climatic heat differently than do adults. Children tolerate temperature extremes less efficiently than adults (26,27,29). They have a lower sweating rate (absolute and per single gland) that potentially lowers capacity to evaporate heat loss (30,31). In addition, a child experiences a greater heat production in exercise and has less ability to transfer heat from the muscles to the skin.

TABLE 15.4   Physiologic Responses of Children to Exercise in the Heat: Comparison with Adults

Characteristic	Typical for Children versus Adults
Metabolizing heat of locomotion	Higher
Sweating rate per m^2 skin	Lower
Sweating rate per gland	Much lower
Sweating threshold	Higher
Density of HASG	Higher
Cardiac output/L O$_2$ uptake	Lower
Blood flow to skin	Higher
Sweat NaCl content	Lower
Sweat lactate and H$^+$	Higher
Exercise tolerance time	Shorter
Acclimatization to heat	Slower
Increasing core temperature with dehydration	Faster

HASG = heat-activated sweat glands

Source: Courtsey of Gatorade Sports Science Institute, Chicago, Illinois

Relative surface area is greater for a child compared to an adult. For example, for an 8-year-old child the ratio of surface area to mass is 360 to 380 cm^2/kg compared to 240 to 260 cm^2/kg for an adult of medium size (26). This results in excessive heat gain in extreme heat and heat loss in the cold. Children also have a lower cardiac output at given metabolic level, which potentially lowers capacity for heat convection from core to periphery during strenuous exercise (26).

The above morphologic and functional characteristics do not interfere with the exercising child's ability to adequately dissipate heat in a neutral or mildly warm climate (26). However, children are at a disadvantage when exposed to extreme heat or cold. The greater the temperature gradient between the air and the skin, the greater the effect on the child.

Acclimatization to exercising in the heat is more gradual in children compared to adolescents or adults (32). A child may require five to six sessions to achieve the same degree of acclimatization acquired by an adult in two to three sessions in the same environment. From a practical standpoint, the intensity and duration of exercise should be restrained during the first 4 to 5 days of beginning an exercise program, particularly in the heat. Over a period of 1 to 1¹/2 weeks, activity can be slowly increased (26). The major physiologic changes that occur during heat acclimatization include a reduction in heart rate and body temperature, an increase in sweat rate, and a decreased concentration of salt in the sweat (26,33).

Dehydration and Heat Disorders

Because children sweat less, have a lower cardiac output, do not tolerate temperature extremes, and acclimate to heat more slowly than young adults (26,31), they are at increased risk for dehydration. As little as a 2% decrease in body weight from fluid loss (eg, 1.2-lb loss for a 60-lb athlete) can lead to a significant decrease in muscular strength and stamina (34).

The progressive effects of dehydration are serious. As an individual becomes dehydrated, heart rate increases, blood flow to the skin decreases, and body temperature can rise steadily to dangerous levels (34). Coaches need to be familiar with the symptoms of heat distress and procedures for obtaining and providing immediate treatment.

Certain groups of children are at particularly high risk of heat illness due to certain diseases and medical conditions (27,33). One common underlying factor among these conditions is that they may induce hypohydration, either through excessive fluid loss or insufficient intake. Excessive fluid loss may be observed in the following conditions: bulimia, congenital heart disease, diabetes mellitus, diabetes insipidus, gastroenteritis, fever, obesity, and vomiting. Insufficient fluid intake may occur in anorexia nervosa, cystic fibrosis, mental retardation, and renal failure.

Obese children are at a disadvantage when exercising in the heat. Rectal temperature and heart rate increased more quickly in mildly obese boys (31.2% body fat) compared to leaner controls during 70 minutes of intermittent exercise and rest (31). According to Bar-Or (27), possible reasons for the deficient thermoregulation in the obese include:

- A relatively small amount of heat is needed to increase the temperature of a given mass of fat.
- Hypohydration denotes a relatively higher percentage of water loss in obese individuals.
- Fat contains less water than most other tissues.
- When obese children exercise at the same intensity, compared to nonobese children, their relative effort is greater (and the rise of core temperature is higher) due to a low maximal aerobic capacity.

The type of clothing worn during exercise affects the body's ability to cool itself. Heavy clothing can be a contributing factor to heat stress. Therefore, children who participate in certain sports may be at an increased risk for dehydration and heat illness. For example, football and hockey players wear protective gear, which reduces the ability of the body to cool itself.

Swimmers may not recognize that they are losing body water through sweat in the pool. They can also become dehydrated by sitting around the pool in a hot, humid environment between exercise sessions. Figure skaters may not realize the importance of fluid replacement because they are in a cool environment. In addition, their typical sports attire—gloves, tights, and body suits and/or sweats—reduces the ability of the body to cool itself.

Athletes in sports that have weight categories for competition, such as wrestling or light-weight rowing, may purposefully restrict fluid and/or food intake in an effort to lose weight, thus increasing the risk of dehydration (35-37). Athletes in sports where appearance and leanness are critically evaluated by judges and audiences, such as gymnasts, ballet dancers, and figure skaters, may also be at increased risk for dehydration if fluid and/or food deprivation are used to control weight (37-40).

To prevent dehydration and reduce the risk of heat injury, adjust the timing of practice depending on weather conditions. Workouts should be scheduled for the coolest time of the day (before 10 AM, after 6 PM), especially in warm, humid weather conditions. Extreme heat and humidity are valid reasons to cancel practice or competition.

Fluid Guidelines

Heat stroke ranks second to head injury among reported causes of death in secondary school athletes. Through education and establishing healthy fluid intake habits at an early age, heat illness can be prevented. Because a substantial level of dehydration can be reached before the body ever feels "thirsty," special emphasis should be placed on ensuring adequate fluid intake in children before, during, and after physical activity. Guidelines for fluid replacement are shown in *Box 15.2*

BOX 15.2   Fluid Guidelines for Active Children

- To prevent dehydration, encourage children to drink cool fluids before, during, and after physical activity.
- Since thirst is not an accurate measure of the body's need for fluid, encourage children to drink on a schedule — every 15 minutes. Once children are thirsty, dehydration has already started.
- Children should be given a squeeze bottle and reminded to drink 3 to 4 oz every 15 minutes during activity.
- Children should be weighed before and after exercise. For every pound of weight lost, make sure they drink 16 to 24 oz of fluid.
- Although plain water is the most economical source of fluid to hydrate the body, children are more likely to drink sufficient amounts if they are given flavored fluids such as a sport drink. A sport drink will supply energy and encourage drinking by "turning on" thirst.
- Avoid beverages that are higher in sugar, like fruit juices and soft drinks, because they are absorbed more slowly and may increase the chance of stomach cramps or nausea.

Children, like adults, do not usually drink enough when offered fluids during exercise in the heat. (26,33). However, one important difference is that for any given level of hypohydration, children's core temperatures increase faster than those of adults (26). During prolonged exercise, children and adolescents may not recognize the symptoms of heat strain and push themselves to the point of heat-related illness (26,29). From a practical standpoint, this suggests that it is important to prevent, or significantly reduce, "voluntary dehydration" in children. This can be accomplished by providing children with a personalized water bottle and encouraging them to drink at regular, frequent intervals beyond thirst. Children less than 10 years old should drink until they do not feel thirsty, and then should drink an additional half a glass of liquid (27). Supervision of fluid intake is essential, particularly for children because they do not instinctively drink enough fluid to replace water losses (26,33).

Children should be weighed before and after exercise to monitor fluid loss. Serial weighing can identify the child who is becoming chronically dehydrated during repetitive training. From a practical standpoint, the young athlete could be weighed during a few training sessions to estimate how much fluid is needed for subsequent workouts.

Fluid losses should be replaced during and after exercise. Children should be allowed to take "fluid breaks" in order to promote adequate hydration. In addition, fluids should be readily available and never be withheld as a disciplinary measure.

Choosing Fluids

Although plain water is the most economical source of fluid to hydrate the body, children may be more likely to drink sufficient amounts if they are given flavored fluids. To enhance a child's willingness to drink, beverages consumed during exercise should be palatable and stimulate thirst (27). Interestingly, prepubertal and early pubertal girls and boys prefer grape-flavored beverages to apple and orange (28). This preference was apparent at rest, following a maximal aerobic test, and during a rehydration stage after prolonged exercise in a hot environment. In a more recent study (41) to further clarify the effect of drink flavor and composition on voluntary drink and hydration, 9- to 12-year-old boys performed three 3-hour exercise sessions (four 20-minute cycling bouts at 50% VO$_2$max followed by 25 minutes rest) in a warm climate. One of three beverages was assigned to each session in a Latin-square sequence: unflavored water, grape-flavored water, and grape-flavored water plus 6% carbohydrate and 18 mmol/L NaCl. Drinking was ad libitum. The results were striking—the children stayed better hydrated when they drank sports drinks (38 oz) compared to drinking plain (20 oz) or flavored water (30 oz). The authors concluded that while flavoring water reduces children's voluntary dehydration, a further addition of 6% carbohydrates and 18 mmol/L NaCl prevents it altogether.

Diluted fruit juice is sometimes used as a fluid replacement beverage during exercise. However, diluted juice may not drive thirst compared to a sports drink (27). More research is needed to identify whether or not diluted fruit juice is a suitable choice for fluid replacement during exercise. Undiluted juice or carbonated soda should not be used during activity since it typically contains too much carbohydrate (10% to 12%) and may cause gastric discomfort and delay gastric emptying. Caffeinated beverages (iced tea, certain soft drinks) should also be avoided since they promote diuresis. Particularly for children, the potential side effects of consuming caffeine—agitation, nausea, muscle tremors, palpitations, and headaches—are not conducive to optimal performance.

Interestingly, sweat sodium and chloride tend to increase with maturation while sweat potassium was lower in young adults compared with prepubescent females and males (28). Because children have a lower sweating rate than young adults, total sodium and chloride losses per kg/BW from sweat were higher in young adults compared with those of the prepubescent and pubescent groups. However, no maturational differences were found in potassium losses. The authors speculate that a protective mechanism may exist in children against excessive salt loss, which accompanies their lower sweating rate. It is not clear whether the lower salt content in children's sweat justifies the use of more dilute beverages for children than for adults. More research is needed.

PRE- AND POSTEXERCISE MEALS

The preevent meal serves two main purposes: first, to prevent athletes from feeling hungry before or during activity; and second, to help supply fuel to the muscles during training and competition. Still, most of the energy needed for any sports event is provided by whatever the child has eaten during the prior week. The most optimal plan is to offer foods 2 to 3 hours before exercise that the child finds pleasing and that are high in carbohydrate, contain low- to moderate-amounts of protein, and are low in fat. In addition, at least 240 mL fluid (water or juice) should be encouraged.

High-fat and high-protein foods should be avoided because they take longer to digest than carbohydrate foods and, if eaten for the preevent meal, can contribute to indigestion and nausea. Children should also avoid eating simple carbohydrates such as sugar, candy, honey, or soft drinks before exercise. They do not provide "quick energy," and some athletes are more sensitive than others to changes in blood glucose levels when simple sugars are eaten. Instead, complex carbohydrates such as breads, cereals, and pasta should be included in the preevent meal. These foods are digested relatively quickly, so that the child's stomach is empty and the blood sugar level is stable before practice or competition.

The child can make choices depending on food availability and preferences based upon the guidelines shown in *Table 15.5*. However, some children prefer not to eat before the event because they feel nervous or excited. Under these circumstances, the child should never be pressured to eat; instead, liquids such as sports drinks or juices should be encouraged.

After exercise, fluids should be offered to promote hydration and carbohydrates encouraged to replenish glycogen stores. Some parents may inappropriately use food as a bribe to encourage a winning performance. Parents should be advised that special treats should not be used to reward a child who does well and withheld if he or she does not do well. Whether the child competed successfully should have no bearing on postexercise food or fluid intake.

TABLE 15.5   Pre-exercise Meal Guidelines

1 to 2 Hours Before	2 to 3 Hours Before	3 or More Hours Before
Fruit or vegetable juices	Fruit or vegetable juice	Fruit or vegetable juices
Sports drinks	Sports drinks	Sports drinks
Fresh fruit (low fiber)	Fresh fruit	Fresh fruit
	Breads, bagels, crackers, English muffins	Breads, bagels, crackers, English muffins
		Peanut butter, lean meat, low-fat cheese
		Low-fat yogurt (regular or frozen)
		Pasta with tomato sauce
		Cereal with low-fat milk

WEIGHT-CONTROL PRACTICES

Sometimes, healthy nutrition practices are disregarded in the pursuit of athletic prowess. The emphasis may be on what will make the child a better athlete, rather than what will make him or her a happy, healthy child. This may be in part because parents and coaches are not well informed about a child's stage of maturation, nutrition needs, emotions, and/or physical ability.

Unfortunately, some parents and coaches have misconceptions about how much the prepubescent child should eat. Some encourage their children to eat excessively, with the erroneous belief that this will build strength and endurance at a faster rate. To the contrary, indiscriminate consumption, in which food intake exceeds the child's caloric requirement, may be the start of a lifelong struggle with being overweight.

At the other extreme are parents and coaches who promote a diet restricted in calories and nutrients that may compromise the health of the child. Given the current focus on lowering cholesterol and fat, some parents inappropriately narrow the child's food choices (eg, excluding red meat, dairy products) in an attempt to control weight or to minimize the future risk of heart disease. Prepubescent children should receive 30% of total calories from fat, since restriction of fat to lower levels may not adequately support growth and development (42). Parents can encourage long-term healthful habits without compromising growth by offering foods with moderate amounts of unsaturated fats and reducing (not eliminating) foods that are high in saturated fats.

Exercise demands by parent or coach to reduce body weight, such as running laps, performing calisthenics, or extra practice time, can be excessive. Especially during hot temperatures, fatigue, heat exhaustion, and illness can be the result. If the child does need to lose fat weight, a medically supervised weight control plan which focuses on weight monitoring, caloric stabilization, and increased activity is recommended (3,4).

Although appropriate weight loss may result in an improvement in athletic performance, there is a point beyond which further weight loss leads to a deterioration in performance and may jeopardize the health of the athlete as well (9). For the young athlete, the effects of weight loss on growth rate, nutritional status, hormone levels, and bone-mineral content are of special concern, in addition to the psychological stress that may result in an eating problem.

While most parents and coaches are supportive of the young child's needs, some are not as well informed about weight control. It is imperative to develop effective strategies to counter a demanding parent or coach who may be exploiting a child for the adult's satisfaction or personal gain. Nutritional requirements for growth and development must be placed before athletic considerations.

ERGOGENIC AIDS AND DIETARY SUPPLEMENTS

Research is lacking on the use of dietary supplements and other performance-enhancing aids by child athletes. However, many older athletes consume a variety of substances, including vitamin and mineral supplements, in an effort to improve performance. Unfortunately, many self-proclaimed "experts" and clever marketing strategies by companies are eager to convince athletes that their product will improve athletic performance by increasing muscle mass, preventing fat gain, enhancing strength, or supplying energy to name just a few.

There is no place in the diet of a healthy child for megadoses of vitamins, minerals, or other ergogenic aids (24). Unsupervised, indiscriminate use of vitamins, minerals, and other substances raises safety concerns (43). Although vitamin and mineral supplementation may improve the nutritional status of individuals consuming marginal amounts of nutrients from food and may improve performance in individuals with deficiencies, no scientific evidence supports the general use of supplements to improve athletic performance (44,45). For the child who consistently is unable to incorporate certain foods into the diet or is chronically restricting intake, a one-a-day multivitamin and multimineral (100% of the RDA) is prudent to ensure adequate intake of micronutrients.

For the young athlete, the key to health and performance cannot be found in any one food or supplement but in a proper combination of foods that provide many different nutrients that the body requires. Variety and moderation are the best strategy to achieve balance.

CASE STUDY

Julia, a talented 10 1/2-year-old figure skater, suffered a disappointing loss in a regional competition. Afterwards, her parents told her that they overheard the judges comment that she was given low artistic marks because "she looked chunky—particularly in her thighs." The coach decided that losing a few pounds would give Julia a "sleek appearance and improve her performance."

She was told to lose weight by her parents and coach by cutting out high-fat foods and snacks. In an effort to improve her appearance, she restricted food and fluid intake and lost 3.0 kg in 12 days. Her weight before dieting was 30.5 kg (25th to 50th percentile). Current measures indicate that she is 27.0 kg (10th to 25th percentile) and 137.0 cm (25th to 50th percentile). She was 88% IBW and 97% ht/age (141.5 cm). She had not started menarche. She was on antibiotics (Augmentin) for a sinus infection.

A 3-day food record revealed that she was consuming an average of 900 kcal per day. Meal patterns showed that she consumed two meals per day—lunch and dinner—and no snacks. She consumed 24 oz of diet soda and 8 oz of water per day. Macronutrient distribution was 53% carbohydrate, 12% protein, and 25% fat. Protein intake was 0.98 g/kg per day and total carbohydrate consumed was 4.3 g/kg per day. The majority of micronutrients were less than two-thirds of the RDAs. Skinfold measures indicate percent body fat of 15% to 16%. Reports of darkened urine suggested that she was dehydrated.

Julia trained 7 days per week. Three hours per day were spent on the ice and 2 hours per week were devoted to ballet. Julia was preoccupied with weight and limiting food intake to improve her performance but did not exhibit a fear of fat or obesity. Upon careful questioning, she denied feeling that she was overweight and had a healthy body image. She acknowledged that dieting made her feel hungry and tired but that she really wanted to please her coach and parents by winning.

Recommendations

- The importance of a healthy body weight and the impact of nutrition on performance were explained to Julia, her parents, and coach. The parents' and coaches' attitude toward her weight and appearance was discussed and appropriate strategies agreed upon. For example, it was resolved that weight was to be discussed only at the appointment with the nutritionist. There would be no weigh-ins by the coach or parents. Skinfold and growth chart measures that showed she was not overweight helped the parents and coaches agree that weight loss was not justified.
- A realistic competitive weight of 29 kg was decided upon. She agreed to stop losing weight and instead focused on increasing calories gradually in an effort to maintain weight. After weight was stable, calories were increased to promote a slow, gradual gain.
- She was encouraged to distribute calories throughout the day with five to six small meals instead of two larger meals. Modification of meal patterns was discussed within the context of feeling less full and helping her to maintain energy levels throughout the day.
- A one-a-day multivitamin/mineral was recommended for 2 months.
- The female athlete triad and the importance of increasing calcium-rich and iron-rich foods were discussed. For example, with calcium, the goal was to include three calcium-rich foods that she liked each day (low-fat yogurt, skim milk with instant breakfast mix, calcium-fortified orange juice).
- The importance of hydration was discussed. For the first week, Julia agreed to increase her water intake to 3 cups a day and to drink 1 cup of a sports drink per hour during practice for hydration and energy. She reduced diet-soda consumption to 12 oz every other day. Since she appeared dehydrated upon assessment, she was informed that the initial weight gain that she would experience was fluid weight, not fat weight. Skinfold measures were taken each week to reassure her that weight gain did not represent fat gain.

- The relationship between fatigue, respiratory infections, performance, and nutrition was discussed.
- Weekly meetings were scheduled until meal patterns and body weight stabilized.

REFERENCES

1. Steen SN. Nutrition for the school-aged child athlete. In: Berning JR, Steen SN, eds. *Nutrition for Sport and Exercise.* Gaithersburg, Md: Aspen Publishing; 1998:217-246.
2. Steen SN. *Sports Nutrition for Young Athletes.* San Marcos, Calif: Nutrition Dimension; 1998.
3. Coleman E, Steen SN. *The Ultimate Sports Nutrition Book.* Palo Alto, Calif: Bull Publishing Co; 1996.
4. Jennings DS, Steen SN. *Play Hard Eat Right: A Parents' Guide to Sports Nutrition for Children.* Minnetonka, Minn: Chronimed Publishing; 1995.
5. Hamill PV, Drizd TA, Johnson CL, Reed RB, Roche AF, Moore WM. Physical growth: National Center for Health Statistics percentiles. *Am J Clin Nutr.* 1979;32:607-629.
6. Chumlea WC. Growth and development. In: Queen PM, Lang CE, eds. Handbook of Pediatric Nutrition. Gaithersburg, Md: Aspen Publishers; 1993:3-25.
7. Garn SM, Rohman CG. Mid-parent values for use with parent-specific age size tables when parental stature is estimated or unknown. *Pediatr Clinics North Am.* 1967;14:283-284.
8. Himes JH, Roche AF, Thissen D, Moore WM. Parent-specific adjustments for evaluation of recumbent length and stature of children. Pediatrics. 1985;75:304-313.
9. Wilmore JH. Body weight standards and athletic performance. In: Brownell KD, Rodin J, Wilmore JH, eds. *Eating, Body Weight and Performance in Athletes: Disorders of Modern Society.* Malvern, Penn: Lea & Febiger; 1992:315-329.
10. Boileau RA, Lohman TG, Slaughter MH, Horswill CA, Stillman RJ. Problems associated with determining body composition in maturing youngsters. In: Brown EW, Banta CF, eds. *Competitive Sports for Children and Youth: An Overview of Research and Issues.* Champaign, Ill: Human Kinetics; 1988:3-16.
11. Lohman TG. *Advances in Body Composition Assessment.* Champaign, Ill: Human Kinetics; 1992.
12. Slaughter MH, Lohman TG, Boileau RA, et al. Skinfold equations for estimation of body fatness in children and youth. *Human Biology.* 1988;60:709-723.
13. Lohman TG. Assessment of body composition in children. *Ped Exerc Sci.* 1989;1:19-30.
14. Tanner JM. *Growth at Adolescence.* 2nd ed. Oxford, England: Blackwell Scientific Publications; 1962.
15. Lucas B. Normal nutrition from infancy through adolescence. In: Queen PM, Lang CE, eds. *Handbook of Pediatric Nutrition.* Gaithersburg, Md: Aspen Publishers; 1993:145-170.
16. Pollitt E, Leibel RL, Greenfield D. Brief fasting, stress, and cognition in children. *Am J Clin Nutr.* 1981;34:1526-1533.
17. Simeon DT, Grantham-McGregor S. Effects of missing breakfast on the cognitive functions of school children of differing nutritional status. *Am J Clin Nutr.* 1989;49:646-653.
18. Ho CS, Gould RA, Jensen LN. Evaluation of the nutrient content of school, sack, and vending lunch of junior high school students. *Sch Food Serv Res Rev.* 1991;15:85-90.
19. National Research Council. *Recommended Dietary Allowances.* 10th ed. Washington, DC: National Academy Press; 1989.
20. MacDougall JD, Roche PO, Bar-Or O, Moroz JR. Maximal aerobic capacity of Canadian school children: prediction based on age-related oxygen cost of running. *Int J Sports Med.* 1983;4:194-198.

21. Frost GJ, Dowling O, Bar-Or O, Dyson K. Contraction in three age groups of children during treadmill locomotion. *J Electromyography Kinesiology*. 1997;7:179-186.

22. Community Childhood Hunger Identification Project. *A Survey of Childhood Hunger in the United States. Executive Summary*. Washington, DC: Food Research Action Center; 1991.

23. *The Kellogg Children's Nutrition Survey. Executive Summary*. Battle Creek, Mich: Kellogg Co; 1991.

24. American Dietetic Association. Timely statement: nutrition guidance for child athletes in organized sports. *J Am Diet Assoc*. 1996;96:610-611.

25. US Dept Agriculture and US Dept Health and Human Services. *Food Guide Pyramid: A Guide to Daily Food Choices*. Washington, DC; 1993.

26. Bar-Or O. Climate and the exercising child—a review. *Int J Sports Med*. 1980:1:53-65.

27. Bar-Or O. Children's responses to exercise in hot climates: implications for performance and health. *Sports Sci Exch*. 1994;7(49).

28. Meyer F, Bar-Or O, MacDougall D, Heigenhauser GJF. Sweat electrolyte loss during exercise in the heat: effects of gender and maturation. *Med Sci Sports Exerc*. 1992;24:776-781.

29. Bar-Or O, Dotan R, Inbar O, Rotshtein A, Zonder H. Voluntary hypohydration in 10- to 12-year-old boys. *J Appl Physiol*. 1980:48:104-108.

30. Drinkwater Bl, Kupprat IC, Denton JE, Crist JL, Horvath SM. Response of pubertal girls and college women to work in the heat. *J Appl Physiol*. 1977;43:1046-1053.

31. Haymes EM, McCormick RJ, Buskirk ER. Heat tolerance of exercising lean and obese prepubertal boys. *J Appl Physiol*. 1975;39:457-461.

32. Wagner JA, Robinson S, Tzankoff SP, Marion RP. Heat tolerance and acclimatization to work in the heat in relation to age. *J Appl Physiol*. 1972;33:616-622.

33. Bar-Or O, Blimkie CJR, Hay JA, MacDougal JD, Ward DS, Wilson WM. Voluntary dehydration and heat intolerance in cystic fibrosis. *Lancet*. 1992;339:696-699.

34. American College of Sports Medicine. Position stand on exercise and fluid replacement. *Med Sci Sports Exerc*. 1996;28:i-vi.

35. Steen SN, McKinney S. Nutritional assessment of college wrestlers. *Phys Sports Med*. 1986;14:100-116.

36. Steen SN, Brownell KD. Patterns of weight loss and regain in wrestlers: has the tradition changed? *Med Sci Sports Exerc*. 1990;22:762-768.

37. Brownell KD, Steen SN. Weight cycling in athletes: implications for behavior, health, and physiology. In: Brownell KD, Rodin J, Wilmore JH, eds. *Eating, Body Weight, and Performance in Athletes: Disorders of Modern Society*. Philadelphia, Penn: Lea & Febiger; 1992:159-171.

38. Steen SN. Nutritional concerns of athletes who must reduce body weight. *Sports Sci Exch*. 1989;2(20).

39. Garner G, Rosen L. Eating disorders among athletes: research and recommendations. *J Appl Sport Sci Res*. 1991;5:100-107.

40. Sherman RA, Thompson RT. *Helping Athletes with Eating Disorders*. Champaign, Ill: Human Kinetics; 1993.

41. Wilk BO, Bar-Or O. Effect of drink flavor and NaCl on voluntary drinking and hydration in boys exercising in the heat. *J Appl Physiol*. 1996;80:1112-1117.

42. Committee on Nutrition, American Academy of Pediatrics. Statement on children, dietary fat and cholesterol. *Pediatrics*. 1992;90:469-474.

43. American Dietetic Association: Position stand on enrichment and fortification of foods and dietary supplements. *J Am Diet Assoc*. 1994;94:661-662.

44. Singh A, Moses FM, Deuster PA. Chronic multivitamin-mineral supplementation does not enhance physical performance. *Med Sci Sports Exerc*. 1992;24:726-732.

45. Haymes EM. Vitamin and mineral supplementation in athletes. *Int J Sports Nutr*. 1991;1:146-149.

16

HIGH SCHOOL ATHLETES

Diane Habash, PhD, RD

Nutrition professionals working with high school athletes must be sensitive to "how teenagers think" and must know something about their athletic "frame of reference" to be effective in promoting good nutrition practices. During this period of growth and maturation, high school athletes may often have a naïve sense of the mental and physical demands of their sport, yet they are very eager to excel. To attain an edge they rely on their own experiences and on advice from many sources, some of which may be misguided.

Often high school athletes, and for that matter teenagers in general, will manipulate whatever is necessary to achieve their goals without worrying about consequences. In general, the goal of most high school male athletes is to get "bigger, faster, and stronger," while most female athletes want to get "leaner and faster." Educating these impressionable athletes about the various factors that can influence their health and sports performance is extremely important and is repeatedly cited in the literature (1-5). Major topics for education in this population are listed in *Box 16.1*.

BOX 16.1   Major Topics for Nutrition Education in High School Athletes

- Typical growth patterns and genetic influence on growth
- Normal changes in body composition
- Physiological requirements of sports
- Normal daily nutrition and hydration requirements
- Impact of nutrition and hydration on performance

However, there are other factors (see *Box 16.2*) which nutrition professionals should keep in mind when educating and counseling high school athletes (6-10). Surveys suggest that while coaches and trainers are the predominant source of nutrition information for high school athletes, the coach's and trainer's knowledge of and attitudes toward nutrition are only average (11-14). Continuing education for coaches and trainers is highly recommended (11-14).

BOX 16.2   High School Athlete Nutrition Counseling Factors

- Socioeconomic status (6)
- Access to food (at home, school, or restaurants) (7)
- Person(s) responsible for buying food and preparing meals (7)
- Use of popular media for advice (8)

---

continued

BOX 16.2   High School Athlete Nutrition Counseling Factors (continued)

- Access to ergogenic aids
- Mental health of parents (9)
- Self-esteem and confidence (10)
- Scheduling demands of family and peers
- Stress and anxiety prior to competition and subsequent impact on food and fluid intake

---

BODY WEIGHT, BODY IMAGE, AND BODY COMPOSITION

One of the most important topics to a teenager is his or her appearance. The sports nutritionist who works with high school athletes will often encounter confusion and unrealistic perceptions of appearance-related issues involving body weight, body image, and body composition. In addition, several sports (gymnastics, cheerleading, dance) add to these unrealistic perceptions by awarding points for the athlete's appearance.

Body Weight

Adolescence is a period of rapid yet unpredictable growth that may worry and frustrate the athlete. To address the issue of body weight, several guides can be used to help the athlete understand "normal" weight and growth during this period (15). The Reference Height-Weight-Age Tables from the National Center for Health Statistics (15) illustrate the relationship between height and weight for each gender (15) as well as the variations that occur with each stage of puberty (16). Teaching the adolescent to calculate body mass index (BMI) would also demonstrate this relationship and, in addition, could serve as a tool for educating him or her about health and obesity risks associated with a high BMI (17). Reviewing standard values for growth curves or BMI with high school athletes will enhance their understanding of appropriate and typical changes in body weight during growth. It can also personalize the message of the nutritionist who demonstrates the comparison to other healthy teens, perhaps even those of the same ethnicity (17), thus providing a realistic framework for growth. Finally, the growth pattern of the athlete's parents can be used to support discussion of typical body weight changes and the expected growth velocity and growth pattern.

During the training and competitive seasons, high school athletes, especially those in weight classification and appearance sports, may try to control their body weight (10,18-20) using some of the practices found in *Box 16.3*. A recent

---

BOX 16.3   Practices Frequently Used by High School Athletes to Control Weight

- Decreased food intake (sometimes severely)
- Binge/purge practices
- Laxatives
- Wearing sweatsuits, using saunas, or other devices to decrease water weight
- Appetite suppressants
- Increased amount or frequency of exercise
- Participation in contests with peers to lose weight

---

study of teenagers in general found that girls who diet to lose weight cut out a variety of foods while teenage boys decrease their intake of dessert (21). Studies of the dietary intake of high school athletes, especially females, reveal that the athletes' nutrition knowledge is often better than their food choices (22,23). When combining poor food choices, a questionable knowledge base, and the behaviors listed above, increased risks of health consequences may be likely. Electrolyte and fluid imbalances can easily result from losing too much weight through excessive sweating or laxative use. As little as a 1% to 3% loss of body weight from water loss has been shown to impair sports performance (24). Weakness, dehydration, fatigue, cardiac abnormalities, decreased sports performance, and increased recovery time may occur. Athletes who participate in such practices during hot, humid weather have elevated risks of heat stroke. Additionally, when weight-loss strategies such as those mentioned in *Box 16.3* are combined with the usual teenage habits of staying up late and eating on the run for weeks or months, the likelihood of a weakened and fatigued immune system may be greatly increased.

Athletes, coaches, trainers, and parents need to be aware of the risks associated with such weight loss practices. The adults most capable of providing support for weight loss (or weight gain) are those who interact with the athlete on a daily basis. Addressing this goal openly and forming a plan and a reasonable goal weight are essential. High school athletes who make plans without supervision are likely to participate in unsafe practices. Suggestions to support a good plan include:

- Promoting open, but private, discussions of weight-related issues with people whom the athlete identifies as his or her support group (ie, parents, coaches, trainers, or friends)
- Setting realistic short-term weight goals 2 to 3 months prior to training when he or she begins to monitor energy and fat intake of the diet
- Learning healthy eating habits and how to obtain a balanced and adequate supply of all nutrients
- Learning about his or her own eating behaviors and how to lose weight slowly (1 to 2 lb per week) if weight loss is necessary
- Incorporating the appropriate type and amount of exercise to burn calories during the months prior to training
- Learning to be realistic about weight maintenance or weight loss during this period of normal growth
- Reconsidering weight classifications, when appropriate

To minimize the loss of lean mass (and perhaps strength) that occurs with weight loss during the wrestling season (25), one study suggested that wrestlers should move to a higher weight classification each year instead of trying to move to a lower weight classification a few weeks before the start of the competitive season (11).

Body Image

Concern for "how they look" or body image is a prevalent and sometimes consummate phenomenon in both adolescents and adults in the United States where the population has an obsession with weight loss (26). Concepts of body image as well as self-esteem play a key role in the development of eating disorders, especially for athletes in appearance-related sports (10, 27). In one study where eating behaviors between athletes and nonathletes of college age were no different, social physique anxiety, gender, and body fat combined to predict 34% of the disordered eating behaviors (28).

The incidence of eating disorders such as anorexia nervosa and bulimia nervosa in the adolescent population is approximately 0.5% and 1% to 5%, respectively (19). For female athletes, it is estimated that from <1% to 39% experience an eating or weight disorder of some type (18). The incidence of subclinical eating disorders is not as well characterized or tabulated (19,29). However, one review suggests that 20% of a randomly selected adolescent female population had abnormal eating behaviors, and 50% to 60% of the high school females surveyed were unhappy with their current weight and were dieting (19). Interestingly, 40% of adult women surveyed admitted to trying to lose weight (30). See numerous reviews (10,18,19,29) and Chapter 28, Eating Disorders in Athletes for an extensive summary of this area and how to work with athletes with these difficulties. Limited information is available about eating disorders in high school wrestlers and males in general (11). However, in a survey of over 700 high school wrestlers, 19% fasted, 25% limited fluid intake, 34% used rubber suits, and 8% engaged in vomiting behaviors to achieve their precompetition weight (31).

Body Composition

The third issue related to physical appearance is body composition. Educating high school athletes about typical ranges for lean and fat masses, sports-specific differences in body composition, and the potential changes attributed to growth, training, weight loss, and gender may help their perception of reality as well as emphasize their nutrition requirements.

During childhood there is minimal gender difference between lean and fat masses. During adolescent growth females gain an average of 6 inches in height and 35 lb in weight while males gain an average of 8 inches in height and 45 lb in weight (31,32). Females tend to gain fat and lean mass while males tend to gain lean mass and lose fat. Explaining these changes and providing typical ranges of healthy body composition (33), as noted in *Table 16.1*, may foster realistic perceptions for the athlete. In addition, since females are often preoccupied with body fat, it may be helpful to discuss their bodies in terms of lean mass and how to improve it, instead of fat mass and how to change it.

TABLE 16.1   Range of Body Composition for High School Athletes (33)

Gender	Average % Lean Body Mass	Average % Body Fat
Male	85%-92%	8%-15%
Female	72%-85%	15%-27%

For detailed information on body composition, refer to Chapter 11, Assessment of Body Size and Composition; however, be aware that much of the body composition data available for athletes have been collected from college-aged athletes.

ENERGY INTAKE AND BALANCE

Total energy needs of high school athletes can be determined by adding caloric requirements for the following:

- Basal energy expenditure of adolescence
- Growth
- Typical daily activities
- Specific sports activities

Charts of sports-specific energy requirements have been established by body weight and can be a useful tool for talking about requirements with doubting teenagers (34). In general, realistic estimates of energy requirements for high school athletes range from 2,200 to 4,000 kcal per day for females and from 3,000 to 6,000 kcal per day for males, depending on the height, weight, and activity of the athlete (35,36).

Other than wrestlers who restrict energy intake to "make weight," energy intake in males between the ages of 11 and 18 meets or exceeds these predictions (35). On the contrary, high school female athletes have reported energy intakes well below both the Recommended Dietary Allowance (RDA) established for healthy nonathletic girls ages 11 to 18 and the theoretical prediction of energy requirements which take their sport into consideration (2,4,23,37,38).

For instance, as noted above, the current recommendation for energy intake in healthy teenage girls (without considering the added energy for sports activity) is approximately 2,200 kcal per day (36). Female gymnasts reportedly consumed about 84% to 86% (2,37), cross-country runners about 81% (23), volleyball players 84% (39), and ballet dancers 72% to 86% (4,38) of this total energy intake without changes in body weight. This decreased level of consumption has also been found for control groups (nonathletes) (4) as well as for the female teenage population in general (40). Additionally, in a 3-year study of cross-country runners who received nutrition education, this type of dietary intake persisted (23). Some explanations for these inconsistencies include an under-reporting of dietary intake, an over-reporting of physical activity, and an adaptation of cellular efficiency perhaps involving lowered resting metabolic rate or increased efficiency of exercise (29).

PROTEIN

The daily recommendation for protein in healthy adolescents, which is based on height and ranges from 0.29 to 0.34 g/cm in males and 0.27 to 0.29 g/cm in females (36), amounts to 0.8 to 1.0 g/kg. Additional protein requirements for athletes of this age group have not been specifically evaluated. Most information has been obtained from young college-aged males and females whose needs may not be similar to the high school athlete. In general, athletes who may require additional protein (>0.8 g/kg per day) include:

- Individuals who are just beginning an exercise or training program. These athletes should consume extra protein (1.2 to 1.7 g/kg per day) and adequate calories to decrease the loss associated with increased protein turnover and nitrogen lost in sweat (41-43).
- Endurance athletes, who require 1.2 to 1.4 g/kg per day (42)
- Resistance training athletes, who require 1.6 to 1.7 g/kg per day (42)
- Athletes who are restricting total calorie intake (42-44)
- Vegans and athletes who restrict meat and dairy foods

Similar to most Americans, the intake of protein in teenagers exceeds the RDA (40). From the limited research conducted on athletes in this age group, protein consumption was greater than the RDA (2,4,22,35) except in athletes who were attempting to meet weight classifications or standards from their coaches (4,37). High school athletes should be reminded to obtain the highest quality proteins including meat, fish, poultry, eggs, and dairy products.

Athletes who are vegetarian should be reminded to incorporate alternative sources of protein, such as soy, in their diet. Some teenagers may believe that vegetarianism is an attractive method for weight reduction and may adopt some of the principles of vegetarianism without fully comprehending the significance of complete proteins. These and other concepts found in Chapter 26, Vegetarian Athletes can be used to educate aspiring vegetarian high school athletes.

IRON

The role of iron in normal metabolism and during the adaptation to exercise has been reviewed in Chapter 5, Vitamins and Minerals for Active People. Adolescents, regardless of their involvement in sports, have a greater risk of developing low blood iron (44). Involvement in physical activity likely increases that risk (45,46) for these reasons:

- Increased growth demands
- Decreased energy and protein intake
- Poor absorptive capacity
- Sports-related hemolysis and blood loss (48)
- Menstruation in females
- Frequent use of nonsteroidal anti-inflammatory agents for injuries (48)
- Inconsistent or faddish dietary intake
- The stress of competition (49)

Various stages of low blood iron have been categorized, but the terminology is not standardized. For the few studies of adolescents, iron deficiency was noted as serum ferritin <12 to 20 µg/L while iron deficiency anemia was represented by the combination of low serum ferritin <12 to 20 µg/L and low hemoglobin— males <13 g/dL, females <12 g/dL (50,51). Endurance performance in adolescents is impaired as a result of iron deficiency anemia; however, iron deficiency without anemia may not have the same effect (50). The effect of iron repletion on performance, which has been studied in older athletes, resulted in mixed responses (51). Endurance performance (specifically time-to-exhaustion while treadmill-running) in repleted runners was increased while maximal oxygen consumption was not affected (51). *Boxes 16.4* and *16.5* give more information on issues related to iron status and suggestions for education.

BOX 16.4   Specific Issues Related to Iron Status of High School Athletes

- Socioeconomic status. Teens who have less access to a variety of foods, especially meat, fish, and poultry, may be at greater risk of developing a low-iron state.
- Risky diet practices that could decrease iron intake or absorption such as fad diets, laxatives, fasting, or poorly maintained vegetarianism. One group of athletes with subclinical eating disorders was found to have adequate dietary iron intake because they consumed fortified cereals and sports drinks and supplements (29).
- Type, length, and intensity of physical activity. Athletes with anemia have decreased endurance performance, and those types of sports with long endurance practices "set the stage" for low-iron status.
- Medical and/or family history of anemia or bleeding diseases.
- Typical menstrual cycle and its length and flow (50).
- Overall diet. Typical dietary intake must support normal daily activity, growth, menstruation (if applicable), repair of tissues worn down by physical activity, and the production of new hemoglobin and/or ferritin to restore or maintain iron status.

BOX 16.5   Suggestions for Discussing Iron with the Adolescent Athlete

- Help the athlete understand some of the consequences of low blood iron such as feelings of fatigue especially upon physical exertion, inability to keep warm, headaches, pallor, susceptibility to infection, cheilosis, glossitis, koilonychia, and impaired ability to concentrate.
- Explain the normal losses of iron and those typical in physical exertion (bleeding associated with the sport, poor absorption with diarrhea, or gastrointestinal disturbances).
- Suggest foods (ie, meat, fish, poultry, and green leafy vegetables) and conditions (ie, meals with low coffee and tea intake or increased sources of vitamin C) which improve absorption of iron. Suggest snacks that would favor iron absorption (dried fruits, orange juice, fortified breakfast cereals).

CALCIUM

Calcium deposition into bone is most critical during adolescence (52); its crucial role in the physiology of a working muscle as well as other important functions are described in Chapter 5, Vitamins and Minerals for Active People. Unlike iron, the effects of low-calcium status may not be apparent without laboratory or bone density tests and may not impair sports performance until stress fractures result.

The high school athlete most at risk for low-calcium status is the female who is predisposed to conditions of the "female-athlete triad." This phenomenon is a combination of excessive training, perfectionist-like expectations of physical appearance, subsequent under-nutrition, and the eventual development of disordered eating, amenorrhea, and bone loss (53).

The recommended intake (DRI) for calcium for adolescents between the ages of 9 and 18 has recently been increased to 1,300 mg per day (54). High school female athletes consume a calcium level that is 1/2 to 2/3 of the 1989 RDA of 1,200 mg per day, (4,23) and nonathletes consume 45% (55). National survey data agree with these smaller studies, suggesting that high school age females consume 400 to 700 mg per day less than the 1989 RDA (56). The national surveys also suggest that high school age males meet their needs for calcium (the exception is African American males) (56); however, a smaller study suggests that males consume only 57% of their requirement for calcium (55).

This low intake of calcium, especially by females, requires special attention from the sports nutritionist. Many adolescent females believe that high-calcium foods are also high-calorie foods and subsequently avoid them. The nutritionist should explain normal conditions for good calcium absorption (ie, the presence of stomach acid, protein, vitamin D, phosphorus, and lactose), food sources with the greatest concentrations of calcium, and the ideal number of servings to meet requirements for calcium. Teenagers are independent of parental supervision for much of their day and may opt for foods that are calorie-dense (candy, soft drinks, cookies, chips) and not nutrient-dense. In addition, lactose intolerance may be a contributing factor. Describing immediate consequences of low bone density (ie, stress fractures) may be the ideal example to convince active teens about the importance of calcium nutrition (57).

OTHER VITAMINS AND MINERALS

Much of the sports literature suggests that there is no performance benefit from vitamin and mineral supplementation in athletes who have normal vitamin and mineral status (58,59). Athletes who are deficient or subclinically deficient in a vitamin or mineral may experience improvements when nutrient levels are restored.

Low dietary intake was reported for zinc, iron, calcium, folacin, and magnesium in the few studies completed with various groups of high school athletes (2,4,35). The intake of nonathletic adolescents was not much better. These teens consumed vitamins A and E, calcium, magnesium, and zinc below recommended levels, and fat, saturated fat, and sodium at levels above the recommendation (6). Fortified food products, such as cereals, will enhance a teen's intake of many of these nutrients and are ideal snacks for this population.

SUPPLEMENT USE

Approximately 40% to 50% of the high school athletes surveyed have used nutritional supplements of some kind (not including sports drinks) (1,60). Although a limited number of surveys have been conducted, the data suggest that males use nutritional supplements (including steroid alternatives) more frequently than females but that females have a higher use of vitamin or mineral supplements (1,60). The use of steroids in high school male athletes ranges from 6% to 7% of those surveyed (1,61), which may be an underestimation. Many school systems are now beginning to require random drug testing in their athletes.

Emphasis on winning and peak performance has increased the use of nutritional supplements; however, increased knowledge of nutrition in high school athletes was significantly associated with decreased use of supplements (1). Interestingly, the mean knowledge score for nutrition in this recent survey of high school athletes was only 65% (1).

Nutrition information and education are warranted; however, getting access to high school athletes is a significant challenge. Numerous directives for obtaining access to this population have been discussed (62), such as getting to know the coaches and trainers, setting up speaking engagements with coaches and trainers at continuing education meetings, or speaking with parents and athletes. Some access may be achieved by working with parents who are feeding the athletes prior to the athletic event. The need for communication and education about nutrition in this population is grave and cannot be underestimated for both improved sports performance and especially for lifelong health and wellness issues.

HYDRATION

All athletes need to know and practice good hydration habits before, during, and after practices and competition. The necessity of water, its intricate functions in exercise, and the suggested levels of intake prior to, during, and after events are covered in Chapter 6, Fluid and Electrolytes. Adequate fluid intake cannot be stressed enough to the high school athlete, and often those who have experienced the fatigue associated with dehydration can assist the sports nutritionist in describing the ill-effects and decreased performance to teammates. Adolescents often feel invincible and do not appreciate how much their bodies require this essential nutrient.

Several reminders can be used to teach high school athletes how to gauge their hydration status. First, it is important to help them understand how much weight they may lose during practice or a game when they are not hydrating properly and whether this weight loss is significant enough to affect performance. Second, they should be told that by the time they feel thirsty, it is too late and they are dehydrated. Third, they should be taught to note the color of their urine as an indicator of their hydration and to drink enough fluid during the day to keep the urine color very pale. Fourth, as with any athlete, teenagers will search for a performance "edge" which often includes the use of caffeine and caffeine products. The dehydrating effect of these substances must be fully explained and the use of caffeinated products discouraged. Finally, many high school athletes want to do everything "perfectly" and the sports nutritionist should be careful to provide guidelines. Some athletes may need to have an explanation of what is too much to drink, as they often go to extremes to excel in their sport.

REFERENCES

1. Massad SJ, Shier NW, Koceja DM, Ellis NT. High school athletes and nutritional supplements: a study of knowledge and use. *Int J Sport Nutr.* 1995;5:232-245.
2. Lindholm C, Hagenfeldt K, Hagman U. A nutrition study in juvenile elite gymnasts. *Acta Paediatr.* 1995;84:273-277.
3. Benardot D. Working with young athletes: views of a nutritionist on the sports medicine team. *Int J Sport Nutr.* 1996;6:110-120.
4. Loosli AR, Benson J. Nutritional intake in adolescent athletes. *Ped Clin N Am.* 1990;37:1143-1152.
5. Harvey JS. Nutritional management of the adolescent athlete. *Clin Sports Med.* 1984;3:671-678.
6. Johnson RK, Johnson DG, Wang MQ, Smiciklas-Wright H, Guthrie H. Characterizing nutrient intakes of adolescents by sociodemographic factors. *J Adolescent Health.* 1994;15:149-154.
7. Schoonen JC. Adolescence. In: Benardot D, ed. *Sports Nutrition: A Guide for the Professional Working with Active People.* 2nd ed. Chicago, Ill: American Dietetic Association; 1993:113-121.
8. Guillen EO, Barr SI. Nutrition, dieting, and fitness messages in a magazine for adolescent women, 1970-1990. *J Adolescent Health.* 1994;15:464-472.
9. Su LJ, Story M, Su SS. Effect of parental mental health status on adolescents' dietary behaviors. *J Adolescent Health.* 1997;20:426-433.
10. Lindeman AK. Self-esteem: its application to eating disorders and athletes. *Int J Sport Nutr.* 1994;4:237-252.
11. Sossin K, Gizis F, Marquart LF, Sobal J. Nutrition beliefs, attitudes, and resource use of high school wrestling coaches. *Int J Sport Nutr.* 1997;7:219-228.
12. Graves KL, Farthing MC, Smith SA, Turchi JM. Nutrition training, attitudes, knowledge, recommendations, responsibility, and resources of high school coaches and trainers. *J Am Diet Assoc.* 1991;91:321-324.
13. Murphy A. Youth sports coaches: using hunches to fill a blank page. *Phys Sports Med.* 1985;12:136-144.
14. Bedgood BL, Tuck MB. Nutrition knowledge of high school athletic coaches in Texas. *J Am Diet Assoc.* 1983;83:672-677.
15. National Center for Health Statistics. Height and weight of youths 12-17 years, United States. *Vital and Health Statistics. Series 11-No. 124.* Health Services and Mental Health Administration. Washington, DC: United States Government Printing Office; 1973.
16. National Center for Health Statistics. *Executive Summary of the Growth Chart Workshop 1992.* Hyattsville, Md: US Dept of Health and Human Services; 1994.
17. Rosner B, Prineas R, Loggie J, Daniels S. Percentiles for body mass index in US children 5 to 17 years of age. *J Pediatrics.* 1998;132:211-222.
18. Sundgot-Borgen J. Eating disorders in female athletes. *Sports Med.* 1994;17:176-188.
19. Fisher M, Golden NH, Katzman DK, et al. Eating disorders in adolescents: a background paper. *J Adolescent Health.* 1995;16:420-437.
20. Beals KA, Manore MM. The prevalence of consequences of subclinical eating disorders in female athletes. *Int J Sport Nutr.* 1994;4:174-195.
21. Middleman AB, Vasquez I, Durant RH. Eating patterns, physical activity, and attempts to change weight among adolescents. *J Adolescent Health.* 1998;22:37-42.
22. Douglas PD, Douglas JG. Nutrition knowledge and food practices of high school athletes. *J Am Diet Assoc.* 1984;84:1198-1202.
23. Wita BG, Stombaugh IA. Nutrition knowledge, eating practices, and health of adolescent female runners: a 3-year longitudinal study. *Int J Sport Nutr.* 1996;6:414-425.
24. Armstrong LE, Costill DL, Fink WJ. Influence of diuretic-induced dehydration on competitive running performance. *Med Sci Sports Exerc.* 1985;17:456-461.

25. Roemmich JN, Sinning WE. Sport-seasonal changes in body composition, growth, power, and strength of adolescent wrestlers. *Int J Sports Med*. 1996;17:92-95.

26. Rodin J. Cultural and psychosocial determinants of weight concerns. *Ann Intern Med*. 1993;11:643-645.

27. Thompson RA, Sherman RT. *Helping Athletes with Eating Disorders*. Champaign, Ill: Human Kinetics; 1993.

28. Cox LM, Lantz CD, Mayhew JL. The role of social physique anxiety and other variables in predicting eating behaviors in college students. *Int J Sport Nutr*. 1997;7:310-317.

29. Beals KA, Manore MM. Nutritional status of female athletes with subclinical eating disorders. *J Am Diet Assoc*. 1998;98:419-425.

30. Horm J, Anderson K. Who in America is trying to lose weight? *Ann Intern Med*. 1993;119:672-676.

31. Oppliger RA, Landry GL, Foaster SW, Lambrecht AC. Bulimic behaviors among interscholastic wrestlers: a statewide survey. *Pediatrics*. 1993;91:826-831.

32. Forbes GB. Growth of lean body mass in man. *Growth*. 1972;36:325-330.

33. Mitchell KM. Nutrition during adolescence. In: Mitchell KM, ed. *Nutrition Across the Life Span*. 1st ed. Philadelphia, Penn: WB Saunders Co; 1997:159-188.

34. McArdle WD, Katch FI, Katch VL. *Exercise Physiology: Energy, Nutrition, and Human Performance*. 3rd ed. Philadelphia, Penn: Lea & Febiger; 1991:804-811.

35. Hickson JF, Duke MA, Risser WL, Johnson CW, Palmer R, Stockton JE. Nutritional intake from food sources of high school football athletes. *J Am Diet Assoc*. 1987;87:1656-1659.

36. Food and Nutrition Board. *Recommended Dietary Allowances*. 10th ed. Washington, DC: National Academy Press; 1989.

37. Loosli A, Benson J, Gillien D, Bourdet K. Nutrition habits and knowledge in competitive adolescent female gymnasts. *Phys Sports Med*. 1986;14:118-130.

38. Calabrese LH, Kirkendall DT, Floyd M. Menstrual abnormalities, nutritional patterns, and body composition in female ballet dancers. *Phys Sports Med*. 1983;11:86-98.

39. Perron M, Endres J. Knowledge, attitudes, and dietary practices of female athletes. *J Am Diet Assoc*. 1985;85:573-576.

40. *Nationwide Food Consumption Survey, Nutrient Intakes: Individuals in 48 States, Year 1977-1978*. Report No. 1-2. Hyattsville, Md: US Dept of Agriculture; 1984.

41. Todd KS, Butterfield GE, Calloway DH. Nitrogen balance in man with adequate and deficient energy intake at three levels of work. *J Nutr*. 1984;114:2107-2118.

42. Lemon PWR. Effect of exercise on dietary protein requirements. *Int J Sport Nutr*. 1998;8:426-447.

43. Paul GL. Dietary protein requirements of physically active individuals. *Sports Med*. 1989;8:154-176.

44. Dallman PR. Iron deficiency and related nutritional anemias. In: Nathan DG, Oski FA, eds. *Hematology of Infants and Childhood*. 3rd ed. Philadelphia, Penn: W B Saunders Co; 1987:288-300.

45. Clarkson PM. Minerals: exercise, performance, and supplementation in athletes. *J Sport Sci*. 1991;9(suppl):91-116.

46. Position of The American Dietetic Association. Nutrition guidance for adolescent athletes in organized sports. *J Am Diet Assoc*. 1996;96:611-612.

47. Robertson JD, Maughan RJ, Davidson RJL. Faecal blood loss in response to exercise. *BMJ*. 1987;295:303-305.

48. Eichner ER. Sports anemia, iron supplements, and blood doping. *Med Sci Sports Exerc*. 1992;24:S315-S318.

49. Diehl DM, Lohman TG, Smith SC, Kertzer R. Effects of physical training and competition on the iron status of female field hockey players. *Int J Sport Med*. 1986;7:264-270.

50. Raunikar RA, Sabio H. Anemia in the adolescent athlete. *Sports Med*. 1992;146:1201-1205.
51. Garza D, Shrier I, Kohl HW, Ford P, Brown M, Matheson GO. The clinical value of serum ferritin tests in endurance athletes. *Clin J Sport Med*. 1997;7:46-53.
52. Matkovic V. Calcium intake and peak bone mass. *N Engl J Med*. 1993;327:119-121.
53. Eichner ER, Johnson M, Loucks AB, Steen SN. Roundtable: the female-athlete triad. *Sports Sci Exch*. 1997;27(8).
54. Food and Nutrition Board. *Institute of Medicine, National Academy of Sciences Dietary Reference Intakes: Recommended Intakes for Individuals*. Washington, DC: National Academy of Sciences; 1998.
55. Harel Z, Riggs S, Vaz R, White L, Menzies G. Adolescents and calcium: what they do and do not know and how much they consume. *J Adolescent Health*. 1998;22:225-228.
56. Eck LH, Hackett-Renner C. Calcium intake in youth: sex, age, and racial differences in NHANES II. *Preventive Med*. 1992;21:473-482.
57. Myburgh KH, Hutchins J, Fataar AB, Hough SF, Noakes TD. Low bone density is a etiologic factor for stress fractures in athletes. *Ann Intern Med*. 1990;113:754-759.
58. Fogelholm M. Indicators of vitamin and mineral status in athletes' blood: a review. *Int J Sport Nutr*. 1995;5:267-284.
59. Singh A, Moses FM, Deuster PA. Chronic multivitamin-mineral supplementation does not enhance physical performance. *Med Sci Sports Exerc*. 1992;24:726-732.
60. Krowchuk DP, Agnlin TM, Goodfellow DB, Stancin T, Williams P, Zimet GD. High school athletes and the use of ergogenic aids. *Am J Dis Child*. 1989;143:486-489.
61. Buckley WE, Yesalis CE, Friedl KE, Anderson WA, Streit AL, Wright JE. Estimated prevalence of anabolic steroid use among male high school seniors. *JAMA*. 1988;260:3441-3445.
62. Kundrat S. Fostering the sports nutritionist-athletic trainer relationship. *SCAN's Pulse*. 1998;17:7-8.

The author wishes to acknowledge the NIH Grant M01RR00034G for the time to prepare this manuscript.

17

COLLEGE ATHLETES

Christine A. Rosenbloom, PhD, RD and Rob Skinner, RD, CSCS

The National Collegiate Athletic Association (NCAA) reported that in 1996-1997 201,997 males and 129,285 females participated in all divisions of NCAA-sponsored sports (1). Yet, only a handful of college athletic associations use the expertise of dietetics professionals. College athletes who have nutrition concerns turn to athletic trainers, strength and conditioning staff, coaches, or other athletes for advice. The opportunity for dietetics professionals in the college athletic arena has yet to be realized. David Ellis, Director of Performance Nutrition at the University of Nebraska, believes that the NCAA should mandate hiring qualified health professionals to manage body composition, supplement use, and feeding programs for college athletes (2). Suzanne Nelson Steen, sports nutritionist at the University of Washington, believes nutrition professionals should be an integral part of the collegiate athletic association (Personal communication). According to Kristine Clark, Director of Sports Nutrition at Penn State University, "Opportunities for establishing strong sports nutrition positions at major universities are on the horizon" (3). These three sports nutritionists offer tips for working with collegiate athletes in *Box 17.1*. This chapter reviews the nutrition concerns of college athletes and describes how one NCAA Division I school incorporated nutrition into programs for all collegiate athletes.

BOX 17.1   Tips for Working with Collegiate Athletes

From Kristine Clark, PhD, RD, Director of Sports Nutrition, Center for Sports Medicine, Penn State University, University Park, Pennsylvania:

1. You must be considered an "expert" in the field of nutrition. Coaches and trainers have some knowledge of nutrition, but it is up to the nutrition professional to inform and educate athletes on specific nutrition issues. Research in the field is greatly expanding and it is important to read and interpret the literature and translate it into practice.

2. Set your goal to become an integral part of the athletic program. Get involved with the entire sports medicine team—team physicians, athletic trainers, strength and conditioning coaches, physical therapists, and administrators. Provide nutrition handouts and make yourself available for team seminars and recruiting tours.

3. Know that you are ultimately a clinical practitioner. Sports nutrition is not a job for the person fresh out of undergraduate school. A graduate degree and work experience are highly regarded by administrators. Be prepared to help athletes lose or gain weight, eat more healthfully, and understand the effects of alcohol and drugs on performance. Assist the sports medicine team with eating disorders. Stay current on new information on herbs, phytochemicals, neutraceuticals, and performance-enhancing drugs.

continued

CONCERNS OF COLLEGE ATHLETES

Old Habits, Convenience, and Economics

Most college athletes understand the importance of food choices on body composition, athletic performance, and health, but many have grown up in a fast-food culture and arrive at college with little nutrition knowledge (4). Athletes may be conscious of good food habits but old behaviors die hard, especially when fast food is readily available (often in the school's dining hall) and inexpensive. As one college football player said, "I know I should choose grilled chicken over Big Mac's, but the value meals are so much cheaper than the healthy stuff!"

Even if athletes want to make nutritious food choices, they often lack the domestic skills needed to shop and prepare meals. While many college dorm rooms have refrigerators, stoves, and microwave ovens, most college athletes are "cooking impaired."

Unorthodox Sources of Information

Sports nutritionists have observed that athletes often get their nutrition information from the popular press, especially "muscle" magazines that are quick to hype supplementation and unproven diet manipulations as the way to achieve the ideal image. Testimonials about supplements substitute as scientific proof of efficacy, and many young college athletes follow these recommendations. Magazines are getting more sophisticated in the methods used to present information, frequently citing research in reputable professional journals to back up claims. But a search of the references finds much of the cited research is conducted in animals, not humans, and information is misrepresented or taken out of context (5).

As the World Wide Web expands, many athletes get their information from Internet websites. Commercial websites usually sell products and present biased information passed off as "research" to support claims. For example, a search for the word "creatine" conducted in April 1999 on a common search engine found 90,190 web pages. Over 90% were commercial sites selling the supplement and touting its benefits.

Time

College athletes lead very busy lives with many demands on their time. They often take heavy class loads, have mandatory study halls, report for early morning conditioning workouts, participate in team practices, report for team meetings, and participate in media interviews. This demanding schedule leaves little time or opportunity for food preparation and meals (6).

Body Weight and/or Body Composition

Athletes frequently have an "ideal" weight or desired percent body fat in their minds that can conflict with good health practices. Burke (7) found that many athletes have misconceptions about appropriate weight, body composition, and weight loss practices. One study (8) found male athletes were more concerned about rapid weight gain than weight loss; with the exception of wrestlers (8). Forty-three percent of the wrestlers were concerned about quick weight loss to "make weight" for competition or compete in a lower weight class. This same study reported that about 30% of student athletes expressed concern about teammates' quick and inappropriate weight loss.

Health Risks

A multicenter, cross-sectional study of seven major collegiate institutions in the United States with 2,298 male and female athletes found that college athletes are at greater risk for maladaptive lifestyles and risky health behaviors than their nonathletic peers. These athletes are less likely to use seatbelts. They ride more often as a passenger in a vehicle driven by a driver under the influence of alcohol or drugs. They also more frequently use smokeless tobacco and anabolic steroids and are more likely to be involved in physical fights than nonathletic peers.

Athletes at highest risk for these behaviors include males participating in contact sports. Female athletes report a higher prevalence of irregular menses, amenorrhea, and stress fractures compared with female nonathletes (9). Other researchers have found that college athletes consume significantly more alcohol per week and engage in binge drinking more often than nonathletes (10).

EXPERIENCE AT A NCAA DIVISION I COLLEGIATE ATHLETIC ASSOCIATION

In 1988 the Georgia Tech Athletic Association (Georgia Institute of Technology, Atlanta, Georgia) hired a nutrition consultant to work with a few offensive linemen who had body fat percentages >30%. Soon trainers, coaches, and other athletes were requesting nutrition services, so a full-time nutrition position was created. The Nutrition Center retained a consultant dietitian to develop a strategic plan for nutrition services. The three-prong approach implemented is described below.

Nutrition Services for the Student Athlete

Four hundred student athletes playing 16 sports were eligible for nutrition services. Recently, cheerleading was added to the list of student athletes who could receive nutrition services. *Box 17.2* lists all of the nutrition services offered to student athletes. The various nutrition services offered are briefly described below.

BOX 17.2   Nutrition Services Available to Student Athletes at Georgia Tech

- Nutrition screening at yearly physicals
- Blood chemistry
- Lipid profile
- Screening for iron deficiency and iron deficiency anemia
- Body composition assessment using body plethysmography
- Team seminars
- Individual nutrition counseling
- Diet analysis
- Nutrition education at the training table
- Off-season weight control, weight gain, or weight maintenance plans
- Help with off-campus meal selection
- Medical nutrition therapy for specialized problems (injury recovery, diabetes, hypertension, etc)

Nutrition screening. Services usually begin at yearly physicals where nutrition screening is conducted. (A sample nutrition screening form can be found in the Tools section.) This screening is not meant to be comprehensive. Time is limited as athletes rotate through 15 stations, so the purpose of this screening is to establish nutrition as an integral part of the sports medicine services and to introduce the sports nutritionist. The screening form is also used to assess supplement use and knowledge of NCAA-banned substances.

Blood is drawn for routine chemical analysis. A lipid profile is done on all athletes, and anemia is assessed for female athletes and male cross-country athletes. Iron deficiency anemia screening is evaluated using hemoglobin, hematocrit, serum ferritin, and total iron-binding capacity (TIBC). If serum ferritin levels are <25 and TIBC is >300 to 360, the team physician is notified and together the sports nutritionist and physician determine the most appropriate course of action (11).

The sports nutritionist using body plethysmography in the Bod Pod (a body composition technique using air displacement) assesses body composition. (See Chapter 11, Assessment of Body Size and Composition.) Occasionally, skinfold measurements are obtained by an exercise physiologist on staff at the institution.

Team seminars. Nutrition seminars are presented during the preseason to any interested team. The sports nutritionist, the athletic trainer, and the strength and conditioning coach discuss concerns specific to the sport, and the dietitian prepares a series of short lectures delivered to the team before or after a conditioning session or practice. For example, for men's basketball it was determined that five 10-minute mini-lectures would be given after preseason conditioning workouts. In contrast, for women's basketball a series of eight interactive discussions were held, complete with "homework" assignments that were turned in at each session. *Table 17.1* lists the nutrition topics covered in team seminars for men and women's basketball. To reinforce the nutrition seminar content, the sports nutritionist is a frequent visitor to team practices to answer questions or discuss nutrition concerns.

TABLE 17.1   Topics for Nutrition Seminars

Men's Basketball Team	Women's Basketball Team
• Fluids and hydration	• Nutrition basics
• Carbohydrates for fuel and recovery	• Carbohydrate
• Pregame meal choices	• Protein
• Eating at the airport, on the road, and at fast-food restaurants	• Fat
• Maintaining weight throughout the season	• Vitamins
	• Minerals
	• Fluids
	• Supplements

Individual nutrition counseling. Athletes can obtain individualized diet plans through referral by the coach, trainer, or strength staff, or by self-referral to the sports nutritionist. A 3-day diet record is obtained and analyzed with a commercial software package. Nutrient goals are personalized and often differ from the Recommended Dietary Allowances (RDA) because they reflect a higher need for some nutrients. For example, protein requirements for a strength athlete are calculated using 1.6 to 1.7 g/kg per body weight and 1.2 to 1.4 g/kg per body weight for an endurance athlete instead of the RDA of 0.8 g/kg per body weight (12). A personalized "nutrition playbook" is completed and the nutrition plan and goals are reviewed with the athlete. During the nutrition counseling session, proper food selection at the training table, in the dorm room, and in restaurants is emphasized. For some athletes a personal performance contract is utilized. (See the Tools section.)

Education at the training table. Several nutrition education strategies are employed in the dining hall. Pie charts are displayed for each food item served and athletes are taught how to use the information to support their nutrition or body-composition goals. Information is displayed for portion size; calories; percent of calories from carbohydrate, protein, and fat; and fat grams (see *Figure 17.1*). Table tents are developed with timely nutrition messages and rotated weekly. Table tent topics are shown in *Table 17.2*. For a change of pace and a little humor, nutrition cartoons might be used or a holiday theme featured. For example, on Valentine's Day a table tent entitled "Top 10 Reasons to Eat Chocolate on Valentine's Day" was displayed.

A series of 12 sports-nutrition handouts were developed and used in team seminars and counseling sessions, and displayed at the training table. *Box 17.3* lists topics for a sports nutrition handout.

FIGURE 17.1   Training Table Pie Chart

You may have noticed pie charts on the serving line when you are choosing your food. The purpose of these pie charts is to educate and inform you about the foods that you eat. The goal is to have a balanced diet with approximately 55% to 65% carbohydrates, 15% to 20% protein, and 15% to 25% fat.

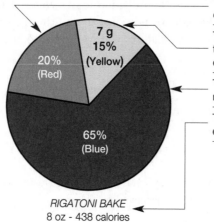

The Red section indicates the percentage of total calories that are derived from protein.

The Yellow section represents the amount of fat in that food item. The amount of fat grams and percentage of calories are shown.

The Blue section represents the percentage of calories derived from carbohydrates.

The name, serving size, and total calories are located at the bottom of the pie chart.

RIGATONI BAKE
8 oz - 438 calories

TABLE 17.2   Table Tent Topics

• Hydration	• The Whole Meal Counts
• Break the Fast with Breakfast	• Fiber Facts
• Best Bets for Mexican Food	• New Year's Resolutions
• Best Bets for Chinese Food	• Exercise and Fuel Systems
• Best Bets for Italian Food	• Pros and Cons of Caffeine
• Best Bets for American Fare	• Electrolytes
• Picking Pizza	• Alcohol, Hydration, and Energy Production
• Smart Shopping	• Energy Bars
• Nutrition Quackery	• Phytochemicals: Plants versus Pills
• Throw Away the Scale	• Complex versus Simple Carbohydrates
• 97 Ways to Have a Healthier 2000	• Supplements: Natural and Dangerous
• Reasons to Eat Chocolate on Valentine's Day	

BOX 17.3 "Fueling Fitness" Sports Nutrition Information Handouts

- Sports Nutrition: The Big Picture
- Lose the Fat—Increase the Performance
- Five Staples = Many Healthy Meals
- Eating Out: Smart Choices
- Smart Snacks
- Healthy Weight Gain
- The Role of Minerals in Sports Performance
- Ergogenic Aids: Help, Hype, or Hope?
- Disordered Eating in Athletes
- Fueling with Carbohydrates
- Gain Control in the Grocery Store and in the Kitchen
- Hydration

Nutrition Consultation to Coaches and Sports Medicine Staff

The sports nutritionist's biggest ally might be the athletic trainer. Often the trainer wears many hats, including team nutritionist, and most are happy to give up the role of nutritionist. At Georgia Tech nutrition services have been well received and even championed by the athletic trainers. It was the director of sports medicine (a certified athletic trainer) who suggested that nutrition screening be part of the yearly physicals. Kundrat (13) suggests several strategies for fostering the relationship between the sports nutritionist and the athletic trainer.

Others who welcome the services of a nutritionist are the strength and conditioning coaches. One nutrition service that has been particularly well received is the evaluation of promotional literature for ergogenic aids. Coaches are bombarded with requests from salespeople (often a well-meaning alumnus or former athlete) to use nutritional supplements or products. The sports nutritionist provides a scientific evaluation of the supplement and a written report of the pros and cons with recommendations for use. Trainers and coaches no longer have the burden of nutritional supplement evaluation. Guidelines for evaluating ergogenic aids have been published (14) and a summary can be found in the Tools section.

The sports nutritionist also takes the lead role in developing a dietary supplement policy. Along with the athletic director, the sports medicine director, and the strength and conditioning coach, a dietary supplement policy can be established and implemented. The NCAA publishes a banned drug class list and updates can be found on the its website (http://www.ncaa.org.html). *Box 17.4* highlights the banned substances that can be found in over-the-counter dietary supplements.

BOX 17.4 Substances Banned by the NCAA and Found in Over-the-counter Dietary Supplements

Stimulants:	Caffeine (if the concentration in the urine exceeds 15 μg/mL)
	Ephedrine (also called Chinese ma huang, ma huang, ephedra, epitonin, sida cordifolia)
Anabolic Agents:	Androstenedione (also called andro)
	Norandrostenedione (also called norandro)

The Sports Science Committee of the NCAA reports athletes may be improving their performance at the cost of their eligibility (15). The NCAA is considering a committee recommendation that would prevent college institutions from providing athletes with supplements that enhance weight gain, including many of the most popular nutrition supplements (16). Sports nutritionists in a college environment must be knowledgeable about the NCAA rules regarding dietary supplements and stay abreast of any changes adopted by the governing body.

The sports nutritionist can also help trainers with pregame meal selection, since they are often responsible for meal selection for away games. The trainer is the person who spends the most time with the athletes and knows what athletes will or will not eat. By reviewing the menus with the sports nutritionist, the most appropriate selections (ie, those appropriate for pregame competition and those which the athlete will eat) can be chosen.

The sports nutritionist also plays a role in the recruitment of future athletes. Often recruits and their families (especially the recruit's parents) are impressed with the nutrition services offered and appreciate that good tasting, healthy food is provided on campus. A brief presentation by the sports nutritionist and a tour of the Nutrition Center is part of the athlete's recruitment visit at Georgia Tech.

Nutrition Consultation and Education for Food Service Staff

The sports nutritionist works closely with the food service director to review menus and make recommendations for recipe modification. Georgia Tech Athletic Association's philosophy is that athletes be offered a wide variety of menu items and be educated on the best choices to meet their individual body composition and performance goals. A policy for meals served at the training table was established and includes the following considerations.

- The food service director submits a cycle menu to the sports nutritionist for review and suggestions.
- The food service director provides recipes to the sports nutritionist for nutrient analysis and production of pie charts containing nutrition information.
- At least two of three entrees served at meals contain <30% of calories from fat.
- The salad bar includes a variety of vegetables (spinach, romaine lettuce, grated carrots, mushrooms, green peppers, onions, sprouts, and canned beans) and reduced-fat and fat-free salad dressings in addition to the full-fat dressings.
- A pasta bar is offered at meals to provide high-carbohydrate food choices.
- Nutrient cards are posted for all items to allow the athlete to make a point-of-purchase decision about the nutrient content of the item.
- The sports nutritionist offers quarterly inservice presentations for training table staff to discuss the goals of the training table and the importance of following recipes to match nutrient cards.

- The food service director plans monthly "theme" meals that are supported by nutrition materials and table tents that coordinate with the theme meal (see *Table 17.3*).

TABLE 17.3   Theme Dinners with Corresponding Nutrition Education Materials

Month	Theme Meal	Nutrition Education Materials
January	Super Bowl bash	Healthy snacks for the big game
February	Valentine's Day	Heart-healthy food quiz
March	Foods from around the world	Best bites from ethnic restaurants
April	Louisiana day	Health benefits of seafood
May	Thai bar	Health benefits of Asian diets
June	Picnic day	Food safety tips for picnics

In 1994 the NCAA implemented a one-meal-per-day rule for training tables (17). At Georgia Tech this means that other students can eat at the training table for breakfast or dinner, but lunch is reserved exclusively to athletes.

FUTURE NEEDS

The sports nutritionist could provide many other services to collegiate athletic associations. At least three areas need to be addressed in the college athlete arena.

1. Research on the best nutritional educational strategies to reach an athletic population
2. Documenting the benefits of nutrition interventions through "outcome" studies
3. A program for "de-training" the athlete who does not go on to play at the professional level

Educational Strategies

Potter and Wood (18) noted that athletes' desire for accurate and practical information is a challenge and a responsibility for dietitians, but there is lack of research on the most effective way to educate athletes. They conducted a study with 46 college athletes (ages 18 to 22 years; 24 females and 22 males) representing the sports of volleyball, wrestling, football, softball, track, basketball, and golf. The athletes were randomly assigned to participate in either group instruction or self-instruction. Four nutrition education modules were developed (basic diet for athletes, pregame meal, fluids, and ergogenic aids) and presented to the athletes in a slide-tape series (group education) or slides with a script to be read at their own pace. The outcome was nutrition knowledge, assessed by pre- and postnutrition questionnaires. The authors found self-instruction resulted in higher gains in nutrition knowledge than group instruction (18).

Updegrove and Johnson (19) used table tents to present sports nutrition information to a college football team. They displayed two table tents per week for 5 weeks on nine different topics. Responses to a follow-up questionnaire showed this approach improved the nutrition knowledge of the players and staff members.

However, as Potter and Wood point out, the goal of nutrition education is to promote positive behavior change, and although gains in knowledge represent a step forward in nutrition education, this does not always result in behavior change (18).

Nutrition Outcomes

Nancy Clark writes about the need for documenting sports nutrition outcomes in Chapter 13, Documenting Sports Nutrition Outcomes. Kristine Clark (20) also writes about the need for documenting sports nutrition outcomes. The reasons athletes seek nutrition counseling should be documented, as well as the effectiveness of nutrition interventions with the entire team (20).

Rosenbloom and Skinner (see *Box 17.5*) recently completed a pilot nutrition outcome study with the Georgia Tech men's basketball team and plan to expand the model to other teams. (A publication of the study is in progress.) The goal of the study was to determine if nutrition interventions resulted in behavior change during the basketball season. The players, strength and conditioning coach, and athletic trainer completed a checklist of nutrition behaviors at the end of the season to assess nutrition behaviors and behavior changes.

"De-training" Programs

Many athletes need to be "de-trained" when their playing days are over. The probability a college football player will go on to a professional football career is only 2 in 100 for student athletes. For men's basketball the number is 3 in 100 (1). Although statistics are not available to support the observation, it has been noted that many college athletes experience an unhealthy weight gain after their college athletic careers end. This seems especially true for sports that encourage higher weights, like football. Millard-Stafford et al (21) noted that overfat college football linemen had significantly higher mean values for systolic blood pressure and triglycerides, and their food records showed that intakes of fat, sugar, cholesterol, and sodium were higher than the recommended levels. Although the importance of continued physical activity and sound nutritional practices for life are frequently discussed with athletes, a formal program targeting the athlete after eligibility has ended could benefit the athlete for life.

BOX 17.5   Outline for Nutrition Outcome Study for Men's Basketball Team

---

Step One: Identify what athletes want/need from nutrition intervention and seek input from players, athletic trainers, and strength and conditioning coaches.

The following outcomes were agreed upon:

- Maintain weight throughout the season.
- Increase fluid consumption during and after practice and games.
- Delay fatigue during games.
- Eat an appropriate pregame meal.
- Increase carbohydrate consumption to supply and replenish muscle glycogen during the season.
- Learn to make more healthful choices while eating out.

Step Two: Develop a series of 10- to 15-minute nutrition education sessions as part of the preseason conditioning workouts.

- Session 1: Fluids

    Strategy: Use sports bottles to show players how much fluid to consume before, during, and after practice and games. Show players how to monitor fluid status by observing urine color and output. Use fruit juice to show color of urine when dehydrated vs well hydrated.

- Session 2: Carbohydrates

    Strategy: At the end of the first session, give players a list of high-carbohydrate foods and ask them to circle their favorites. The sports nutritionist calculates grams of carbohydrates for each athlete (using 7 to10 g/kg per body weight) and gives them a card with their favorite carbohydrate foods in 50 g-portion sizes. Athletes are shown how to use the card to meet their carbohydrate goals. Emphasis is placed on recovery carbohydrates after practices and games.

- Session 3. Pregame meal

    Strategy: Have a general discussion about myths about pregame meals. Review menus for breakfast buffet for 1PM games and dinner menus for 7 and 9 PM games. Menu items are classified as "good, better, and best."

- Session 4: Eating out

    Strategy: At the end of the second session, players are given a list of fast-food establishments and common types of ethnic foods and chain restaurants, and asked to circle their favorites. A handout is developed and given to each player identifying his favorite restaurants with notations indicating the best choices for fueling sports. Suggestions are made for choosing high-carbohydrate foods in airport food courts and take-out establishments. Attention is given to low-cost items, as collegiate athletes have food budgets determined by the NCAA.

- Session 5: Maintaining weight during the season

    Strategy: Athletes are instructed to weigh-in and weigh-out before and after every practice. A weight chart is posted directly above the scale in the locker room and monitored by the strength and conditioning coach. If a trend toward weight loss (versus fluid loss) is seen, the sports nutritionist meets with the player to determine the cause of weight loss and to develop a plan with the player to increase food intake.

Step Three: Measure outcomes.

Outcomes will be measured in two ways:

- At the end of the season, players will complete a checklist of dietary changes that they made as a result of the nutrition interventions.
- At the end of the season, the strength and conditioning coach and athletic trainer will complete a checklist of observations of player's eating behaviors.

REFERENCES

1. NCAA Fact Sheet. http://www.ncaa.org/about/factsheet.html. Accessed June 28, 1998.
2. Hawes K. Creatine boom creates administrative challenges. *The NCAA News.* September 14, 1998;1:16-17.
3. Clark KL. Working with college athletes, coaches, and trainers at a major university. *Int J Sport Nutr.* 1994;4:135-141.
4. Ellis D, Ray R, Hought D, Stephens S, Maglischo E. Roundtable: University sports medicine teams: an interdisciplinary approach. *Sports Sci Exch.* 1993;4:1-4.
5. Lightsey D, Attaway J. Deceptive tactics used in marketing purported ergogenic aids. *Natl Strength Conditioning Assoc J.* 1992;14:26-31.
6. Burke L. Practical issues in nutrition for athletes. *J Sports Sci.* 1995;13:S83-S90.
7. Burke L. Sport and body fatness. In: Hill AP, Wahlqvist ML, eds. *Exercise and Obesity.* Philadelphia, Penn: Lea & Febiger; 1994:128-145.
8. Hoffman C, Logomarsino JV, Minelli MJ. Weight change concerns of collegiate athletes. *Top Clin Nutr.* 1994;10:38-47.
9. Nativ A, Puffer JC, Green GA. Lifestyles and health risks of collegiate athletes: a multi-center study. *Clin J Sport Med.* 1997;7:262-272.
10. Leichliter JS, Meilman PW, Presley CA, Cashin JR. Alcohol use and related consequences among students with varying levels of involvement in college athletics. *J Am Coll Health.* 1998;46:257-262.
11. Ashenden MJ, Martin DT, Dobson GP, Mackintosh C, Hahn AG. Serum ferritin and anemia in trained female athletes. *Int J Sport Nutr.* 1998;8:223-229.
12. Lemon PWR. Effects of exercise on dietary protein requirement. *Int J Sport Nutr.* 1998;8:426-447.
13. Kundrat S. Fostering the sports nutritionist-athletic trainer relationship. *SCAN's Pulse.* 1998;17:7-8.
14. Rosenbloom C, Storlie J. A nutritionist's guide to evaluating ergogenic aids. *SCAN's Pulse.* 1998;17:1-5.
15. Hawes K. Athletes buying trouble with dietary supplements. *The NCAA News & Features.* http://www.ncaa.org/news/19980511/active/3519n03.html. Accessed June 22, 1998.
16. Competitive-safeguards group cites summer medical issues. *The NCAA News.* July 20,1998:11.
17. *1998-99 NCAA Division I Manual.* Overland Park, Kan: National Collegiate Athletic Association; 1998.
18. Potter GS, Wood OB. Comparison of self and group instruction for teaching sports nutrition to college athletes. *J Nutr Ed.* 1991;23:288-290.
19. Updegrove NA, Johnson RM. Using table tents to present sports nutrition facts to collegiate athletes. *J Nutr Ed.* 1987;19:302D.
20. Clark KS. Sports nutrition counseling: documentation of performance. *Top Clin Nutr.* 1999;14:34-40.
21. Millard-Stafford M, Rosskopf LB, Sparling PB. Coronary heart disease: risk profiles of college football players. *Phys Sports Med.* 1989;17:151-163.

18

ELITE AND OLYMPIC ATHLETES

Ann C. Grandjean, EdD and Kristin J. Reimers, MS, RD

Elite athletes are "the best or most skilled." While one can find elite athletes at all levels of competition, most people consider the elite athlete as the one who is successful in national or international competition, such as the Olympics which includes a wider variety of sports than professional, college, or high school athletics (ie, while swimming, basketball, and wrestling are common, sports such as orienteering, team handball, luge, and equestrian are not but are included in the Olympics) (1). Elite athletes approach their sports as professionals and work full-time at developing their skills (2). They may live with their immediate family, a spouse, roommates, or alone. They may be adolescents or parents of adolescents. Elite athletes represent a group of very dedicated and hard-working individuals who are training at the limit of their physical capacity (3), which sets them apart from their less successful counterparts. Even though the "experienced" marathon runner may average 46 km per week (4), the elite runner is training at 90 to 150 km per week (4). Road cyclists may ride 644 to 965 km during a training week.

Elite athletes, among other qualities, possess a positive self-concept, function with a strong sense of personal autonomy, and have a high expectancy of success (5). Winning a gold medal in international competition is a common goal for these athletes.

DIETARY INTAKE

The literature contains studies on elite athletes from several countries. Grandjean and Ruud (6) collected data on 103 Olympians representing a variety of sports (see *Table 18.1*). Daily energy intakes ranged from 2,533 to 4,269 kcal per day for male athletes and from 1,866 to 3,009 kcal per day for female athletes. Considering that the majority of these athletes train heavily on a daily basis, group mean carbohydrate intakes were lower than current recommendations, ranging from 4.2 g/kg BW for male hockey players to 6.5 g/kg BW for male cyclists, and 4.4 g/kg BW for female judo players to 7.1 g/kg BW for female cyclists. Mean protein intakes for male groups ranged from 1.5 g/kg BW for judo players to 2.2 g/kg BW for cyclists, supplying 14% to 19% of energy. For female athletes protein intake ranged from 1.0 g/kg BW in judo players to 1.7 g/kg BW in cyclists, supplying 12% to 15% of energy. Fat intakes as percent of total calories ranged from means of 29% in male distance runners to 41% for male cyclists and 29% for female tennis players to 34% for female judo players.

TABLE 18.1   Nutrient Intake of 103 Olympic Athletes

	Energy			Protein			Carbohydrate			Fat		
	n	kJ per day	kJ/kg	Per day	Per weight	Percent of total energy	Per day	Per weight	Percent of total energy	Per day	Per weight	Percent of total energy
				g/d	g/kg	%	g/d	g/kg	%	g/d	g/kg	%
Males												
Cycling	9	17,861	247	160	2.2	15	471	6.5	43	196	2.7	41
Distance running	11	13,000	188	124	1.8	16	420	6.1	53	106	1.5	29
Figure skating	7	10,598	180	103	1.8	16	336	5.8	52	88	1.5	31
Hockey	8	14,510	180	156	1.9	18	343	4.2	39	155	1.9	39
Judo	7	13,217	176	114	1.5	14	358	4.9	45	127	1.7	36
Weightlifting	21	15,723	172	178	1.9	19	372	4.2	39	165	1.8	38
Females												
Cycling	10	12,590	218	100	1.7	13	409	7.1	53	111	1.9	31
Distance running	9	8,962	176	82	1.6	15	275	5.4	50	74	1.4	30
Figure skating	8	7,807	167	66	1.4	14	248	5.3	52	69	1.5	33
Judo	4	8,226	134	62	1.0	12	264	4.4	53	77	1.2	34
Tennis	9	8,535	146	80	1.4	15	279	4.8	54	68	1.2	29

1 kilojoule (kJ) = 0.239 kilocalories (kcal)

Source: Grandjean AC, Ruud JS. Olympic athletes. In Wolinsky I, Hickson JF, eds. *Nutrition and Exercise in Sport*. 2nd. ed. Boca Raton, Fla: CRC Press Inc; 1994:447. Used with permission.

Mean intakes of vitamins and minerals for all male elite athletes studied by Grandjean and Ruud (6) met or exceeded the Recommended Dietary Allowance (RDA) (7). In contrast, elite female athletes consumed less than 100% of the RDA for iron, calcium, zinc, and vitamin B-6. Vitamin C intakes from food were high in male and female cyclists, representing 586% and 425% of the RDA, respectively. Vitamin B-12 intakes were also high—499% of the RDA for the group of weightlifters.

In 1989 van Erp-Baart et al (8,9) reported food intake data on 419 athletes competing primarily on an international level, including several European, world, and Olympic medal winners. The athletes' eating habits varied greatly with gender and sport. Consistent with data of Grandjean and Ruud (6), energy intakes were highest in male endurance sports athletes and lowest in female athletes concerned with body weight (gymnasts, figure skaters, etc). Only five sport groups (Tour de France cyclists, Tour de l'Avenir cyclists, amateur cyclists, marathon skaters, and runners) reached the level of 55% of total calories from carbohydrate (8). More recent data on elite cyclists have been reported by Garcia-Roves et al (10). This study of 10 males during the Tour of Spain cycling competition showed that they consumed a high carbohydrate intake (60% of calories).

In general, vitamin intakes for the total group studied by van Erp-Baart et al (9) were adequate with the exception of low vitamin B-6 and thiamin intakes in professional cyclists. The authors attributed this to a high intake of refined foods, such as sweets, cakes, or soft drinks. With respect to mineral intake, the authors concluded that calcium and iron may be problematic for young female athletes who are dieting. The major differences in food choices among the sports groups were in meat intake; endurance athletes tended toward a vegetarian diet.

Energy and macronutrient intake of elite soccer players is an area where little data exist. Maughan (11) reported that the dietary intake of two groups of male, Scottish, professional soccer players was surprisingly similar to that of the general population: 2,630 to 3,060 calories, with one group's mean calorie consumption being 2,629 kcal and a second group's being 3,059. This is lower than expected for endurance-type athletes.

Although it is often assumed that most athletes have higher-calorie diets than the general population, this is not always true. Rankinen (12) found that Finnish elite ski jumpers consumed on average only 1,769 kcal per day, compared to the 2,629 kcal intake of age-matched controls.

The available data show that elite athletes are very heterogeneous, sometimes varying significantly from the norm. Each athlete must be assessed based on individual parameters.

DIETARY SUPPLEMENTS

Many elite athletes ingest a variety of nutrient and non-nutrient supplements. Grandjean and Ruud (6) reported that 52% use dietary supplements. Patterns emerge when the data are analyzed by sport (see *Table 18.2*), with male and female cyclists being the largest consumers of nutrition supplements. Similar results were reported by van Erp-Baart et al (9), who found high-supplement use by professional cyclists and bodybuilders. Tour de France cyclists studied by Saris et al (13) used several concentrated vitamin/mineral supplements, particularly iron and vitamin B-12.

TABLE 18.2   Percent of Athletes Reporting Routine Use of Supplements by Sport

Sport	Percent
Males	
Cycling	66
Distance running	54
Weightlifting	47
Judo	42
Hockey	37
Figure skating	4
Females	
Cycling	100
Distance running	66
Tennis	55
Figure skating	37

Source: Grandjean AC, Ruud JS. Olympic athletes. In Wolinsky I, Hickson JF, eds. *Nutrition and Exercise in Sport.* 2nd ed. Boca Raton, Fla: CRC Press Inc; 1994:447. Used with permission.

Although little is known about the rationale for supplement use by Olympic athletes, one would assume it is to improve performance, gain a competitive edge, and "be the best." Burke and Read (14) studied the eating habits of elite Australian football players and found the most frequently reported reasons for taking vitamins were to compensate for poor nutrition and lifestyle or in response to respiratory infections and excess alcohol consumption. Some players also felt dietary supplements would compensate for tiredness and loss of appetite due to heavy training.

DIETARY CONCERNS

Meal Regularity

Many elite athletes are unable to maintain adequate intake or a regular meal schedule. Often, the stress of hard training can suppress appetite, making it increasingly difficult for the athlete to consume adequate calories and carbohydrate on a regular basis. Training for several hours a day leaves little time for preparing and eating meals, a dilemma shared by many professional and collegiate athletes. As a result, small meals and/or snacks contribute significantly to total calorie intake. In a study by Lindeman (15), triathletes ate an average of nine times a day. A survey of the 1997 United States Ski Team by the International Center for Sports Nutrition (personal communication from the International Center for Sports Nutrition) showed that the average frequency of eating was greater than five times a day. An erratic schedule and lack of time to prepare meals are additional reasons why elite athletes use supplements. In fact, many elite athletes' primary nutrition questions are about supplements.

In addition to long training hours, travel is another disruption for athletes who compete on an international level. Food intake often depends on local restaurant facilities and thus access to familiar foods may be limited. This can be a dilemma, especially for athletes with high-calorie requirements who are at risk for weight/strength loss. Eating atypical foods for long periods of time may have negative psychological and physical effects. Consumption of unfamiliar foods and beverages can result in diarrhea, constipation, gas, and/or nausea.

Food Safety

Food-borne illness is a paramount concern for traveling athletes. One report (16) suggests that up to 60% of athletes traveling abroad may be affected by some form of gastroenteritis. Traveler's diarrhea can be caused by food or water that contains bacteria, viruses, or parasites. It is estimated that bacterial enteropathogens cause at least 80% of traveler's diarrhea with *Escherichia coli* and *Shigella* being the two most common agents (17). Clinical features of traveler's diarrhea include frequent loose stools and abdominal cramps, sometimes accompanied by nausea, vomiting, or the passage of bloody stools. Since contaminated food and water can cause traveler's diarrhea, athletes need to be cautious of what they eat and drink and to apply stringent food-hygiene rules. Prevention of the problem involves selecting eating establishments that are well known or recommended by coaches or other individuals who have been to the area before and who are aware of food-safety issues. Using the embassy in the country of destination to identify potential problems in advance can also be valuable. Information on immunization requirements and recommended prophylactic precautions should also be established well in advance of travel. This advice is readily available from travel agents, airlines, and embassies.

Foods such as fruits that can be peeled and vegetables that have been thoroughly washed with boiling water are generally safe food choices. For the most part, athletes should drink only bottled water, juices, or soft drinks from sealed containers. *Box 18.1* provides guidance for foods and beverages generally considered safe for travel. However, when in doubt, remember the phrase: "Boil it, cook it, peel it, or forget it" (18).

Foods and beverages are not the only source of pathogens. If the level of water purity is unknown, athletes should use bottled water to brush their teeth and should not swallow water when bathing. Athletes participating in water sports such as rowing or canoeing need to avoid swallowing lake or river water.

BOX 18.1   Foods Appropriate for Trips

- Sandwiches that do not require refrigeration
- Breads, biscuits, bagels, crackers, chips, pretzels
- Muffins, cookies, cereal bars
- Bottled, canned, or boxed fruit juices or milk-based drinks not requiring refrigeration
- Canned vegetables
- Dried or canned fruits
- Bottled water
- Canned or bottled sports drinks, soft drinks
- Meal-replacement beverages, canned
- Nuts, trail mix
- Ready-to-eat cereal
- Canned meat (tuna, chicken)

DIETARY RECOMMENDATIONS

"If it ain't broken, don't fix it" is the guiding philosophy when working with elite athletes. Olympians are Olympians, in part, because they have found a nutrition program that works for them. The sports nutritionist can assist elite athletes with questions and concerns, but arbitrary manipulation of habitual intake to conform to dogmatic guidelines may not enhance performance and instead may diminish performance and credibility. In other words, elite athletes' diets do not always follow the rules. One example is a distance runner who experienced severe diarrhea several days to a week before a race. The situation kept her from qualifying at the Olympic Trials, even though she was expected to. Her normal diet included a high intake of fresh fruits, vegetables, and whole grains. Changing her dietary intake the week before competition to a diet with only low-fiber, low-residue foods alleviated the diarrhea and her performance improved. Another example is the Olympic ski racer who was convinced she needed to lose weight because she believed that losing body fat was always helpful. However, because she participated in a power sport where more weight can mean more speed, she was encouraged to eat at a level to support her training and not to focus on body weight. In doing so she gained weight and experienced her best season to date.

A wide range of nutrient intakes can meet the individual's nutrient requirements. Sports nutritionists should understand that unless the athlete desires significant dietary changes, and/or unless performance indicates a change is needed, dietary change can be harmful to performance. The body adapts to habitual nutrient intake. For example, one study by Helge et al (19) on untrained males showed similar performance after 4 weeks of training on a high-fat diet (62% of calories) and a high-carbohydrate diet (65% of calories). This study is mentioned not to advocate use of diets providing only 21% of calories as carbohydrate (the high-fat diet was 62% fat plus 21% CHO) because it is unlikely that this regimen is effective (19) or palatable, but to highlight the adaptability of the body to many dietary patterns.

One cannot rely on assessing the diet based on distribution of calories (ie, percentage of calories from carbohydrate, protein, and fat). Nutrient intakes on a per kilogram basis are more meaningful, taking into consideration the athlete's size, sport, period of training and conditioning, nontraining activities, and age. The recommendations for energy and intake of carbohydrate, protein, fat, fluid, and vitamins and minerals provided below are meant to serve as a starting point from which the elite athlete's diet can be "fine tuned."

Energy

The energy intake of elite athletes is highly variable. Because of the variability of energy requirements, depending on period of training, body size, training environment, and genetics, no "formula" or calculations exist that accurately predict the energy needs of individual athletes. The most accurate way to assess energy requirements is to assess energy intake at various times of the year (heavy training, competitive period, recovery period). Energy intake, when weight is stable, represents energy requirements. The innate flaw in most self-reported dietary intake is under-reporting. However, the motivated elite athlete who is warned of this tendency can avoid it. When elite athletes understand that the purpose of the recording is to enhance performance, they will make every effort to provide accurate information.

Carbohydrate

It is well established that dietary carbohydrate contributes directly to the maintenance of muscle glycogen stores and that consumption of high-carbohydrate diets compared to low-carbohydrate may delay fatigue and improve physical performance (20-22). As such, athletes participating in prolonged (>60 minutes), intense exercise (65% to 70% VO_2max) are advised to consume a diet containing approximately 7 to 10 g of carbohydrate/kg BW (23). This amount of dietary carbohydrate has been shown to adequately restore skeletal glycogen within 24 hours (24). However, it is unknown whether athletes consuming less than this amount will have impaired performance. For athletes training aerobically for durations less than 60 minutes daily, performance can likely be maintained with a lower carbohydrate intake (25). Although optimal carbohydrate intake will vary depending on body size, sport, and training routine, a minimum of 200 g of carbohydrate per day is required to maintain liver glycogen.

Protein

Research suggests that athletes have increased protein requirements compared to the general population. Factors that increase athletes' protein requirements include growth, muscle hypertrophy, training, the biological value of protein, and calorie intake. According to Lemon (26), both endurance- and strength-training athletes benefit from diets providing more protein than the current RDA of 0.8 g/kg BW per day. Strength athletes may require up to 1.8 g/kg BW and endurance athletes up to 1.4 g/kg BW (26). In most cases the additional amount of protein can be easily covered by a normal, varied diet as long as adequate amounts of food are consumed. Energy intake is a primary consideration, as protein requirement increases as energy intake decreases. Thus, weight-conscious athletes may require a more protein-dense diet to cover needs. The strict vegetarian also needs to consume higher levels of protein to maintain nitrogen balance than athletes who eat meat, dairy products, or eggs. This is due primarily to differences in the digestibility and amino-acid composition of plant protein compared to animal protein.

Fat

The USDA's *Dietary Guidelines for Americans* (27) recommends that individuals consume no more than 30% of total calories from fat. However, this recommendation targets sedentary Americans and is meant to decrease the risk of heart disease and some cancers. Disease risk attributed to fat based on clinical studies of sedentary individuals may not apply to elite athletes. For example, Leddy et al (28) studied 25 runners and found those who consumed 42% fat in their diets maintained favorable coronary heart disease (CHD) risk factors, but a 16% fat diet lowered apoprotien Al and high-density lipoprotein (HDL) cholesterol and raised the total cholesterol to HDL ratio. Thus, dietary fat guidelines for elite athletes must consider the athletes' health, current eating habits, and performance goals.

In a review of the nutrition habits of elite athletes, Economos (29) reported that during training, total fat intake for male endurance athletes ranged from 20% to 40% and for elite female endurance athletes, 26% to 38% of total calories. Among athletes with high calorie needs, fat intakes greater than 30% are sometimes necessary to meet high caloric needs. The Committee on Nutrition of the United Nations (30), of which the World Health Organization is a member, recommends that the lower limit of fat intake be 15% of energy for most adults, with women of reproductive age consuming at least 20% of their calories as fat. The upper limit of fat intake recommended is 30% of energy for sedentary individuals and 35% for active people.

Fluids

As is the case for all athletes, adequate hydration is essential for optimal performance. Most elite athletes are keenly aware of the importance of hydration. The major additional hurdles for them are travel and change of climate. Reliance on bottled water and unfamiliar foods during travel can reduce fluid intake. In addition, the dry cabin air on flights can increase the risk of dehydration.

Environment is also a factor in adequate fluid consumption. The athlete might be training in a temperate, dry climate and then travel to a country with intense heat and humidity. Most coaches and athletes travel to the country of a major competition a few weeks before so they can become acclimated. Additionally, most will try to replicate conditions of competition while at home.

During periods of heavy sweating, encouraging consumption of fluids regardless of thirst and monitoring body weight are important for any athlete. Elite athletes must also focus on adequate electrolyte replacement, usually through a variety of foods and beverages. Low-salt diets are not recommended during periods of heavy sweating.

Vitamins and Minerals

Taken in excess, vitamins and minerals provide no advantage, can be toxic, and may interfere with the absorption and metabolism of other nutrients. On the other hand, vitamin and mineral deficiencies impair performance. The United States Olympic Committee's (USOC) Sports Medicine Committee has developed supplementation guidelines (see *Table 18.3*). It should be noted that these are currently under revision, and revisions will eventually be distributed via the USOC system.

USOC Guidelines on Dietary Supplementation

The primary goal of any nutrition program for athletes is for an athlete to consume a diet that meets nutritional requirements. The use of nutrition supplements may be indicated in some circumstances. However, nutrition supplements are just that—supplements, not substitutes for a good diet.

There are a variety of conditions in which nutrition supplementation may be indicated. These include a time of heavy menstrual bleeding, women prior to conception and during pregnancy, individuals with low-calorie intakes, and other physiological, environmental, or religious factors that interfere with adequate intake or increase nutrient and/or weight loss. In such cases, a supplement may be used to "rescue" an inadequate diet.

The USOC supplementation guidelines are based on keeping the athlete healthy in order to train adequately. There is no scientific evidence that intakes of vitamins and minerals greater than the recommended amounts will enhance performance. Additionally, optimizing nutrition will not overcome other deficits in training.

The use of supplements is indicated only after dietary inadequacies have been identified via dietary evaluation. If dietary evaluation is not possible and cursory review of the athlete's dietary habits indicates possible reason for concern, prophylactic supplementation may be desirable. The following guidelines for supplementation have been established when considering such situations.

TABLE 18.3 USOC Supplement Guidelines

Nutrient	Supplement Range	Other Considerations
Beta-carotene	3-20 mg (5,000-33,340 IU)	No data on individuals under 18 years
Vitamin C	250-1,000 mg	No data on individuals under 18 years
Vitamin E	100-400 IU	No data on individuals under 18 years

Iron

    Males: Recommended for males only if a medical work-up indicates a problem with iron deficiency. A medical work-up is recommended only as indicated by disease or symptoms. Diet analysis and appropriate lab tests should be included as part of the work-up.

    Females: A medical work-up is recommended yearly, including a diet analysis and appropriate lab tests. The recommendation is 100% RDA unless medical work-up indicates a need for higher supplementation.

    NOTE: Iron and calcium supplements should be taken at least 4 hours apart to maximize the absorption of iron.

Nutrient	Supplement Range	Other Considerations
Multivitamin/mineral	100% RDA, or Estimated Safe & Adequate Daily Dietary Intake (ESADDI). See the Tools section.	
Protein	1.2-2.0 g/kg BW per day	This is a total intake recommendation which assumes adequate calories and a diet containing some foods of high biological protein value. If a supplement is needed to meet these levels, a low-fat milk-based product is recommended.
B-complex		Refer to Recommended Dietary Allowance (RDA) for ages 11 to 60 and Military Recommended Dietary Allowance (MRDA) for 17 and older (see the Tools section and Chapter 41, Military Training).
Calcium	500-1,000 mg	A 2:1 calcium to magnesium ratio is recommended.
Zinc	14-20 mg	14-20 mg is the zinc level found in most multivitamin/mineral products. Total zinc intake should not exceed this range due to risk of toxicity.

CAUTIONS AND CONSIDERATIONS

Nutrient	Comments
Vitamin B-6	Supplementing above 500 mg per day may be toxic. Some individuals may experience adverse side effects at lower levels (eg, 100 mg).
Niacin	Large doses may impair performance. Individuals using high doses to reduce blood cholesterol levels should do so only under medical supervision.
Garlic	Garlic will not enhance performance. While some studies have shown that it may decrease cholesterol levels, research is equivocal and no conclusions can be made.
Medium-chain triglycerides (MCTs)	Increase ketone formation. May lead to acidosis, cause stomach upset, and impair endurance performance.

continued

TABLE 18.3   USOC Supplement Guidelines (continued)

CAUTIONS AND CONSIDERATIONS	
Carnitine	Further research is needed, particularly on acetyl carnitine.
Amino acids (eg, arginine, ornithine, phenylalanine, tryptophan, isoleucine, valine, etc)	Not recommended
Choline	Not recommended
Chromium	Research does not support intakes above the ESADDI for chromium.

Source: United States Olympic Committee, Sports Medicine Committee; Colorado Springs, Colo; 1994.

REFERENCES

1. Butts K. Profile of elite athletes: physical and physiological characteristics. In: Butts NK, Gushiken TT, Zarins B, eds. *The Elite Athlete*. Jamaica, NY: Spectrum Publications; 1985:183-207.
2. McDonald M. Pushing the envelope. *Civilization*. 1996;May-June:20-47.
3. Holmich P, Darre E, Jahnsen F, Hartvig-Jense T. The elite marathon runner: problems during and after competition. *Br J Sports Med*. 1988;22:19-21.
4. Nieman DC, Butler JV, Pollett LM, Dietrich SJ, Lutz RD. Nutrient intake of marathon runners. *J Am Diet Assoc*. 1989;89:1273-1278.
5. Parsons TW, Bowden D, Garrett M, et al. Profile of the elite athlete. *Coaching Rev*. 1986;9:62-65.
6. Grandjean AC, Ruud JS. Olympic athletes. In: Wolinsky I, Hickson JF, eds. *Nutrition and Exercise in Sport*. Boca Raton, Fla: CRC Press Inc; 1994:447-454.
7. Food and Nutrition Board. *Recommended Dietary Allowances*. 10th ed. Washington, DC: National Academy Press; 1989.
8. van Erp-Baart AMJ, Saris WHM, Binkhorst RA, Vos JA, Elvers JWH. Nationwide survey on nutritional habits in elite athletes. Part I. Energy, carbohydrate, protein, and fat intake. *Int J Sports Med*. 1989;10:S3-S10.
9. van Erp-Baart AMJ, Saris WHM, Binkhorst RA, Vos JA, Elvers JWH. Nationwide survey on nutritional habits in elite athletes. Part II. Mineral and vitamin intake. *Int J Sports Med*. 1989;10:S11-S16.
10. Garcia-Roves PM, Terrados N, Fernandez SF, Patterson AM. Macronutrient intake of top level cyclists during continuous competition — change in the feeding pattern. *Int J Sports Med*. 1998;19:61-67.
11. Maughan RJ. Energy and macronutrient intakes of professional football (soccer) players. *Br J Sports Med*. 1997;31:45-47.
12. Rankinen T, Lyytikainen S, Vanninen E, Penttila I, Rauramaa R, Uusitupa M. Nutritional status of the Finnish elite ski jumpers. *Med Sci Sports Exerc*. 1998;30:1592-1597.
13. Saris WHM, van Erp-Baart MA, Brouns F, Westerterp KR, ten Hoor F. Study on food intake and energy expenditure during extreme sustained exercise: the Tour de France. *Int J Sports Med*. 1989;10:S26-S31.
14. Burke LM, Read RSD. A study of dietary patterns of elite Australian football players. *Can J Sport Sci*. 1988;13:15-19.
15. Lindeman AK. Eating and training habits of triathletes: a balancing act. *J Am Diet Assoc*. 1990;90:993-995.

16. Grantham P. Traveler's diarrhea in athletes. *Phys Sports Med*. 1983;11:65-70.
17. DuPont HL, Ericsson CD. Prevention and treatment of traveler's diarrhea. *N Engl J Med*. 1993;328:1821-1827.
18. Mayo Clinic Health Letter. Traveler's diarrhea. January 1997;1:6.
19. Helge JW, Wulff B, Kiens B. Impact of a fat-rich diet on endurance in man: role of the dietary period. *Med Sci Sports Exerc*. 1998;30:456-461.
20. Akermark C, Jacobs I, Rasmusson M, Karlsson J. Diet and muscle glycogen concentration in relation to physical performance in Swedish elite ice hockey players. *Int J Sport Nutr*. 1996;6:272-284.
21. Balsom PD, Wood K, Olsson P, Ekblom B. Carbohydrate intake and multiple sprint sports: with special reference to football (soccer). *Int J Sports Med*. 1999;20:48-52.
22. Karlsson J, Saltin B. Diet, muscle glycogen, and endurance performance. *J Appl Physiol*. 1971;31:203-206.
23. Sherman WM, Wimer GS. Insufficient dietary carbohydrate during training: does it impair athletic performance? *In J Sport Nutr*. 1991;1:28-44.
24. Costill DL, Sherman WM, Fink WJ, Maresh C, Witten M, Miller JM. The role of dietary carbohydrate in muscle glycogen resynthesis after strenuous running. *Am J Clin Nutr*. 1981;34:1831-1836.
25. Sherman WM, Doyle JA, Lamb DR, Strauss RH. Dietary carbohydrate, muscle glycogen, and exercise performance during 7 days of training. *Am J Clin Nutr*. 1993;57:27-31.
26. Lemon PWR. Effects of exercise on dietary protein requirements. *Int J Sport Nutr*. 1998;8:426-447.
27. *Nutrition and Your Health: Dietary Guidelines for Americans*. 4th ed. Washington, DC: US Depts of Agriculture and Health and Human Services; 1995. Home and Garden Bulletin No. 252.
28. Leddy J, Horvath P, Rowland J, Pendergast D. Effect of a high or a low fat diet on cardiovascular risk factors in male and female runners. *Med Sci Sports Exerc*. 1997;29:17-25.
29. Economos CD, Bortz SS, Nelson ME. Nutritional practices of elite athletes. *Sports Med*. 1993;16:381-399.
30. WHO and FAO Joint Consultation: Fats and oils in human nutrition. *Nutr Rev*. 1995;53:202-205.

19

PROFESSIONAL ATHLETES

Leslie J. Bonci, MPH, RD

The majority of dietetics professionals see clients in a traditional health care setting—a hospital, an office, an outpatient clinic, or a physician's office. Making the transition to working with professional athletes requires a paradigm shift. Counseling settings and client goals are often very different as is the clients' mindset regarding nutrition. *Table 19.1* delineates the differences between outpatient clients and professional athlete clients.

TABLE 19.1 Differences between Outpatient Clients and Sports Clients

Variables	Outpatients	Professional Athletes
Time issues	You control.	They control.
Flexibility	You determine.	They determine.
Assertiveness	Not always necessary	Critical
Education format	Instructions can be lengthier.	Instructions must be short and to the point.
Creativity	Can be helpful	Essential
Communication	With patients and other health care professionals	With players, coaches, trainers, and team physicians
Business savvy	Usually not a high priority	Number one priority

SURVIVAL TACTICS

If you are interested in cultivating a relationship with professional athletes as individuals or as a team, consider learning and applying these survival tactics.

- **Know the sport.** It is absolutely essential to understand the nature of the game, energy expenditure, time of day games are played, travel schedule, nutritional requirements specific to positions, conditioning regimen, in-season vs off-season variations in activity, tapering schedules, altitude considerations, climate changes, time zone changes, injury and rehabilitation issues affecting nutritional status, and sports-specific supplement use (1-6).
- **Be assertive.** You are the expert in nutrition and need to hold your ground, especially against the multitude of salespeople who try to lure the athlete with various supplements.
- **Be creative and innovative**. You have the knowledge base; the trick is to apply your knowledge in a practical and unique way that the athlete will buy into and believe. One size does not fit all, and different sports will require different approaches.

- **Be flexible.** The professional athlete's job is not 9 to 5. If you want to work with athletes, be prepared to work weekends, holidays, and late nights. It is not unusual to make a late night trip to a health food store to locate a supplement for a player because the team physician is unavailable. You might also find yourself spending holidays away from your family to meet a player's nutrition needs.
- **Compromise.** As an expert in nutrition, you know what is best for athletes, but you need to make it work for them by considering their goals, food preferences, beliefs, schedules, eating habits, cooking abilities, living arrangements, and activity levels. As you develop a plan, realize that your goals may not always be the same as the athlete's. To the athlete performance comes before health, and he or she is more interested in short-term performance than long-term health.
- **Change the expectations.** As clinicians, dietitians are interested in outcome measures as well as disease prevention and health promotion. When working with professional athletes, there are times when you feel less like a dietitian and more like a mother or a hired hand. You may have to go to the store to buy fiber supplements, low-calorie snack foods, or a vitamin supplement for a player even though this is not in the job description. The athletes appreciate the extra effort, and you will get positive feedback from the coaching and training staff and be seen as a team player.
- **Set goals.** As the sports nutritionist and the athlete set goals, make them realistic and tangible, anticipating what outcomes are expected. For example, goals might include:
  — Change in energy levels
  — Weight changes
  — Quicker recovery postexercise
  — Improved sleep patterns
  The goal is to get the athlete to value and adopt the recommendations, so the more practical, the better.
- **Speak in lay terms, not like a clinician.** These are the questions that athletes will ask, so keep these points in mind as you work with the athlete.
  — Why should I try that?
  — How will it benefit me?
  — Give me examples of how to do it.
  — What if it doesn't work?
- **Be a good resource.** Professional athletes have limited time and rely on you to tell them what foods to buy, how to order out, or how to prepare foods and meals (3). Be knowledgeable about the wide variety of energy bars and sports drinks on the market and prepare a list of those you recommend. Visit the restaurants frequented by athletes and obtain a copy of the menu. Highlight the best choices on the menu. Take the athlete grocery shopping and conduct a nutrition education session while selecting food. Identify local chefs who are willing to cook for the athlete.

- **Maintain a sense of humor.** Competitive athletes are focused, goal-oriented, and quite serious about the sport which is their livelihood. Even though nutrition is a science and a serious subject, a sense of humor may make nutrition goals easier to achieve. When discussing the use of supplements, illustrate the danger to the ridiculous to make a point and to encourage interaction. Athletes who want the quick fix to lose weight, such as herbal products, may find themselves frequenting the restroom due to the diuretic and cathartic effects of the products. When athletes are in training, learning new plays or drills, and also trying to make dietary changes, the less of a chore it is, the more favorable the reaction will be.

GETTING STARTED

1. **Network wherever you are and whenever you can.** If you are interested in a particular sport, find out who provides the health care. Call the National Athletic Training Association (NATA) to identify athletic trainers for specific teams. Put together an educational handout or brochure on the sport you are interested in and send it to the team physician or athletic trainer and follow up with a phone call (7).
2. **Get some experience under your belt.** Start at the high school or college level, or offer to give a talk to a health club. Write for a local fitness magazine or get involved in a road race, offering to develop educational materials for the runners. You will be surprised who picks up materials, especially when they are free (4).
3. **Persevere.** If at first you don't succeed, try and try again. Talk to a different person; try a different angle. You might have luck talking with caterers who are involved with professional sports teams. You never know where your "in" will be.
4. **Become business savvy.** Write a business plan on what you envision your role to be. Know the team and how it operates. Know the goals of the team's organization and propose ways that you can assist the team in attaining its goals. Be detailed, listing every possible nutrition service you feel you can provide. A team may not want you to do individual counseling, but if you present team seminars, players may tell the coach or trainer they would like to have an individual nutrition plan (8).
5. **Win over the coach and/or trainers.** They are your staunchest allies or worst enemies. Offer your nutrition services to the team's coaches and trainers. This raises your credibility and gives them a first-hand opportunity to see what their players are getting.
6. **Do not be afraid to speak your mind.** Many sports nutritionists work in a male-dominated industry. Be assertive, take an active role, and if you disagree, say so. The coaches, trainers, and athletes appreciate working with someone who has an opinion, and although they may not always agree with you, this can lead to a more trusting and productive relationship in the long run.

7. **Manage your time well.** If you want to work with professional athletes, your time is their time. You need to be flexible to accommodate a last-minute meeting or unexpected travel. Flexibility is key in working with professional athletes where schedules can and often do change on a day-to-day basis (9).

FREQUENTLY ASKED QUESTIONS AND GUIDELINES

Nutrition can be a very confusing and overwhelming topic for the professional athlete who is being asked to train, compete, attend functions, and learn new drills and skills in addition to finding the time to fuel his or her body properly. *Box 19.1* highlights the most frequently asked nutrition questions. Guidelines for nutrition knowledge the athlete should possess are presented in *Box 19.2*. *Box 19.3* details information the sports nutritionist should know about the professional athlete.

BOX 19.1   Frequently Asked Questions

- What are acceptable methods of weight control?
- How much dietary fat should I get? What foods contain fat? How do I count fat grams?
- What foods can I eat to increase energy?
- What foods will speed recovery from injury?
- What about supplement use?
- What foods are good snacks and when should I snack?
- What guidelines are available for eating out?

BOX 19.2   What Does the Professional Athlete Need to Know about Nutrition?

- Energy requirements for specific sports, including modifications for injury, off-season, training, and competition (2)
- Energy, nutrient, and fluid requirements for the sport (2)
- Meal/snack timing and composition
- Eating while injured and during recovery
- Guidelines for supplement use
- Heat-related illness concerns: dehydration, cramping
- Dealing with gastrointestinal complaints: gastritis, nausea, vomiting, diarrhea, constipation
- Guidelines for weight management
- Guidelines for body fat goals and nutrition recommendations to achieve goals
- Fueling during travel (3,5,9)
- Guidelines for eating out (3)
- Guidelines for food purchases

BOX 19.3   What Does the Sports Nutritionist Need to Know about
the Professional Athlete?

- Time is at a premium.
- Meals are often eaten out.
- Food preparation skills may be nonexistent or rudimentary.
- Money is not always an issue and more money may be spent on expensive supplements than on food.
- Independence and wealth can be a problem in making appropriate food choices.
- Many professional athletes are used to being taken care of. When they need to make their own decisions (grocery shopping, meal planning), they can become overwhelmed.
- They need guidance regarding dietary supplements

Additional challenges that may arise in working with professional athletes include the following:

- **Product endorsements.** Professional athletes are often given products or paid to endorse an energy bar, sports drink, or supplement. The safety and legality of the supplement are critical issues. Be flexible and compromising in this area and make your recommendations based upon fact, not personal belief. At times you may strongly advise an athlete to stop using a product because of safety concerns. But be aware of the sport governing body's position on supplement use. You may think it is unnecessary for an athlete to use a product based upon his or her diet, but if it is not harmful or banned, let the athlete experiment.

- **Superstitions.** Some athletes will eat only certain foods before games, not eat at all, or eat strange combination of foods. Be flexible, be empathetic, and adopt the attitude that as long as it is not harmful, do not worry about it. For example, for athletes who will not eat anything the day of a game, encourage them to eat something 3 to 4 hours before the game. Set it up as a challenge and dare them to eat. Start with small goals and build from there. A professional athlete needs to be able to see the added value from a recommendation.

- **Athletes' motivation and level of interest.** Some athletes will show up at your door only at the coach's or trainer's insistence. Assess the athlete's readiness and willingness to modify his or her diet and plan accordingly. Do not be afraid to let the coach or trainer know if you feel it is not time for the athlete to work on nutrition goals. Forcing change will not work for you or the athlete.

Working with professional athletes can be rewarding but also demanding (10). You must always be the investigator, researching the latest supplements, finding out what other athletes are using, and reading the magazines they read. Not all of your recommendations may be implemented, but if one athlete values your advice and sees personal benefits, that is the best advertisement. If you do not feel comfortable with the business angle, enlist help or become more knowledgeable. Professional athletes have agents who handle their business deals and sports teams have a business department. Do not sell yourself short. One of the advantages of working with individual professional athletes or with a team is that they can pay. Keep in mind that many athletes are used to having things given to them for free, so negotiate your fees very clearly from the outset. Contact other dietitians who work with sports teams and discuss fee structure. Plan for the long haul. Whatever program you market to the athlete and/or teams, tailor it based upon seasons and needs.

As the nutrition consultant to the National Football League Pittsburgh Steelers, I have included a scope of services that I provide as an example of the types of programs that can be offered. I have worked with this team since 1992, and my involvement has expanded yearly due in part to aggressive marketing as well as the players' interest in a more comprehensive program.

COMPONENTS OF THE PITTSBURGH STEELERS' NUTRITION PROGRAM

Off-season (January-April)

- Development of nutrition education materials for the conditioning manual
- Monthly mailings to players on nutrition topics of interest (eg, dietary supplements)
- Individual player consultations as needed
- Individual coach/staff consultations as requested

Spring (Mini-camp: May-June)

- Nutrition lectures to the rookies
- Individual player/staff consultations
- Menu development in conjunction with the trainers, conditioning coach, and food service staff for training camp

Summer (July-August)

- Weekly visits to training camp to meet with individual players
- Weekly consultations with food service staff
- Serving as a resource on dietary supplements
- Serving as a liaison to the conditioning coach in scheduling players for body fat analysis

In-season (Late August-January)

- Weekly consultation with players
- Finding a personal chef for players who request the service
- Taking players to the grocery store
- Conducting cooking demonstrations
- Serving as a media resource on nutrition issues related to the team
- Helping players' spouses prepare healthful meals

- Working with the player development staff on programs for players, web site development, and programs for high school athletes
- Working with the coaches and trainers to develop protocols for supplementation use
- Development of in-service education curricula on nutrition topics
- Working with the food service personnel who provide meals during the season
- Consulting with airline food service staff on foods served in-flight for away games
- Development of menus for away games in conjunction with the conditioning coach and the hotel food service department

End of Season

- Development of nutrition materials on maintaining the edge in the home stretch
- Troubleshooting—addressing weight issues with individual players, reviewing supplement use to ensure safety and legality, addressing any new health concerns or change in living arrangements that may impact diet
- Goal setting for off-season

POSITIONING FOR THE LONG HAUL

In an effort to secure my position with the team, I have tried to develop new and innovative programs for the players. These include:

- A closed circuit video on hydration and supplement use which will be shown during training camp
- A quick self-assessment nutrition analysis program for the rookies and other interested players
- Cooking classes with local chefs and three or four players
- Working with players, local grocery stores, and schools to develop nutrition programs for children

Final Words of Wisdom

If you have made the decision that being employed as a sports nutritionist who works with professional athletes is your dream, consider these words of advice to assist you in your endeavors.

- Go for it.
- Dream and aim high.
- No idea is too outlandish.
- Have fun, sell yourself, know your stuff, and believe in what you do.
- Make connections wherever you can and learn from others who have already paved the path.

This can be a very rewarding but demanding career choice, but at the same time one definitely worth pursuing.

REFERENCES

1. Marquart LF, Cohen EA, Short SH. Nutrition knowledge of athletes and their coaches and surveys of dietary intake. In: Wolinsky I, ed. *Nutrition in Exercise and Sport.* 3rd ed. Boca Raton, Fla: CRC Press; 1998:559-596.

2. Murray R, Horswill CA. Nutrient requirements for competitive sports. In: Wolinsky I, ed. *Nutrition in Exercise and Sport.* 3rd ed. Boca Raton, Fla: CRC Press; 1998:521-558.

3. Berning JR. Eating while traveling. In: Berning JR, Steen SN, eds. *Nutrition for Sport & Exercise.* 2nd ed. Gaithersburg, Md: Aspen Publishing; 1998:247-259.

4. Peterson M. The problem athlete. In: Peterson MS, ed. *Eat to Compete.* 2nd ed. St. Louis, Mo: Mosby; 1996:189-202.

5. Jehue R, Street D, Huizenga R. Effect of time zone and game time changes on team performance: National Football League. *Med Sci Sports Exerc.* 1993;25:127-131.

6. Van Dinter NR. Introduction: competitive vs. recreational athletes—an American recreational and cultural perspective. In: Jackson CGR, ed. *Nutrition for the Recreational Athlete.* Boca Raton, Fla: CRC Press; 1995:1-18.

7. Burns J, Dugan L. Working with professional athletes in the rink: the evolution of a nutrition program for an NHL team. *Int J Sport Nutr.* 1994;4(2):132-134.

8. Kleiner S. Nutrition and the NFL: experiences of a registered dietitian. In: Bernardot D, ed. *Sports Nutrition: A Guide for the Professional Working with Active People.* 2nd ed. Chicago, Ill: American Dietetic Association; 1993:321-323.

9. Mielcarek J, Kleiner S. Time zone changes. In: Bernardot D, ed. *Sports Nutrition: A Guide for the Professional Working with Active People.* 2nd ed. Chicago, Ill: The American Dietetic Association; 1993:195-196.

10. Manore MM, Berning JR, Clark K, Engelbert-Fenton K. Roundtable: consulting in sports nutrition. *Int J Sport Nutr.* 1996;6:198-206.

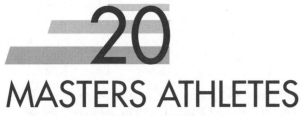

MASTERS ATHLETES

Christine A. Rosenbloom, PhD, RD

On a hot summer day in Atlanta, Georgia 100 men gathered and took turns running a mile each and broke the 100-mile relay race record by more than 6 1/2 minutes. The race was capped off with a blistering 4:39-minute mile. What makes this race remarkable is that it was undertaken by men all at least 40 years of age or "Masters athletes." The Masters runners averaged 5:23 minutes per mile, 3.4 seconds faster than the previous world record.

WHO ARE MASTERS ATHLETES?

Many sports have "Masters" divisions defined by the rules of the governing body (eg, USA Track and Field governs Masters Track and Field) or a separate organization designed to meet the needs of older athletes (eg, Golf Senior Tour or Seniors Tennis Tour for older professional athletes). The age at which an athlete becomes a "Master" ranges according to the sport and can be as young as 19 years (swimming) or 50 years (Golf Senior Tour). Some sports have different ages for female Masters, and within the Masters competition, age grouping is common. *Table 20.1* summarizes the differences between some sports.

TABLE 20.1   Defining Masters Athletes (1-5)

Sport	Governing Organization	Age of a "Masters Athlete"
Baseball	Men's Senior Baseball League (MSBL) and Men's Adult Baseball League (MABL)	Age groups: 18 years and older, 30 years and older, and 40 years and older
Golf	Golf Seniors Tour	Professional males, 50 years and older
Orienteering	International Orienteering Federation	35 years and older with 5-year age intervals up to age 70
Swimming	US Masters Swimming	19 years and older with 5-year intervals up to age 95 years and older
Tennis	Seniors Tennis Tour	Professional males, 35 years and older
Track & Field	USA Track & Field	"Submasters" 30-39 years are eligible to compete in national competitions. Masters men 40 years and older; Masters women 35 years and older

Track and Field

In track and field Masters are 40 years and older for men and 35 years and older for women (1). Governed by USA Track and Field (USATF), athletes compete in many sanctioned meets including the nationals in running, jumping, and throwing events. "Submasters" (ages 30 to 39) are allowed to compete in the National Track and Field championships. Senior meets (including the Senior Olympics and Senior Sports Classics) are limited to Masters age 50 years and older. Although exact figures are not available, it is estimated that 50,000 athletes call themselves Masters in track and field (1). In addition to events sanctioned by USATF, the World Association of Veteran Athletes (WAVA), subsidized by the International Amateur Athletics Federation (IAAF), holds world Masters championships every 2 years (1). In July 1997 the world championships were held in Durban, South Africa with more than 53,000 athletes from 79 nations competing.

The National Senior Olympics (also called National Senior Sports Classic) are not regulated by the USATF or WAVA and are held every 2 years. Athletes over the age of 50 years must qualify in local or state events to participate in the event. The USATF reports that discussion is underway to merge some of the Masters events because too many major meets are currently scheduled in close proximity to each other (1).

Many countries have their own organization for Masters track and field athletes as interest in competing at older ages grows. For example, the Canadian Masters Athletic Association (CMMA) promotes and coordinates events in track and field, cross country, road racing, and race walking (2).

Swimming

Masters swimming is an organized program of swimming for adults in events from lap swimming to international competition (3). Anyone 19 years or older is eligible to join Masters swimming and US Masters Swimming Inc, which provides the organizational structure for the sport. The organization claims to have over 30,000 members (some members are in their 90s and even 100s) (3). There are over 450 local Masters Swim Clubs and it is estimated that about 30% of members compete in swimming meets on a regular basis. Events include "short course" (25 yd and 25 m) and "long course" (50 m) as well as pool meets, lake and ocean open water swims, and international competitions (3). Competitions are organized by age groups with 5-year increments (19-24, 25-29, 30-34, 35-39, etc to 95 and over.) A recent US Masters Swimming national championship meet drew 2,400 participants (3).

Baseball

The Men's Senior Baseball League (MSBL)/Men's Adult Baseball League (MABL) are national organizations with more than 40,000 members playing on 3,000 teams (4). Started in 1986 with 60 members, MSBL/MABL provides the opportunity for nonprofessional baseball players 18 years and older to compete in a professional environment. Age categories include 18 years and over; 30 years and over; and 40 years and over. The MSBL/MABL World Series is held in November in Arizona. The rules for the game conform to standard baseball rules, complete with major league-style uniforms. Nine-inning games are usually played once a week on Sundays (4).

Orienteering

Orienteering is an endurance sport that involves running through a forest with a map and compass to find certain features of the terrain. Enthusiasts call it "running with cunning." Top athletes navigate the course without stopping and the distance covered in the event demands a 1 to 2 hours running time (5). Masters are defined as 35 years and over, with 5-year interval age classes up to the age of 70 (5).

AGING IN THE UNITED STATES

When the 20th century began, average life expectancy in the United States was 42 years (6). Today, the average person in the United States lives twice as long as 100 years ago (7). By the year 2000, about 35 million (one of every eight Americans) will be over the age of 65 (7). Future demographic projections indicate that in the year 2030 about 70 million people will be over the age of 65 (6). By the year 2040, one of every four Americans will be 65 years of age or older (7). How many of these older people will be competing at a Masters level in athletics is unknown, but growth in Masters competition in recent years bodes well for increasing numbers in the future. Dychtwald (8) points out that baby boomers (those 79 million born between 1946 and 1964) are more likely to be active. Seventeen percent of "boomers" belong to health clubs compared to only 8% of "nonboomers" (8). Surveys of baby boomers reveal that 26% say they jog on a regular basis, 29% bicycle, and 23% say they perform regular calisthenics (8).

Benefits of Exercise

In 1996 the Surgeon General issued a first of its kind report, *Physical Activity and Health* (9). The physical and mental benefits of a physically active lifestyle are summarized in *Table 20.2*. The report concludes that regular physical activity induces higher cardiopulmonary fitness which decreases overall mortality, reduces risk of coronary heart disease and high blood pressure, reduces risk of colon cancer, protects against development of type 2 diabetes mellitus, builds bone mass, increases muscle strength and balance, helps to control body weight, helps relieve symptoms of depression and anxiety, and improves mood (9). The report recommends that "all Americans accumulate at least 30 minutes or more of moderate-intensity physical activity on most, or preferably all, days of the week" (9).

TABLE 20.2   Benefits of a Physically Active Lifestyle (9)

Physiological Responses

↓ Resting blood pressure

↑ Cardiac output

↑ Blood flow to skeletal muscles and skin

↑ Maximal oxygen uptake (VO_2max)

↑ Certain components of immune system (natural killer cells, circulating T- and B-lymphyocytes)

↑ Bone mass

↑ High-density lipoprotein cholesterol levels (HDL-C)

↑ Strength and balance

Health Benefits

↓ Overall mortality

↓ Risk of cardiovascular disease

↓ Risk of hypertension

↓ Risk of thrombosis

↓ Risk of colon cancer

↓ Risk of type 2 diabetes

↓ Risk of falls and fractures in elderly persons

↓ Obesity

↓ Symptoms of depression and anxiety

↑ Psychological well-being

Aging and Exercise

It is common to classify aging based on chronological age—young adulthood (20 to 35 years), young middle-age (35 to 45 years), later middle-age (45 to 65 years), early old-age (65 to 75 years), middle old-age (75 to 85 years), and very old-age (>85 years) (10). Yet chronological age is a poor predictor of functional age. A Masters athlete at 65 years may out-perform a sedentary person 25 years old on measures of maximal oxygen intake, muscle strength, and flexibility (10).

Astrand (11) reviewed both laboratory data and statistics of world records and noted that personal best performances declined after the age of 30 to 35. At this age range, there is a decline in maximal aerobic power even in those athletes who were well conditioned and trained (11).

Peak performance in a sport depends on the key functional element that is required for success. For example, in sports such as gymnastics where flexibility is crucial, top athletes are usually in their teens (10). In aerobic sports, competitors usually peak in their mid-20s when training improvements and competition experience help the athlete before decrease in VO_2max negates those gains. In sports like golf, the best athletes are in their 30s or 40s (10).

Maximal oxygen uptake declines by about 5 mL/kg per minute per decade, beginning at age 25 years. Researchers note that it is hard to know how much of this loss is a normal age change or the extent to which it is related to adoption of a more sedentary lifestyle. Even athletes who train regularly see a rate of decrease as they age that is just slightly slower than the general population (10).

Muscle strength peaks around 25 years of age, plateaus through ages 35 or 40, and then declines, with 25% loss of peak strength by 65 years (10). The decline in muscular strength seems to parallel decreases in muscle mass (11). The age-related loss of skeletal muscle mass is called sarcopenia (12). Forty percent of women between 55 and 64 years, 45% between 65 and 74 years, and 65% between 75 and 84 years cannot lift 10 lb (12). But, muscle strength can be improved in as little as 10 weeks with resistance training, even in frail nursing-home residents (13).

Research on Masters Athletes

Research on Masters athletes is usually conducted based on cross-sectional studies of competitive athletes of various ages. Longitudinal data are less frequently reported (5).

Shephard et al (14) examined the health benefits of endurance exercise in Masters competitors (N = 750, 551 males and 199 females, mean age 58 years) over a 7-year period. The majority of subjects had initial maximal exercise tests and completed questionnaires about their health at the end of a 7-year period. Their weekly training time ranged from 10 to 30 hours. During the 7-year follow-up, only 0.6% had a nonfatal heart attack and 0.6% required coronary bypass surgery (14). Ninety percent said they were very interested in maintaining good health, 76% considered themselves to be less vulnerable to viral infections than their sedentary peers, and 68% reported their quality of life as much better than their sedentary peers. There were some former smokers in the group, but most had stopped smoking before they were regular exercisers. Thirty-seven percent of the former smokers reported that exercise helped them with the effects of withdrawal from tobacco. Fifty-nine percent reported getting regular medical check-ups, and 88% reported sleeping very well. The authors concluded that participation in Masters competition appears to carry very real health benefits, but the gains may in part reflect an overall healthy lifestyle (14).

Morgan and Costill (15) reported on health behaviors and psychological characteristics of 15 male marathon runners who were first tested in 1969 (N=8) and in 1976 (N= 7) with an average age of 50 years at the time of follow-up. The health behaviors in this sample of men were uniformly positive—all reported moderate use of alcohol, no insomnia, few physical health problems, and good overall mood (15).

Seals et al (16) studied 14 endurance-trained Masters athletes (mean age 60 years), 12 untrained men who were not lean (mean age 62 years), 9 untrained men who were lean (mean age 61 years), 15 young endurance-trained men (mean age 26 years), and 15 untrained young men (mean age 28 years) to determine if Masters athletes have a more favorable lipid profile than younger men. None of the subjects had heart disease or ECG abnormalities. Diet was not assessed, but alcohol intake was recorded and no subjects ingested more than 2 oz of alcohol per day. While the total cholesterol (TC) and low-density lipoproteins (LDL) were higher in the Masters athletes than in the young athletes, the high-density lipoproteins (HDL) were significantly higher in the Masters athletes than in the other groups (66 mg/dL versus 55 mg/dL in young athletes; 50 mg/dL in young, untrained men; 45 mg/dL in older untrained men who were lean; and 42 mg/dL in older untrained lean men). The total cholesterol/high-density lipoprotein ratios (TC/HDL) were lower for both the young and the older groups of athletes compared with the older untrained men. This study indicates that the older

Masters athletes have significantly higher HDL cholesterol levels than their sedentary peers, which could confer a reduced risk for coronary artery disease (16).

A longitudinal study on coronary heart disease (CHD) risk factors in older track athletes was reported by Mengelkoch et al (17). Three evaluation points (initial, 10-year, and 20-year) were conducted on 21 subjects, ages 60 to 92 years. Nine of the subjects remained in the high fitness category, as evidenced by participation in national and international competition; 10 subjects were classified in the moderate-intensity group; and only two subjects had greatly reduced their training volume and intensity. Measurements included smoking history, blood pressure, resting ECG, total cholesterol level, plasma glucose, body weight, percent body fat, body mass index (BMI), waist-to-hip ratio (WHR), and VO$_2$max. All CHD risk factors remained low, and even after 20 years all values for variables measured were within normal limits. Thus, in this study, the prevalence of CHD risk factors remained low into old age in Masters athletes (17).

Seals et al (18) studied endurance-trained Masters athletes (N=14, mean age 60 years) with older untrained men (N=12, mean age 60 years) and older untrained lean men (N=9, mean age 61 years) to obtain information on glucose tolerance. Each subject underwent an oral glucose tolerance test. Both groups of untrained older men had an almost two-fold greater area under the glucose curve compared to the Masters athletes. In addition, the Masters athletes had a significantly blunted insulin response compared to the untrained subjects. These data suggest that regular, vigorous, physical activity can prevent the deterioration of glucose tolerance and insulin sensitivity that are seen in some people as they age (18).

Although there is not abundant research of the benefits of physical activity in Masters athletes and not all types of sports are studied, it is clear from the research reviewed that physical health benefits are conferred upon people who maintain a very active lifestyle. Chronic diseases such as cardiovascular disease, hypertension, and diabetes are rarely seen in Masters athletes. Age changes that have come to be seen as "normal," such as reduced muscle mass and strength, reduced aerobic capacity, and bone loss, might be minimized in Masters athletes. These athletes might very well "use it and not lose it" when compared to their sedentary peers.

NUTRITION CONCERNS

Energy Intake

While there is evidence to suggest that energy needs decline with age, with about a third of the decrease related to a decline in basal metabolic rate (BMR) and the rest to decreases in physical activity (19), these data do not include individuals who vigorously exercise.

Energy needs and endurance exercise. Bunyard et al (20) studied the energy requirements of 14 lean sedentary men (mean age 58 years), 18 obese sedentary men (mean age 56 years), and 10 endurance-trained Masters athletes (mean age 59 years). The authors hypothesized that energy requirements of sedentary middle-aged men would increase to be comparable to Masters athletes' energy requirements after 6 months of aerobic training (or aerobic training plus weight loss). At baseline, VO$_2$max, BMI, WHR, and percent body fat were determined. The obese subjects received weight-loss counseling from registered dietitians and participated in regular aerobic exercise sessions three times per week. The lean subjects participated in the aerobic sessions three times a week. The Masters athletes were asked to "decondition" by stopping all endurance activities for 4 weeks to decrease their VO$_2$max by 10%. The authors found that the usual age-related decline in VO$_2$max could be attenuated as much as 50%, suggesting that the decline in VO$_2$max with aging can be partially prevented in healthy older men if regular aerobic exercise is pursued. The average increase in daily energy needs was 184 kcal per day or roughly equivalent to the energy expended in walking 1.75 miles (20).

Poehlman et al (21) studied 22 young endurance-trained men (mean age 24 years), 11 older endurance-trained men (mean age 66 years), 20 untrained young men (mean age 28 years), and 15 older untrained men (mean age 68 years) to assess age, maximal aerobic capacity, body composition, resting metabolic rate (RMR), and hormone levels. They found RMR to be about 6% higher (normalized for fat-free weight) in endurance-trained young and older men compared to untrained men. VO$_2$max and fat-free mass accounted for a significant portion of the variation in RMR. An increase in energy expenditure by exercise and an associated higher RMR allow for greater food consumption without an increase in body fat mass (21).

Energy needs and strength training. Campbell et al (22) studied the effects of 12 weeks of progressive resistance training on energy balance in sedentary, healthy older adults (8 men and 4 women, ages 56 to 80 years). Subjects were given adequate calories to maintain body weight and randomly assigned to either 0.8 or 1.6 g/kg/protein per day. At the end of 12 weeks, muscular strength increased, fat-free mass increased, fat mass decreased, and mean energy intake needed to maintain body weight increased by approximately 15% during the resistance-training program (22). The amount of protein did not influence the energy requirements in this study (22).

Exercise and the thermic effect of food. Studies have reported that exercise training increases the thermic effect of food (TEF) in older subjects. Lundholm et al (23) studied 10 active, well-conditioned men (average age 70 years) participating in aerobic exercise three to five times a week for at least 1 hour. Case controls were used for comparison. Subjects were fed a liquid formula containing 500 kcal (56% carbohydrate, 24% protein, 20% fat) and BMR was measured. Higher oxygen uptake was found in the well-trained men compared to the sedentary controls, but the TEF was significantly elevated (~56%). The authors concluded that in this study physical activity appeared to have a potentiating effect on TEF in older subjects.

Poehlman et al (24) assessed the difference in RMR and TEF in subjects of younger and older men who were either sedentary or physically active. The study design was similar Lundholm's study (23), but Poehlman included younger subjects. They found that TEF was significantly elevated (~40%) in the active subjects, regardless of age, compared to the sedentary subjects. The results of these two studies suggest that exercise confers benefits in energy expenditure beyond what is expected from an increase in RMR with physical activity (23,24). An increase in TEF in active older people could help negate the weight gain commonly experienced by older sedentary individuals.

Carbohydrate, Protein, and Fat

Carbohydrate should provide the major source of energy in any athlete's diet (25). While no ideal level of carbohydrate consumption has been defined for older, active people, the guidelines used for younger athletes should be recommended. Hawley and Burke (25) point out that using a percentage of total energy requirements to calculate carbohydrate needs might shortchange the athlete's need for carbohydrate. They correctly note that an active person's fuel needs and carbohydrate needs are not always synchronized; for example, an athlete may be receiving only 45% of his or her total calories as carbohydrate, but when calculated on a per kilogram basis, it might be adequate to meet his or her needs (25). They suggest using flexible guidelines to establish carbohydrate goals, recognizing that individual training and competition schedules may necessitate adjustment of carbohydrate intake. Hawley and Burke recommend 7 to 10 g/kg/BW as a carbohydrate target to maximize daily muscle glycogen recovery to support prolonged endurance training. To meet fuel needs and general nutrition goals for athletes who exercise less than an hour a day with moderate-intensity activity or several hours with low-intensity exercise, 5 to 7 g/kg/BW is the target. For recovery after exercise, 1.0 to 1.5 g/kg/BW of carbohydrate is recommended within an hour of exercise, with the goal of consuming 1 g/kg/BW every 2 hours (25). For more information on carbohydrate intake, see Chapter 2, Carbohydrate and Exercise.

Debate about protein needs of exercising individuals is not new, but when aging is thrown into the equation it begs the question of what are the dietary protein requirements of Masters athletes? While the question cannot be answered with precision, several researchers have looked at protein requirements in active, older people. Meredith et al (26) studied 12 physically active men (N=12; 6 men, ages 22 to 30 years and 6 men, ages 48 to 59 years). Subjects lived in a metabolic research unit during three, separate, 10-day study periods to accurately assess nitrogen balance. Subjects maintained activity and body weight for the duration of the study. They consumed diets with adequate energy intake and protein intakes of 0.6 g/kg, 0.9 g/kg, or 1.2 g/kg on three separate occasions. All subjects were in negative nitrogen balance with a protein intake of 0.6 g/kg. The authors estimated the protein needs to be 0.94 g/kg + 0.05 g/kg per day for older subjects (26).

Campbell et al (27) looked at the effect of 12 weeks of strength training in 12 older subjects (8 men and 4 women, ages 56 to 80 years). Nitrogen balance, fed-state leucine kinetics, and urinary 3-methylhistidine excretion were assessed before and after strength training. Diets provided either 0.8 or 1.62 g/kg per day and energy intake was individualized to maintain baseline body weight. The results showed that whole-body protein was significantly changed with strength training, and nitrogen retention was related to the anabolic stimulus of strength training. The efficiency of nitrogen retention was greater with the lower protein intake (0.8 g/kg per day) than with the higher protein (1.62 g/kg per day) intake. This study demonstrates that the anabolic stimulus of strength training enhances nitrogen retention when protein requirements are based on nitrogen balance studies (27).

It is reasonable to assume that the protein needs of Masters athletes are similar to younger athletes. It is important to remember that in research studies, energy intake is usually adequate to support protein intake. Athletes who ingest low-calorie diets, less than recommended carbohydrate intakes, or are in the beginning stages of an endurance- or strength-training program need more protein than those who get sufficient calories and carbohydrate, or are well trained (28). Therefore, individual assessment of protein needs is suggested for Masters athletes. Using guidelines suggested by Lemon (28), endurance athletes need 1.2 to 1.4 g/kg per day, while strength-training athletes might need as much as 1.6 to 1.7 g/kg per day.

Fat intake for older active people does not differ from that of younger people (19). A minimum of 10% of kcal from fat ensures adequate intake of essential fatty acids with 30% of kcal from fat as the upper limit recommended by most public health organizations (19).

Vitamins and Minerals

Ideal vitamin and mineral requirements for older individuals have yet to be established. The Dietary Reference Intakes (DRIs) (to date, published only for nutrients for bone health and the B vitamins) recognize the need for increased intakes of some micronutrients (29). A comprehensive review of vitamin and minerals for active people is found in Chapter 5, Vitamins and Minerals for Active People. Little research has been conducted on the micronutrient needs of active older individuals. Deficiencies in micronutrients can impair exercise tolerance, but little is known about the dietary intakes or requirements for Masters athletes. *Table 20.3* highlights the effect of nutrient deficiencies on exercise tolerance (30).

It has been assumed that an active older person's increased need for calories would ensure an increase in nutrient intakes as well, but caution is warranted as there is no guarantee that nutrient-dense food choices will be made when energy needs are increased (31). A few micronutrients have been studied and the pertinent research is discussed in this section.

TABLE 20.3 Nutrient Deficiencies that Impair Exercise Tolerance

Deficiency	Physiological Consequence	Primary Exercise Capacity Affected
Thiamin	Nerve conduction impairment, myopathy, cardiac dysfunction	Aerobic capacity, muscle strength, power, and endurance
Vitamin B-12	Central and peripheral nervous system dysfunction	Muscle strength and power
Vitamin D	Muscle contractile dysfunction and atrophy	Aerobic capacity, muscle strength, power, and endurance
Calcium	Muscle contractile dysfunction, cardiac conduction disturbance	Aerobic capacity, muscle strength, power, and endurance
Iron	Decreased oxygen-carrying capacity	Aerobic capacity
Magnesium	Muscle contractile dysfunction, cardiac conduction disturbance	Aerobic capacity, muscle strength, power, and endurance
Potassium	Muscle contractile dysfunction, cardiac conduction disturbance	Aerobic capacity, muscle strength, power, and endurance

Adapted with permission from: Fiatarone-Singh MA. The geriatric exercise prescription: nutritional implications. In: Chernoff R, ed. *Geriatric Nutrition: The Health Professional's Handbook.* 2nd ed. Gaithersburg, Md: Aspen Publishers; 1999:366-381.

Riboflavin requirements in active older women were studied by Winters et al (32). Fourteen women, ages 50 to 67 years, were found to have significant changes in markers of riboflavin deficiency when the riboflavin intake was 0.6 mcg/kcal (1989 Recommended Dietary Allowance). The authors point out that riboflavin did not improve exercise performance, only that older women who exercised appear to have higher dietary requirements for this B vitamin (32).

Vitamin D recommendations were increased in 1998 (29), but no studies to date have assessed vitamin D requirements in active older persons (31). The recommendations for vitamin D were increased from 5 to 10 mcg per day for men and women 51 to 70 years and 15 mcg for men and women over age 70 years (31). The tolerable upper intake level (UL) for vitamin D is 50 mcg.

Vitamin E is best known as a potent fat-soluble antioxidant, but it also helps to stabilize cell membranes and regulate their fluid nature, and regulates protein synthesis; it also affects nucleic acid metabolism (31). Vitamin E intakes decline with age, but alpha-tocopherol blood concentrations are better indicators of vitamin E status than dietary intakes. Blumberg et al (31) observed blood levels of vitamin E to increase into the seventh decade of life and then decline. Vitamin E has been suggested to protect against exercise-induced oxidative injury, based on studies of younger people. Vitamin E has also been reported to have a role in the prevention of atherosclerosis, certain cancers, cataract formation, and Alzheimer's disease (33). To date, there is no scientific proof that these conditions can be prevented by taking vitamin E supplements. In the United States many people are taking vitamin E supplements in the range of 100 to 400 IU, even though the RDA is 30 IU per day. Data from animal and human studies indicate that this level of supplementation is safe (34). Older athletes who choose to take vitamin E supplements are advised to inform their health care provider of supplement use, especially if taking anticoagulant medication.

Dietary calcium recommendations were increased in 1998 to 1,200 mg for men and women over 51 years of age (29). The UL for calcium is 2,500 mg per day. Athletes have higher bone density that nonathletes, and when previously sedentary women begin an exercise program, there is a small gain in bone mass (35). Suleiman et al (36) found that healthy, older, active postmenopausal women who had the highest calcium intake (>700 mg per day) and the highest physical activity (>50 hours per week) had the highest bone-mineral density when compared to women of similar age who were less active and consumed less calcium (36).

Much remains to be learned about the effect of aging and activity on micronutrient intakes. Blumberg and Meydani (31) point out that there is little evidence to support an ergogenic effect of increased intakes of vitamin or minerals; however, optimal intakes of nutrients show promise to reduce tissue injury resulting from exercise. Rock (37) suggests that for those older athletes concerned about adequate micronutrient intake, a balanced and varied diet coupled with a low-dose multivitamin mineral supplement (one that does not exceed 2 to 10 times the RDA) is usually appropriate.

FLUIDS

There are several reasons to be concerned about fluid requirements in older athletes. First, older people have less body water. Body water declines to about

60% to 70% in older persons, from a high of 80% in infancy (38). Second, thirst sensation declines in older people. Body water regulation relies on thirst to control water intake (38). Third, after the age of 40, renal mass declines with a subsequent decrease in renal blood flow. The ability of the older kidney to concentrate urine declines, meaning more water is needed to remove waste products (38). Normal age changes in thirst and fluid requirements, coupled with the increased need for fluids in the exercising individual, make this topic of paramount concern to a Masters athlete.

Kenney and Anderson (39) conducted several studies on the effect of exercise in older persons and fluid needs. In 1988 they studied 16 women (8 older women, mean age 56 years and 8 younger women, mean age 25 years) exercising in hot, dry environments and warm, humid environments. Subjects were exercised on a motor-driven treadmill for 2 hours at 35% to 40% VO_2max and were not allowed to consume fluids during the trials. Four of the older women were unable to complete either the hot-dry or warm-humid exercise trials. In the warm-humid environment, older women sweat at a rate equal to young women, but in the hot-dry environment the older women sweat less. The authors suggest that older women retain the ability to produce high sweat rates, but the sweat rate may be altered if adequate hydration is not available (39).

Zappe et al (40) studied 12 men (6 active older men, 62 to 70 years and 6 young men, 17 to 34 years) to see if older active men showed an expansion of fluid volume after repeated exercise, as is seen in younger men (40). Subjects exercised with a cycle ergometer at 50% VO_2max for 90 minutes on 4 successive days. No fluids were given during exercise, but 3 mL/kg of sports drinks was given at the end of exercise. Over the 4 days of exercise, the older subjects were able to maintain body fluid and electrolyte balance similar to the younger subjects. However, the older subjects did not increase their plasma volume compared to the younger men. The older men had a blunted thirst effect in the face of loss of body water (40).

Kenney (41) notes that older athletes can exercise in hot environments and can tolerate the heat stress as well as younger athletes of similar VO_2max, acclimatization state, body size, and composition. However, there are subtle, age-related differences in the blood flow to the skin and body fluid balance. He offers these tips to older athletes exercising in hot or humid conditions:

- **Acclimate.** Perform about 1/2 of your usual exercise on the first few days of hot weather.
- **Hydrate.** Drink as much fluid as tolerable 30 to 45 minutes before exercise and at least 8 oz every 15 minutes during exercise. After exercise, force fluid consumption and drink more than that which satisfies your thirst over a 2-hour period. Eat foods with high water content. Use a sports drink to restore lost electrolytes.
- **Use common sense.** If you are concerned that it is too hot to exercise, it probably is.
- **Maintain a high fitness level.** The best predictor of toleration to the heat is maximal aerobic capacity.
- **Learn about exercise in the heat.** Pay attention to warning signs and symptoms of dehydration, heat exhaustion, and heat stroke.

- **Know about medications.** Many prescription drugs can affect thermoregulation in hot environments. Ask your health provider about the effects of medication. (41).

The "graying" of the population brings challenges and opportunities to athletes. Today, "old" people run marathons, climb mountains, sky dive, swim competitively, and hike the 2,160-mile Appalachian Trail. In Schenectady, New York the "Seventy-Plus Ski Club" boasts 14,000 members—400 of them in their 90s (42). The evidence is clear that a vigorous lifestyle can be maintained by many older people.

CASE STUDY

Rich is a 51-year-old Masters competitor in running events from 1 mile to half-marathons. He is 67.5" tall and weighs 140 lb (63.6 kg). His body fat percentage (using body plethysmography) was 11%. He was an Olympic athlete who competed in the Montreal games in 1976. He is a former indoor mile world record holder with a time of 3:54, set in 1978. One year ago he competed in the Masters division of a national 10-K road race and won the event with a time of 32:50. Recently, he ran a mile (outdoor track) with a time of 4:39.

Rich feels he tires easily and doesn't recover as quickly as he did in his younger days. He kept a detailed food diary and training log for 2 weeks. The records showed that he eats three meals a day with three small snacks. He runs about 50 miles a week. The training logs showed that on some days he runs 3 or 4 miles, with occasional longer runs of 10 to 12 miles. One day he ran 36 miles.

Analysis of his diet revealed that he eats a "wheat-free" diet and avoids all simple sugars. He believes he is a binge eater and is "addicted to sugar" and wishes to avoid sugar and wheat in his diet. He substitutes "sprouted wheat" bread for white, wheat, or whole-grain breads. The complex carbohydrate in his diet comes from oatmeal, millet cereal, cream of rice cereal, baked potatoes, corn, brown rice, and black bean soup. He eats apples, bananas, and pineapples, and drinks orange juice.

A computerized analysis of his food diary revealed the following energy and nutrient averages:

Energy intake	2,670 kcal	(~42 kcal/kg/BW)
Carbohydrate	404 g	(~6.3 g/kg/BW and 59% of total kcal)
Protein	110 g	(~1.7 g/kg/BW and 16% of total kcal)
Fat	75 g	(~1.2 g/kg/BW and 25% of total kcal)
Vitamin A	744 RE	(74% of RDA)
Calcium	946 mg	(78% of RDA)

All other nutrients were >100% of RDAs.

Recommendations

Based on Rich's training, his carbohydrate intake may be too low to support adequate muscle glycogen stores. His diet also lacked variety as he tended to eat the same types of foods at every meal. Diet modifications included the following suggestions:

- Increase carbohydrate intake to 7 to 10 g/kg/BW or 445 to 636 g carbohydrate per day.
- Add more variety in grains such as couscous, wild rice, lentils, black beans, corn tortillas, kidney beans, black-eyed peas, and green peas.
- Increase fruit consumption to include more carbohydrate- and vitamin A-rich sources such as apricots, peaches, cantaloupe, and tangerines.
- Increase carbohydrate- and vitamin A-rich vegetables such as sweet potatoes, acorn squash, broccoli, carrots, collard and turnip greens, spinach, and tomatoes.
- Include carbohydrate-rich snacks such as homemade trail mix with dry corn or rice cereal, nuts (almonds, peanuts, cashews, or walnuts) and dried fruit (raisins, apricots, apples, dates, or figs).
- Add sports drinks as a fluid replacement beverage.
- Protein intake at 1.7 g/kg/BW is slightly higher than recommended for endurance athletes. If carbohydrate intake increases, protein levels could be lowered to 1.2 to 1.4 g/kg/BW. Most of the protein came from chicken breast. Suggest adding variety to protein by including fish, canned tuna or salmon, and lean red meat.
- Calcium intake was lower than RDA. Suggest using calcium-fortified orange juice and adding an additional serving of fat-free or 1% milk.
- Rich was not taking any dietary supplements. Discuss increasing antioxidant-rich fruits and vegetables and adding a multivitamin-mineral supplement to the meal plan to increase vitamin A, calcium, and antioxidant nutrients.
- Provide education about binge eating and the relationship of sugar to energy production.

REFERENCES

1. Frequently asked questions about masters track and field. http://www.members.aol.com/trackceo/fqu.html. Accessed August 23, 1998.
2. The Canadian Masters Athletic Association. http://www.cadivision.com.html. Accessed May 4, 1999.
3. United States Masters Swimmers frequently asked questions. http://www.usms.org/fqa.html. Accessed January 17, 1999.
4. Don't go soft—play hardball. http://www.msblnational.com/Pages/cgenfo.html. Accessed March 3, 1999.
5. Saltin B. The aging endurance athlete. In: Sutton JR, Brock RM, eds. *Sports Medicine for the Mature Athlete*. Indianapolis, Ind: Benchmark Press Inc; 1986:59-80.
6. Chernoff R. Demographics of aging. In: Chernoff R, ed. *Geriatirc Nutrition: The Health Professional's Handbook*. 2nd ed. Gaithersburg, Md: Aspen Publishers; 1999:1-12.
7. Hurley BF, Hagberg JM. Optimizing health in older persons: aerobic or strength training? In: Holloszy JO, ed. *Exercise and Sports Science Reviews*. Vol 26. Baltimore, Md: Williams and Wilkins; 1998:61-89.
8. Dychtwald K. Introduction: healthy aging or Tithonius' revenge? In: Dychtwald K, ed. *Healthy Aging: Challenges and Solutions*. Gaithersburg, Md: Aspen Publishers; 1999:1-16.
9. US Dept Health and Human Services. *Physical Activity and Health: A Report of the Surgeon General*. Atlanta, Ga: US Dept Health and Human Services, Centers for Disease Control and Prevention, National Center for Chronic Disease Prevention and Health Promotion; 1996.
10. Shephard RJ. Aging and exercise. In: Fahey TD, ed. *Encyclopedia of Sports Medicine and Science*. Internet Society for Sport Science. http://www.sport sci.org.html. Accessed June 25, 1998.
11. Astrand PO. Exercise physiology of the mature athlete. In: Sutton JR, Brock RM, eds. *Sports Medicine for the Mature Athlete*. Indianapolis, Ind: Benchmark Press; 1986:3-13.
12. Evans WL. Effects of aging and exercise on nutrition needs of the elderly. *Nutr Reviews*. 1996;54:S35-S39.
13. Fiatarone MA, O'Neill EF, Ryan ND, et al. Exercise training and nutritional supplementation for physical frailty in very elderly people. *N Engl J Med*. 1994;330:1769-1775.
14. Shephard RJ, Kavanagh T, Mertens DJ, Qureshi S, Clark M. Personal health benefits of Masters athletic competition. *Br J Sports Med*. 1995;29:35-40.
15. Morgan WP, Costill DL. Selected psychological characteristics and health behaviors of aging marathon runners: a longitudinal study. *Int J Sports Med*. 1996;17:305-312.
16. Seals DR, Allen WK, Hurley BF, Dalsky GP, Ehsani AA, Hagberg JM. Elevated high-density lipoprotein cholesterol levels in older endurance athletes. *Am J Cardiol*. 1984;54:390-393.
17. Mengelkoch LJ, Pollock ML, Limacher MC, et al. Effects of age, physical training, and physical fitness on coronary heart disease risk factors in older track athletes at twenty-year follow-up. *J Am Geriatrics Soc*. 1997;45:1446-1453.
18. Seals DR, Hagberg JM, Allen WK, Dalsky GP, Ehsani AA, Holloszy JO. Glucose tolerance in young and older athletes and sedentary men. *J Appl Physiol*. 1984;56:1521-1525.
19. Carter WJ. Macronutrient requirements for elderly persons. In: Chernoff R, ed. *Geriatric Nutrition: The Health Professional's Handbook*. 2nd ed. Gaithersburg, Md: Aspen Publishers; 1999;13-26.
20. Bunyard LB, Katzel LI, Busby-Whitehead MJ, Wu Z, Goldberg AP. Energy requirements of middle-aged men are modifiable by physical activity. *Am J Clin Nutr*. 1998;86:1136-1142.
21. Poehlman ET, McAuliffe TI, Van Houten DR, Danforth E. Influence of age and endurance training on metabolic rate and hormones in healthy men. *Am J Physiol*. 1990;259:E66-E72.

22. Campbell WW, Crim MC, Young VR, Evan WJ. Increased energy requirements and changes in body composition with resistance training in older adults. *Am J Clin Nutr*. 1994;60:167-175.

23. Lundholm K, Holm G, Lindmark L, Larrson B, Sjostrom L, Bjorntop P. Thermogenic effect of food in physically well trained elderly men. *Eur J Appl Physiol*. 1986;55:486-492.

24. Poehlman ET, Melby CL, Badylak SF. Relation of age and exercise status on metabolic rate in younger and older adults. *J Gerontol*. 1991;46:B54-B58.

25. Hawley J, Burke L. *Peak Performance: Training and Nutritional Strategies for Sport*. Sydney, Australia: Allen and Unwin; 1998.

26. Meredith CN, Zacklin WR, Frontera WR, Evans WJ. Dietary protein requirements and body protein metabolism in endurance-trained men. *J Appl Physiol*. 1989;66:2850-2856.

27. Campbell WW, Crim MC, Young VR, Joseph LJ, Evans WJ. Effects of resistance training and dietary protein intake on protein metabolism in older adults. *Am J Physiol*. 1995;268:E1143-E1153.

28. Lemon PWR. Effects of exercise on dietary protein requirements. *Int J Sport Nutr*. 1998;8:426-447.

29. Food and Nutrition Board. *Dietary Reference Intakes: Recommended Intakes for Individuals*. Washington, DC: National Academy Press; 1998.

30. Fiatarone-Singh MA. The geriatric exercise prescription: nutritional implications. In: Chernoff R, ed. *Geriatric Nutrition: The Health Professional's Handbook*. 2nd ed. Gaithersburg, Md: Aspen Publishers; 1999:366-381.

31. Blumberg JB, Meydani M. The relationship between nutrition and exercise in older adults. In: Lamb DR, Gisolfi CV, Nadal E, eds. *Perspectives in Exercise Science and Sports Medicine: Exercise in Older Adults*. Vol 8. Carmel, Ind: Cooper Publishing Group; 1995:353-394.

32. Winters LRT, Yoon JS, Kalkwarf HJ, et al. Riboflavin requirements and exercise adaptation in older women. *Am J Clin Nutr*. 1992;56:526-532.

33. Suter P. Vitamin status and requirements of the elderly. In: Chernoff R, ed. *Geriatric Nutrition: The Health Professional's Handbook*. 2nd ed. Gaithersburg, Md: Aspen Publishers; 1999:27-62.

34. Bendich A, Machlin LJ. Safety of oral intake of vitamin E. *Am J Clin Nutr*. 1988;48:612-619.

35. Drinkwater BL. Osteoporosis and the female Masters athlete. In: Sutto JR, Brock RM, eds. *Sports Medicine for the Mature Athlete*. Indianapolis, Ind: Benchmark Press; 1986:353-339.

36. Suleiman S, Nelson M, Li F, Buxton-Thomas M, Moniz C. Effect of calcium intake and physical activity level on bone mass and turnover in healthy, white, postmenopausal women. *Am J Clin Nutr*. 1997;66:937-943.

37. Rock CL. Nutrition of the older athlete. *Clin Sports Med*. 1991;10:445-457.

38. Chernoff R. Thirst and fluid requirements. *Nutrition Reviews*. 1994;52(suppl):S3-S5.

39. Kenney WL, Anderson RK. Responses of older and younger women to exercise in dry and humid heat without fluid replacement. *Med Sci Sports Exerc*. 1988;20:155-160.

40. Zappe DH, Bell GW, Swartzentruber H, Wideman RF, Kenney WL. Age and regulation of fluid and electrolyte balance during repeated exercise sessions. *Am J Physiol*. 1996;270:R71-R79.

41. Kenney WL. The older athlete: exercise in hot environments. *Sports Sci Exch*. 1993;(3).

42. Parker L. Too old? Yeah, right. *USA Today*. Oct 23-25, 1998:1A-2A.

The author wishes to thank graduate student Katja Minak for her help in gathering research for this chapter.

21

PHYSICALLY DISABLED ATHLETES

Jayanthi Kandiah, PhD, RD

According to the Developmental Disabilities Assistance and Bill of Rights Act (1), the term "developmental disability" means a severe, chronic disability that is:

- Attributable to mental or physical impairment or a combination of mental and physical impairments
- Manifested before the person attains age 22
- Likely to continue indefinitely
- Results in substantial functional limitations in three or more of the following areas of major life activity:
  1. Self-care
  2. Receptive and expressive language
  3. Learning
  4. Mobility
  5. Self-direction
  6. Capacity for independent living
  7. Economic sufficiency
- Reflects the person's need for a combination and sequence of special, interdisciplinary, or generic care, treatment, or other services which are of life-long or extended duration and which are individually planned or coordinated

An estimated 2 to 3 million athletes with developmental disabilities are involved annually in athletic competition in the United States. The range of activities for these athletes includes archery, athletics, badminton, basketball, boccie, cycling, fencing, swimming, kayaking, lawn bowling, shooting, table tennis, tennis, volleyball, water polo, weightlifting, skiing, and other recreational sports (2). With developmentally disabled athletes participating in competitive games in growing numbers, the current focus needs to address and find solutions to problems so that athletic performance will improve. Although extensive research has been conducted on able-bodied athletes and the role of nutrients in athletic performance, very limited nutrition research is available on developmentally disabled athletes (3). This chapter reviews the health and nutritional considerations of a subgroup of developmentally disabled athletes—the physically disabled athlete participating in national and international games.

GENERAL HEALTH CONCERNS

Individuals with physical disabilities are faced with many obstacles. Some of these stem from functional inabilities to perform tasks such as writing or eating, while others may be caused by the environment, such as maneuvering problems encountered while trying to shop at the grocery store. Together these hurdles may have a negative impact on the health and well-being of the individual (4,5).

The dietetics professional working with physically disabled athletes needs to keep in mind that many of these athletes are at increased nutritional risk. Neuromuscular dysfunction as well as the absence of appropriate body and motor control may interfere with self-feeding and obtaining/preparing food. The ability to chew and swallow may be affected. Because of the complex causes of feeding problems, a feeding assessment team is needed to evaluate the situation in order to maximize the athlete's ability to eat or self-feed to meet nutrition needs. Metabolic disorders, drug/nutrient interactions, altered growth patterns, and inappropriate quality care further increase nutritional risks.

Obtaining a nutrition history from these athletes may be difficult because their oral and/or written communication skills may be impaired. A communication device such as computerized artificial speech may be necessary. Caregivers or family members may be important secondary sources of information about food habits.

Currently, no reference standards exist for the assessment of anthropometric data for physically disabled athletes. Thus, a combination of measurements is used and comparisons are made to norms developed for physically healthy individuals (see *Box 21.1*). Most often, the prevention and treatment of nutrition problems in this population require an individualized approach. Since much of the research is centered on two groups of physically disabled athletes, the following sections discuss the causes, nutrition assessment, and concerns of athletes with cerebral palsy and spinal cord injury.

BOX 21.1   Anthropometric Measurements of Ambulatory and Nonambulatory Athletes with Cerebral Palsy or Spinal Cord Injury

---

Estimation of height: Knee height measurement, stadiometer

Estimation of growth: Compare weight for height, height for age, weight for age.

Estimation of linear growth: Upper arm and lower leg lengths

Estimation of weight: Digital electronic scale, sling scale or wheel chair scale

Body frame size: Elbow width or wrist measurement

Additional measurements: Skinfold thickness, upper arm circumference

---

ATHLETES WITH CEREBRAL PALSY

Cerebral palsy (CP) is a group of neuromuscular conditions caused by damage to the neurons in the brain that control and coordinate muscle tone, reflexes, and action. *Box 21.2* classifies the various types of CP. CP occurs either during the prenatal (prematurity, maternal illness, or blood incompatibilities), natal (trauma), or postnatal (infections, poisoning, malnutrition) stages of life (6).

> **BOX 21.2   Classification of Cerebral Palsy (6)**
>
> Cerebral palsy disorders might be unilateral or bilateral (involving one or both sides of the body) and are associated medical classifications such as:
>
> - **Spastic:** 70% of cerebral palsied individuals are spastic. Muscles are taut causing limited activity.
> - **Athetoid:** 20% to 30% of cerebral palsied individuals have athetoid involvement. The muscles are in constant motion. Muscle movements often increase with stress and emotion.
> - **Ataxia:** 10% of cerebral palsied individuals have ataxia. These indivuals have poor balance and difficulty in fine and rapid movements due to cerebellar disturbance.
> - **Mixed:** This form of cerebral palsy is the most common form. It is a combination of two or more of the above.

Energy Requirements

Caloric needs vary depending on the medical classification of CP. For example, differences in the level of physical activity and motor dysfunction dictate different energy needs for individuals with spastic or athetoid CP. Because of limited energy expenditure, obesity is often an issue with nonambulatory spastic individuals, while an increase in energy requirements is observed in athetoid CP individuals (7). When the condition requires drug therapy, lethargy may ensue which may decrease motor activity and further alter caloric needs. Energy recommendations based on kcal/cm of height may be a more useful reference than kcal/kg of body weight, since physical growth often varies from one type of CP to another (6).

Continuous involuntary movement in athetosis has been shown to increase the resting metabolic rate by approximately 500 kcal per day (7). Often times, open-circuit indirect calorimetry is used to measure resting energy expenditure and the doubly-labeled water method with deuterium is used to measure total energy expenditure (8).

Nutrient Needs

Individuals who are severely affected with CP often have metabolic bone disease such osteopenia and fractures. Causes of deficient bone mineralization include oral motor dysfunction which makes feeding difficult, low calorie intake, medications, or the physical handicap which inhibits normal bone mineralization. Calcium intake of less than 500 mg per day has been shown to affect the proximal parts of the femora and the lumbar spine.

Female CP athletes tend to have lower intakes of calcium, zinc, folate, and iron than other athletes. (8). This low intake of calcium often results from drinking less than 2 cups of milk per day, resulting in a mean intake of 364 ± 160 mg of calcium per day (8). Such a low calcium intake predisposes females to premature fractures that could hinder athletic performance. Decreased consumption of all types of animal protein and seafood, and limited intake of dark-green leafy vegetables also cause female CP athletes to have lower dietary intakes of various nutrients (8).

Like able-bodied female athletes, CP athletes may also have low iron intakes. Mean intake of dietary iron among female athletes is 10.3 mg per day (8). Even though female CP athletes assessed in one study were not vegetarians, they generally consumed less than 3 oz of meat, fish, or poultry per day (8). As a result, only 11% to 14% of dietary intake was from animal flesh (4% to 6% heme iron). Since the foods generally high in iron are also good sources of zinc, females were also found to have inadequate intakes of this trace mineral (8). Such iron deficiency anemia can be addressed with iron supplementation. It should also be noted that copper deficiency decreases iron absorption while ascorbic acid increases nonheme iron absorption.

The Paralympic Games are a biennial event for elite athletes with any disability. They follow the Olympic Games every two years, with both summer aand winter games. In 1996 in Atlanta, 3,500 disabled athletes from 120 nations competed in sports like wheelchair tennis, basketball, and road racing (9). In elite Paralympic CP athletes, dietary fat intake was greater than 30% of total calorie intake, with saturated fat contributing 14% and 12% in the diets of males and females, respectively (8). Mean intake of dietary cholesterol for males was 349.0 ± 191 mg per day. Generally, studies have demonstrated that able-bodied athletes involved in physically active sports like swimming and running have higher fat intakes than weight-conscious athletes such as figure skaters and gymnasts (10,11). This was found to be true with the CP swimmers and track and field athletes who consumed high amounts of fat (8).

Anthropometric Measurements

In assessing CP athletes, it is necessary to select appropriate standards for comparison and to use good clinical judgment when making recommendations. Measurements such as length, arm span, body circumferences, and skinfolds should be used as needed to determine body size (12). It is recommended that skinfold measurements be taken from seven sites (triceps, axilla, subscapular, chest, abdomen, thigh, supra ilium) with professional metal calipers that apply pressure of 10 g/mm^2. For athletes who have bilateral involvement, skinfold measurements should be taken on the least affected side. Since growth retardation is often a problem and tends to persist with age and activity, upper-arm and lower-leg lengths are used to measure linear growth. Body weight is measured to the nearest 0.5 kg using an appropriately calibrated scale. Nonambulatory CP athletes should be weighed in a preweighed wheelchair, and the weight of the wheelchair subtracted from the total (7,10).

Drug-nutrient Interactions

Anticonvulsant drugs, such as phenobarbital, phenytoin, and primidone, are often used to treat seizures in CP athletes. Since constipation is a common side effect of anticonvulsant drugs, increased dietary fiber and fluids (1.5 to 2.0 L per day) can address this problem. Long-term use of anticonvulsant drugs also interferes with vitamin D and bone metabolism, causing altered folic acid metabolism and connective tissue disorders (gum hypertrophy).

Vitamin D deficiency contributes to osteomalacia, reduced serum calcium and phosphorus levels, and elevated alkaline phosphatase levels (13). Folate deficiency may decrease serum ferritin and total iron-binding capacity resulting in megaloblastic and microcytic hypochromic anemia. These deficiencies can be off-set by eating foods rich in folate, requiring increased exposure to sunlight, and taking therapeutic doses of these nutrients.

Medications may further affect the bioavailability of nutrients by causing anorexia, nausea, and diarrhea. Frequent nutrient supplements or planning meal-times to coincide with the time that the drug is causing the least amount of side effects may help alleviate problems.

ATHLETES WITH SPINAL CORD INJURY (WHEELCHAIR ATHLETES)

Wheelchair confinement may be required due to spinal cord injury/disease, mus-cular dystrophy, cerebral palsy, multiple sclerosis, or stroke. Spinal cord injury (SCI) is categorized by the level of injury to the root of the spinal cord nerve. The vertebrae are coded from top to bottom, cervical or C1-8, thoracic or T1-12, lum-bar or L1-5, and coccyx, Coc-1. Injury between C-3 (3rd cervical bone in the neck) and T-1 (1st thoracic bone in the spine) causes quadriplegia; injury below T-1 causes paraplegia. Depending on the extent of injury to the vertebrae, damage can range from lack of head control to poor bowel and bladder function (4).

Nutrient Needs

Decreases in lean tissue with associated increases in body fat have been observed in paraplegic athletes (14). Although controversy exists in the percent distribution of body fat and lean muscle mass from atrophy of the lower limbs in wheelchair athletes, Kofsky et al (15) found that a large sample of wheelchair-confined men and women had body mass and body fat figures in the normal range (15).

Work by other researchers has shown that newly diagnosed SCI athletes are at greater risk of cardiovascular disease due to low high-density lipoprotein (HDL) levels caused by decreased mobility. This decrease in activity warrants reduction in dietary fat to less than 20% of total calories. With regular endurance activity, an increase in HDL levels is observed, with a decreased risk for the development of cardiovascular disease (4,16).

Generalized osteoporosis is commonly noted in this group of athletes as a result of high intakes of fat and increased urinary losses of calcium associated with insufficient activity (12). Increasing dietary intake of calcium or recommend-ing calcium supplementation should rectify this problem. However, caution is required in choosing a calcium supplement because SCI athletes are known to retain an increased concentration of calcium in their kidneys and bladder that can lead to renal stone formation. Because they are well absorbed, calcium phosphate dibasic, calcium citrate malate, calcium carbonate, calcium lactate, or calcium glu-conate are all good choices for supplementation. Studies have shown that calcium citrate malate is a more bioavailable calcium source than the others (4). Orange juice is the best means of delivering the calcium citrate supplement, since it increases calcium bioavailability. Increased fluid intake is also helpful in the pre-vention of renal stone formation (4).

Daniel and Gorman (17) suggest that wheelchair athletes' diets be composed of 20% fat, 68% carbohydrate, and 12% protein. Of the 20% of caloric intake consumed as fat, they suggest that 15% should be from mono- and polyunsaturated fats with only 5% from saturated fat. If trauma occurs, protein intake should be increased to 15% (17). Nutrient inadequacies observed among the SCI population include iron, calcium, vitamin C, beta carotene, thiamin, folate, and copper (15).

Since spinal cord-injured athletes are susceptible to hypo- and hyperthermia during moderate temperature variations, adequate hydration is recommended. Dehydration can be prevented by drinking plenty of water or cool fluid replacement beverages before, during, and after exercise. Alcoholic and caffeinated beverages are not recommended. Increased consumption of fluids will also help reduce the incidence of bladder infections.

Anthropometric Measurements

In ambulatory SCI athletes, knee height appears to be a good measure to estimate height, but one needs to be cautious that contractures and/or the inability to hold the arms, shoulders, or body upright do not interfere with measurements (18). In nonambulatory persons, an assistant may be required to hold the body in position and to limit involuntary muscle movements. Photogrammetric measurement techniques may be useful to reduce the need for body manipulation. Any measurement method must be able to be exactly replicated to obtain reliable measurements. Weight may be measured with a sling scale or wheelchair (weight of equipment subtracted). Weight should be measured at the same time of the day with an empty urine collection bag and in the same wheelchair with the same accessory equipment. For estimation of energy needs in SCI individuals, the Harris-Benedict equation (4) is usually used as a reference tool.

Other Health Issues

Issues facing the sports nutritionist when dealing with wheelchair athletes include dehydration, minor respiratory infections, gastrointestinal disorders, bladder infections, development of pressure sores, thermoregulatory dysfunction, and severe osteoporosis (19).

Thermoregulatory dysfunction caused by hypo- or hyperthermia at relatively moderate temperatures of 50° to 60°F could be overcome by adequate hydration and protecting the athlete from extreme temperatures by removing him or her from the environment. Long-term immobilization of the lower extremities may cause severe osteoporosis. Since this condition makes the athlete vulnerable to fracture risk from even minor trauma or muscle spasm, adequate dietary calcium intake is recommended and wheelchairs should be well padded. To reduce the incidence of dehydration and bladder infections, nonambulatory athletes who use urine bags to collect fluid should be encouraged to drink plenty of liquids. Decubitus ulcers and thrombosis may also be caused by the paralyzed limbs (20).

Since the normal body contains approximately 60% water, dehydration affects the body in a variety of ways. Adverse effects of loss of water weight range from a decrease in work capacity (1% loss of body weight or 1.7% loss of total body water), to dry mouth and reduction in urinary output (3% loss of body weight or 5% loss of total body water), to serious problems which could cause the athlete to collapse (7% loss of body weight or 10% loss of total body water) (21).

Like with able-bodied athletes, appropriate replacements of fluids, nutrients, and electrolytes will prevent dehydration and gastrointestinal disorders in disabled athletes. For activities lasting less than 1 hour (eg, football, basketball, cycling, track), with exercise intensity ranging from 75% to greater than 100% VO$_2$max, a preactivity beverage should contain 6% to 8% carbohydrate (volume of 300 to 500 mL). This will enhance performance in the event of glycogen depletion. During the activity it is recommended that 500 to 1,000 mL of cool water (5° to 15°C) be provided to replace fluids lost in sweat and to address the rise in core temperature.

In events that last 1 to 3 hours (eg, soccer, most marathons) where exercise intensity is between 60% to 90% VO$_2$max, the preactivity beverage should be 300 to 500 mL of plain water. During the activity, 800 to 1,600 mL per hour of cool (5° to 15°C), 6% to 8% carbohydrate solution containing 10 to 20 mEq of sodium/L is recommended. Sodium is needed to enhance palatability, prevent hyponatremia, and promote carbohydrate and fluid absorption, while chloride, an anion, is required for fluid absorption.

Although the amount of water and the composition of chloride and carbohydrate solutions are similar preactivity and during activities lasting 1 to 3 hours, endurance activities over 3 hours require 20 to 30 mEq of sodium/L to avoid the onset of hypovolemia, dehydration, glycogen depletion, and possibly hyponatremia. Due to excessive sweating, adding 3 to 5 mEq of potassium to a sports drink may also be beneficial to replace potassium lost in sweat and to stimulate rehydration of the intracellular fluid compartment.

Postactivity fluid and electrolyte must be replaced during the first 2 hours of recovery to enhance performance in subsequent athletic competitions. To promote glycogen resynthesis and fluid and electrolyte replacement, the recovery beverage should contain 30 to 40 mEq of sodium and chloride along with 25 g of carbohydrate per hour (22).

Medications

Prescribing medications to SCI athletes is very common, but many of these medications may have side effects that could interfere with proper nutrition. Skeletal muscle relaxants, antibiotics, and urinary antispasmodics are often prescribed and may cause constipation, nausea, vomiting, loss of appetite, and dry mouth.

REFERENCES

1. Developmental Disabilities Assistance and Bill of Rights Acts, Pub L No. 95-602, Sec. 03, Sec. 102 (1978).
2. Tiessen K. Sports opportunities for athletes with disabilities. In: DePauw KP, Gavron SJ, eds. *Disability and Sport*. Champaign, Ill: Human Kinetics; 1995:83-90.
3. Kandiah J. Nutrition and the physically disabled athlete. In: Wolinsky I, ed. *Nutrition in Exercise and Sport*. Boca Raton, Fla: CRC Press; 1998:515-529.
4. Rice HB, Ponichtera-Mulcare JA, Glase RM. Nutrition and the spinal cord injured individual. *Clin Kinesiol*. 1995;54:21-27.
5. Shepard RJ. Benefits of sport and physical activity for the disabled: implications for the individual and for the society. *Scand J Rehab Med*. 1991;23:51-59.
6. Sherrill C, Mushett C, Jones JA. Cerebral palsy and the CP athlete. In: Jones JA, ed. *Training Guide to Cerebral Palsy Sports*. Champaign, Ill: Human Kinetics; 1988:9-13.
7. Johnson RK, Goran MI, Ferrara MS, Poehlman ET. Athetosis increases resting metabolic rate in adults with cerebral palsy. *J Am Diet Assoc*. 1995;95:145-148.
8. Kandiah J. Nutritional assessment of US paralympic athletes with cerebral palsy. *Int J Biosocial Med Research*. 1996;14:133-141.
9. What are the Paralympics? http://www.canoe.com/Paralympics/what.html. Accessed September 20, 1999.
10. Brotherhood JR. Nutrition and sports performance. *Sports Med*. 1984;1:350-389.
11. Short SH, Short WR. Four-year study of university athletes' dietary intake. *J Am Diet Assoc*. 1983;82:632-645.
12. Chumela WC, Roche AF. Nutritional anthropometric assessments of non-ambulatory persons using recumbent techniques. *Am J Phys Anthrop*. 1984;63:146-149.
13. Rice BL. Nutritional problems of developmentally disabled children. *Ped Nurs*. 1981;7:15-18.
14. Coldwell LL, Squires WG, Raven PB. Benefits of aerobic exercise for the paraplegic: a brief overview. *Med Sci Sports Exerc*. 1986;18:501-508.
15. Kofsky PR, Shepard RJ, Davis GM, Jackson RW. Fitness classification tables for lower limb disabled individuals. In: Sherrill C, ed. *Sports and Disabled Athletes*. Champaign, Ill: Human Kinetics; 1986:147-156.
16. Peck DM, McKeag DB. Athletes with disabilities: removing medical barriers. *Phys Sports Med*. 1994;22:59-62.
17. Daniel M, Gorman D. Nutritional considerations for the wheelchair athlete. *Sport N Spokes*. 1983;9:8-13.
18. Chumela WC. Methods of assessing body composition in nonambulatory persons. *Body Composition Assessment in Youth and Adults*. Columbus, Ohio: Ross Laboratories; 1984:86-88.
19. Shephard RJ. Sports medicine and the wheelchair athlete. *Sports Med*. 1988;4:226-247.
20. Curtis KA, Dillon DA. Survey of wheelchair athletic injuries—common patterns and prevention. In: Sherrill C, ed. *Sports and Disabled Athletes*. Champaign, Ill: Human Kinetics; 1986:211-216.
21. Sawka MA, Greenleaf JE. Current concepts concerning thirst, dehydration, and fluid replacement. *Med Sci Sports Exerc*. 1992;24:643-647.
22. Gisolfi CV, Duchman SM. Guidelines for optimal replacement beverages for different athletic events. *Med Sci Sports Exerc*. 1992;24:672-679.

NUTRITIONAL CONSIDERATIONS DURING INJURY AND REHABILITATION

Jean Storlie, MS, RD and Nancy Clark, MS, RD, FADA, FACSM

Very little research has been published about the nutrition needs of injured athletes; however, the medical literature yields substantial evidence to document the importance of nutrition during wound healing. Classic studies in the 1970s brought this issue into focus and led to the development of procedures and protocols to screen for malnutrition in surgical patients and to provide various forms of nutrition support for hospitalized patients (1-3). Since athletes do not fit the profile of the typical patient at risk for hospital malnutrition—older, frail patients with chronic illnesses—they may not get the scrutiny required to detect suboptimal nutritional status. Further, injuries not requiring surgery are typically treated in an outpatient setting where minimal, if any, nutrition intervention is offered. Thus, borderline malnutrition—and the underlying dietary causes—may go undetected and can prolong the rehabilitation process. This chapter reviews the role of nutrition in wound healing, examines two case studies that illustrate how poor eating habits can impair healing, and provides practical guidelines for managing athletes' nutrition care during rehabilitation.

NUTRITION-INJURY CONNECTION

There are three stages in the healing response: inflammation, proliferation, and maturation (1). The inflammation stage begins at the time of injury and continues for 4 to 6 days. The proliferation stage, which begins on the third or fourth day postinjury and lasts up to 2 weeks, is characterized by synthesis of epithelial cells, fibroblasts, and collagen. Maturation involves tapering of the regenerative process as the tensile strength of the wound increases; it begins in the second or third week after injury and can continue for up to 2 years.

Malnutrition adversely affects healing at each of these stages. Deficiencies of key nutrients impair critical healing functions (eg, vitamin C and collagen formation, vitamin A and epithelialization, zinc and cell proliferation). In addition, malnutrition causes an array of metabolic alterations that disrupt energy and protein metabolism, compounding the deleterious effects of trauma. Studies show that even mild forms of protein-calorie malnutrition impair the healing process (4). Athletes who adhere to calorie- and protein-restricted diets may develop subclinical malnutrition and be at greater risk of complications if they become injured and require surgery.

Trauma and Metabolic Stress

Starvation, surgery, infection, major injury, burns, and shock impose a trauma or physical stress on the body (2). During trauma the body organs must work harder to compensate for the damage. The degree of stress depends on the severity of the trauma and how well a person is prepared to meet the increased needs. A person who is well-nourished and healthy before the trauma will be more likely to recover quickly. But a person who has been weakened by other stressors, such as disease, infection, previous injury, or starvation, may take longer to heal and need more medical and nutrition intervention.

Trauma and stress alter metabolic and nutrition needs, in particular protein and calories. While the body must continue to meet basal metabolic needs, additional metabolic demands are imposed by the stress. The body becomes hypermetabolic; in some types of trauma such as major surgery or severe burns, the metabolic rate may increase by 50% or more (5).

Starvation. Unlike other forms of stress, during starvation the metabolic rate actually decreases in an effort to compensate for the lack of food (5). But even though metabolism is depressed, protein turnover is high as the body breaks down muscle for energy. Starvation on top of other traumas can be a very serious combination—the body is being deprived of nutrients at a time when needs are especially high. A person who is malnourished before an injury or surgery is more likely to develop complications and take longer to recover.

Surgery. Most surgery is considered a minor trauma. It involves the shock of anesthesia, trauma to the organ itself, open tissue with risk of infection, and demands associated with recovery from the surgery as well as the problem that caused the surgery (5). Minor surgery raises resting metabolism by about 15%, major surgery by 20% to 50%. Since food restrictions are imposed prior to and immediately after surgery, a patient may go without eating for as long as 48 hours. During this time without food, the body must rely on its own stores of carbohydrate, protein, and fat to meet the increased calorie requirements. Carbohydrate stores provide 800 to 1,200 calories which is less than 1 day's need; when they are depleted, muscle protein becomes a major source of energy. This is one reason why optimal nutritional status—sufficient energy and protein stores—is so important prior to surgery.

Injuries. Minor athletic injuries can cause local and systemic elevations in metabolic rate which increase calorie needs slightly. Serious injuries that involve major trauma and shock or severe burns may increase energy needs by 20% to 45% (5). The extremely high energy and protein needs in these situations can severely compromise immune function, making infection likely. Aggressive medical and nutritional support is needed in these situations.

Nutrients Involved in Healing

Protein, fat, carbohydrates, vitamins, and minerals are needed for complete and timely wound healing (3). Even if one of the essential nutrients is not present, healing can be delayed. *Table 22.1* lists some of the key nutrients, their role in healing, signs of deficiency, and food sources.

TABLE 22.1   Nutrients Involved in Healing

Nutrient	Healing Function(s)	Deficiency Signs/Symptoms
Protein	Growth, maintenance, repair of tissues	Decreased serum albumin and other serum proteins
	Immune function	Anemia
	Enzyme and hormone formation	Hair loss (also brittle and dull)
		Brittle, ridged nails
	Energy	Frequent infections
		Impaired wound healing
Calories	Energy for normal metabolism	Chronic dieting
	Energy for increased metabolism associated with stress and trauma	Eating disorders
		Starved appearance
		Muscle wasting
		Subcutaneous fat loss
		Increased infections
		Poor wound healing
Carbohydrates	Energy	Fatigue
	Leukocyte functioning	Dizziness
		Headache
Essential fatty acids	Energy	Flaky, itchy skin
	Component of cell membrane	Sores on scalp
		Diarrhea
Calcium	Growth and maintenance of bones and teeth	Stunted growth in children
	Regulation of muscle contraction	Osteoporosis in adults
		Poor bone healing
	Transmission of nerve impulses	
Iron	Transportation of oxygen	**Depletion (subclinical)**
	Synthesis of myoglobin and hemoglobin	Lowered serum ferritin
	Energy metabolism	Normal hemoglobin
		Possible decrease in endurance performance
		Deficiency (clinical)
		Lowered serum ferritin
		Lowered hemoglobin
		Impaired aerobic metabolism
		Fatigue and lethargy
		Impaired coordination
Zinc	Physical growth	**Clinical/subclinical deficiency**
	Injury healing	Low plasma zinc
		Poor wound healing
		Infertility
		Short stature/poor growth
Copper	Collagen formation	Anemia
		Low white blood cell (neutrophil) count
		Bone loss
		Increased serum cholesterol levels
		Poor growth

continued

TABLE 22.1   Nutrients Involved in Healing (continued)

Nutrient	Healing Function(s)	Deficiency Signs/Symptoms
Vitamin C	Collagen formation — Scar tissue — Bone growth/repair Iron absorption Antioxidant Strengthens resistance to infection	**Early deficiency** Bleeding gums Bruising Frequent infections **Advanced deficiency** Rough, scaly, dry skin Poor wound healing Weakened bones/joint pain Loose teeth Anemia

Vitamin A	Epithelial cell formation
	Supporting immune function
	Promoting growth and bone
	    remodeling
		Deficiency
		Impaired bone growth
		Cracks in teeth
		Frequent respiratory and GI
		    infections
		Dry, rough, scaly skin
		Lumps around hair follicles

Vitamin K	Blood clotting Preventing hemorrhage	Hemorrhage
B-complex vitamins	Energy metabolism Cofactors for cellular development	Smooth tongue Dermatitis
Folacin	Maturation of red and white blood cells	Inflammation of tongue Diarrhea Poor growth Mental confusion Problems with nerve function
Pyridoxine (vitamin B_6)	Cellular immunity	**Mild** Weakness Irritability Insomnia **Advanced** Growth failure Impaired motor function Convulsions

Sources:

Storlie J. Eating with an injury. *Train Condition.* 1997;VII(5):19-31.

Trujillo EB. Effects of nutritional status on wound healing. *J Vasc Nurs.* 1993;11:12-18.

Macronutrients. Protein is the most important macronutrient for wound healing. It plays several special roles in the body:

1. Growth, maintenance, and repair of body tissues
2. Support for the immune functions in the body
3. Synthesis of enzymes and hormones

Protein also serves as a back-up energy source. When determining protein needs, the metabolic interactions between protein, carbohydrate, and fat must be considered. Carbohydrates are the favored fuel, while protein is an expensive, reserve fuel. When carbohydrates are not available, protein is converted to carbohydrate and burned as a fuel. During energy-demanding states if calorie intake is insufficient, protein can become a significant source of fuel. The shunting of proteins into the energy pool will bypass the primary functions of protein, leaving the body without the building blocks to repair tissue, fight infection, and perform regulatory functions. During recovery from trauma, an adequate intake of carbohydrates and calories is especially important to preserve protein for its crucial functions.

Protein needs range from 1.0 to 1.5 g/kg per day during recovery from minor traumas. Recovery from major traumas, like a severe burn, could boost the protein needs to 2 to 3 g/kg per day. Meeting the calorie and protein needs during major traumas usually requires some form of nutrition supplementation, usually provided via tube feeding. On the other hand, the protein needs during minor trauma easily can be met with food sources (eg, 2 to 3 servings of meat, fish, or poultry and 2 to 3 servings of milk products per day). Eating these foods with plenty of breads, cereals, fruits, and vegetables will provide the carbohydrates to spare protein and balance the diet. Fat provides energy and essential fatty acids, which are a core component of cell membranes and important for tissue repair. Moderate fat intakes are advised during rehabilitation, as in healthy living.

Minerals. There is some evidence that clinical and subclinical mineral deficiencies are linked to higher injury rates and prolonged healing times. For example, athletes with injuries took in 25% to 40% less calcium and zinc than noninjured athletes (4). Twice the injury rate was observed in athletes who had lower serum ferritin levels (5).

As athletes strive for low intakes of fat and cholesterol, many of them eliminate red meat and practice vegetarian diets. These dietary patterns place athletes at risk for iron and zinc deficiencies, since nonmeat sources of iron and zinc are poorly absorbed and not as concentrated. This practice may also result in insufficient protein intake if the athlete is not careful about eating enough high-quality vegetable proteins, such as legumes, to replace meat protein.

Similarly, many athletes restrict their intake of milk products, either to avoid fat or for intolerances or personal preferences. This habit can compromise calcium intake and lead to weakened bones which are more susceptible to stress fractures.

Vitamins. Several vitamins play key roles in the healing process (4). Vitamin C is especially important because it aids in the synthesis of collagen, a core component of scar tissue. Vitamin A enhances the inflammatory response, moderates collagen turnover, stimulates epithelial cell formation, and supports immune function. Vitamin K indirectly affects tissue repair by aiding in the formation of blood clots and preventing hemorrhage. The hypermetabolic state associated with trauma and stress increases B vitamin needs. Specific B vitamins play more precise roles in healing: Folacin facilitates the maturation of red and white blood cells and pyridoxine aids in antibody formation.

DETECTING NUTRITIONAL RISK FACTORS

Screening

Table 22.2 lists several nutritional "red flags" that should be explored when an athlete appears to be recovering slowly from an injury or surgery. Evidence of eating disorders frequently signals impaired nutritional status; appropriate referrals to medical and psychological professionals should be considered. The other red flags are more subtle indicators and may not necessarily indicate a dietary problem. However, if an athlete reveals two or three of them (eg, no red meat, no milk, and chronic dieting), there is a good possibility of dietary inadequacies or imbalances. In these situations, a comprehensive nutrition assessment is indicated.

TABLE 22.2   Identifying Possible Nutrition Problems

Red Flag	Possible Nutrition Problems
Eating disorders — Obsessed with appearance — Obsessed with eating — Overly restrictive eating habits — Not eating much — Excessive exercise — Eating and disappearing	Starvation (protein-calorie malnutrition) Vitamin and mineral inadequacies Electrolyte imbalances (if bulimic)
Chronic dieting and weight restriction	Inadequate calories Inadequate protein Vitamin and mineral inadequacies/imbalances
Restricting red meat	Inadequate protein intake Inadequate iron and zinc intake
Vegetarian diet	Inadequate protein intake Inadequate iron and zinc intake
Very-high-carbohydrate, very-low-fat diet	Inadequate protein intake Inadequate iron and zinc intake Inadequate intake of essential fatty acids Nutrient imbalances
No milk or dairy products	Inadequate protein intake Inadequate calcium intake

Nutrition Assessment

Comprehensive nutrition assessment involves collection and interpretation of anthropometric, biochemical, clinical, and dietary data. The procedures and protocols for conducting such an assessment are discussed elsewhere (4,6). *Table 22.3* summarizes the data that might be used in a comprehensive nutrition assessment.

TABLE 22.3   Comprehensive Nutrition Assessment

Type of Data	Data
Anthropometric	Weight change Triceps skinfold Midarm muscle circumference
Biochemical	Serum albumin Transferrin Prealbumin Retinol-binding protein Total lymphocyte count Nitrogen balance
Clinical	Medical history Physical examination
Diet history	Recent changes in weight, appetite, food intake Food aversions, intolerances, or allergies Chewing or swallowing problems History of nausea/vomiting or diarrhea Use of medication or dietary supplements Usual energy and nutrient intake

MANAGING WEIGHT DURING REHABILITATION

Another major nutrition consideration during rehabilitation is weight management. Calorie needs for many athletes will drop during the early phase of rehabilitation, then slowly build back up.

Acute Recovery

During the acute phase of recovery when athletes are bedridden, they usually will be in a hypermetabolic state due to the trauma of the injury or surgery, so risk of weight gain is minimal. However, in rare cases when the injury results in prolonged immobility, such as a back injury or paralysis, long-term weight management strategies are important. Once athletes begin rehabilitation, they will be expending calories through their rehabilitation exercise and daily living. Current rehabilitation practices involve relatively brief periods of bedrest. For example, patients recovering from anterior cruciate ligament (ACL) knee reconstruction might be involved in some form of rehabilitation 2 to 4 days postoperation (6).

Rehabilitation

Exercise during the first month of rehabilitation usually consists of stretching, low-level strength training, range of motion work, and low-level biking (50% maximal heart rate) for warm-up purposes. The calorie cost of this low-level exercise is minimal. But within a month most rehabilitation protocols involve some form of weight-supported aerobic exercise at 60% to 80% maximal heart rate for 30 to 40 minutes. A workout at this level would expend approximately 300 to 500 calories. Within 3 months, sports-specific activities are incorporated and an athlete gradually increases caloric expenditure (9).

Some athletes may not compensate for the decreased energy expenditure with a decreased food intake and gain excess fat weight. Extra body fat places stress on injured joints and hampers sports performance. This scenario is most likely with endurance athletes whose previous calorie expenditure from exercise alone was extremely high (eg, 1,500 to 2,000 per day) and when the rehabilitation process is long. Due to the metabolic cost of trauma and healing, loss of appetite which usually occurs posttrauma and the relatively brief period of inactivity and low caloric expenditure (about 1 month), excess weight gain is not that common. Athletes are not likely to gain more than 5 to 10 lb during rehabilitation.

Some athletes overreact to lack of exercise and severely restrict their calories for fear of gaining weight. This tendency is more problematic than a little extra body fat. Calorie restriction during recovery from the stress and trauma of an injury and/or surgery will deprive the body of the protein needed to heal and fight infection. This approach could impair healing, slow recovery, and increase the likelihood of future injuries. To help athletes cope with the changes in their calorie balance, it is useful to calculate the caloric difference between the preinjury training program and the rehabilitation exercise program. A dietetics professional can use this information to develop a realistic target for how many food calories to decrease.

PSYCHOLOGICAL CONSIDERATIONS

During rehabilitation athletes may experience mood disturbances and lowered self-esteem due to withdrawal from their sport and the sense of failure brought on by the injury. The extent to which these issues are evident will depend to a large degree on how the athlete defines himself or herself in relation to the sport. Those who are "all-consumed" by their sport and athletic prowess will suffer more emotionally than those who lead more balanced lives. Two coping strategies have been observed when people are depressed: Some athletes throw themselves too aggressively into rehabilitation and overdo it; others become lethargic, lacking the motivation to comply (9).

When working with athletes during rehabilitation, it helps to be aware of how the athlete is coping psychologically and how his or her emotions may affect food intake and performance during rehabilitation. Some athletes use "food as a drug" for coping with stressful emotions and overeat in response to their feelings of loss and depression. Of greater concern, however, are athletes who become overly concerned with body weight and severely restrict calorie intake. Quantifying energy needs and discussing the role of rehabilitation exercise in curtailing excess weight gain are important intervention strategies. Other strategies that keep recovering athletes close to their sports, such as attending practice sessions and competitive events and eating with the team, will help to alleviate the social withdrawal that can compound depression.

CASE STUDIES

Recurrent Stress Fractures

Sheree, a 25-year-old, injured female recreational runner, sought nutrition counseling because she was concerned about recurring stress fractures and afraid that her diet was contributing to the impaired healing. At the time of the initial consultation, she was unable to run due to a stress fracture, but she hoped to be recovered in time to train for a marathon that was 7 months away. The key findings from her initial consultation are presented in *Box 22.1*

Sheree represents an all too common case of an athlete whose obsession with body weight leads to severely restrictive eating habits and a series of nutrition problems. Although she was unsuccessful at restricting her calorie intake, she limited her food choices, which resulted in an inadequate intake of key nutrients involved in healing: protein, fat, calcium, iron, and zinc. These eating patterns may have played a role in weakening her bones, making her more susceptible to the original stress fracture (8). Continuing with these poor eating habits, she did not have the building materials to repair the injury, so her bone became even weaker and prone to subsequent injuries. Helping her to understand the role of specific nutrients and healing is a core strategy in her care plan.

Her obsession with thinness caused other problems. By attempting to restrict her calorie intake by 40%, she was nagged with hunger and food cravings that led to binge eating on sugary and starchy foods like jelly beans and bagels. Since she felt like a failure every time she binged, this behavior pattern caused frustration, guilt, and lowered self-esteem. Sheree was taught that her sweet cravings were related to hunger, stemming from her inadequate calorie intake, as well as restriction of protein and fat.

With 16% body fat, Sheree had no real need to lose weight. Her postcollege weight gain was due to increased muscle resulting from her strength-training program. After gaining this insight she acknowledged that she could be at peace with her body, knowing that she "wasn't fat."

Her preference for vegetarianism narrowed her food choices and contributed to an inadequate intake of high-quality protein sources. Although appropriately planned vegetarian diets are healthful and nutritionally adequate (7), Sheree did not consume alternate sources of the nutrients found in meat protein, iron, and zinc. Since she is committed to a vegetarian style of eating, nonmeat sources of these nutrients need to be included in her regular eating patterns.

Her desire to eat a very low-fat diet presents a final problem. Sheree needs to understand that eating some fat can help to solve her nutritional problems (ie, satiety, essential fatty acids, and healing) and that performance improvements can occur when fat is included in the diet of endurance runners (8).

BOX 22.1   Recurrent Stress Fractures

Subjective

- "Three years ago, I got a stress fracture in my leg and I have had two more since then in the same spot. I'm probably not eating well enough for it to heal."
- "I want to lose weight. I'm eating a low-fat diet, but I'm not being successful. In fact, I've gained 12 lb since I graduated from college."
- Tries to restrict calories to less than 1,500 per day
- Currently leaner than other family members
- Vegetarian—no red meat or chicken for 8 years; eats one serving of dairy foods about four times per week; occasionally eats fish, eggs, tofu, or beans
- Calls herself as a "bagel-aholic," eating two to three large bagels a day
- Hopes to improve her first marathon time of 3 hours and 45 minutes
- Appears motivated to make dietary changes that would enhance healing

Objective

- 25-year-old physical therapist and recreational runner
- 5'5" (165 cm)
- 132 lb (60 kg)
- 16% body fat (skinfold calipers)
- Requires approximately 2,100 calories to maintain her weight without running and 2,500+ calories with running
- Nutrient analysis:

Total calories:	2,500
Carbohydrates:	540 g (86%)
Protein:	75 g (12%), <10 g of high-quality protein
Fat:	5 g (2%)
Calcium, iron, and zinc intake:	<50% RDA

- Training program:

Strength training:	Two times/week
Running:	4 to 10 miles a day when not injured

Assessment

- Obsession with body weight and fat
  — Narrow food choices
  — Avoids protein-rich foods and dairy products
- Low intakes of protein, iron, zinc, and calcium
- Unsuccessful attempts to severely restrict calories
  — Hunger cravings
  — Binge eating
- Unbalanced vegetarian pattern of eating
- Desire to eat a fat-free diet

Plan

1. Set aside thoughts about dieting and focus on the benefits of healthy eating:
   - Food is not "fattening."
   - Food provides an important source of nutrients that enhance health.
   - Food provides fuel for running.

2. To enhance healing of stress fractures:
   - Boost intake of calcium-rich foods (at least 3 to 4 servings per day of low-fat milk, yogurt, cheese, calcium-fortified orange juice).
   - Boost protein intake protein to 90 g of protein per day with at least 60 g of high-quality protein.*
   - Boost intake of iron- and zinc-rich foods.
   - Consider a multivitamin and mineral supplement.

3. To decrease sweet cravings and enhance satiety:
   - Eat enough calories—target 2,100 to 2,500 calories per day, depending on level of activity.
   - Gradually increase fat intake to 45 to 55 g per day, emphasizing polyunsaturated and monounsaturated fats.
   - Distribute the calories evenly, eating at least every 4 hours.

4. Incorporate nonmeat source of protein, iron, and zinc.

* Based on 1.0 to 1.5 g protein per kilogram of body weight

continued

BOX 22.1   Recurrent Stress Fractures (continued)

Self-reported Food Intake

Time	Food	Calories
7:30 AM	Large bagel with jam Coffee, black	450
9:30 AM	Fat-fee muffin	250
Noon	Salad with fat-free dressing Bagel	100 400
3:00 PM	Candy	200+
5:00 PM	Fat-free frozen yogurt	200+
6:00 PM	Salad with fat-free dressing Bagel	100 400
8:00 PM	Fat-free frozen yogurt	400+

2,500+ calories, 540 g CHO (86%), 75 g PRO (12%), 5 g FAT (2%)

Modified Food Plan

Time	Food	Calories
6:00 AM (before run)	Yogurt	200
7:30 AM	Cereal with milk Calcium-fortified orange juice	550
9:30 AM	Banana	100
Noon	Bagel with peanut butter Salad	700
3:00 PM	Yogurt Trail mix with nuts	300
6:00 PM	Salad Tuna Calcium-fortified orange juice Bagel	700

2,550 calories, 442 g CHO (70%), 97 g PRO (15%), 38 g FAT (15%)

Knee Surgery

Nora, a 39-year-old female avid exerciser, sought nutrition advice to quell her fears of weight gain during recovery from her upcoming knee surgery. The key findings from her consultation are presented in *Box 22.2.*

Coping with the loss of exercise during rehabilitation is hard for committed athletes; Nora's fears and frustrations are normal. Addressing these fears before they manifest in overly restrictive eating habits is ideal.

After discussing the calorie costs of surgery, trauma, and rehabilitative exercise, Nora recognized that the risk of excess weight gain is minimal. Teaching her how to calculate and adjust her calorie needs during rehabilitation empowered her to take a responsible approach to weight management.

Maximizing her intake of healing nutrients through consumption of nutrient-dense foods and possibly supplementation with vitamins C and E and zinc can boost her nutritional status before and after surgery. Since Nora is going into surgery in a well-nourished state, these strategies serve as a "health insurance policy" to enhance her potential for rapid recovery and return to exercise.

BOX 22.2   Nutrition Consultation

Subjective

- "I tore my ACL and am having surgery in 2 weeks. What should I eat to enhance healing?"
- "I'm so afraid I'm going to gain weight because I'm not able to exercise as much as I used to."
- "I feel so depressed now that I can't run an hour every day...."

Objective

- 39-year-old female avid exerciser
- 5'5" (165 cm)
- Preinjury weight: 120 lb
- Weight at time of initial consult: 121 lb
- 17% body fat (skinfold calipers)

Assessment

- Health-conscious, weight-conscious exerciser
- Well-balanced diet, including a variety of fruits, vegetables, grains, proteins, and dairy foods
- Increased need for healing nutrients
- Fear of weight gain could catalyze poor eating habits.
- Struggling with loss of exercise

Plan

1. To promote healing:
   - Be well-nourished going into surgery.
   - Focus on intake of the nutrient-dense, "powerhouse foods" (see below).
   - Consider a supplement of vitamin C plus zinc (250 mg C; 25 mg zinc) and a supplement of vitamin E (200 to 400 IUs) for "health insurance."
2. To manage weight and loss of exercise
   - Take into account the calorie needs of trauma and stress.
   - Adjust calorie intake for recovery and rehabilitation.
   - Stay in tune to body's cues of hunger and satiety.
   - Enjoy alternative forms of exercise (eg, swimming, stationery cycling, rehabilitation exercises).
   - Manage "stress-eating":
     — Keep a food journal to monitor eating habits; learn from each day to prevent the problem from happening again.
     — Focus on the real problem, not on food.

	Powerhouse Foods
Vitamin C	Fruits: oranges/orange juice, melon, strawberries, kiwi, grapefruit Vegetables: broccoli, spinach, tomatoes, peppers
Protein, iron, and zinc	Lean beef (2-4 times per week) Chicken thigh (without skin) Light-meat tuna, salmon
Protein and calcium	Low-fat dairy: low-fat milk and yogurt (3 to 4 servings per day)

CONCLUSION

Many promising athletic careers have been struck down by chronic and acute injuries. Athletes who push themselves to their physical limits in training and competition are likely to encounter injury and be forced to deal with rehabilitation. Fortunately, orthopedic surgery and physical therapy techniques have become very sophisticated, helping athletes quickly return to their sports. Despite these technical advances, some athletes encounter delays in wound healing and experience subsequent injuries that eventually cripple their athletic goals. Although wound healing is a complex process that is affected by a number of factors, nutritional status plays a key role.

Through nutrition screening and counseling, dietetics professionals can support the rehabilitation process. First, they can educate coaches and athletic trainers to detect nutrition risk factors and make appropriate referrals. Second, sports nutritionists can help athletes understand the role of nutrition in wound healing and manage their weight during rehabilitation. When athletes become obsessed with their body weight and pursue severely restrictive eating habits, they can jeopardize their nutritional status and impair healing. As the first case study illustrated, Sheree's eating problems and poor wound healing stemmed from her obsession with her body weight (*Figure 22.1*). Unfortunately, this situation is not uncommon; many athletes follow restrictive eating habits in pursuit of the "perfect physique." Sports nutritionists need to educate athletes, as well as trainers and coaches, about the potential dangers associated with weight restriction, especially during rehabilitation.

FIGURE 22.1   Nutrition-related Problems Stemming from Obsession with Body Weight

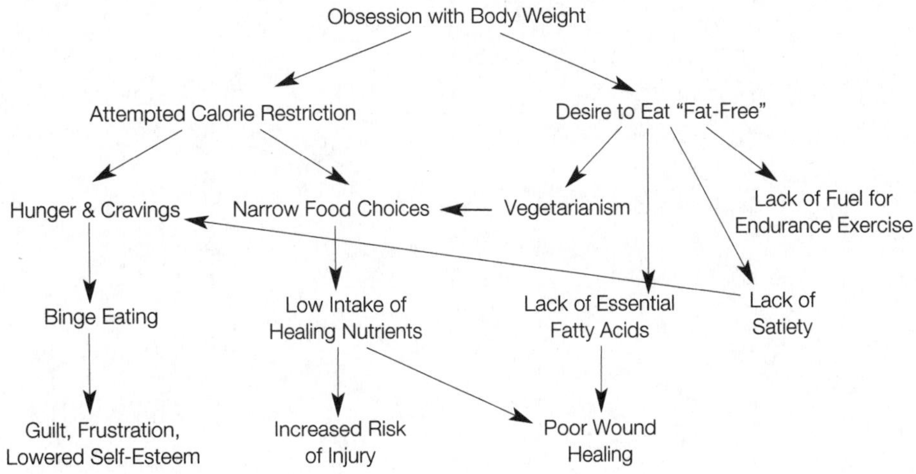

REFERENCES

1. Bistrian BR, Blackburn GL, Hallowell E, Heddle R. Protein status of general surgical patients. *JAMA*. 1974;230:858-860.

2. Bristrian BR, Blackburn GL, Vitale J, Cochran D, Naylor J. Prevalence of malnutrition in general medical patients. *JAMA*. 1976;235(15):1567-1570.

3. Blackburn GL, Bistrian BR, Maini BS, Schlamm HT, Smith MF. Nutritional and metabolic assessment of the hospitalized patient. *JPEN J Parenter Enteral Nutr*. 1977;1(1):11-22.

4. Trujillo EB. Effects of nutritional status on would healing. *J Vasc Nurs*. 1993;11:12-18.

5. Holman SR. *Essentials of Nutrition for the Health Professions*. Philadelphia, Penn: J B Lippincott Co; 1987:360-368.

6. Osak MP. Nutrition and wound healing. *Plast Surg Nurs*. 1993;13(1):29-36.

7. Updegrove NA. Highlights of the 9th Annual SCAN Symposium: winning strategies in sports nutrition. *Nutrition Today*. 1992;July/August:34-36.

8. Loosli AR. Reversing sports-related iron and zinc deficiencies. *Phys Sports Med*. 1993;21(4):70-78.

9. Storlie J. Eating with an injury. *Train Condition*. 1997;VII(5):19-31.

10. The American Dietetic Association. Position of The American Dietetic Association: vegetarian diets. *J Am Diet Assoc*. 1997;97(11):1317-1321.

11. Muoio D, Leddy J, Horvath P, Awad A, Pendergast D. Effect of dietary fat on metabolic adjustments to maximal VO_2 and endurance in runners. *Med Sci Sports Exerc*. 1994;26(1):81-99.

23

HYPERTENSION, DIET, AND EXERCISE

Satya S. Jonnalagadda, PhD

Approximately 50 million adult Americans have hypertension, one of the major risk factors associated with the development of cardiovascular disease (CVD) (1). The risk of disease is directly related to blood pressure level, sometimes even at relatively normal blood pressure (BP) levels (ie, 120 mm Hg of systolic BP (SBP) and 80 mm Hg of diastolic BP (DBP)) (2). Morbidity and mortality risk increases curvilinearly with rising levels of SBP and DBP. Risk increases progressively and incrementally when SBP and DBP are >120 mm Hg and >80 mm Hg, respectively. The most recent definition of high blood pressure is a SBP of ≥140 mm Hg and a DBP of ≥90 mm Hg (see *Table 23.1*) in individuals who are not taking antihypertensive medications and who have no acute illness (3). To lower the morbidity and disability associated with hypertension, it is necessary to shift the entire blood pressure distribution to lower levels. A change of even a few millimeters of Hg would lower both the extent and severity of disease in the population. It has been established that a 2 mm shift downward in the entire distribution of SBP may lower the annual mortality from stroke, coronary heart disease, and all-cause mortality by 6%, 4%, and 3% respectively (4). An intervention that would lower DBP by 1 to 3 mm Hg could lower the incidence of hypertension by as much as 20% to 50% (4).

TABLE 23.1 Classification of Blood Pressure for Adults Age 18 and Older*

Category	Systolic (mm Hg)		Diastolic (mm Hg)
Optimal**	<120	and	<80
Normal	<130	and	<85
High-normal	130-139	or	85-89
Hypertension†			
Stage 1	140-159	or	90-99
Stage 2	160-179	or	100-109
Stage 3	≥180	or	≥110

* Not taking antihypertensive drugs and not acutely ill.

** Unusually low readings should be evaluated for clinical significance.

† Based on the average of two or more readings taken at each of two or more visits after an initial screening

Adapted from: National High Blood Pressure Education Program, National Institutes of Health, National Heart, Lung and Blood Institute. *The Sixth Report of the Joint National Committee on Prevention, Detection, Evaluation and Treatment of High Blood Pressure*. Bethesda, Md: NIH Publication No. 98-4080; 1997.

FACTORS AFFECTING HYPERTENSION

Hypertension is an inherited, multifactorial trait (5). Blood pressure levels are influenced by genetics, age, obesity, and dietary factors. Blood pressure tends to increase with age and levels appear to be correlated among family members, probably due to common genetic, lifestyle, and environmental backgrounds (6).

The prevalence of hypertension increases with age. It is ≥50% prevalent in individuals over the age of 55, and ≥60% prevalent in individuals between the ages of 65 and 74. A decline in renal function commonly observed with increasing age has been suggested as a potential cause of this age-associated increase in BP (5). Lifestyle modification (see *Box 23.1*) has been shown to prevent or delay the expected rise in BP in susceptible individuals. Lifestyle modifications can not only lower BP, but can also prevent other CVD risk factors. These lifestyle modifications can also assist with a reduction in the number and dosage of antihypertensive medications (7).

BOX 23.1   Lifestyle Modifications for Hypertension Prevention and Management

- Lose weight if overweight.
- Limit alcohol intake to no more than 1 oz ethanol per day or 0.5 oz ethanol per day for women and lighter-weight people.
- Include aerobic physical activity (30 to 45 minutes most days of the week).
- Reduce sodium intake to ≤100 mmol per day (2.4 g sodium or 6 g sodium chloride).
- Maintain adequate intake of dietary potassium, calcium, and magnesium.
- Reduce intake of dietary saturated fat and cholesterol.
- Stop smoking.

Adapted from: National High Blood Pressure Education Program, National Institutes of Health, National Heart, Lung and Blood Institute. *The Sixth Report of the Joint National Committee on Prevention, Detection, Evaluation and Treatment of High Blood Pressure.* Bethesda, Md: NIH Publication No. 98-4080; 1997.

Weight Reduction

In the United States, obesity and weight gain are the most important determinants of the elevation in blood pressure. Weight loss is one of the most successful methods for lowering BP levels among both normotensive and hypertensive individuals. Additionally, the distribution of body fat also appears to affect BP. For example, visceral obesity is a strong risk factor for hypertension and consequently increased risk of CVD. A body mass index (BMI) of >27 is strongly correlated with elevated BP. Visceral or abdominal fat distribution (waist circumference of >34 in for females and >39 in for males) has been associated with risk of hypertension, dyslipidemia, diabetes, and coronary heart disease (CHD) mortality. Weight loss, as little as 10 lb, in overweight individuals can enhance the BP-lowering effect of antihypertensive agents and also lower other CVD risk factors (7,8).

Alcohol Consumption

Increased alcohol consumption is an important risk factor for high blood pressure, causing resistance to antihypertensive therapy (9,10). Epidemiological studies suggest that elevated BP in heavy drinkers can be normalized within a week upon abstinence from alcohol (11). Alcohol consumption should be limited to 1 oz of ethanol per day (12) which translates into:

- 24 oz of beer
- 10 oz of wine
- 2 oz of 100-proof whiskey

Females and lower-weight/lean individuals are more susceptible to the effects of alcohol because the absorption rate is increased; therefore, these individuals should limit their ethanol intake to 0.5 oz per day (13). Changes in intracellular sodium metabolism, effect on smooth muscle, insulin resistance, and an overactive sympathetic nervous system have all been suggested as potential mechanisms for the role of alcohol in hypertension (10).

Physical Activity

Moderate physical activity via aerobic exercise can increase weight loss, improve functional health status, and lower the risk of CVD and all-cause mortality. Risk of hypertension is increased 20% to 50% in sedentary individuals compared to their active counterparts (14). Moderate physical activity can be achieved with brisk walking for 30 to 45 minutes each day, which can also help lower elevated blood pressure (14). However, individuals with CVD and other related health problems require a thorough evaluation, such as a cardiac stress test, before embarking on an exercise program.

Exercise is an effective nonpharmacological way to lower BP. Walking, running, and exercising on a cycle ergometer have all been shown to be associated with lowering BP. The overall goal of exercise is to increase total energy expenditure. The benefits of exercise/physical activity in lowering BP disappear within 2 weeks after exercise cessation and, therefore, physical activity must be sustained over time (14). The mechanism of exercise-induced reduction in BP is unclear, but it may be associated with a reduction in peripheral vascular resistance and an increase in cardiac output. A recent meta-analysis on the effects of regular exercise on BP revealed that aerobic exercise training can lower resting SBP and DBP by approximately 4 to 5 mm Hg and 3 to 4 mm Hg, respectively (15). Long-term prospective studies on the impact of BP-lowering effects of exercise on CVD morbidity and mortality have not been conducted. However, pharmacological interventions have shown that a reduction in DBP of 5 to 6 mm Hg is associated with a 42% reduction in the incidence of stroke and a 14% reduction in CHD (16,17), thereby suggesting that exercise could also have a potentially similar impact on overall morbidity and mortality.

This relationship between exercise intensity and BP reduction needs to be further investigated. Exercise-induced reductions in BP have been observed to be more prominent in hypertensive individuals, as opposed to normotensive individuals (18). Additionally, lower intensity exercises have been found to be as effective or more effective than higher intensity exercises. Typically, lower intensity exercises, such as walking, cycling, and swimming, are associated with greater compliance, adherence, and lower risk of CVD and are easier to implement. In addition to lowering BP, regular exercise can also favorably influence dyslipidemia, insulin resistance, body weight, left ventricular hypertrophy, risk of stroke, and other CVD events.

Dietary Sodium

Epidemiological studies have demonstrated a positive association between sodium intake and blood pressure (19). Cutler et al (20) in a meta-analysis of clinical trials observed that reducing dietary sodium to 75 to 100 mmol (1 mmol sodium = 23 mg sodium; to convert sodium to sodium chloride multiply by 2.54) lowered BP over several weeks to several years. However, individual response to sodium restriction varies considerably, with certain groups of populations being more sensitive than other groups (21). Typically, a reduction in dietary sodium is also associated with reduction in antihypertensive medication, reduction in diuretic-induced potassium wasting, regression in left ventricular hypertrophy, protection from osteoporosis, and reduction in renal stones (7,22-25).

The average North American consumption of sodium is >150 mmol per day. Current recommendations are to lower sodium intake to <100 mmol per day (6 g sodium chloride or 2.4 g sodium per day). Approximately 75% of dietary sodium intake is derived from processed foods; therefore, individuals should be educated on reading food labels and selecting low-sodium foods.

The most recent estimates of sodium intake are provided by the Third National Health and Nutrition Examination Survey (NHANES III) which reported higher intakes by males than by females (26). Although in adults the mean sodium intake was similar among race and ethnic groups, African American children were observed to have higher intakes than Caucasian children (3.2 g versus 2.9 g in 6 to 11 years, 3.6 g versus 3.4 g in 12 to 15 years, respectively). In males sodium intake decreased with increasing age, which was 4.7 g in 20 to 29 years, 3.96 g in 40 to 49 years, and 3.1 g in 70 to 79 years. In females a similar trend was observed, with sodium intakes of 3.0 g in 20 to 29 years, 2.9 in 40 to 49 years, and 2.4 g in 70 to 79 years. Although these intakes parallel reductions in total energy intakes, the nutrient density of sodium in the diet increased with age. This may be due to the increased use of discretionary salt by the elderly to compensate for the alteration in taste.

See *Box 23.2* for additional discussion of low-salt diets.

BOX 23.2   Low-salt Diets

Salt-sensitivity

Individuals vary in their responses to change in salt intake, extracellular fluid balance, and blood pressure. The term "salt-sensitivity" identifies individuals who respond to high-salt intake with an increase in BP and others who do not (salt resistant). Salt-sensitivity has been observed more frequently in hypertensive individuals, African Americans, and older individuals. The definition of salt-sensitivity remains arbitrary; a clinically useful definition and a practical means to identify salt-sensitivity are yet to be established.

Morris CD. Effect of dietary sodium restriction on overall nutrient intake. *Am J Clin Nutr*. 1997; 65(suppl):687S-691S.

Adverse effects of very-low-salt diets

In hypertensive individuals, severe (1 g sodium chloride per day) and moderate (4 to 6 g sodium chloride per day) salt restriction can lower BP. However, modest salt restriction combined with antihypertensive therapy can raise BP in some individuals because of an active rennin-angiotensin system. Typically with salt restriction, intake of energy, fat, and sugar is lowered. Adherence with low-salt diets is variable. Salt restriction also reduces the intake of other micronutrients. Three food groups are the main sources of dietary sodium: meats, poultry, and fish; grain products; milk and dairy products. These food groups are also good sources of dietary calcium, iron, magnesium, and vitamin B-6. Therefore, a decrease in the intake of these foods will also influence the intake of these micronutrients. Sodium restriction can therefore have both a positive and a negative impact on intake of ceratin nutrients. Proper measures need to be taken to prevent any detrimental effects that can result due to alterations in other micronutrients.

Adapted from: Egan BM, Stepniakowski KT. Adverse effects of short-term, very-low-salt diets in subjects with risk-factor clustering. *Am J Clin Nutr*. 1997;65(suppl):671S-677S.

Maintaining compliance to a low-salt diet

- Hands-on educational programs
- Careful assessment of client and risk factors
- Specific implementation plan
- Repetitive educational efforts
- Built-in monitoring system

Adapted from: Luft FC, Morris CD, Weiberger MH. Compliance to a low-salt diet. *Am J Clin Nutr*. 1997;65(suppl):698S-703S.

Chloride Intake

An increase in dietary chloride alone, similar to an increase in dietary sodium alone, fails to produce hypertension, whereas high amounts of chloride in the form of sodium chloride can produce hypertension (27). Expansion of extracellular fluid volume may be responsible for the development of hypertension in this case.

Potassium Intake

The amount of potassium in the diet contributes to blood pressure levels (ie, high potassium intake can lower BP, as well as the risk of CVD). Inadequate dietary potassium intake can raise BP, and therefore adequate potassium intake of approximately 90 mmol per day (1 mmol potassium = 40 mg potassium) from fresh fruits and vegetables should be achieved. Meta-analysis of randomized controlled trials observed a significant reduction in SBP and DBP with potassium supplements (3.11 mm Hg and 1.97 mm Hg, respectively), and this effect was enhanced in individuals with high sodium intakes (25). However, potassium-containing salt substitutes, potassium supplements, and potassium-sparing diuretics should be used with caution especially in individuals susceptible to hyperkalemia and those with renal insufficiency.

Calcium Intake

Low calcium intake (<800 mg per day) has been associated with an increased prevalence of hypertension (28). However, only a minimal reduction in hypertension has been observed with an increased calcium intake. It has been postulated that the BP-lowering effects of both potassium and calcium may be related to their ability to increase the excretion of sodium salts, thereby lowering the negative impact of sodium on BP, especially in salt-sensitive individuals. Additionally, deficiencies of potassium and calcium have been observed to increase individuals' sensitivity to salt, which can adversely impact BP (27). Although currently no rationale exists for recommending calcium supplements to lower BP, it is the general recommendation that all individuals meet the daily recommended intakes for dietary calcium in order to reduce their risk of sodium chloride-induced hypertension.

Magnesium Intake

Although cohort studies suggest an association between low dietary magnesium intake and hypertension, the mechanism of action is unclear and therefore does not justify an increase in magnesium intake above the recommended intakes as a therapeutic intervention (9).

Dietary Fat

There is little substantive evidence that dietary fat plays a role in blood pressure regulation (9,29). Of the many ways that dietary fat and fatty acids can affect risk factors for CHD, it is clear from epidemiological and clinical studies that this is not due to any appreciable change in BP. There is little consistent evidence from experimental studies that the type and amount of fat significantly affect BP. High doses of omega-3 fatty acids (3 to 15 g per day) have been shown to have a modest lowering effect on SBP and DBP, especially in individuals with elevated BP, but the long-term treatment effect of omega-3 fatty acids remains to be elucidated. One of the key questions that is unanswered is whether total fat affects BP independent of body weight. In practice, this has been difficult to address because higher fat diets are associated with a higher body weight, which is clearly a major risk factor for hypertension.

Caffeine

Caffeine may raise blood pressure but tolerance to this effect develops rapidly (9). With chronic caffeine consumption a blunted response to individual challenge doses has been observed. A small but significant drop in BP (1.5 mm Hg SBP and 1.0 mm Hg DBP) was observed in normotensive individuals when caffeinated coffee was substituted with decaffeinated coffee (30). Additionally, a reduction in heart rate response to mental stress was observed with abstinence from caffeinated coffee (31). However, no direct relationship has been reported between caffeine consumption and BP and the mechanism of action is unclear at the present time.

Cigarette Smoking

Cigarette smoking is a major modifiable risk factor of CVD which is associated with a significant increase in blood pressure. Smoking cessation has been associated with reduction in BP and CVD risk. Additionally, appropriate counseling is required with smoking cessation to prevent or minimize weight gain (32).

THE DASH DIET PLAN

Dietary Approaches to Stop Hypertension (DASH) was a multicenter clinical trial funded by the National Institutes of Health (NIH) to examine the influence of dietary modification on hypertension. The results of this study demonstrated that a reduction in BP (5.5 mm Hg SBP and 3.0 mm Hg DBP) can be achieved with a combination diet similar in magnitude to that observed in monotherapy and antihypertensive drug trials, suggesting that this diet combination could be an effective alternate for individuals with Stage 1 hypertension (see *Table 23.1*) and could potentially prevent or delay the initiation of drug therapy (33). This combination diet is rich in fruits, vegetables, and low-fat dairy foods; low in total fat, saturated fat, and cholesterol; high in dietary fiber, potassium, calcium, and magnesium; and moderately high in protein (see *Table 23.2*).

TABLE 23.2   The DASH Diet Plan

Food Groups	Daily Servings	Serving Sizes	Examples	Nutritional Significance
Grains and grain products	7-8	1 slice bread 1/2 cup dry cereal	Whole-wheat bread, bagels	Major source of energy and fiber
Vegetables	4-5	1 cup raw leafy vegetables 6 oz vegetable juice	Tomatoes, spinach, beans	Rich sources of K, Mg, and fiber
Fruits	4-5	1 medium fruit 6 oz fruit juice	Bananas, melons, raisins	Important sources of K, Mg, and fiber
Low-fat or nonfat dairy foods	2-3	8 oz milk 1 cup yogurt	Skim or 1% milk, low-fat, nonfat yogurt	Major sources of Ca and protein
Meats, poultry, and fish	2 or less	3 oz cooked meats, poultry, or fish	Select only lean, trim visible fat; broil, roast, or boil; remove skin from poultry.	Rich sources of protein and Mg
Nuts, seeds, and legumes	4-5 per week	1/3 cup nuts 1/2 cup cooked legumes	Almonds, peanuts, kidney beans, lentils	Rich sources of energy, Mg, K, protein, and fiber

Key: K=potassium, Mg=magnesium, Ca=calcium

Adapted from: National High Blood Pressure Education Program, National Institutes of Health, National Heart, Lung and Blood Institute. *The Sixth Report of the Joint National Committee on Prevention, Detection, Evaluation and Treatment of High Blood Pressure.* Bethesda, Md: NIH Publication No. 98-4080; 1997.

EXERCISE PRESCRIPTION

In addition to the nonpharmacological treatments for hypertension, such as weight loss, alcohol restriction, and sodium restriction, aerobic activity is also commonly prescribed for individuals with hypertension. The recommended exercise program for individuals with moderate hypertension includes large muscle activities at moderate intensity (50% to 85% VO$_2$max), low-resistance and dynamic aerobic activities, such as cycling, walking on a treadmill, dancing, or gardening, three to five times per week for 20 to 60 minutes (37-39). Lower intensity exercise (40% to 70% VO$_2$max) may also be effective in lowering BP, especially in the elderly (39). The exercise program for hypertensive individuals should be initiated at a comfortable pace and increased gradually by 5 minutes every week until individuals can perform the activity comfortably for at least 45 minutes (38).

This endurance exercise training has been observed to lower SBP and DBP by 10 mm Hg in individuals with mild elevations in BP, but these benefits can be observed only as long as the endurance training is maintained (39). Hypertensive individuals who are active in athletics should include moderate, dynamic activities and should increase their level of activity gradually. Additionally, athletes and active individuals with Stage 3 hypertension (see *Table 23.1*) should add endurance exercise training only after the initiation of pharmacological therapy (37,39,40). All hypertensive individuals participating in some kind of a regular activity program should have their BP measured every 2 to 4 months to monitor the impact of exercise training. It should also be recognized that certain individuals with essential hypertension may not respond to endurance exercise training and may require pharmacological intervention. Unlike endurance exercise, resistive or strength training exercises have not been shown to lower BP and are not recommended for hypertensive individuals unless they are a component of a comprehensive fitness program (39). Overall, endurance exercise not only lowers BP, but can also favorably modify the risk factors of CVD.

REFERENCES

1. Burt VL, Whelton P, Roceklla EJ, et al. Prevalence of hypertension in the US adult population: results from the Third National Health and Nutrition Examination Survey, 1988-1991. *Hypertension*. 1995;25:305-313.
2. Kannel WB. Blood pressure as a cardiovascular risk factor: prevention and treatment. *JAMA*. 1996;275:1571-1576.
3. National High Blood Pressure Education Program, National Institutes of Health, National Heart, Lung and Blood Institute. *The Sixth Report of the Joint National Committee on Prevention, Detection, Evaluation and Treatment of High Blood Pressure.* Bethesda, Md; 1997. NIH Publication No. 98-4080.
4. Stamler J, Neaton JD, Wentworth DN. Blood pressure (systolic and diastolic) and risk of fatal coronary heart disease. *Hypertension*. 1989;13:I2-I12.
5. Preuss HG. Diet, genetics and hypertension. *J Am Coll Nutr*. 1997;16:296-305.
6. Ward R. Familial aggregation and genetic epidemiology of blood pressure. In: Laragh JH, Brenner BM, eds. *Hypertension: Pathophysiology, Diagnosis, and Management*. New York, NY: Raven Press; 1990:81-100.
7. Neaton JD, Grimm RH, Prineas RJ, et al. Treatment of Mild Hypertension Study: final results. *JAMA*. 1993;270:713-724.
8. Trials for Hypertension Prevention Collaborative Research Group. Effects of weight loss and sodium reduction intervention on blood pressure and hypertension incidence in overweight people with high-normal blood pressure: the Trials of Hypertension Prevention, Phase II. *Arch Intern Med*. 1997;157:657-667.
9. Stamler J, Caggiula AW, Grandits GA. Relation of body mass and alcohol, nutrient, fiber, and caffeine intakes to blood pressure in the special intervention and usual care groups in the Multiple Risk Factor Intervention Trial. *Am J Clin Nutr*. 1997;65(suppl):338S-365S.
10. Puddey IB, Parker M, Berlen LJ, Vandongen R, Masarei JRL. Effects of alcohol and caloric restrictions on blood pressure and serum lipids in overweight men. *Hypertension*. 1992;20:533-541.
11. Klatsky AL. Alcohol, coronary heart disease and hypertension. *Ann Rev Med*. 1996;47:149-160.
12. US Dept of Agriculture and US Dept of Health and Human Services. *Nutrition and Your Health: Dietary Guidelines for Americans*. 4th ed. Washington, DC: US Dept of Agriculture; 1995. Home and Garden Bulletin No. 232.
13. Frezza M, di Padova C, Pozzato G, Terpin M, Baraona E, Lieber CS. High blood alcohol levels in women: the role of decreased gastric alcohol dehydrogenase activity and first-pass metabolism. *N Engl J Med*. 1990;322:95-99.
14. US Department of Health and Human Services. *Physical Activity and Health: A Report of the Surgeon General*. Atlanta, Ga: Centers for Disease Control and Prevention, National Center for Chronic Disease Prevention and Health Promotion; 1996.

15. Halbert JA, Silagy CA, Finucane P, Withers RT, Hamdorf PA, Andrews GR. The effectiveness of exercise training in lowering blood pressure: a meta-analysis of randomized trials of four weeks or longer. *J Human Hypertension*. 1997;11:641-649.

16. Psaty BM, Smith NL, Siscovick DS, et al. Health outcomes associated with antihypertensive therapies used as first-line agents: a systemic review and meta-analysis. *JAMA*. 1997;277:739-745.

17. Collins R, Peto R, MacMahon S, et al. Blood pressure, stroke and coronary heart disease. Part 2: Short-term reductions in blood pressure: overview of randomized drug trials in their epidemiological context. *Lancet*. 1990;335:827-838.

18. van Baak MA. Exercise and hypertension: facts and uncertainties. *Br J Sports Med*. 1998;32:6-10.

19. Elliott P, Stamler J, Nichols R, et al. Intersalt revisited: further analyses of 24 hour sodium restriction and blood pressure within and across populations. *BMJ*. 1996;312:1249-1253.

20. Cutler JA, Follmann D, Allender PS. Randomized trials of sodium restriction: an overview. *Am J Clin Nutr*. 1997;65(suppl):643S-651S.

21. Luft FC, Weinberger MH. Heterogeneous responses to changes in dietary salt intake: the salt-sensitivity paradigm. *Am J Clin Nutr*. 1997;65(suppl):612S-617S

22. Singer DRJ, Markander ND, Cappuccio FP, Miller MA, Sagnella GA, MacGregor GA. Reduction of salt intake during converting enzyme inhibitor treatment compared with addition of a thiazide. *Hypertension*. 1995;25:1042-1044.

23. Devine A, Criddle RA, Dick IM, Kerr DA, Prince RL. A longitudinal study of the effect of sodium and calcium intakes on regional bone density in post-menopausal women. *Am J Clin Nutr*. 1995;62:740-745.

24. Antonios TF, MacGregor GA. Salt—more adverse effects. *Lancet*. 1996;348:250-251.

25. Whelton PK, He J, Cutler JA, et al. Effects of oral potassium on blood pressure: meta-analysis of randomized controlled clinical trials. *JAMA*. 1997;277:1624-1632.

26. McDowell MA, Briefel RR, Alaimo K, et al. Energy and macronutrient intake of persons ages 2 months and over in the United States: Third National Health and Nutrition Examination Survey, Phase I, 1988-1991. *Advance Data from Vital and Health Statistic No. 255*. Hyattsville, Md: National Center for Health Statistics; 1994.

27. Kotchen TA, Kotchen JM. Dietary sodium and blood pressure: interactions with other nutrients. *Am J Clin Nutr*. 1997;65(suppl):708S-711S.

28. McCarron DA. Role of adequate dietary calcium intake in the prevention and management of salt-sensitive hypertension. *Am J Clin Nutr*. 1997;65(suppl):712S-716S.

29. Sacks FM. Dietary fats and blood pressure: a critical review of evidence. *Nutr Rev*. 1989;47:291-300.

30. van Dusseldorp M, Smits P, Thien T, Katan MB. Effect of decaffeinated versus regular coffee on blood pressure. A 12-week, double-blind trial. *Hypertension*. 1989;14:563-569.

31. van Dusseldorp M, Smits P, Lenders JW, Temme L, Thien T, Katan MB. Effects of coffee on cardiovascular responses to stress: a 14-week controlled trial. *Psychosom Med*. 1992;54:344-353.

32. US Dept of Health and Human Services. *The Health Benefits of Smoking Cessation: A Report of the Surgeon General*. Rockville, Md: Centers for Disease Control, Center for Chronic Disease Prevention and Health Promotion, Office of Smoking and Health; 1990. DHHS Publication (CDC):90-8416.

33. Appel LJ, Moore TJ, Obarzanek E, et al. A clinical trial of the effects of dietary patterns on blood pressure. DASH Collaborative Research Group. *N Engl J Med*. 1997;336:1117-1124.

34. Egan BM, Stepniakowski KT. Adverse effects of short-term, very-low-salt diets in subjects with risk-factor clustering. *Am J Clin Nutr*. 1997;65(suppl):671S-677S.

35. Morris CD. Effect of dietary sodium restriction on overall nutrient intake. *Am J Clin Nutr*. 1997;65(suppl):687S-691S.

36. Luft FC, Morris CD, Weiberger MH. Compliance to a low-salt diet. *Am J Clin Nutr*. 1997;65(suppl):698S-703S.

37. National High Blood Pressure Education Program. *Working Group Report on Primary Prevention of Hypertension*. Washington, DC: National Heart, Lung, and Blood Institute, National Institutes of Health, Public Health Service, US Dept of Health and Human Services; 1993. NIH Publication No. 93-2669. http://www.nhlbi.nih.gov/nhlbi/cardio/hbp/prof/pphbp.htm. Accessed February 17, 1999.

38. Yeater RA, Ullrich IH. Hypertension and exercise. Where do we stand? *Postgrad Med*. 1992;91:429-434.

39. American College of Sports Medicine Position Stand. Physical activity, physical fitness, and hypertension. *Med Sci Sports Exerc*. 1993;25:i-x.

40. Kaplan NM, Deveraux RB, Miller HS. Systemic hypertension. *Med Sci Sports Exerc*. 1994;26(10 suppl):S268-S270.

24

CARDIOVASCULAR DISEASE AND EXERCISE

Satya S. Jonnalagadda, PhD

Cardiovascular disease (CVD) is a general term that encompasses many different diseases of the heart and circulatory system. In the United States coronary heart disease (CHD), or ischemic heart disease (IHD), is the most prevalent form of CVD and accounts for over 50% of all CVD deaths (1). Other major CVDs include hypertensive heart disease and cerebrovascular disease.

ATHEROSCLEROSIS AND CHD RISK

CHD occurs as a result of atherosclerosis of the coronary arteries. Atherosclerosis is the result of a complex biological process initiated by chronic endothelial injury or damage. The earliest lesion is referred to as a fatty streak. By puberty, flat or slightly raised fatty streaks are present in most children, although in some the lesion is more advanced (atheroma). Some fatty streaks appear to regress while others progress and evolve into a fibrous plaque (2). Fibrous plaques are formed particularly in coronary arteries and abdominal aorta as a result of continuous lipid deposition, chronic inflammation, and repair (Figure 24.1).

FIGURE 24.1   Development of Atherosclerosis

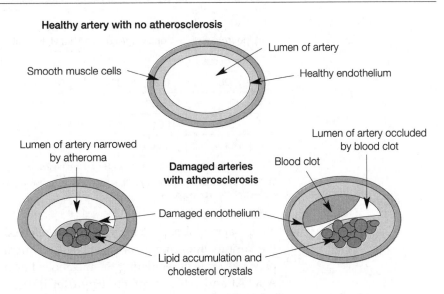

Typically, this fibrous plaque first appears during early adulthood and progresses with age (2). During middle age, fibrous plaques undergo changes that reflect an alteration in their content of lipids, smooth muscle cells, connective tissue, calcium, and vessel involvement. The progression of lesions to enlarged atherosclerosis plaques is especially rapid in persons with coronary risk factors (3).

As atherosclerosis progresses, fibrous plaques increase in size, protrude into the arterial lumen, and thereby impede blood flow (2). Usually by this time the plaques are covered with a dense cap of connective tissue that contains embedded smooth muscle cells, which typically overlay a core of lipid and necrotic debris. This sequence of events can result in the ulceration of connective tissue and smooth muscle cap, thereby exposing blood to the lipid layer and necrotic debris and precipitating thrombosis. Hemorrhage into the plaque and subsequent swelling are another serious complication which may also induce ulceration and thrombosis. If atherosclerosis affects the cerebral arteries, the clinical outcome is a stroke that results from a cerebral infarct or a cerebral hemorrhage. CHD occurs as a result of atherosclerosis of the coronary arteries and affects the cardiac muscle. Blood flow to the heart is interrupted, which can eventually result in death.

LIPOPROTEIN AND CHD RISK

Lipoproteins are macromolecular complexes composed of different lipids and proteins. The major lipids are triacylglycerol (TAG), sometimes still referred to as triglycerides, cholesterol, and phospholipids; the proteins in these lipids are referred to as apolipoproteins. The lipoprotein classes are chylomicrons, very-low density lipoprotein (VLDL), intermediate-density lipoprotein (IDL), low-density-lipoprotein (LDL), and high-density lipoprotein (HDL). Chylomicrons and VLDL are TAG-rich particles, IDL and LDL are rich in cholesterol, and HDL is a smaller, dense particle containing proportionally more protein than lipid. The physical and chemical characteristics of major lipoprotein classes are shown in *Table 24.1A*.

TABLE 24.1A   Characteristics of Major Lipoproteins

Lipoprotein	Density (g/dL)	Percent Lipid*		
		Triacylglycerol	Cholesterol	Phospholipids
Chylomicron	0.95	80 – 95	2 – 7	3 – 9
VLDL	0.95 – 1.006	55 – 80	5 – 15	10 – 20
IDL	1.006 – 1.019	20 – 50	20 – 40	15 – 25
LDL	1.019 – 1.063	5 – 15	40 – 50	20 – 25
HDL	1.063 – 1.21	5 – 10	15 – 25	20 – 30

* Percent composition of lipids; apolipoproteins make up the rest.

VLDL = very-low density lipoprotein; IDL = intermediate-density lipoprotein; LDL = low-density lipoprotein; HDL = high-density lipoprotein

Nine major apolipoproteins, commonly referred to as "apo" and associated with the various lipoprotein classes, provide structural stability to the particles and play a key role in regulating the metabolic fate of these lipoproteins (*Table 24.1B*). Apo AI and AII are affected by diet-induced changes in HDL cholesterol (HDL-C), whereas apo B usually changes in parallel with LDL cholesterol (LDL-C). In addition to the major lipoprotein classes, a genetic variant of LDL,

TABLE 24.1B   Characteristics of Major Apolipoproteins

Apolipoprotein	Lipoprotein	Metabolic Functions
Apo AI	HDL	Component of HDL
	Chylomicrons	LCAT activator
Apo AII	HDL	Unknown
	Chylomicrons	
Apo AIV	HDL	Unknown
	Chylomicrons	
Apo B48	Chylomicrons	Needed for assembly and secretion of chylomicrons from small intestine
Apo B100	VLDL	Needed for assembly and secretion of VLDL from liver
	IDL	Structural protein of VLDL, IDL, and LDL
	LDL	Ligand for LDL receptor
Apo CI	All major lipoproteins	Unknown
Apo CII	All major lipoproteins	Activator of lipoprotein lipase
Apo CIII	All major lipoprotiens	Inhibitor of lipoprotein lipase
		May inhibit hepatic uptake of chylomicrons and VLDL remnants
Apo E	All major lipoproteins	Ligand for binding of several lipoproteins to the LDL receptor and possibly to separate hepatic apo E receptor

LCAT = lecithin cholesterol acyl transferase; VLDL = very-low density lipoprotein; IDL = intermediate-density lipoprotein; LDL = low-density lipoprotein; HDL = high-density lipoprotein

namely Lipoprotein (a) [Lp(a)], is produced from LDL and apoprotein (a). This apoprotein (a) portion of the Lp(a) molecule has a structural resemblance to plasminogen and can prevent the plasminogen from dissolving blood clots. Although the physiological functions of Lp(a) are not clearly understood, current evidence suggests that it may

- Bind to the fibrin clots thereby delivering cholesterol to the site of injury
- Result in the blockage of blood vessels
- Lead to a myocardial infarction (MI)

Plasma total cholesterol (TC) which correlates with LDL-C levels, the major atherogenic lipoprotein, is measured to assess CHD risk status. The National Cholesterol Education Program (NCEP) Adult Treatment Panel II (ATP II) guidelines (4) recommend that plasma TC and HDL-C be measured initially, and a lipoprotein analysis be conducted subsequently if individuals have desirable or borderline high blood cholesterol and low HDL-C (<35 mg/dL) or a high blood cholesterol level. *Table 24.2* presents the risk assessment based on blood lipid levels (5). Currently, plasma TAG is also measured to clarify CHD risk assessment in individuals with a desirable blood cholesterol level but the presence of two or more CHD risk factors or in patients with disorders associated with elevated TAG levels, such as diabetes, which are also related to an increase in CHD risk.

TABLE 24.2 Risk Assessment Based on Blood Lipid Levels and Comparable Levels for Serum Total Cholesterol and LDL Cholesterol

Total Cholesterol		LDL Cholesterol	
Level	Category	Level	Category
<200 mg/dL	Desirable	<130 mg/dL	Desirable
200 – 239 mg/dL	Borderline	130 – 159 mg/dL	Borderline high
≥240 mg/dL	High	≥160 mg/dL	High

RISK FACTORS OF CVD

Cardiovasular disease is progressive, and develops silently over decades, and is the result of chronic exposure to both modifiable and nonmodifiable risk factors (*Box 24.1*). The major modifiable risk factors for CVD are an elevated blood cholesterol, specifically LDL cholesterol, hypertension, cigarette smoking, and obesity. Other risk factors include low HDL cholesterol (<35 mg/dL) and diabetes mellitus. Important nonmodifiable CVD risk factors are family history of premature CHD, age, and gender.

BOX 24.1 Risk Factors of Cardiovasular Disease

Major Risk Factors

- **Modifiable Risk Factors**
  — High blood cholesterol levels
  — High blood pressure (Hypertension)
  — Obesity
  — Cigarette and tobacco use
  — Low HDL-cholesterol levels
  — Physical inactivity
  — Diabetes mellitus

- **Nonmodifiable Risk Factors**
  — Heredity
  — Increasing age
  — Male gender
- **Other Risk Factors**
  — Small LDL particles
  — Elevated Lp(a) levels
  — Elevated blood total homocysteine levels
  — Abnormalities in coagulation factors
  — Stress

Diet is important because it can favorably affect CHD risk factors such as blood cholesterol, blood pressure level, and obesity. It is considered the cornerstone for both the prevention and treatment of CVD.

The major risk factors also play a role in the development of fibrous plaques. For example, cigarette smoking and elevated TC may play a role in unstable plaque formation, whereas hypertension may play a role in plaque enlargement. Determining the relative risk (ie, the likelihood of developing CHD in individuals with and without a given risk factor or a given intensity of a risk factor) plays an important role in both primary and secondary prevention of CHD. Additionally, the absolute risk (ie, the probability of developing CHD in a given time period) can also be lowered by identifying these risk factors. Therefore, primary prevention is characterized by an effort to modify risk factors or prevent their development with the aim of delaying or preventing new onset CHD. Secondary prevention involves intervention to reduce recurrent CHD events and lower coronary mortality in patients with established CHD. Secondary prevention is aimed at both control of risk factors and direct therapeutic protection of coronary arteries from plaque eruption.

Results of the National Cholesterol Education Program (NCEP) and the Framingham Heart Study have established strategies to prevent CHD. *Table 24.3* presents comprehensive risk assessment guidelines recommended by the American Heart Association (6). In addition, the Framingham Heart Study (7) has helped develop a simple coronary disease prediction algorithm based on current guidelines for blood pressure, total cholesterol, and LDL-C. This algorithm allows physicians to predict multivariate CHD risk in clients without overt CHD and can be found in Wilson et al (7). The individual risk factors are discussed briefly below.

TABLE 24.3   Guide to Primary Prevention of Cardiovascular Diseases

Risk Intervention	Recommendations	
Smoking *Goal:* Complete cessation	Ask about smoking status as part of a routine evaluation. Reinforce nonsmoking status. Strongly encourage client and family to stop smoking. Provide counseling, nicotine replacement, and formal cessation programs as appropriate.	
Blood Pressure Control *Goal:* ≤140/90 mm Hg	Measure blood pressure in all adults at least every 2¹/2 years. Promote lifestyle modification: weight control, physical activity, moderation in alcohol intake, moderate sodium restriction. If blood pressure ≥140/90 mm Hg after 3 months of life-habit modification or if initial blood pressure is >160/100 mm Hg, add blood pressure medication; individualize therapy to client's other requirements and characteristics.	
Cholesterol Management *Primary goal:* LDL <160 mg/dL if 0-1 risk factors *or* LDL <130 mg/dL if 2 or more risk factors *Secondary goals:* HDL >35 mg/dL TG <200 mg/dL	Ask about dietary habits as part of routine evaluation. Measure total and HDL cholesterol in all adults ≥20 years of age and assess positive and negative risk factors at least every 5 years. For all persons: Promote AHA Step I diet (≤30% fat, <10% saturated fat, <300 mg/day cholesterol), weight control, and physical activity. Measure LDL if total cholesterol ≥240 mg/dL or ≥200 mg/dL with 2 or more risk factors or if HDL is <35 mg/dL.	

If LDL is:
≥160 mg/dL with 0-1 risk factors or ≥130 mg/dL on two occasions with 2 or more risk factors, then:
 	
• Start Step II diet (≤30% fat, <7% saturated fat, <200 mg/day cholesterol) and weight control.
• Rule out secondary causes of high LDL (LFTs, TFTs, UA).
 	
If LDL is:
  ≥160 mg/dL plus 2 risk factors; *or*
  ≥190 mg/dL; *or*
  ≥220 mg/dL in men <35 years or in premenopausal women, then:
 	
• Consider adding drug therapy to diet therapy for LDL levels greater than those listed above that persist despite Step II diet.
 	
Suggested drug therapy for high LDL levels (≥160 mg/dL) (drug selection priority modified according to TG level):
	Risk factors: age (men ≥45 years, women ≥55 years or postmenopausal), hypertension, diabetes, smoking, HDL <35 mg/dL, family history of CHD in first-degree relatives (in male relatives <55 years, female relatives <65 years).
	If HDL ≥60 mg/dL, subtract 1 risk factor from the number of positive risk factors.

TG <200 mg/dL	TG 200 – 400 mg/dL	TG >400 mg/dL	
Statin Resin Niacin	Statin Niacin	Consider combined drug therapy (niacin, fibrates, statin).	HDL <35 mg/dL: Emphasize weight management and physical activity, avoidance of cigarette smoking. Niacin raises HDL. Consider niacin if client has 2 or more risk factors and high LDL (except clients with diabetes).

If LDL goal not achieved, consider combination drug therapy.

continued

TABLE 24.3   Guide to Primary Prevention of Cardiovascular Diseases (continued)

Risk Intervention	Recommendations
Physical Activity *Goal:* Increase amount Exercise regularly three to four times per week for 30 minutes.	Ask about physical activity status and exercise habits as part of routine evaluation.
	Encourage 30 minutes of moderate-intensity dynamic exercise three to four times per week as well as increased physical activity in daily life habits for persons who are inactive.
	Encourage regular exercise to improve conditioning and optimize fitness level.
	Advise medically supervised programs for those with low functional capacity and/or comorbidities.
	Promote environmental factors conducive to health (ie, golf courses that permit walking).
Weight Management *Goal:* Achieve and maintain desirable weight (BMI 21-25 kg/m²)	Measure client's weight and height, BMI, and waist-to-hip ratio at each visit as part of routine evaluation.
	Start weight management and physical activity as appropriate. Desirable BMI range: 21-25 kg/m².
	BMI of 25 kg/m² corresponds to percentage desirable body weight of 110%; desirable waist-to-hip ratio for men, <0.9; for middle-aged and elderly women, <0.8.
Estrogen	Consider estrogen replacement therapy in postmenopausal women, especially those with multiple CHD risk factors.
	Individualize recommendations consistent with other health risks.

TG = triglycerides; LFTs = liver function tests; TFTs = thyroid function tests; UA = uric acid; CHD = coronary heart disease; BMI = body mass index

Reproduced with permission. Guide to primary prevention of cardiovascular disease. *Circulation.* 1997;95:2329-2331. © American Heart Association.

Age

Because of the progressive nature of coronary atherosclerosis, the risk of CHD increases with age in both males and females (more so in females); therefore, primary prevention should start early in life. Although primary prevention is justifiable in those aged 65 to 75 years, the initiation of cholesterol-lowering therapy in individuals older than 75 years for primary prevention is under debate. The general recommendation is that preventive therapy should be started early and continued throughout life.

Cigarette and Tobacco Use

Smoking accelerates plaque development and is a risk factor for angina pectoris and MI. Individuals who smoke a pack of cigarettes a day are four times more likely to have CHD than those who do not smoke (8). Smoking cessation can lower risk of MI, with a major reduction in risk occurring within the first year of smoking cessation. Additionally, smoking is a major risk factor for peripheral arterial disease and stroke; however, with smoking cessation the risk reduces dramatically (8).

Hypertension

Elevated blood pressure (BP) is a strong risk factor for CVD in both men and women. Proper BP control can help prevent strokes, a major outcome of elevated BP.

Serum Cholesterol

NCEP (4) defines a total cholesterol of <200 mg/dL as desirable. However, based on the results of the Framingham Heart Study, CHD risk has been observed to be lower at levels <160 mg/dL. NCEP also suggests that lowering LDL-C should be the primary target of cholesterol-lowering therapy. *Table 24.2* shows an approximate relationship between TC and LDL-C levels as developed by NCEP. TC levels can be used in the initial detection of elevated blood cholesterol; however, serum LDL-C should be used for risk assessment and evaluation of responses to therapy. According to NCEP, individuals with LDL >190 mg/dL or >160 mg/dL and two other major CHD risk factors should be immediately started on cholesterol-lowering medications.

Low HDL-C

A strong inverse association between HDL-C level and CHD risk has been established. HDL-C may potentially lower the atherogenecity of LDL-C. Additionally, low HDL-C may also be associated with elevated levels of VLDL remnants, small LDL particles, and insulin resistance, thereby increasing risk of disease. NCEP has identified three levels of HDL-C:

1. Low HDL-C   <35 mg/dL   Major risk factor
2. Normal HDL-C   35 to 60 mg/dL   Goal
3. High HDL-C   >60 mg/dL   Protective factor

Smoking cessation, weight control, and regular exercise have been shown to raise HDL-C levels. Hormone replacement therapy in postmenopausal women tends to raise plasma HDL-C levels and therefore may be beneficial in women with low HDL-C levels.

Diabetes Mellitus

Individuals with diabetes are at increased risk for CHD. Hyperglycemia is an independent risk factor for CHD. Improved glycemic control can reduce microvascular complications commonly observed in these individuals. Typically, these individuals have other CHD risk factors such as hypertension, low HDL-C, and elevated TAG levels.

Obesity

It is estimated that approximately 97 million adults (55% of the population) in the United States are overweight or obese, which can increase risk of chronic disease including CVD. The American Heart Association has reclassified obesity as a major, modifiable risk factor for CHD (9). A modest weight reduction of 5% to 10% has been show to lower BP and TC, and improve glucose tolerance in individuals with diabetes. Recently released clinical guidelines (10) consider everyone with a BMI >25 kg/m² at risk of disease (*Table 24.4*). A BMI 25 to 29.9 kg/m² is considered overweight and a BMI of >30 kg/m² is considered obese. Although treatment of overweight individuals is recommended only when two or more risk factors are present, it is generally recommended that treatment of obese individuals focuses on weight loss over a prolonged period. Weight loss can result in improvement of CVD risk factors (ie, lowers BP, TAG, TC, and LDL-C, and raises HDL-C). In addition to body weight, waist circumference, which is strongly associated with abdominal fat, is considered an independent predictor of disease risk.

TABLE 24.4 Classification of Overweight and Obesity by BMI, Waist Circumference, and Associated Disease Risks

	BMI (kg/m²)	Obesity Class	Disease Risk* Relative to Normal Weight and Waist Circumference	
			Men ≤102 cm (≤40 in) Women ≤88 cm (≤35 in)	>102 cm (>40 in) >88 cm (>35 in)
Underweight	<18.5		—	—
Normal⁺	18.5 – 24.9		—	—
Overweight	25.0 – 29.9		Increased	High
Obesity	30.0 – 34.9	I	High	Very high
	35.0 – 39.9	II	Very high	Very high
Extreme obesity	≥40	III	Extremely high	Extremely high

* Disease risk for type 2 diabetes, hypertension, and CVD

⁺ Increased waist circumference can also be a marker for increased risk even in persons of normal weight.

Clinical guidelines suggest that waist circumference is a better predictor of disease risk than the waist-to-hip ratio. A waist circumference of >40 inches in males and >35 inches in females signifies increased risk in those who have a BMI of 25 to 34 kg/m². *Figure 24.2* represents the treatment algorithm proposed by the NIH Expert Panel for the treatment of overweight individuals (10).

FIGURE 24.2   Treatment Algorithm for the Assessment of Overweight and Obesity

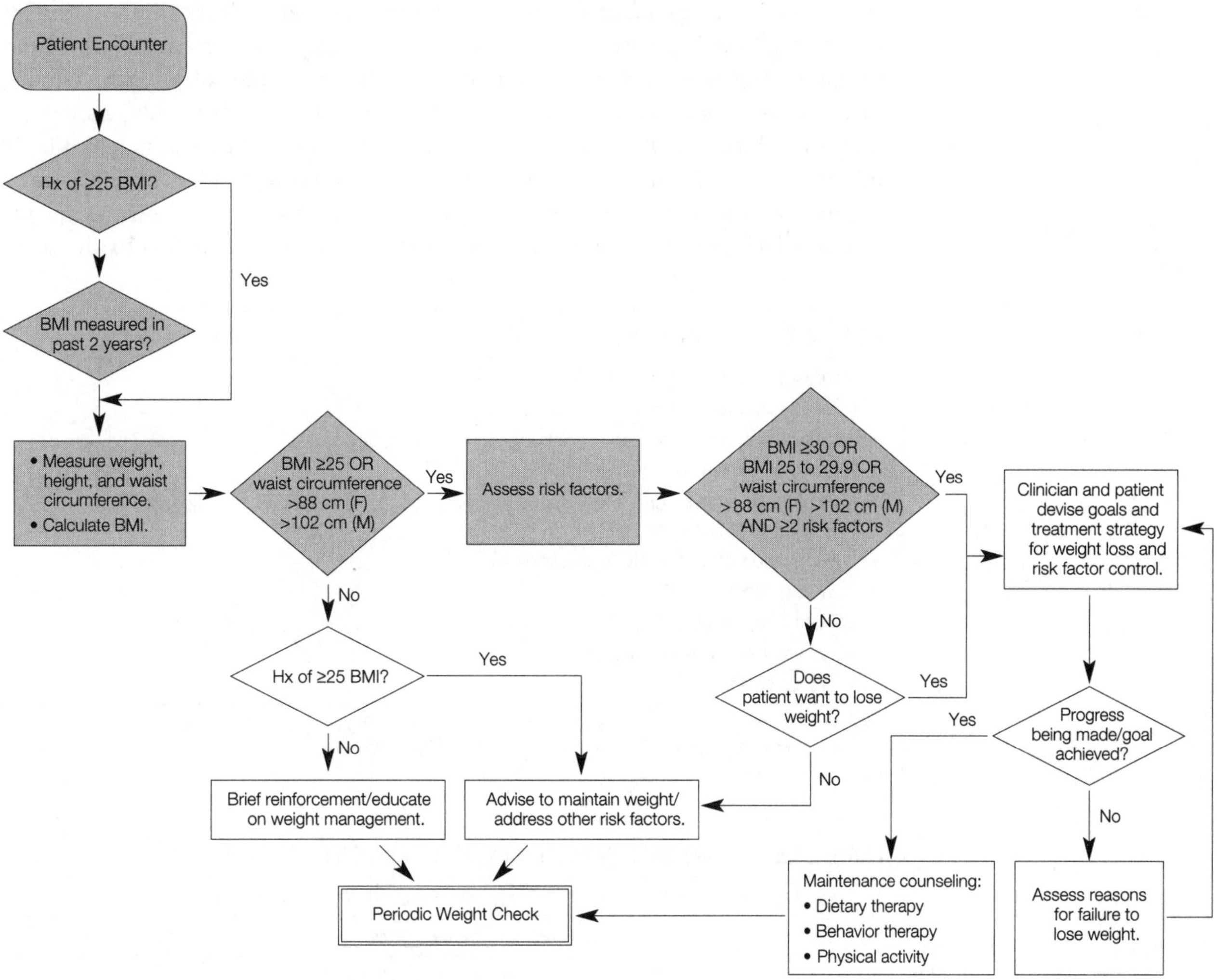

Exercise

Physical inactivity is an independent risk factor for CVD (11). Regular aerobic physical activity plays a role in primary and secondary prevention of CVD by increasing cardiovascular functional capacity and decreasing myocardial O_2 demand. Exercise helps control elevated blood lipids, glucose, blood pressure, and obesity (*Box 24.2*). Exercise capacity is defined as the point of maximum ventilatory O_2 uptake or the highest work intensity that can be achieved. Low-intensity activities at a range of 40% to 60% of maximum capacity include walking for pleasure, gardening, yard work, house work, dancing, and prescribed home exercises (*Table 24.5*). To promote good health, 30 to 60 minutes of physical activity, three to six times weekly is recommended (*Box 24.3*). Additionally, moderate-intensity exercise (60% to 75% of maximal capacity) for approximately 5 to 20 minutes (for a total of 30 minutes on most days) is recommended. Strength-training exercise alone has been shown to have only a modest effect on risk factors compared to aerobic exercise; however, resistance training using 8 to 10 different

---

BOX 24.2   Benefits of Physical Activity

- Increases maximum ventilatory O_2
- Increases cardiac output
- Increases ability of muscle to extract and use O_2 from blood
- Reduces myocardial O_2 demand
- Encourages beneficial changes in hemodynamic, hormonal, metabolic, neurological, and respiratory functions
- Lowers blood lipids and blood glucose
- Increases blood HDL-C
- Lowers body weight
- Alters adipose tissue distribution
- Improves flexibility and quality of life

Adapted from: Fletcher GF, Balady G, Blair SN, et al. Statement on exercise: benefits and recommendations for physical activity programs for all Americans. *Circulation*. 1996;94:857-862.

TABLE 24.5   Examples of Activities at Various Intensities

Less vigorous, More time	Washing and waxing car for 45 to 60 minutes
	Washing windows or floors for 45 to 60 minutes
	Gardening for 30 to 45 minutes
	Wheeling self in wheelchair for 30 to 40 minutes
	Walking 1 3/4 mile in 30 minutes (20 minutes/mile)
	Bicycling 5 miles in 30 minutes
	Raking leaves for 30 minutes
	Walking 2 miles in 30 minutes (15 minutes/mile)
	Water aerobics for 30 minutes
	Swimming laps for 20 minutes
	Bicycling 4 miles in 15 minutes
	Running 1 1/2 miles in 15 minutes (10 minutes/mile)
	Shoveling snow for 15 minutes
More vigorous, Less time	Stair walking for 15 minutes

Note: With the increasing intensity of the activities, from top to bottom, the time spent is decreased.

Adapted from: US Department of Health and Human Services. *Physical Activity and Health: A Report of the Surgeon General.* Atlanta, Ga: US Dept Health and Human Services, Centers for Disease Control and Prevention, National Center for Chronic Disease Prevention and Health Promotion; 1996.

BOX 24.3   Exercise Recommendations for Primary and Secondary Prevention of CVD

Primary Prevention

- 30 to 60 minutes, four to six times per week *or* 30 minutes on most days of the week
- End point of exercise is subjective.
    1. Breathlessness
    2. Fatigue levels such as "Somewhat hard" or "Hard" in Borg Perceived Exertion Scale

Aerobic activities such as:
    1. Bicycling—stationary or routine
    2. Walking, jogging
    3. Swimming

Resistive exercise:
    1. Two to three times per week
    2. 8 to 10 exercise sets
    3. 10 to 15 repetitions per set
    4. Moderate intensity
    5. Use of free weights (15 to 30 lb)

Secondary Prevention

Initial activity: Walking
    1. Gradual increase in duration
    2. Active, nonresistive range of motion of upper extremities
    3. Should be supervised

Long-term activity:
    1. Symptom-limited exercise test after stabilization
    2. Regular conditioning program
        —Large muscle group activities for 20 minutes
        —Warm-up and cool down

---

exercise sets with 10 to 15 repetitions each at moderate to high intensity for a minimum of 2 days per week is recommended for the maintenance of muscle mass, strength, flexibility, functional capacity, bone-mineral density, prevention, and/or rehabilitation of musculoskeletal problems (11).

Multiple mechanisms may contribute to the protective effects of physical activity to combat CVD. Endurance-exercise training, along with other CVD risk factor interventions, has been shown to prevent progression and reduce the severity of atherosclerosis (12,13). Exercise training increases HDL-cholesterol which acts as a lipid scavenger and removes the extra hepatic cholesterol. Exercise training can also increase lipoprotein lipase activity, which helps remove cholesterol and fatty acids from the circulation and can lower plasma TAG levels. Exercise increases coronary blood flow and improves the efficiency of O_2 exchange. Endurance training reduces thrombosis by increasing the breakdown of blood clots and decreasing platelet adhesiveness and aggregation. Stefancik et al (14) observed a significant reduction in plasma LDL cholesterol (9%) with aerobic exercise combined with a Step II diet (see *Table 24.6A*) in postmenopausal women and men with elevated LDL-C and low HDL-C. A dose-response association has been observed between amount of exercise performed and all-cause mortality, and CVD mortality in middle-aged and elderly populations (15,16).

Diet and physical activity are the most effective primary and secondary means of preventing CVD. Also effective are changes in unhealthy habits (such as cigarette smoking) or behaviors (such as a high-stress lifestyle) in addition to hypolipidemic drugs. Diet and exercise in combination have the most significant impact on several CVD risk factors. Because of the additive nature of these risk factors and the presence of multiple risk factors, there is a growing need to identify individuals with these factors and initiate a multilevel intervention program as early as possible.

CHOLESTEROL-LOWERING THERAPY

Table 24.3 represents the current recommendations of the American Heart Association for the primary prevention of CHD. NCEP recommends an intensive cholesterol-lowering therapy for individuals with any form of atherosclerotic disease. Recent clinical trials (eg, Scandinavian Simvastatin Survival Study (17) and Cholesterol and Recurrent Events Study (18)) have demonstrated a marked reduction in major coronary events, coronary mortality, and total mortality with aggressive cholesterol-lowering therapy. These studies have also demonstrated that risk reduction can be achieved within 2 years after initiation of cholesterol-lowering therapy. However, up to two-thirds of clients with CHD do not receive any cholesterol-lowering therapy. The goal of therapy in these patients is to lower LDL-C to <130 mg/dL. The major cholesterol-lowering drugs are statins, bile acid sequestrants, and nicotinic acid. The choice and dose of the drug therapy are dependent on the individual's LDL-C level and lipoprotein profile, and combined drug therapy may be indicated for some individuals. The dietary guidelines suggested by various health care organizations are shown in *Box 24.4.* Having a dietetics professional individualize a diet therapy program should improve dietary adherence. However, even with the use of cholesterol-lowering drugs diet therapy should be continued since it can enhance the drugs', actions and lower the risk of recurrent events.

BOX 24.4   Dietary and Lifestyle Recommendations for the Population at Large*

- Consume a nutritionally adequate diet; include a variety of foods.
- Lower consumption of total fat to ≤30% of total calories, SFA ≤10% of total calories, MUFA 10% to 15% of total calories, PUFA up to 10% of total calories, and cholesterol <300 mg/day.
- Increase consumption of complex carbohydrate to 55% to 60% of total calories.
- Decrease consumption of sodium to ≤2.4 g/day.
- If alcohol is not contraindicated, limit to ≤2 drinks/day (1 to 2 oz of ethanol).
- Achieve and maintain appropriate body weight.
- Eliminate cigarette smoking.
- Consume appropriate calories and maintain physical activity to prevent obesity; lower body weight in obese individuals.

---

* These are a summary of the general recommendations by various health organizations.

Dietary Interventions

Diet is the primary therapeutic approach for individuals at risk for CHD due to elevated cholesterol levels (>200 mg/dL). Based on epidemiological and clinical intervention trials, NCEP and The American Heart Association have established the Step I and Step II diets to lower saturated fatty acids (SFA) and dietary cholesterol to lower plasma total cholesterol and LDL-C levels (4,5,19) (*Tables 24.6A and 24.6B*). The Step I diet has been shown to lower LDL-C by approximately 7% to 9% and Step II can lower LDL-C by approximately 10% to 20%. However, because of genetic and individual variation in lipid and lipoprotein responses, responsiveness to dietary interventions will vary from individual to individual (20). The role of some of the individual dietary components in the management of CHD are briefly discussed below.

TABLE 24.6A Step I and Step II Dietary Recommendations

	Step I	Step II
Total fat	≤ 30% of total calories	
Saturated fatty acids (SFA)	8% to 10% of total calories	Less than 7% of total calories
Polyunsaturated fatty acids (PUFA)	Up to 10% of total calories	
Monounsaturated fatty acids (MUFA)	Up to 15% of total calories	
Carbohydrate	55% or more of total calories	
Protein	Approximately 15% of total calories	
Cholesterol	Less than 300 mg/day	Less than 200 mg/day
Total calories	To achieve and maintain desirable weight	

TABLE 24.6B Maximum Daily Intake of Fat and Saturated Fat to Achieve the Step I and Step II Dietary Recommendations*

	Total Calorie Level							
	1,600	1,800	2,000	2,200	2,400	2,600	2,800	3,000
Total Fat, g**	53	60	67	73	80	87	93	100
Saturated Fat, Step I, g†	18	20	22	24	27	29	31	33
Saturated Fat, Step II, g†	12	14	16	17	19	20	22	23

* Average daily energy intake for women is 1,800 kcal and for men is 2,500 kcal.

** Total fat content of both diets = 30% of calories (estimated by multiplying calorie level of the diet by 0.3 and dividing the product by 9 kcal/g).

† Recommended intake of saturated fat on the Step I diet is 8% to 10% of total calories. It is less than 7% of the total calories for the Step II diet.

Adapted from: National Cholesterol Education Program. *Report of the Expert Panel on Detection, Evaluation, and Treatment of High Blood Cholesterol in Adults (ATP II).* Bethesda, Md: National Heart, Lung, and Blood Institute, US Dept of Health and Human Services. NIH Publication No. 93-3095.

Total fat. Diets providing approximately 25% of calories from total fat have been shown to lower plasma TC and LDL-C by approximately 9% to 11%, which is primarily associated with a reduction in dietary SFA content.

Saturated fatty acids (SFA). Epidemiological studies, such as the Seven Countries Study, were the first to show a significant relationship between serum cholesterol and SFA intake and between the incidence of CHD and serum cholesterol. SFA are commonly found in animal fats, coconut oil, palm kernel oil, and palm oil. The main contributors to the dietary intake of SFA are meat, poultry, eggs, and dairy products. Clinical trials have consistently shown SFA to raise blood cholesterol levels approximately twice as much as polyunsaturated fatty acids (PUFA) lower them. Among the SFA, myristic acid is the most potent hypercholesterolemic long-chain SFA (LCSFA), followed by palmitic acid and then lauric acid. Interestingly, stearic acid is a unique LCSFA which appears to have no effect on plasma TC and lipoprotein cholesterol levels.

Monounsaturated fatty acids (MUFA). Epidemiological studies have demonstrated a negative association between MUFA intake and CHD incidence when SFA and cholesterol intake are controlled. The major component of olive oil is MUFA. Meat, poultry, and fish contribute substantially to the MUFA intake. Clinical studies have shown MUFA to elicit either a neutral or a hypocholesterolemic effect, and to be a more potent hypocholesterolemic fatty acid than polyunsaturated fatty acids.

Polyunsaturated fatty acids (PUFA). PUFA intake has been shown to be negatively correlated with CHD mortality. n-6 PUFA have been shown to lower TC and LDL-C levels, and linoleic acid may have a more potent blood cholesterol-lowering effect than oleic acid. Grain products such as yeast breads, rolls, cakes, cookies, and pastries are main contributors of linoleic acid intake. n-3 fatty acids include alpha-linolenic acid (LNA), eicosapentaenoic acid (EPA), and docosahexaeoic acid (DHA). LNA, found in soybean and canola oil, tofu, and nuts, is an important plant-based n-3 fatty acid for vegetarians. EPA and DHA are long-chain polyunsaturated fatty acids mainly from marine sources, namely fish and shellfish. There is little evidence on the effect of n-3 fatty acids on serum TC. Studies with the Greenland Eskimos were the first to implicate the protective role of marine lipids, especially n-3 fatty acids, in lowering CHD incidence in this population by lowering plasma TAG. These n-3 fatty acids lower TAG especially in individuals with hypertriglyceredemia and influence cellular responses in platelets, monocytes, and endothelial cells by decreasing platelet aggregation and prolonging bleeding time. Fish oil supplements are generally not recommended except in individuals with severe, treatment-resistant hypertriglyceredemia because of their potential side effects such as fishy odor, gastrointestinal upset, increased bleeding time, increased nosebleed, easy bruising, increased TC in individuals with hyperlipidemia, increased caloric intake with increased weight gain, and increased oxidation potential (21). Typically, high PUFA (>10% calories) diets are not recommended because they can make LDL more susceptible to oxidation.

***Trans* fatty acids.** *Trans* fatty acids have been observed to raise blood cholesterol levels compared to *cis* MUFA fatty acids. Major sources of *trans* fatty acids are margarine and hydrogenated fats. *Trans* MUFA raise LDL-C about two-thirds as much as palmitic acid and may have a HDL-C lowering effect and potentially raise Lp(a).

Table 24.7 summarizes the effects of the individual fatty acids on various CVD risk factors.

TABLE 24.7   Summary of Effects of Individual Fatty Acids on CVD Risk Factors

	Atherosclerosis			Thrombosis	Blood Pressure
	TC/LDL-C	HDL-C	TG		
Saturated Fatty Acids (SFA)					
Lauric acid	↑	↑	NE	NE/↑	NE
Myristic acid	↑	↑	NE	NE/↑	NE
Palmitic acid	↑	↑	NE	NE/↑	NE
Stearic acid	NE	NE	NE	NE/↑	NE
Monounsaturated Fatty Acids (MUFA)					
cis C18:1	NE/↓	↑	NE	NE	NE
trans C18:1	↑	↓	↑	ND	ND
Polyunsaturated Fatty Acids (PUFA)					
n-6 fatty acids	↓	↑/NE	↓	↑/↓	NE
n-3 fatty acids	NE	NE	↓	↓	↓

↑=raises; ↓=lowers; NE=no effect; ND=no data

Dietary cholesterol. Dietary cholesterol raises plasma TC, primarily LDL-C, although this hypercholesterolemic effect is less than SFA (20,22). A linear relationship is observed up to approximately 500 mg/day, above which only a small incremental increase is observed. An increase of approximately 4 mg/dL in plasma TC has been observed for every 100 mg increase in dietary cholesterol in a 2,500-calorie diet. Individual variation in response to dietary cholesterol is quite substantial. A diet high in SFA has been shown to elicit a greater hypercholesterolemic response to dietary cholesterol, whereas a diet high in PUFA attenuates the response.

Randomized fats. Randomization is a process by which fatty acids on the triacylglycerol molecule are rearranged, thereby affecting the absorption and function of the TAG molecule. Mixed results have been observed with these randomized fats on blood cholesterol levels (20).

Fat substitutes. Because of inadequate information on long-term health effects and overall health benefits, the American Heart Association discourages use of these products (20). Additionally, it believes that an emphasis on low-fat or reduced-fat foods may make individuals overlook total calorie intake. Therefore, adequate nutrition education is required when recommending these products to individuals attempting to lower total fat intake.

High-carbohydrate diets. Typically, low-fat diets are high in carbohydrates which have been shown to raise VLDL and TAG. However, if these high-carbohydrate diets are rich in fiber and complex carbohydrates, low in simple sugars, and are accompanied with weight loss, then the elevation in TAG can be minimized and can result in the lowering of blood lipid levels (20,23).

Dietary protein. The amount and type of dietary protein have been shown to affect TC and LDL-C. The difference between animal and vegetable protein has been attributed to the essential amino acids—lysine and methionine—which are in higher concentrations in animal protein and have been observed to have a hypercholesterolemic effect; however, arginine, which is high in plant proteins, appears to be hypocholesterolemic. Additionally, soy protein has been observed to have a hypocholesterolemic effect, probably because of its isoflavonoid content (22).

Dietary fiber. Dietary fiber that includes components of vegetables and fruits that are resistant to human digestive enzymes encompasses polysaccharides (like cellulose, hemicellulose, pectin, gums) and nonpolysaccharides, (like lignin and other indigestible plant components). Properties such as fermentability, viscosity, and bile acid-binding capacity have been attributed to the physiological functions of dietary fiber. *Table 24.8* and *Box 24.5* provide examples of the sources of major types of dietary fiber and some of their proposed physiological functions.

TABLE 24.8   Sources of Dietary Fiber

Insoluble Fiber	Soluble Fiber	Lignin
Wheat	Oats	Carrots
Rye	Legumes	Wheat
Rice	Beans	Fruit with edible seeds
Most whole grains	Peas	
Bran	Fruits and vegetables	
	Guar gum	
	Carrots	

BOX 24.5   Physiological Functions of Dietary Fiber

- Increases fecal bulk
- Increases frequency of defecation
- Increases postprandial satiety
- Decreases intraluminal pressure
- Increases bile acid excretion
- Reduces intestinal transit time
- Delays gastric emptying
- Reduces glucose and cholesterol absorption
- Binds with minerals, altering mineral balance
- Is a substrate for colon bacteria

In regard to CVD, dietary fiber has been shown to have a cholesterol-lowering effect. Several mechanisms have been proposed for this effect:

- Viscous polysaccharides that may prevent a rise in blood cholesterol by lowering dietary cholesterol and fatty acid absorption and by lowering absorption of biliary cholesterol or bile acids
- Dietary fiber that can alter serum hormone and short-chain fatty acid concentrations thereby altering fatty acid and cholesterol metabolism

Clinical studies have observed a 10% to 15% reduction in TC with oats, beans, and psyllium (24,25). Fiber supplements such as pectin and guar gum have also been shown to produce marked reductions in plasma TC by approximately 10%. However, with the increasing usage of fiber supplements, gastrointestinal side effects and reduction in mineral absorption are commonly observed; therefore, obtaining dietary fiber from natural sources is preferable. Observational studies have also shown an inverse association between total dietary fiber intake and both CVD and all-cause mortality (26). Typically, with a high-fiber diet total dietary fat and cholesterol are significantly lowered, thereby contributing to the overall reduction in mortality (27). In addition to lowering total cholesterol, dietary fiber has been shown to lower blood pressure and improve glycemic response. Based on current evidence the American Heart Association recommends that individuals consume 25 to 30 g of total dietary fiber per day from natural sources (ie, food not supplements) to ensure nutrient adequacy and maximize the cholesterol-lowering impact of a fat-modified diet (28).

ANTIOXIDANTS, PRO-OXIDANTS, AND CVD

Antioxidants

Oxidation of LDL-C *in vitro* has been observed to promote the deposition of cholesterol esters in macrophages and arterial smooth muscle cells (29-31). Oxidized LDL is thought to promote adhesion of blood monocytes to the endothelium which could lead to a narrowing of the artery. Additionally, oxidized LDL may also induce endothelial damage, promoting atherosclerosis by increasing the entry of blood components and platelet aggregation at the site of injury, and may interfere with the response of arteries to endothelial-derived relaxation factors (nitric oxide). Therefore, antioxidants, especially those derived from the diet, may aid in inhibiting or lowering LDL oxidation and in preventing the atherogenesis process. Several naturally occurring compounds in foods contain antioxidant properties which may play a role in retarding the development of atherogenesis (*Table 24.9*). Generally, fruits and vegetables are good sources of these antioxidants and also contain additional compounds that together may inhibit the development of atherosclerosis. Some of the well-known, naturally occurring antioxidants are briefly discussed below.

TABLE 24.9   Sources of Dietary Antioxidants

Antioxidant	Dietary Source
Vitamin E	Vegetable oils, nuts, whole grains (germ), butter, liver, egg yolk, some fruits and vegetables
Carotene	Orange fruits and vegetables, spinach, broccoli, green beans, peas, and peppers
Beta-carotene	Carrots, cantaloupe, broccoli, spinach
Lycopene	Tomatoes and tomato products
Lutein	Spinach, greens, broccoli, corn, green beans, peas
Ascorbic acid	Fresh fruits, cruciferous vegetables, potatoes and other vegetables
Flavonoids	Colored fruits and vegetable skins, apples, citrus fruits, onions, potatoes, tea
Ubiquinone-10	Soybean oil, meats, sardines, nuts, wheat germ, beans, garlic, spinach
Selenium	Grains, meat, fish, garlic

Adapted from: Diplock AT. Antioxidant nutrients and disease prevention: an overview. *Am J Clin Nutr.* 1991;53:189S-193S.

Vitamin E (tocopherols and tocotrienols). Tissue, plasma, and LDL-cholesterol contain alpha-tocopherol, a lipid-soluble antioxidant. Vitamin E traps the free radicals, a chain-breaking reaction, thereby providing protection against lipid peroxidation. Additionally, vitamin E is the predominant antioxidant found in the core of LDL-cholesterol. Despite this protective effect, human intervention studies with vitamin E supplements have not provided any conclusive evidence about the role of vitamin E in protecting against CVD. The Nurses Health Study (32) and the WHO/MONICA Project (33) observed an inverse relationship between vitamin E and CVD mortality. However, there are no placebo-controlled clinical trials examining the effects of vitamin E therapy on CVD events and mortality.

Carotenoids. Approximately 600 carotenoid compounds have been identified in plants, some of which are beta-carotene, alpha-carotene, lycopene, beta-cryptoxanthin, and crocetin. Of all these varied compounds, beta-carotene has been the most studied. Beta-carotene is a lipid-soluble antioxidant that traps free radicals and quenches singlet oxygen, suggesting a potential protective role against the development of atherosclerosis by inhibiting oxidative modification of LDL. Although prospective cohort studies have demonstrated an inverse association between plasma beta-carotene, MI, and CVD (33,34), the Physicians Health Study (35) and the ATBC Trial (36) have not demonstrated any protective effect of beta-carotene supplementations.

Ascorbic acid. Ascorbic acid is a water-soluble antioxidant which reacts directly with superoxide, hydroxyl radicals, and singlet oxygen in a chain-breaking reaction (31). Ascorbic acid also plays a role in regenerating reduced tocopherol, although *exvivo* and epidemiological evidence suggests that ascorbic acid may prevent LDL oxidation and is inversely associated with CHD mortality. Its exact role and the amount required to provide a protective role against CVD are unclear.

Ubiquinone-10. Ubiquinone is a lipid-soluble antioxidant that plays a major role in the electron transport chain and also protects vitamin E and LDL against oxidation. However, its antiatherogenic effects have not been well studied.

Selenium. Selenium is a trace element that enhances the cells' defenses against the cytotoxic effects of oxidized LDL. The potential protective role of selenium in atherosclerosis is not well studied.

Although it is not possible to make recommendations about consumption of antioxidant supplements, a balanced, low-fat diet rich in fruits, vegetables, legumes, and fiber may have an overall protective role (30).

Pro-oxidants

Iron. Recent evidence suggests that high intakes of iron and copper may be atherogenic because of their pro-oxidant properties, especially in individuals with elevated LDL-cholesterol levels (37,38).

Homocysteine. A metabolite of methionine, elevated total homocysteine levels have been shown to potentially be an independent risk factor of CVD by promoting LDL-oxidation and by proliferation of smooth muscle cells affecting endothelial cell function. An increase in total homocysteine of 5 mmol/L has been estimated to raise the risk of CVD by as much as an increase of 20 mg/dL in cholesterol concentration (39).

PHYTOCHEMICALS AND CVD

A strong protective association has been observed between fruit and vegetable consumption and CHD (40). Current evidence suggests that certain components of fruits and vegetables (ie, plant sterols, flavonoids, and sulphur-containing compounds) may play a significant role in their protective effect (41). Some of these compounds are briefly discussed below.

Plant Sterols

Plant sterols include compounds that are structurally related to cholesterol. The main plant sterols in the US diet are sitosterol, stigmasterols, and campesterol; the most predominant one is beta-sitosterol. Recent clinical trials have shown beta-sitosterol to have a significant cholesterol-lowering effect of approximately 10% or more (42), potentially lowering dietary cholesterol absorption.

Flavonoids

Flavonoids are found in fruits, vegetables, nuts, and seeds. This group includes flavanols, flavones, catechins, flavanones, and anthocyanins, which in the US diet are commonly provided by tea, onions, soy, and wine. Epidemiological studies have shown an inverse association between flavonoid intake and CHD; however, the exact nature of this relationship is unclear. It has been suggested that some flavonoids may possess antioxidant properties preventing LDL-oxidation, which is one of the mechanisms proposed for the cholesterol-lowering effects of the phenolic compounds found in red wine. Compounds such as quercetin inhibit macrophage-mediated LDL-oxidation and potentially block the cytotoxic effects of oxidized LDL. Phenolic compounds found in red wine and olives may also protect against LDL oxidation, which may explain the reduction in CVD observed in individuals consuming wine (43). Nigdikare et al (44) observed that the polyphenolic compounds in red wines could potentially change the chemical properties of plasma components making them more resistant to oxidation. Similar findings have been observed with tea and grape juice. Additionally, isoflavones, found in high concentration in soy foods, have also been observed to lower cholesterol (45). However, it is premature to suggest that consumption of these compounds will benefit human health.

Sulphur Compounds

Plants containing sulphur compounds, namely the allium family, have been shown to lower plasma TC. Garlic in various forms has been shown to have a hypocholesterolemic effect (approximately 9%), potentially by inhibiting cholesterol synthesis.

In spite of these potential effects, it should be recognized that all these compounds are effective in their natural forms and excess intake of individual supplements of these compounds may have such adverse toxic effects as gastrointestinal disturbances and allergic reactions in some individuals. Therefore, it is more prudent and cost-effective to consume a balanced diet containing a variety of fruits, vegetables, and whole-grain products than to consume individual supplements (22).

ALCOHOL AND CVD

Extensive observational studies suggest that total mortality may be reduced in individuals consuming one to two alcoholic drinks per day. This protective effect could be attributed to the rise in HDL-C levels observed in these individuals or by alcohol's influence on tissue plasminogen activator, a major component of the fibrinolytic system, thereby activating the antithrombotic mechanism (46). However, this association between alcohol intake and mortality has a J-shaped curve suggesting that with high-alcohol intake (>3 drinks per day), mortality increases (47,48). Additionally, in the "French paradox," which is associated with the low rates of CHD in the French attributed to widespread red wine consumption, a high rate of alcohol addiction and alcohol-induced diseases is observed in spite of the lowered CHD mortality, thereby making it difficult to make any recommendations to the general public regarding alcohol consumption and CHD. General recommendations for counseling about alcohol consumption are listed in *Box 24.6*.

Some of the components of red wine could explain the favorable effects on blood lipids. Flavonoids with antioxidant properties are found in peels or skin and outer layers of the flesh of flowers, fruits, and berries. These flavonoids are thought to prevent oxidation of lipoproteins by conserving the alpha-tocopherol content of lipoproteins and delaying the lipid peroxidation. Polyphenols in red wine inhibit both cyclo-oxygenation and lipo-oxygenation of platelets and therefore may potentially decrease thrombosis tendencies (48).

BOX 24.6   Recommendations for Counseling Regarding Alcohol Consumption

- Conduct an alcohol consumption history assessment.
  - Determine amount, frequency, and pattern.
  - Alcohol intake >1 to 2 oz/day is associated with increased health risk.
- Question about dependence on alcohol and/or drinking problem.
- Counsel to avoid alcohol consumption if working or operating vehicles or other mechanical objects where functions can be impaired.
- Recommend complete abstinence for individuals with conditions such as liver or pancreatic diseases, hypertension, hypertriglyceredemia, congestive heart failure, cerebral hemorrhage, etc.
- Allow alcohol consumption of <1 oz/day but no more than 3 drinks/day in absence of known risk factors.
  - Should be monitored regularly
- Identify patterns of excess consumption, drinking problems, and other consequences in follow-up visits.
- Alter recommendations as needed.

Adapted from: Pearson TA, Terry P. What to advise patients about drinking alcohol: the clinician's conundrum. *JAMA.* 1994;272:967-968.

CAFFEINE AND CVD

Caffeine in coffee, tea, and cola soft drinks is the most widely consumed stimulant in the United States. Fifty-six percent of the adult population consumes an average of 3.4 cups of coffee per day. It has been suggested that coffee consumption alters blood lipids, which may be associated with factors such as the method of coffee brewing, diet, body fat, or smoking. Boiled coffee has been observed to increase serum cholesterol, probably due to cafestol, a lipid compound in coffee which is typically removed when coffee is brewed using paper filters (50-52).

LIFESTYLE MODIFICATION AND CVD

Lifestyle modification, such as low-fat vegetarian diets, moderate aerobic exercise, weight loss, stress management, smoking cessation, and social group support, has been shown to result in regression of arterial stenosis and delay in the progression of atherosclerosis (12). Additionally, reduction in plasma TC and LDL-C can be achieved along with an improvement in functional status. Although these lifestyle modifications may be more cost-effective than lipid-lowering medications, client adherence is a major obstacle to the widespread adoption of these modifications. A comprehensive assessment of the client's motivation, dedication, and commitment is required prior to prescription of these changes.

Athletes

Athletes' aerobic training provides an advantage with respect to cardiovascular fitness by widening the arterial lumen and changing the tone of the smooth muscles of the arteries. Additionally, aerobic training enhances the arteries' response to the vasodilating factors and inhibits their response to vasoconstrictive factors. Although an inverse relationship exists between the level of activity and the incidence of CHD, it should be recognized that even among athletes exercise does not provide immunity from the disease and they should be monitored on a regular basis. Recently, many sudden and unexpected deaths of young, trained athletes have occurred (53-56). However, these occur in only about 1 in 200,000 individual student athletes per year (53-55) and should not deter young individuals from participating in sports. Cardiovascular lesions, such as ruptured aortic aneurysm, aortic valve stenosis, and myocarditis, account for <5% of the total causes of death in the trained athlete (53).

About one-third of the deaths in young athletes are attributed to hypertrophic cardiomyopathy associated with sudden and unexpected cardiac death, usually occurring after moderate to severe exertion. This risk of sudden death may be compounded by alterations in blood volume, dehydration, and electrolyte imbalance commonly encountered in the competitive athlete. Another common cause of sudden death in athletes is congenital abnormalities of the coronary arteries. Additionally, African-American male athletes seem to be more susceptible to sudden death on the athletic field. Therefore, in the presence of risk factors, intense physical activity may act as a trigger to and precipitating factor of the sudden death of an athlete, especially in sports such as football and basketball. It may be prudent for athletes and individuals with hypertrophic cardiomyopathy to withdraw from competitive sports. The American Heart Association recommends obtaining a personal and family medical history and physical exam to target detection of cardiovascular lesions in athletes (56).

In individuals above the age of 30, the major cause of death during or soon after exercise is attributed to CHD, which is mainly associated with rupturing of the plaque and/or thrombosis (53,55). Therefore, active individuals should be aware of the symptoms of exercise intolerance, such as chest discomfort, unusual dyspnea, and physical or verbal manifestation of severe fatigue, and seek medical attention promptly (55).

Diet Prescription

Although both dietary modification and physical activity have been observed to modify the risk of CVD, the exact mechanism of the interaction between diet, physical activity, and CVD remains unclear. Dietary modification and physical activity in combination can lower body weight and prevent other CVD risk factors from emerging. At the present time there are no specific dietary recommendations for active individuals with CVD. However, dietary modifications in accordance with the principles of the Food Guide Pyramid and the US Dietary Guidelines can result in a significant reduction in known CVD risk factors and improve the response to exercise training in active individuals (57,59). Therefore, a prudent dietary intake and physical activity pattern will play a major role in the prevention and treatment of CVD regardless of the individual's age, gender, or physical fitness (59).

REFERENCES

1. American Heart Association. *1998 Heart and Stroke Facts: Statistical Update.* Dallas, Tex: American Heart Association; 1998.
2. Ross R. The pathogenesis of atherosclerosis: a perspective for the 1990s. *Nature.* 1993;362:801-809.
3. Fuster V, Badimon L, Badimon JJ, Chesebro JH. The pathogenesis of coronary artery disease and the acute coronary syndrome. *N Engl J Med.* 1992;326:242-250.
4. National Cholesterol Education Program. *Second Report of the Expert Panel on Detection, Evaluation and Treatment of High Blood Cholesterol in Adults (Adult Treatment Panel II).* Bethesda, Md: National Heart, Lung and Blood Institute, National Institutes of Health, US Dept of Health and Human Services; 1993. NIH Publication No. 93-3095.
5. Grundy SM, Balady GJ, Criqui MH, et al. When to start cholesterol-lowering therapy in patients with coronary heart disease. A statement for healthcare professionals from the American Heart Association Task Force on Risk Reduction. *Circulation.* 1997;95:1683-1685.
6. Grundy SM, Balady GJ, Criqui MH, et al. Pimary prevention of coronary heart disease: guidance from Framingham. A statement for health care professionals from the AHA Task Force on Risk Reduction. *Circulation.* 1998;97:1876-1887.
7. Wilson PWF, D'Agostino RB, Levy D, Belanger AM, Silbershatz H, Kannel WB. Prediction of coronary heart disease using risk factor categories. *Circulation.* 1998;97:1837-1847.
9. Eckel RH, Krauss RM for the AHA Nutrition Committee, American Heart Association. Call to action: obesity as a major risk factor for coronary heart disease. *Circulation.* 1998;97:2099-2100.
10. Obesity Education Initiative. *Clinical Guidelines on the Identification, Evaluation and Treatment of Overweight and Obesity in Adults: The Evidence Report.* Bethesda, Md: National Institutes of Health, National Heart, Lung and Blood Institute; 1998. http://www.nhlbi.nih.gov/nhlbi/cardio/obes/prof/guidelns/ob_home.htm. Accessed June 15, 1998.
11. Fletcher GF, Balady G, Blair SN, et al. Statement on exercise: benefits and recommendations for physical activity programs for all Americans. *Circulation.* 1996;94;857-862.
12. Ornish D, Brown SE, Scherwitz LW, et al. Can lifestyle changes reverse coronary heart disease? The Lifestyle Heart Trial. *Lancet.* 1990;336:129-133.
13. *Physical Activity and Health: A Report of the Surgeon General.* Atlanta, Ga: US Dept of Health and Human Services, Center for Disease Control and Prevention, National Center for Chronic Disease Prevention and Health Promotion; 1996.
14. Stefanick ML, Mackey S, Sheehan M, Ellsworth N, Haskell WL, Wood PD. Effects of diet and exercise in men and post-menopausal women with low levels of HDL cholesterol and high levels of LDL cholesterol. *N Engl J Med.* 1998;339:12-20.
15. Lee IM, Hsieh CC, Paffenbarger RS. Exercise intensity and longevity in men: the Harvard Alumni Health Study. *JAMA.* 1995;273:1179-1184.

16. Blair SN, Kohl HW, Barlow CE, Paffenbarger RS, Gibbons LW, Macera CA. Changes in physical fitness and all-cause mortality: a prospective study of healthy and unhealthy men. *JAMA*. 1995;273:1093-1098.

17. Scandinavian Simvastatin Survival Study (4S) Group. Randomized trial of cholesterol lowering in 4444 patients with coronary heart disease: Scandinavian Simvastatin Survival Study (4S). *Lancet*. 1994;344:1383-1389.

18. Sacks FM, Pfeffer MA, Moye LA, et al. The effect of pravastatin on coronary events after myocardial infarction in patients with average cholesterol levels. Cholesterol and Recurrent Events Trial investigators. *N Engl J Med*. 1996;335:1001-1009.

19. Grundy SM, Balady GJ, Criqui MH, et al. Guide to primary prevention of cardiovascular diseases. A statement for healthcare professionals from the Task Force on Risk Reduction. *Circulation*. 1997;95:2329-2331.

20. Stone NJ, Nicolosi RJ, Kris-Etherton P, Ernst ND, Krauss RM, Winston M. Summary of the scientific conference on the efficacy of hypocholesterolemic dietary interventions. *Circulation*. 1996;94:3388-3391.

21. Stone NJ. Fish consumption, fish oil, lipids and coronary heart disease. *Circulation*. 1996;94:2337-2340.

22. Krauss RM, Deckelbaum RJ, Ernst N, et al. Dietary guidelines for healthy American adults. A statement for health professionals from the Nutrition Committee, American Heart Association. *Circulation*. 1996;94:1795-1800.

23. Jacobs DR, Meyer KA, Kushi LH, Folsom AR. Whole-grain intake may reduce the risk of ischemic heart disease death in postmenopausal women: the Iowa Women's Health Study. *Am J Clin Nutr*. 1998;68:248-257.

24. Ripsin CM, Keenan JM, Jacobs DR, et al. Oat products and lipid lowering: a meta-analysis. *JAMA*. 1992;267:3317-3325.

25. Anderson JW, Smith BM, Gustafson NJ. Health benefits and practical aspects of high-fiber diets. *Am J Clin Nutr*. 1994;59(suppl):1242S-1247S.

26. Anderson JW, Garrity TF, Wood CL, Whitis SE, Smith BM, Oeltgen PR. Prospective, randomized, controlled comparison of the effects of low-fat and low-fat plus high-fiber diets on serum lipid concentrations. *Am J Clin Nutr*. 1992;56:887-894.

27. Rimm EB, Ascherio A, Giovannucci E, Spiegelman D, Stampher MJ, Willett WC. Vegetables, fruit and cereal fiber intake and risk of coronary heart disease among men. *J Am Diet Assoc*. 1996;275:447-451.

28. Van Horn L. Fiber, lipids and coronary heart disease. A statement for healthcare professionals from the Nutrition Committee, American Heart Association. *Circulation*. 1997;95:2701-2704.

29. Duell PB. Dietary antioxidants and atherosclerosis. *Curr Op Endocrinol Diabetes*. 1994;1:251-259.

30. Duell PB. Prevention of atherosclerosis with dietary antioxidants: fact or fiction? *J Nutr*. 1996;126:1067S-1071S.

31. Kwiterovich PO. The effect of dietary fat, antioxidants and pro-oxidants on blood lipids, lipoproteins and atherosclerosis. *J Am Diet Assoc*. 1997;97(suppl):S31-S41.

32. Stampfer MJ, Hennekens CH, Manson JE, Colditz GA, Rosner B, Willett WC. Vitamin E consumption and the risk of coronary heart disease in women. *N Engl J Med*. 1993;328:1444-1449.

33. Nyyssonen K, Porkkala E, Salonen R, Korpela H, Salonen JT. Increase in oxidation resistance of atherogenic serum lipoproteins following antioxidant supplementation: a randomized double-blind placebo-controlled clinical trial. *Eur J Clin Nutr*. 1994;48:633-642.

34. Bolton-Smith C, Woodward M, Tunstall-Pedoe H. The Scottish Heart Health Study. Dietary intake by food frequency questionnaire and odds ratios for coronary heart disease risk. II. The antioxidant vitamins and fibre. *Eur J Clin Nutr*. 1992;46:85-93.

35. Gaziano JM, Hatta A, Flynn M, et al. Supplementation with beta-carotene in vivo and in vitro does not inhibit low density lipoprotein oxidation. *Atherosclerosis.* 1995;112:187-195.

36. The Alpha-Tocopherol, Beta Carotene Prevention Cancer Prevention Study Group. The alpha-tocopherol beta-carotene lung cancer prevention study: initial results from a controlled trial. *N Engl J Med.* 1994;330:1029-1035.

37. Salonen JT, Nyyssonen K, Korpela H, Tuomilehto J, Seppanen R, Salonen R. High stored iron levels are associated with excess risk of myocardial infarction in Eastern Finnish men. *Circulation.* 1992;86:803-811.

38. Ascherio A, Willett WC, Rimm EB, Giovannucci ECL, Stampfer MJ. Dietary iron intake and risk of coronary disease among men. *Circulation.* 1994;89:969-974.

39. Boushey CJ, Beresford SAA, Omenn GS, Motulsky AG. A quantitative assessment of plasma homocysteine as a risk factor for vascular disease. Probable benefits of increasing folic acid intakes. *JAMA.* 1995;274:1049-1057.

40. Hertog MG, Feskins EJ, Hollman PC, Katan MB, Kromhout D. Dietary antioxidant flavonoids and risk of coronary heart disease: the Zupthen Elderly Study. *Lancet.* 1993;342:1007-1011.

41. Howard BV, Kritchevsky D. Phytochemicals and cardiovascular disease. A statement for health professionals from the American Heart Association. *Circulation.* 1997;95:2591-2593.

42. Miettinen TA, Puska P, Gylling H, VanHanen H, Vartiainens E. Reduction of serum cholesterol with sitostanol-ester margarine in a mildly hypercholesterolemic population. *N Engl J Med.* 1995;333:1308-1312.

43. Waterhouse AL, German JB, Walzem RL, Hansen RJ, Kasim-Karakas SE. Is it time for a wine trial? *Am J Clin Nutr.* 1998;68:220-221.

44. Nigdikar SV, Williams NR, Griffin BA, Howard AN. Consumption of red wine polyphenols reduces the susceptibility of low-density lipoproteins to oxidation in vivo. *Am J Clin Nutr.* 1998;68:258-265.

45. Lichtenstein AH. Soy protein, isoflavones and cardiovascular risk. *J Nutr.* 1998;128:1589-1592.

46. Ridker PM, Vaughan DE, Stampfer MJ, Glynn RJ, Hennekens CH. Association of moderate alcohol consumption and plasma concentration of endogeneous tissue-type plasminogen activator. *JAMA.* 1994;272:929-933.

47. Pearson TA, Terry P. What to advise patients about drinking alcohol: the clinician's conundrum. *JAMA.* 1994;272:967-968.

48. Gronbaek M, Deis A, Sorense TIA, Becker U, Schnohr P, Jensen G. Mortality associated with moderate intakes of wine, beer or spirits. *BMJ.* 1995;310:1165-1169.

49. Constant J. Alcohol, ischemic heart disease and the French Paradox. *Clin Cardiol.* 1997;20:420-424.

50. Bak AAA, Grobbee DE. The effect of serum cholesterol levels of coffee brewed by filtering or boiling. *N Engl J Med.* 1989;321:1432-1437.

51. Weusten-Van der Wouw MP, Katan MB, Viani R, et al. Indentity of the cholesterol-raising factor from boiled coffee and its effects on liver function enzymes. *J Lipid Res.* 1994;35:721-733.

52. Urgert R, Meyboom S, Kuilman M, et al. Comparison of effect of cafetiere and filtered coffee on serum concentrations of liver aminotransferases and lipids: six month randomised controlled trial. *BMJ.* 1996;313:1362-1366.

53. Maron BJ. Cardiovascular risks of young persons on the athletic field. *Ann Intern Med.* 1998;129:379-386.

54. Sharma S, Whyte G, McKenna WJ. Sudden death from cardiovascular disease in young athletes: fact or fiction? *Br J Sports Med.* 1997;31:269-276.

55. Thompson PD. Athletes, athletics and sudden cardiac death. *Med Sci Sports Exerc.* 1993;24:981-984.

56. Maron BJ, Thompson PD, Puffer JC, et al. Cardiovascular preparticipation screening of competitive athletes. A statement for health professionals from the Sudden Death Committee (clinical cardiology) and Congenital Cardiac Defects Committee (cardiovascular disease in the young), American Heart Association [published addendum appears in *Circulation.* 1998;97:2294]. *Circulation.* 1996;94:850-856.

57. Gambera PJ, Schneeman BO, Davis PA. Use of the Food Guide Pyramid and US dietary guidelines to improve dietary intake and decrease cardiovascular risk in active-duty Air Force members. *J Am Diet Assoc.* 1995;95:1268-1273.

58. Blair SN, Horton E, Leon AS, et al. Physical activity, nutrition and chronic disease. *Med Sci Sports Exerc.* 1996;28:335-349.

59. von Duvillard SP. Symposium on lipids and lipoproteins in diet and exercise: introduction. *Med Sci Sports Exerc.* 1997;29:1414-1415.

25

DIABETES MELLITUS AND EXERCISE

Charlotte Hayes, MMSc, MS, RD, CDE

Physical activity plays a cornerstone role in diabetes management (1). The important health benefits of activity for people with diabetes include a reduction in cardiovascular risk factors, lowered body weight, reduced body fat, and a heightened sense of well-being (1-4). Exercise also significantly affects blood glucose (BG) control (3,4). It increases peripheral insulin sensitivity, lowers insulin requirements, and improves glucose tolerance (3). Metabolic adaptations to exercise improve glycemic control for individuals with type 2 diabetes (4,5). However, these same adaptations can lead to significant BG fluctuations and result in management challenges for individuals with type 1 diabetes (6,7).

The casual exerciser, as well as the athlete with diabetes, often faces the need to adjust management in order to maintain euglycemia with activity. Adjustments may be necessary in medications, meal planning, and in the exercise regimen itself. The need for multiple, complex adjustments may require input from a specialized diabetes team. The registered dietitian (RD), whether a member of such a team or not, plays a central role in integrating diabetes nutrition management and activity. The desired outcome of nutrition intervention is the achievement of optimal glycemic control with exercise, so that the individual with diabetes can realize the many health benefits of an active lifestyle.

TYPE 2 DIABETES

Type 2 diabetes, previously called noninsulin-dependent diabetes mellitus (NIDDM) or Type II diabetes, is the predominant form of diabetes. It is characterized by defects in insulin secretion and by reduced insulin-mediated glucose uptake due to insulin resistance (8). Risk factors for developing type 2 diabetes are multiple (8) (see *Box 25.1*). Lack of physical activity should be noted as a considerable risk factor for its development. Potential benefits of exercise to the individual with type 2 diabetes are numerous (1) (see *Box 25.2*). Because exercise reduces insulin resistance and improves insulin action, it is considered an important modality for prevention as well as treatment of the disorder. The benefit of exercise in improving the metabolic abnormalities associated with type 2 diabetes appears to be greatest early in the progression of the disease (1).

BOX 25.1   Risk Factors for Development of Type 2 Diabetes

- Age
- Family history
- Obesity
- Abdominal fat distribution
- Hypertension

- Dyslipidemia
- Lack of physical activity
- History of gestational diabetes
- Racial/ethnic group

Adapted from: The Expert Committee on the Diagnosis and Classification of Diabetes Mellitus. The report of the expert committee on the diagnosis and classification of diabetes mellitus. *Diabetes Care.* 1998;21:S5-S19.

BOX 25.2   Potential Health Benefits of Exercise in Type 2 Diabetes

- Improved glycemic control
- Reduced cardiovascular risk factors
- Improved lipid profile: ↓VLDL ↓LDL ↑HDL
- Lower blood pressure
- Increased fibrinolytic activity
- Greater success with weight loss and maintenance

Adapted from: American Diabetes Association. Position statement: Diabetes mellitus and exercise. Diabetes Care. 1998;21:S40-S44.

Diabetes Medical Nutrition Therapy (MNT) is an equally integral part of type 2 diabetes management. Desired outcomes of MNT include achievement and maintenance of glucose, lipid, and blood pressure goals (9). Weight loss is often an important aspect of management as well. A moderate loss of 10 to 20 lb is sufficient to considerably improve glycemic control, blood lipids, and blood pressure (9). The combination of diet plus exercise has been shown to optimize weight loss (10), decrease the reductions in lean body mass and resting metabolic rate which accompany weight loss (11), and improve cardiovascular risk factors to a greater degree than either therapy alone (12). Thus, diet and exercise should be considered adjunctive therapies in type 2 diabetes management.

Diabetes MNT and Exercise for Optimal Glycemic Control

When advising individuals with type 2 diabetes, it is important to emphasize that the combined therapies of meal planning plus exercise can lead to an optimal BG-lowering effect in addition to other health benefits. In contrast, the consumption of unnecessary, extra food and calories when exercising can easily counter the energy deficit and BG-lowering effect created by activity, especially if an individual's physical capacity is limited and the energy deficit created is small.

Individuals controlled only by diet and exercise are not at increased risk of hypoglycemia when active (7). Extra food for exercise is unnecessary and should certainly be avoided if weight management is a goal. Moderate exercise performed by those on oral antidiabetes medication(s) typically leads to a gradual lowering in BG that is unlikely to result in hypoglycemia. However, with certain medications hypoglycemia is still possible (13-15) (see *Table 25.1*), and prolonged activity increases the possibility of BG levels falling too low (7). If the BG falls

TABLE 25.1 Oral Antidiabetes Agents and Associated Hypoglycemia Risk

Medication	Potential for Hypoglycemia
First-generation sulfonylreas	Moderate
(chlorpropamide)	
(tolazamide)	
(tolbutamide)	
Second-generation sulfonylureas	Moderate
(glyburide)	
(glipizide)	
(glimepiride)	
Alpha glucosidase inhibitors* **	Low
(acarbose)	
(miglitol)	
Biguanides (metformin)	Low
Thiazolidinediones (troglitazone)*	Low
Repaglinide (prandin)	Low - Moderate

* Can contribute to hypoglycemia if used as combination therapy with insulin or sulfonylureas

** Glucose must be used as treatment for hypoglycemia; alpha glucosidase inhibitors prevent the conversion of sucrose to metabolically available sugars.

Adapted from: Setter SM. New drug therapies for the treatment of diabetes. *On the Cutting Edge.* 1998;19(2):3-5.

Sharp AR. Nutrition implications of new medications to treat diabetes. *On the Cutting Edge.* 1998;19(2):8-10.

Brodows R. Repaglinide (Prandin): a new therapy for type 2 diabetes. *Practical Diabetology.* 1998;17(2):32-36.

below a desirable range, a reduction in the dosage of medication(s) should be discussed with the diabetes team. Extra food to maintain adequate BG values should be used conservatively. Individuals treated with insulin are at risk of experiencing exercise-related BG fluctuations and hypoglycemia. To maintain euglycemia with activity, the principles of adjusting insulin, carbohydrates, and exercise that guide individuals with type 1 diabetes should be applied to type 2 diabetes management (7).

Postmeal exercise may reduce blood glucose response to food consumed (16). Individuals who experience postprandial hyperglycemia may benefit from exercising 1 to 2 hours after eating. Exercise at this time may reduce postmeal blood glucose rise and certainly will reduce risk of exercise-related hypoglycemia.

Exercise Recommendations for Type 2 Diabetes

The Surgeon General's Report on Physical Activity and Health recommends that all Americans accumulate 30 minutes of moderate activity on most days of the week. The report encourages individuals to begin by taking small steps each day to informally increase activity levels (17). These general recommendations are safe and effective for most people with type 2 diabetes. The emphasis on daily activity is important. Since the beneficial metabolic effects of exercise on glycemic control last only a few days (3,18,19), to achieve an optimal reduction in BG, exercise must be performed regularly and consistently. Planned exercise 5 to 7 days per week for 20 to 45 minutes per session may offer additional health benefits and greater improvement in glycemic control (3). Prior to beginning such exercise, a thorough medical evaluation to screen for macrovascular and microvascular complications of diabetes (see *Box 25.3*) is indicated (1). This will minimize exercise risk and assure appropriateness of an exercise prescription.

BOX 25.3   Macrovascular and Microvascular Complications of Diabetes

Macrovascular:
- Coronary artery disease
- Peripheral vascular disease
- Cerebrovascular disease

Microvascular:
- Retinopathy
- Neuropathy
- Nephropathy

Adapted from: The Expert Committee on the Diagnosis and Classification of Diabetes Mellitus. The report of the expert committee on the diagnosis and classification of diabetes mellitus. *Diabetes Care.* 1998;21:S5-S19.

TYPE 1 DIABETES

Type 1 diabetes, previously called insulin-dependent diabetes mellitus (IDDM) or Type I diabetes, accounts for 5% to 10% of all cases of diabetes and is characterized by the loss of insulin production by the pancreatic islet cells (20). Individuals with this type of diabetes must overcome considerable obstacles during exercise because for them metabolic adjustments to maintain fuel homeostasis (see *Table 25.2*) are lacking (6,7). The result can be a mismatch between hepatic glucose production and muscle glucose utilization, and significant deviation from euglycemia (21). Exercise must be carefully integrated into the diabetes management regimen so that optimal BG levels can be maintained with activity. Many variables influence BG response to exercise (1,7,21,22) (see *Box 25.4*). Those that can most readily be modified are circulating insulin levels and nutritional status. Insulin adjustments and carbohydrate supplementation can be used independently or together to maintain optimal BG levels during activity. The individual with type 1 diabetes must monitor BG regularly with exercise in order to understand glycemic response to activity, learn to make appropriate exercise-related management decisions, and evaluate the effectiveness of these decisions.

Self-monitoring of Blood Glucose and Pattern Management

Self-monitoring of blood glucose (SMBG), careful record keeping, and recognition of BG patterns with activity are important skills which enhance the ability of the individual with type 1 diabetes to self-adjust management for increased exercise safety and optimal, competitive performance (1). SMBG should be conducted regularly pre-exercise, postexercise, and during prolonged or "unusual" activity.

TABLE 25.2   Hormonal Adjustments to Maintain Fuel Homeostasis

Hormone	Response to Exercise	Metabolic Effect
Insulin	Decreases	Restricts use of glucose by nonexercising skeletal muscle; increases hepatic glycogenolysis; facilitates lipolysis
Glucagon	Increases	Stimulates hepatic glycogenolysis and gluconeogenesis
Epinephrine	Increases	Stimulates glucose production during prolonged exercise Increases muscle glycogenolysis Increases adipose tissue lypolysis
Norepinephrine	Increases	Modulates initial hepatic glucose release
Cortisol	Increases	Increases hepatic glucose production

Adapted from: Young JC. Exercise prescription for individuals with metabolic disorders, practical considerations. *Sports Med.* 1995;19:43-45.

Wasserman DH, Zinman B. Fuel homeostasis. In: Ruderman N, Devlin JT, eds. *The Health Professional's Guide to Exercise and Diabetes.* Alexandria, Va: American Diabetes Association; 1995:29-47.

Franz MJ. Exercise and diabetes mellitus. In: Powers MA, ed. *Handbook of Diabetes Nutritional Management.* Rockville, Md: Aspen Publishers; 1987:73-89.

BOX 25.4   Variables That Influence the Effect of Exercise on Blood Glucose Levels in Type 1 Diabetes

- Level of training and fitness
- Intensity of exercise
- Duration of exercise
- Time of exercise
- Type of exercise
- Metabolic control
- Nutritional status and glycogen stores
- Circulating insulin levels

Adapted from: American Diabetes Association. Position statement: diabetes mellitus and exercise. *Diabetes Care.* 1998;21:S40-S44.

Wasserman DH, Zinman B. Fuel homeostasis. In: Ruderman N, Devlin JT, eds. *The Health Professional's Guide to Exercise and Diabetes*. Alexandria, Va: American Diabetes Association; 1995:29-47.

Richter EA, Turcotte L, Hespel P, Kiens B. Metabolic responses to exercise: effects of endurance training and implications for diabetes. *Diabetes Care.* 1992;15:1767-1776.

Walsh J, Roberts R. Exercise. In: *Pumping Insulin.* 2nd ed. San Diego, Calif: Torrey Pines Press; 1995:83-95.

Frequent monitoring helps to anticipate the onset of hypoglycemia or hyperglycemia occurring during or after exercise and thus reduces risk of these acute complications. Data from monitoring, when carefully recorded and analyzed, become the basis for decision making about adjustments in management for subsequent exercise (7) (see *Figure 25.1*). Pattern management, the methodical process of data collection, analysis, and decision making (see *Box 25.5*), is the foundation of successful BG control with activity.

FIGURE 25.1   Sample Blood Glucose Flow Sheet

Name: _____   For: Month _____   Year _____

Address: _____   Home Phone: _____   Work: _____

City: _____   State: _____   Zip: _____

Blood Glucose Target Range: 70 – 150 mg/dL

TIME	2-4 AM	PRE-BREAKFAST				NOON				PRE-SUPPER				BEDTIME		REMARKS
DATE	BG	BG	Reg	Sup		BG	Reg	Sup		BG	Reg	Sup		BG	NPH	* Reaction # Exercise Record Wt. Weekly
1/14	98	126	6	0	11:00 (52) (59)	59	6	0	4:00 (63)# (70)	70	6	0		77	6	* Vaccumed house a.m. # Aerobics class 2:00-3:00
1/15	97	121	4	0	[174]	174	4	1		112	6	0		136	6	
1/16	133	132	4	0		132	4	2	3:00 (59)#	102	6	0		[171]	6	*Aerobics class 2:00-3:00
1/17	129	104	4	0	10:30 (61)	115	4	0		127	6	0		(62)	6	# Dog-walked 30 min. a.m.
1/18	141	110	4	0	10:30 72	131	4	0		111	4	0		[74]	6	
1/19	137	[152]	4	1		141	4	0	4:30 (48)#	122	4	0		133	6	#Stairmaster 45 min. (2:30)
1/20	104	97	4	0		75	4	0	3:00 (67)#	132	4	0		[151]	6	#Aerobics class 2:00-3:00
1/21	147	128	4	0	10:00 (57)	159	4	1		149	4	0		86	6	*Scrubbed kitchen floor a.m.

◯ = BG <70 mg/dL

▢ = BG >150 mg/dL

BOX 25.5   Pattern Management: A Six-step Process

Step 1. Record blood glucose readings.

Step 2. Study the recorded information.

Step 3. Find and interpret blood glucose patterns.

Step 4. Make adjustment decisions based on identified patterns.

Step 5. Implement adjustments (modified management strategies).

Step 6. Evaluate blood glucose response.

Adapted from: Daly A, Barry B, Gillespie S, Kulkarni K, Richardson M. *Carbohydrate Counting: Moving On*. Chicago, Ill: American Dietetic Association; 1995.

Management of diabetes: self-monitoring of blood glucose. In: Holler HJ, Pastors JG, eds. *Diabetes Medical Nutrition Therapy*. Chicago, Ill: American Dietetic Association; 1997:43-49.

Carbohydrate Supplement

Carbohydrate supplement, though useful in a number of exercise situations, should be used conservatively. When deciding about the need for additional carbohydrate during exercise, a number of factors should be considered (1) (see *Box 25.6*). Unnecessary or immoderate carbohydrate intake can quickly neutralize the beneficial BG-lowering effects of exercise and can supply excessive calories.

BOX 25.6   Factors That Influence Carbohydrate Supplement and Insulin Adjustment Decisions

- Blood glucose level pre-exercise
- Planned exercise intensity
- Planned exercise duration
- Level of training
- Time of day for planned exercise
- Time of last meal
- Insulin therapy
- Previously measured metabolic response to exercise

American Diabetes Association. Position statement: diabetes mellitus and exercise. *Diabetes Care*. 1998:21:S40-S44.

Wasserman DH, Zinman B. Fuel homeostasis. In: Ruderman N, Devlin JT, eds. *The Health Professional's Guide to Exercise and Diabetes*. Alexandria Va: American Diabetes Association; 1995:29-47.

Carbohydrate supplement is useful when activity is spontaneous or unplanned and is typically necessary during long-duration exercise or competitive events when energy expenditure is high. Carbohydrate can be consumed before, during, or after such exercise. As a general rule, intake of supplemental carbohydrate is indicated pre-exercise whenever the BG is ≤100 mg/dL prior to the start of activity (1). Individuals who participate in long-duration activities or competitive events which last longer than 40 minutes may need to consume carbohydrate during exercise to maintain optimal BG control and delay fatigue. Muscle efficiency is greatest and performance is best when BG values are maintained between 70 and 150 mg/dL, or as near normal as possible, during exercise (22). Enough carbohydrate should be consumed during exercise to keep the BG in this optimal range. Intake of 15 to 30 g of carbohydrate every 15 to 30 minutes of exercise is a general, safe starting guideline for supplementing carbohydrate (23). Sports drinks and diluted juices serve to replace fluid, as well as to provide carbohydrate, and are certainly appropriate for individuals with diabetes. Additional insulin should not be taken to cover carbohydrate consumed for the purpose of maintaining target range BG levels with activity (24). Because numerous variables can influence BG response to exercise, strategies for supplementing carbohydrate must be highly individualized (1,7). SMBG and pattern management allow the individual to draw on prior exercise experience, fine-tune carbohydrate supplementation strategies, and achieve optimal BG levels for peak performance.

Endurance athletes with diabetes may employ strategies of manipulating carbohydrate intake to optimize muscle and liver glycogen stores prior to long-endurance events. Frequent SMBG and insulin adjustment is necessary for maintenance of glycemic control when carbohydrate intake and training are altered prior to an event. Carbohydrate loading can be used with caution and meticulous care by athletes with diabetes (25). Extra carbohydrate may be needed after exercise when insulin sensitivity is increased and glycogen synthesis is enhanced (3,7,22,23). Intake of additional carbohydrate at this time can promote glycogen storage and reduce the likelihood of hypoglycemia. SMBG should be performed every 1 to 2 hours postexercise to assess the BG response to activity and make necessary adjustments in food intake and insulin dosages (23).

Insulin Adjustment

Because insulin sensitivity and responsiveness change with exercise, significant blood glucose fluctuations can occur if circulating insulin levels are too high or too low (3,7,22) (see *Table 25.3*). Pre-exercise insulin adjustment to lower the usual dosage and thus reduce circulating insulin levels is often necessary especially before long-duration or competitive activity. Insulin adjustment to reduce insulin can also be used by those who exercise for weight management purposes and therefore wish to minimize the need to supplement carbohydrate (24). Elevated pre-exercise BG can indicate insulin deficiency. Supplemental insulin may be necessary to correct low insulin levels and improve metabolic control before exercise is undertaken. Adjustment decisions should always be made with consideration of several significant variables (see *Box 25.6*). SMBG, careful record keeping, and evaluation of BG patterns are crucial for determining successful adjustment strategies.

TABLE 25.3 Metabolic Response to Exercise Based on Insulin Status

Insulin Level	Liver Glucose Output	Muscle Glucose Uptake	Metabolic Effect
Low	↑↑	↑	↑ BG, ↑ FFA, ↑ ketones
Desirable	↑↑	↑↑	Stable BG
High	↑	↑↑	↓ BG, hypoglycemia

↑↑ = large increase　　↑ = moderate increase　　↓ = decrease

Adapted from: Young JC. Exercise prescription for individuals with metabolic disorders, practical considerations. Sports Med. 1995;19(1):45.

A number of guidelines for reducing insulin dosages prior to planned exercise have been suggested (7,22-24,26). A 30% to 50% reduction in the dosage of insulin acting during the time of exercise is generally accepted as a safe starting guideline. Greater reductions may be needed for prolonged or extreme exercise (26). Because adjustment decisions require recognition of the insulin acting during the time of exercise, familiarity with the time course of insulin action (see *Figure 25.2*) is important.

FIGURE 25.2   Approximate Time Course of Insulin

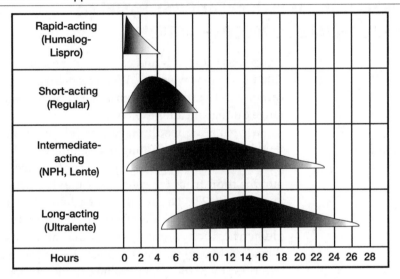

Adapted with permission from: Nutrition Dimensions Inc. Pastors JG. *Nutrition Care of Diabetes*. 2nd ed. San Marcos, Calif: *Nutrition Dimensions*; 1995.

Intensive insulin therapy, either multiple daily injections (MDI) or continuous subcutaneous insulin infusion (CSII), is considered standard treatment for type 1 diabetes (26). The advantage of intensive therapy is that it offers multiple opportunities to adjust insulin dosages throughout the day. Adjustments for exercise can thus be made with great precision. Conventional, or twice daily insulin therapy, offers fewer opportunities to manipulate dosages to reflect changes in insulin requirements. Therefore, adjustments for exercise tend to be less precise. Dosages of intermediate or long-acting insulin are significantly higher in conventional therapy than in intensive therapy, which predominately uses rapid or short-acting insulin. Longer-acting insulin(s) can cause sustained hyperinsulinemia and therefore impede glycemic control during and after intense or prolonged activity (26). For these reasons intensive therapy is more likely to allow safe and optimal exercise performance and is certainly the therapy of choice for athletes with type 1 diabetes.

Dosages of insulin may need to be modified for an extended time after extreme or prolonged activity, when insulin sensitivity and muscle glycogen repletion are increased. The period of heightened sensitivity to insulin can last for up to 36 hours after extreme or unusual exercise. Reduction in insulin dosages during this period may be necessary to prevent postexercise hypoglycemia, which can be quite severe. Frequent SMBG, including monitoring during the night (eg, at 3:00 AM) is an advisable precautionary measure. In contrast, high-intensity, short-duration activity can result in postexercise hyperglycemia due to counter-regulatory hormone release and excessive hepatic glucose production (21,26). BG elevation in this situation is usually transient, and use of supplemental insulin as a corrective measure is not indicated. Extra insulin could cause hypo-glycemia if its action should coincide with an increase in insulin sensitivity postexercise (26).

INTERPRETATION OF BLOOD GLUCOSE PATTERNS AND APPROPRIATE CORRECTIVE ACTIONS

Pre-exercise BG levels and changes that occur during and after exercise reflect circulating insulin levels (22). When diabetes medications are properly adjusted and carbohydrate intake appropriate, BG levels should remain in a desired target range during and after exercise.

If circulating insulin levels are elevated, glucose will enter the exercising muscle cell rapidly, resulting in a significant fall in BG (21). Too much circulating insulin also restricts glucose production by the liver and reduces free fatty acid mobilization from fat cells, thus making other important fuels for exercise unavailable (22). The result can be hypoglycemia. The appropriate corrective action is to reduce the dosage of insulin or oral antidiabetes medication and supplement carbohydrate in controlled amounts at the next exercise session. Whenever hypoglycemia is suspected, exercise must be delayed until the BG level is verified by SMBG. A BG value ≤70 mg/dL indicates hypoglycemia. This must be treated appropriately before exercise is resumed (27) (see *Figure 25.3*).

If circulating insulin levels are too low, glucose has difficulty entering exercising muscle cells. Glucose production and release from the liver, and fatty acid mobilization are increased. The result can be significant hyperglycemia and keto-sis (4,7,21,22). If pre-exercise BG is ≥250 mg/dL, urine ketones should always be tested. The combination of a BG value ≥250 mg/dL and positive ketones or ≥300 mg/dL with or without ketones indicates insulinopenia and poor metabolic control (1). Supplemental insulin should be administered and exercise should be delayed until improved metabolic control is achieved (7). Intake of noncaloric fluids should be encouraged to prevent dehydration associated with hyperglycemia and to help clear ketones. Moderate hyperglycemia in the absence of ketones is often due to factors such as prior dietary indiscretion or psychological stress. If such is the case, exercise will usually result in a reduction in BG and improved control.

FIGURE 25.3   Carbohydrate Supplement Use during Exercise

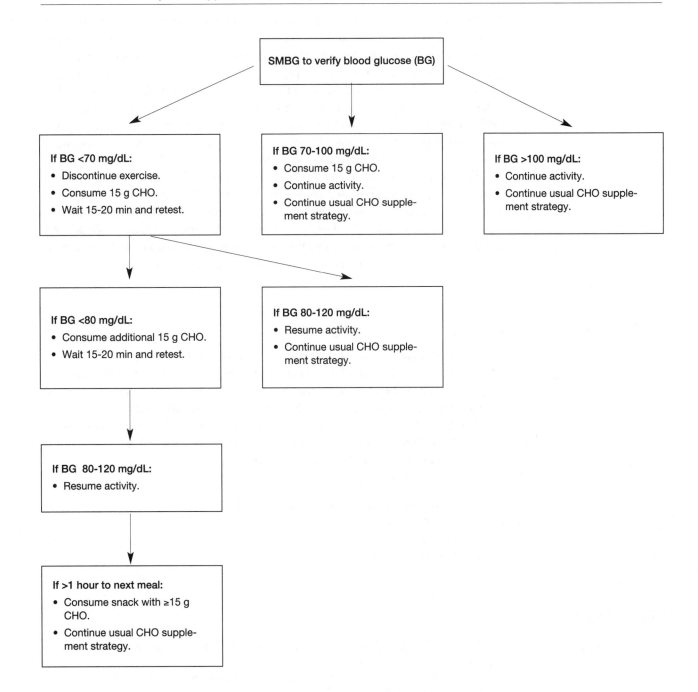

CONCLUSION

For individuals with type 2 diabetes, regular physical activity can improve BG control and may even alleviate symptoms of the disease. However, for individuals with type 1 diabetes, exercise does not have the same tendency to improve glycemic control. Rather, it has the potential to cause significant BG fluctuations and considerable management challenges (7). Even so, all individuals with diabetes should be encouraged to live active lifestyles in order to achieve the many health benefits of vigorous living. The athlete with diabetes, who is striving for competitive performance, should be offered the support and self-management training needed to achieve optimal performance.

This chapter presents general guidelines and strategies for adapting diabetes medications and MNT to accommodate exercise. The information presented should be considered a starting point. Strategies must be modified and individualized based on uniqueness of each client and each exercise situation. SMBG and pattern management allow successful strategies to be developed and fine-tuned, in order to minimize exercise risk while maximizing performance.

RESOURCE

The International Diabetic Athletes Association (IDAA)
This nonprofit service association is dedicated to encouraging an active lifestyle for people with diabetes. Members include individuals with diabetes who participate in fitness activities at all levels, health care professionals, and everyone interested in the relationship between diabetes and exercise. IDAA's mission is to enhance the quality of life for people with diabetes through exercise.

For more information about IDAA contact:

International Diabetic Athletes Association
1647 West Bethany Home Road Suite B
Phoenix, AZ 85015-2507
Tel: (602) 433-2113
Fax: (602) 433-9331

REFERENCES

1. American Diabetes Association. Position statement: Diabetes mellitus and exercise. *Diabetes Care*. 1998;21:S40-S44.
2. Barnard RJ, Jung T, Inkeles SB. Diet and exercise in the treatment of NIDDM. *Diabetes Care*. 1994;17:1469-1472.
3. Young JC. Exercise prescription for individuals with metabolic disorders, practical considerations. *Sports Med*. 1995;19:43-45.
4. Martin IK, Wahren J. Glucose metabolism during physical exercise in patients with non-insulin-dependent (Type II) diabetes. *Adv Exp Med Biol*. 1993;334:221-223.

5. Vanninen E, Uusitupa M, Siitonen O, Laitinen J, Lansimies E. Habitual physical activity, aerobic capacity, and metabolic control in patients with newly diagnosed type 2 (non-insulin-dependent) diabetes mellitus: effect of 1-year diet and exercise intervention. *Diabetologia*. 1992;35:340-346.

6. Raguso CA, Coggan AR, Gastadelli A, Sidossis LS, Bastyr EJ III, Wolfe RR. Lipid and carbohydrate metabolism in IDDM during moderate and intense exercise. *Diabetes*. 1995;44:1066-1074.

7. Wasserman DH, Zinman B. Fuel homeostasis. In: Ruderman N, Devlin JT, eds. *The Health Professional's Guide to Exercise and Diabetes*. Alexandria, Va: American Diabetes Association; 1995:29-47.

8. The Expert Committee on the Diagnosis and Classification of Diabetes Mellitus. The report of the expert committee on the diagnosis and classification of diabetes mellitus. *Diabetes Care*. 1998;21:S5-S19.

9. American Diabetes Association. Nutrition recommendations and principles for people with diabetes mellitus. *Diabetes Care*. 1998;21:S32-S35.

10. King AC, Tribble DL. The role of exercise in weight regulation in nonathletes. *Sports Med*. 1991;11:331-349.

11. Bouchard C, Depres JP, Tremblay A. Exercise and obesity. *Obes Res*. 1993;1:133-147.

12. Wood PD, Stefanick ML, Williams PT, Haskelll WL. The effects on plasma lipoproteins of a prudent weight-reducing diet, with or without exercise, in overweight men and women. *N Engl J Med*. 1991;325:461-466.

13. Setter SM. New drug therapies for the treatment of diabetes. *On the Cutting Edge*. 1998;19(2):3-5.

14. Sharp AR. Nutrition implications of new medications to treat diabetes. *On the Cutting Edge*. 1998;19(2):8-10.

15. Brodows R. Repaglinide (Prandin): a new therapy for type 2 diabetes. *Practical Diabetology*. 1998;17(2):32-36.

16. Rassmussen OW, Lauszus FF, Hermansen K. Effects of postprandial exercise on glycemic response in IDDM subjects. *Diabetes Care*. 1994;17:1203-1205.

17. US Department of Health and Human Services. *Physical Activity and Health: A Report from the Surgeon General*. Atlanta, Ga: US Dept Health and Human Services, Centers for Disease Control and Prevention, National Center for Chronic Disease Prevention and Health Promotion; 1996.

18. Dela F, Larsen JJ, Mikines KJ, Plough T, Petersen LN, Galbo H. Insulin-stimulated muscle glucose clearance in patients with NIDDM: effects of one-legged physical training. *Diabetes*. 1995;44:1010-1020.

19. Yamamouchi K, Shinokazi T, Chikada K, et al. Daily walking combined with diet therapy is a useful means for obese NIDDM patients not only to reduce body weight but also to improve insulin sensitivity. *Diabetes Care*. 1995;18:775-778.

20. Centers for Disease Control and Prevention. *National Diabetes Fact Sheet: National Estimates and General Information on Diabetes in the United States*. Atlanta, Ga: US Dept Health and Human Services, Centers for Disease Control and Prevention; 1997.

21. Richter EA, Turcotte L, Hespel P, Kiens B. Metabolic responses to exercise: effects of endurance training and implications for diabetes. *Diabetes Care*. 1992;15:1767-1776.

22. Exercise. In: Walsh J, Roberts R, eds. *Pumping Insulin*. 2nd ed. San Diego, Calif: Torrey Pines Press; 1995:83-95.

23. Franz MJ. Nutrition, exercise, and diabetes. In: Ruderman N, Devlin JT, eds. *The Health Professional's Guide to Exercise and Diabetes*. Alexandria, Va: American Diabetes Association; 1995:101-108.

24. Zinman B. Exercise and the pump. In: Fredrickson L, ed. *The Insulin Pump Therapy Book*. Los Angeles, Calif: Minimed Inc; 1995:106-115.

25. Sherman WM, Ferrara C, Schneider B. Nutritional strategies to optimize athletic performance. In: Ruderman N, Devlin JT, eds. *The Health Professional's Guide to Exercise and Diabetes*. Alexandria, Va: American Diabetes Association; 1995:91-98.

26. Berger M. Adjustment of insulin therapy. In: Ruderman N, Devlin JT, eds. *The Health Professional's Guide to Exercise and Diabetes*. Alexandria, Va: American Diabetes Association; 1995:116-122.

27. Special topics in meal planning. In: Holler HJ, Pastors JG, eds. *Diabetes Medical Nutrition Therapy*. Chicago, Ill: The American Dietetic Association; 1997:83-92.

28. Franz MJ. Exercise and diabetes mellitus. In: Powers MA, ed. *Handbook of Diabetes Nutritional Management*. Rockville, Md: Aspen Publishers; 1987:73-89.

29. Daly A, Barry B, Gillespie S, Kulkarni K, Richardson M. *Carbohydrate Counting: Moving On*. Chicago, Ill: The American Dietetic Association; 1995.

30. Management of diabetes: self-monitoring of blood glucose. In: Holler HJ, Pastors JG, eds. *Diabetes Medical Nutrition Therapy*. Chicago, Ill: The American Dietetic Association; 1997:43-49.

26

VEGETARIAN ATHLETES

D. Enette Larson, PhD, RD

An increasing number of athletes and active individuals are adopting vegetarian diets for health, ecological, religious, spiritual, economical, and ethical reasons. Vegetarian diets—except fruitarian and strict macrobiotic diets—can easily provide the nutritional requirements for all types of athletes if they contain a variety of plant foods. Vegetarian athletes, like most athletes, may benefit from education on food choices that provide adequate nutrients for promoting optimal performance and good health.

SPORTS NUTRITION CONSIDERATIONS

Energy and Macronutrient Requirements

Energy. The energy needs of active vegetarians vary considerably and depend on the athlete's body size, body composition, gender, training regimen, and activity pattern. Energy expenditure, assessed by doubly labeled water, is shown to vary from ~2,600 kcal per day in female swimmers to ~8,500 kcal per day in male cyclists participating in the Tour de France bicycle race (1). The energy requirements of smaller or less active individuals may be slightly less.

In clinical practice an athlete's daily energy expenditure (DEE) must be estimated since methods like doubly labeled water are expensive and not practical. Daily energy expenditure can be approximated by directly estimating DEE or by estimating the components of DEE which include resting energy expenditure, energy cost of occupational and spontaneous physical activity (nontraining physical activity), and energy cost of training or organized physical exercise. (Refer to the Tools section for specifics on estimating the energy cost of physical activities.) It is interesting to note, however, that resting energy expenditure is acutely elevated after exercise (2) and is shown to be ~11% higher in vegetarians compared to nonvegetarians. This appears to be partially mediated by the habitual high-carbohydrate composition of the diet in combination with increased basal sympathetic nervous system activity (3). Any effects of habitual exercise or diet on resting energy expenditure are not accounted for in predictive equations. While the estimation of DEE from its components may be more cumbersome, it accounts for more variation in activity patterns and can also serve as an educational tool when calculated in the athlete's presence. Estimating DEE is useful when developing meal plans and when evaluating adequacy of energy intake (along with body weight changes and dietary intake assessments).

It is reported that athletes who follow vegetarian and especially vegan diets have difficulty meeting energy requirements due to the energy density of plant-based diets (4). While this may be true in some cases, nutritionists are likely to encounter active vegetarians with a variety of energy needs. Some will need to consume 6 to 8 meals/snacks per day to meet energy needs. Others may require weight loss for health and/or performance reasons. The Vegetarian Pyramid (see *Figure 26.1*) or eating plans, such as those developed by Houtkooper (5) and Messina and Messina (6), are helpful for educating vegetarian and vegan athletes. *Box 26.1* contains sample menus for a 3,000 kcal vegetarian diet and a 4,500 kcal vegan diet.

FIGURE 26.1   Food Guide Pyramid for Vegetarian Meal Planning

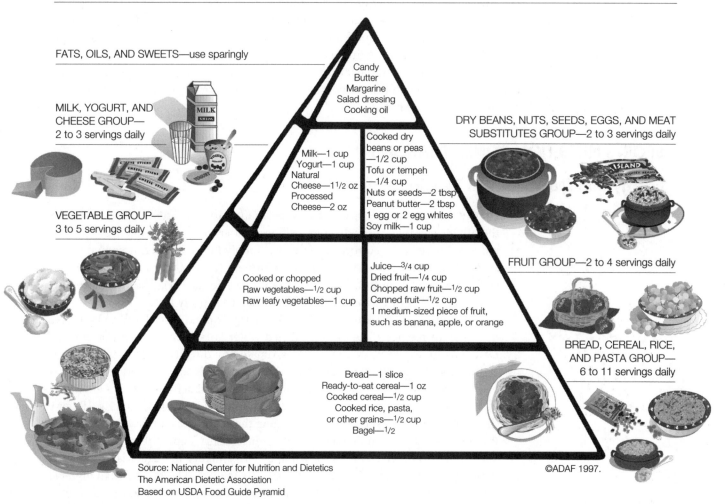

FATS, OILS, AND SWEETS—use sparingly

Candy
Butter
Margarine
Salad dressing
Cooking oil

MILK, YOGURT, AND CHEESE GROUP—
2 to 3 servings daily

DRY BEANS, NUTS, SEEDS, EGGS, AND MEAT
SUBSTITUTES GROUP—2 to 3 servings daily

Milk—1 cup
Yogurt—1 cup
Natural
Cheese—1 1/2 oz
Processed
Cheese—2 oz

Cooked dry
beans or peas
—1/2 cup
Tofu or tempeh
—1/4 cup
Nuts or seeds—2 tbsp
Peanut butter—2 tbsp
1 egg or 2 egg whites
Soy milk—1 cup

VEGETABLE GROUP—
3 to 5 servings daily

Cooked or chopped
Raw vegetables—1/2 cup
Raw leafy vegetables—1 cup

Juice—3/4 cup
Dried fruit—1/4 cup
Chopped raw fruit—1/2 cup
Canned fruit—1/2 cup
1 medium-sized piece of fruit,
such as banana, apple, or orange

FRUIT GROUP—2 to 4 servings daily

BREAD, CEREAL, RICE,
AND PASTA GROUP—
6 to 11 servings daily

Bread—1 slice
Ready-to-eat cereal—1 oz
Cooked cereal—1/2 cup
Cooked rice, pasta,
or other grains—1/2 cup
Bagel—1/2

Source: National Center for Nutrition and Dietetics
The American Dietetic Association
Based on USDA Food Guide Pyramid

©ADAF 1997.

BOX 26.1   Sample 3,000 and 4,500 Calorie Vegetarian Menus

3,000 calorie	4,500 calorie
Breakfast	**Breakfast**
1 cup raisin bran	1 1/2 cups raisin bran
1 cup skim milk	1 cup fortified soy milk
2 slices mixed-grain toast	3 slices mixed-grain toast
2 t soy margarine	3 t soy margarine
1 medium banana	1 medium banana
8 oz fruit juice	8 oz fruit juice
Lunch	**Lunch**
Veggie whole-wheat pita stuffed with shredded spinach, sliced tomato, 2 oz feta cheese, 2 t olive oil	Tofu salad on a 4 oz hoagie roll (1 cup firm tofu, 2 t mustard, 2 t soy mayonnaise, lettuce, tomato)
1 large apple	1 large apple
2 small oatmeal cookies	3 small oatmeal cookies
Snack	8 oz carrot juice
Sesame seed bagel	**Snack**
1 T peanut butter	Sesame seed bagel
1 T jam	1 T peanut butter and 1 T jam
Dinner	1 cup fortified soy milk
Lentil spaghetti sauce (1 cup cooked lentils, 1/2 onion, 1 1/2 cups canned tomatoes, 1 T olive oil)	**Dinner**
3 oz dry pasta, cooked	Lentil spaghetti sauce (1 1/2 cups cooked lentils, 1/2 onion, 1 1/2 cups canned tomatoes, 1 T olive oil)
1 T parmesan cheese	4 oz dry pasta, cooked
2 (1 oz) slices french bread dipped in 1 T olive oil	3 (1 oz) slices french bread dipped in 2 T olive oil
1 cup steamed broccoli	1 1/2 cups steamed collards
Snack	**Snack**
1 cup fruit yogurt	1 cup fruit sorbet
	1 oz toasted almonds

3,066 kcal, 106 g protein, 469 g carbohydrate, 85 g fat (14% protein, 25% fat, 61% carbohydrate), 1,600 mg calcium, 29 mg iron, 14 mg zinc

Note: Both menus assume grain products are made from enriched flour.

Carbohydrate. Carbohydrates should make up the bulk of the athlete's diet. High-carbohydrate diets optimize muscle and liver glycogen stores (7,8) and optimize performance during prolonged, moderate-intensity exercise (ie, distance running and cycling) (9-12) and during intermittent and short-duration, high-intensity exercise (13-15), which includes sprinting performance at the end of an endurance bout of exercise (16). Thus, for many athletes and active vegetarians this translates into a longer playing (or exercising) time before fatigue and faster sprinting potential at the end of a race or event. The benefit of carbohydrate consumption, however, may not be limited to maintenance of glycogen stores; it may also be related to maintenance of Krebs cycle intermediates (12) and preservation of the bioenergetic state of exercising muscle (15), factors also related to muscle fatigue.

While carbohydrate needs of active individuals can be easily met on a vegetarian diet, active individuals at all levels may benefit from education on carbohydrate recommendations and dietary carbohydrate sources. Active vegetarians should strive for the recommended 60% to 65% of total energy as carbohydrates (17). College, elite, or other competitive athletes in heavy training may benefit from following the recommended 7 to 10 g/kg of body weight (18). In practice, however, 6 to 8 g/kg are more appropriate guidelines for smaller female athletes. Carbohydrate exchanges and label-reading exercises are useful in all cases and are usually well received. Knowledge of carbohydrate sources is also useful in planning carbohydrate intake before, during, and after exercise.

Protein. Protein needs of athletes vary according to the type of activity and level of training. Protein needs of active vegetarians who perform light to moderate activity several times a week are very likely met by the Recommended Dietary Allowances (RDA) of 0.8 g/kg of body weight while protein requirements of more heavily training athletes may be considerably higher than the RDA. The American and Canadian Dietetic Associations recommend that athletes consume 1.5 g of protein/kg of body weight (17). These recommendations are no different for vegetarian athletes. Lemon (19) suggests that protein requirements are approximately 1.2 to 1.4 g/kg per day for endurance athletes and as high as 1.6 to 1.7 g/kg per day for strength athletes. The rationale for the additional required protein in endurance and strength training results from increased protein utilization as an auxiliary fuel during exercise and, to a lesser degree, protein deposition during muscle development. Inadequate intakes of carbohydrate and total energy also increase protein needs. During prolonged endurance activity, athletes with low glycogen stores metabolize twice as much protein as those with adequate stores primarily due to increased gluconeogenesis (20). There is currently no evidence to suggest that adult vegetarian and vegan athletes need more protein than omnivorous athletes to account for the general "lower biological" value of plant proteins, as implied by Lemon (19), as long as the diet provides adequate energy and contains a variety of protein-containing plant foods (21). However, research specifically focusing on the protein requirements of heavily training vegetarian athletes is needed.

Vegetarian athletes can easily achieve adequate protein providing their diet is adequate in energy and contains a variety of plant-based protein foods such as legumes, grains, nuts, and seeds. As reviewed by Young and Pellett (21), vegetarians need not be concerned with eating "complementary proteins" at each meal, but with choosing a variety of protein over the course of a day. Vegetarian diets generally contain 12.5% of energy from protein while vegan diets contain 11% (6). An 80-kg male athlete consuming 3,600 kcal would receive 1.41 g/kg of protein from the average vegetarian diet and 1.2 g/kg of protein from the average vegan diet. A 50-kg female gymnast consuming 2,200 kcal would receive 1.38 g/kg from a vegetarian diet and 1.21 g/kg from a vegan diet. Thus, most vegetarian athletes meet the requirements for endurance training without special meal planning. Strength-trained athletes (weightlifters, football players, wrestlers) or those with high training levels or low energy intakes may need to include more protein-rich foods. This is easily accomplished by encouraging the athlete to add one to three servings of protein-rich vegetarian foods (eg, soy milk shake to breakfast, lentils to spaghetti sauce, tofu to stir-fry, or garbanzo beans to salad). *Table 26.1* provides a list of commercially available protein-rich vegetarian foods.

TABLE 26.1   Nutrient Content of Selected Whole and Commercially Available Protein Foods

Food	Protein (g)	Fat (g)	CHO (g)	Kcal	Calcium (mg)	Iron (mg)	Zinc (mg)
Legumes*							
Black beans, 1 cup	15	1	41	227	46	3.6	1.9
Chickpeas, 1 cup	14.5	4	45	270	80	4.7	2.5
Kidney beans, 1 cup	15	1	40	225	50	5.2	1.9
Lentils, 1 cup	18	1	40	230	38	6.6	2.5
Pinto beans, 1 cup	14	1	44	234	90	4.5	1.9
Tempeh, 1 cup	16	6	14	165	85	1.9	1.5
Tofu, firm, 1 cup	20	11	5	183	258	13	1
Tofu, soft, 1 cup	10	6	2	94	130	6	2
Vegetarian Patties							
Advantage/10 Southwestern	8	1	24	140	40	4.2	na
Amy's Organic Vegetables, Texas [†]	12	2.5	15	130	40	1.8	na
Boca Burger, Vegan Original	12	0	9	84	50	1.4	na
Gardenburger, Original [†]	8	3	18	130	80	tr	na
Gardenburger, Classic Greek [†]	6	3	17	120	80	1.1	na
Gardenburger, Hamburger Style [†]	16	2.5	7	110	100	1.8	na
Gardenburger, Vegan	11	0	23	140	20	0.7	na
Lightlife, BBQ Grilles [†]	10	3.5	11	120	20	1.8	na
Lightlife, Tamari Grilles [†]	11	5	9	120	40	1.8	na
Morningstar Grillers [†]	14	6	5	140	40	1.4	na
Morningstar Garden Veggie Patty [†]	10	2.5	9	100	40	0.7	na
Vegetarian Dogs							
Morningstar Veggie Dogs [†]	11	0.5	6	80	0	2.7	na
Yves Tofu Wieners	9	0.5	2	45	20	1.1	na
Protein Crumbles							
Marjon Tofu Crumbles, 2.5 oz	6	3	2	55	60	1.6	na
Morningstar Protein Granules, 3 T	10	1	6	70	40	1.8	4.5
Morningstar Crumbles, 2/3 cup	10	3	4	90	1.5	na	na
Meatless Slices							
Lightlife, Turkey Style, 3 slices	9	0	1	40	20	2.7	na
Lightlife, Country Ham Style	10	0	2	50	0	5.4	na

* Legumes are cooked. Boiled values obtained from Pennington JAT. *Bowes and Church's Food Values of Portions Commonly Used.* 16th ed. Philadelphia, Penn: JB Lippincott; 1994.

† Vegetarian but not vegan. Ingredients include eggs, dairy products, or honey.

Fat. Dietary fat should make up the remainder of energy intake after carbohydrate and protein needs are met. The American and Canadian Dietetic Associations recommend that no more than 30% of total energy intake should come from fat (17). An athlete's diet, however, should not be too low in fat as certain quantities are needed not only for absorption of fat-soluble vitamins, but also to maintain intramuscular triglyceride stores. Researchers have become interested in intramuscular triglycerides as a fuel during exercise (22) and have speculated that a certain amount of fat may be required to maintain intramuscular triglycerides (23) which may serve as an important fuel during moderate to heavy exercise (24).

Some vegetarian athletes, particularly endurance-trained groups (runners and triathletes), may go overboard with the desire to consume a high-carbohydrate diet and consume too little fat. Similarly, while the extremely low-fat (<10%) vegetarian diets recommended by Ornish et al (25) may be beneficial to those with a personal or family history of cardiovascular disease (ie, the postmyocardial infarction (MI) recreational athlete), they may be too restrictive for athletes during heavy training. Incorporating high-fat foods (particularly those high in mono- and polyunsaturated fats) such as nuts and seeds, nut butters, tahini, avocados, olives, olive oil, and sesame oil may make it easier for vegetarian athletes to meet energy and nutrient needs, and ensure that intramuscular triglycerides are not compromised (26). On the other hand, nutritionists can still expect to encounter vegetarian athletes and active persons with diets that are lacking in carbohydrate and too rich in saturated fat, mainly from full-fat dairy products or processed foods.

Minerals and Vitamins

Calcium. Regular exercise has not been shown to increase calcium requirements above the RDA. Recently, however, a study by Klesges et al (27) found that large amounts of calcium were lost in sweat during intense training in male basketball players, suggesting that additional calcium may be required to offset dermal loss. While of interest to sports nutritionists, the methodology used in this study and the validity of the results were severely criticized (28,29), suggesting that further research is needed before nutritionists recommend additional calcium to athletes. Nevertheless, other research has found that females with low circulating estrogen may require an intake of 1,500 mg per day to retain calcium balance (30). Thus, higher calcium intake may be required for postmenopausal and amenorrheic female athletes. On the other hand, there is evidence to suggest that vegans (and likely vegetarians who consume few dairy products) have lower calcium requirements than suggested by the RDAs due to their lower intake of animal protein, total protein, and/or sodium, all of which stimulate calcium loss in the urine (6). The mechanism for the calciuric effect of protein is not known but is thought to be dependent on the quantity of sulfur-containing amino acids (31). (For an extensive review of this topic see reference 6.) Until more is known about calcium requirements in this group, however, it is prudent that vegetarian athletes at least meet the RDA for calcium. Low calcium intake has been associated with an increased risk of stress fractures (32), decreased bone mineral content (27), and decreased bone density, particularly in anemorrheic athletes (33).

Eumenorrheic athletes can meet calcium requirements by including several servings of dairy products and/or calcium-containing plant foods daily. Plant foods that are rich in well-absorbable calcium include low-oxalate green leafy vegetables (collard, mustard, and turnip greens), calcium-set tofu, fortified soy and rice milks, textured vegetable protein, tahini, certain legumes, fortified orange juice, almonds, and blackstrap molasses. With the exception of legumes, calcium in these foods is absorbed as efficiently as, if not better than, dairy products (34). From their extensive laboratory analysis, Weaver and Plawecki (34) have estimated that fractional absorption (adjusted for calcium load in a typical serving size) is between 31% to 68% for the aforementioned plant foods, 32% for milk, and 17% for legumes. However, foods with a high oxalate or phytate content such as spinach, swiss chard, beet greens, and rhubarb are not well-absorbed sources of calcium. *Table 26.2* lists the calcium content of selected vegetarian foods. Depending on their energy intake and food choices, female vegans may need to use fortified foods or calcium supplements to meet calcium requirements, particularly when amenorrhea is evident. Well-absorbed and inexpensive calcium supplements such as calcium carbonate are appropriate when the athlete does not have access to or cannot afford calcium-fortified foods (eg, college athletes). Recent evidence has suggested that long-term supplementation with calcium carbonate does not compromise iron status in iron-replete adult onmivores and vegetarians (35), but it is preferable that calcium supplements be consumed at bedtime rather that with iron-containing meals (36).

TABLE 26.2   Calcium Content of Selected Foods

Food	Calcium (mg)
Vegetables (1/2 cup cooked)	
Bok choy	79
Broccoli	36
Cabbage, green	30
Collard greens	74
Dandelion greens	73
Kale	90
Mustard greens	75
Turnip greens	99
Legumes (1/2 cup cooked)	
Chickpeas	40
Great northern beans	61
Navy beans	64
Pinto beans	45
Soybeans	86
Tempeh	85
Tofu (calcium-set)	258
Vegetarian baked beans	64
Nuts and Seeds	
Almonds, 1/4 cup	94
Almond butter, 2 T	86
Brazil nuts, 1/4 cup	62
Tahini, 2 T	128

continued

TABLE 26.2   Calcium Content of Selected Foods (continued)

Food	Calcium (mg)
Milks (1 cup)	
Cow's milk	300
Rice milk, fortified	240
Soymilk	20-80
Soymilk, fortified	200-500
Other Foods	
Yogurt, 1 cup	400
Soy cheese, 1 oz	200-300
Blackstrap molasses, 2 T	274
Calcium-fortified cereal (eg Total), 1 oz	200-250
Orange juice, calcium-fortified, 6 oz	240
Cheddar cheese, 1 oz	204
Figs, 5 medium	135
Hummus, 1/2 cup	62
Orange, 1 medium	56
Bread, whole-wheat, 2 slices	25-40

Source: Vegetarian Nutrition Dietetic Practice Group. *Calcium in Vegetarian Diets*. Chicago, Ill: The American Dietetic Association; 1995.

Iron. All athletes, particularly female endurance athletes, are at risk for iron depletion and iron deficiency anemia. Iron loss may be increased in some athletes, particularly heavily training endurance athletes, due to gastrointestinal bleeding (37), heavy sweating (38), and hemolysis (39). Insufficient iron intake or reduced absorption, however, are the most probable causes of poor iron status. Snyder et al (40) found that female vegetarian runners had a similar iron intake but lower iron status than nonvegetarian runners, a finding that has been well documented in nonathletes (6). Most of the iron in a vegetarian diet is nonheme iron which has a relatively low absorption rate (2% to 20%) compared with heme iron (15% to 35%) (41). This may be of significance since low iron stores, even without anemia, have been associated with decreased endurance (42) and maximal oxygen uptakes (43).

In most cases vegetarian athletes can achieve proper iron status without iron supplementation. However, these athletes should be educated on plant sources of iron (see *Table 26.3*) and factors that enhance and interfere with nonheme iron absorption (see *Box 26.2*) (41). For example, an athlete who consumes milk or tea with legumes at a meal could be advised to replace the beverage with citrus fruit juice to enhance the iron absorbed from that meal. In some cases active individuals may require supplements to replenish or maintain iron stores. However, iron status (serum ferritin level or serum iron-binding capacity) should be determined before iron supplementation is considered. Athletes taking iron supplements should have iron status monitored due to the prevalence of hemochromatosis in the United States and the potential association between iron status and chronic disease (44).

TABLE 26.3 Iron Content of Plant Foods

Food	Iron (mg)
Legumes (1/2 cup cooked)	
Soybeans	2.7
Lima beans	2.0
Red kidney beans	1.8
Lentils	1.6
Peas	1.5
Grains and Pasta (1 cup cooked)	
Oatmeal	1.7
Spaghetti, enriched	1.4
Macaroni, enriched	1.4
Brown rice	0.8
Whole-wheat bread, 1 slice	0.8
Vegetables	
Collards, 1/2 cup cooked	1.0
Tomato, medium	0.8
Broccoli, 1/2 cup cooked	0.7
Potato, medium	0.7
Nuts and Seeds (1 oz)	
Sunflower seeds	2.2
Almonds	1.3
Peanuts	1.0
Fruits and Dried Fruits	
Prunes, 5 large	1.7
Dates, 5 medium	1.5
Watermelon, 1 slice (15 cm x 2 cm)	1.5
Strawberries, 5 large	1.0
Raisins (1 oz)	1.0
Orange juice, 1 cup	1.0
Figs, 5 medium	0.9
Pineapple juice, 1 cup	0.8
Orange, medium	0.6

Source: Craig W. Iron content of plant foods. *Am J Clin Nutr*. 1994;59(suppl):1233S-1237S.

BOX 26.2   Factors that Influence the Absorption of Nonheme Iron

Substances that inhibit nonheme-iron absorption:

- Phytates
- Plant polyphenolics
- High dietary amounts of zinc and other divalent cations
- Soy protein
- Bran
- Egg
- Milk
- Tea and coffee
- Calcium-rich antacids
- Calcium phosphates

continued

BOX 26.2   Factors that Influence the Absorption of Nonheme Iron (continued)

Substances that enhance nonheme-iron absorption

- Ascorbic acid
- Meat, poultry, and fish
- Citric, malic, lactic, and tartaric acids, and other organic aids
- Fermentation products of soybean
- Other factors:
  — Low iron stores of individuals
  — Low iron content of meals
  — Iron in ferrous form

Source: Craig W. Factors that influence the absorption of nonheme iron. *Am J Clin Nutr*. 1994;59(suppl):1233S-1237S.

Zinc. Several studies have reported altered zinc status in athletes during heavy training (45). This finding, coupled with the reportedly low zinc intakes in athletes, has stimulated some concern that active persons may be at risk for compromised zinc status. Manore et al (46), however, has cautioned that apparent changes in zinc status due to exercise may be transient and that measurement of plasma zinc during heavy training periods may not reflect zinc status. Although more research is needed in this area, published studies have found that zinc supplementation does not influence zinc levels during training (46,47) and has no benefit on athletic performance (47).

Little is known regarding the zinc status of vegetarian athletes. Concern has been expressed, however, about the adequacy of zinc provided by vegetarian diets since the absorption of this mineral from plant foods is somewhat lower than from animal products due to higher phytate concentrations of plant foods (48). A recent study from the US Department of Agriculture found that women consuming a lacto-ovo-vegetarian diet containing legumes and whole grains for 8 weeks maintained zinc status within normal limits, even though the diet was lower in total zinc and higher in phytate and fiber than a control omnivorous diet (49). The authors advised that legumes and whole grains be consumed regularly, which is a wise suggestion for active vegetarians and athletes in heavy training. Plant sources of zinc include legumes, hard cheeses, whole-grain products, wheat germ, fortified cereals, nuts, tofu, and miso. The zinc content of selected protein-containing plant foods is shown in *Table 26.1*.

B Vitamins. Vegetarian diets can easily provide the requirements for most B vitamins. Depending on the type of vegetarian diet, however, riboflavin and B-12 are potential exceptions. Several studies have suggested that riboflavin needs are increased in individuals who begin an exercise program, particularly if riboflavin status is marginal (50,51). This could also be applicable to athletes who suddenly increase their training status. Since riboflavin intakes are reportedly low in some vegans (4), active vegetarians who avoid dairy products should be educated on the plant sources of riboflavin to ensure adequate intake. Plant sources of riboflavin include whole-grain and fortified cereals, soybeans, dark green leafy vegetables, avocado, nuts, and sea vegetables (sea weed, kombu, arame, sulse).

Vitamin B-12 has been of interest in athletic populations possibly due to its role in maintaining the cells of the hemopoietic and nervous systems. In fact, injections of B-12 are still used by some athletes and coaches because of the belief that the vitamin will increase oxygen and thereby enhance endurance performance. In the absence of actual deficiency, however, studies have failed to demonstrate any benefit of this practice (52) or of high-dose supplementation with a multivitamin (47). Since cobalamin, the active form of B-12, is found exclusively in animal products (53), vegan athletes need to regularly consume B-12–fortified foods which include Redstar brand nutritional yeast (T6635) and those brands of soymilk, breakfast cereals, and meat analogs that are B-12 fortified. While there is some evidence that large quantities of Nori and Chorella seaweeds can supply bioavailable B-12, sea vegetables should currently not be considered a reliable dietary source of this vitamin (54). Vegetarians who consume eggs, cheese, milk, or yogurt receive an ample supply of B-12 (53). Selected food sources of B-12 are listed in *Table 26.4*.

TABLE 26.4 Vitamin B-12 Content of Fortified Plant Foods

Food	B-12 (µg)
Commercial Cereals	
Grapenuts (1/4 cup)	1.5
Nutrigrain (2/3 cup)	1.5
Kellogg's Raisin Bran, (3/4 cup)	1.5
Meat Analogs (1 serving as listed by the package)	
Loma Linda "Chicken" Nuggets	3
Morningstar Farms Grillers	6.7
Loma Linda Sizzle Franks	2
Worthington Stakelets	5.2
Green Giant Harvest Burgers	1.5
Fortified Soymilk/Vegetable Milks (1 cup)	
Better Than Milk (soymilk)	0.6
Edensoy Extra	3
Insta-Soy	1.5
Sno E (soymilk)	1.2
Soyagen	1.5
Take Care (soymilk)	0.9
Vegelicious (vegetable milk)	0.6
White Tofu Drink	0.9
Other	
Nutritional Yeast, Red Star Brand T6635, 1 T	4

Source: Vegetarian Nutrition Dietetic Practice Group. *Vitamin B-12 in Vegan Diets.* Chicago, Ill: The American Dietetic Association; 1996.

Supplements

Vegetarian athletes, like other athletes, may inquire about nutritional supplements or ergogenic aids to assist their athletic training and performance. While a discussion of supplements is beyond the scope of this chapter, several supplements including protein, antioxidants, creatine, and carnitine may be of particular interest to vegetarian athletes.

Protein. As discussed above, the protein needs of vegetarian and vegan athletes can be met by diet alone. For convenience, liquid sports nutrition beverages (eg, Go, Boost, Carnation Instant Breakfast) or bars (eg, Tiger Sport, Genisoy) can be used occasionally to supplement the diet, but the athlete should understand that these products are not necessary and are not a replacement for food. Protein or amino acid supplements beyond the requirement do not improve performance or stimulate greater lean muscle gain (55).

Antioxidants. Increasing evidence is suggesting that vitamins C and E, and ß-carotene, and other phytochemicals may protect against exercise-induced "oxidative stress." Several recent reviews have summarized current knowledge of the potential benefits of anitoxidant supplements for protection against free radical production and lipid peroxidation (56,57). In brief, supplementation with antioxidants appears to reduce lipid peroxidation but has not been shown to enhance exercise performance. Whereas regular training is also found to augment endogenous antioxidant systems, athletes who train sporadically (ie, "weekend athletes") may particularly benefit from dietary antioxidants since it is not known if these athletes have the augmentation produced through continued training. While it remains controversial whether athletes or recreational exercisers could benefit from antioxidant supplements, there is no doubt that athletes should ingest foods rich in antioxidants. Vegetarian athletes may have an advantage because antioxidants are readily obtained from a diet rich in fruits, vegetables, nuts, seeds, and vegetable oils. One study has noted favorable values of prooxidative-antioxidative parameters in vegetarians compared to nonvegetarians, which was associated with a reduced risk of lipoperoxidations (58).

Creatine. Double blind, placebo-controlled studies have shown that creatine supplementation increased muscle concentrations of creatine by about 20% (59) and improved performance during repeated bouts of high-intensity activity (60-63) which includes strength-training (64,65). Most of the creatine found in the body is in skeletal muscle where it exists mostly as creatine phosphate (66), an important storage form of energy that buffers adenosine triphosphate (ATP) and thus serves to maintain the bioenergetic state of exercising muscle. The average dietary intake is about 2 g per day in omnivores (66) and negligible amounts in vegetarians since it is found primarily in muscle tissue. Even though creatine can be synthesized extramuscularly from amino acid precursors (66), serum (67), and skeletal muscle (59), creatine concentrations have been found to be lower in vegetarians compared to nonvegetarians. Thus, there is some thought that vegetarian athletes in particular may benefit from creatine supplementation. The one study that compared the effects of creatine supplementation in vegetarian compared to nonvegetarian athletes, however, did not report a greater benefit in the vegetarian group (68). According to the manufacturers, creatine is not synthesized using animal derivatives.

Carnitine. Carnitine plays a central role in the metabolism of fatty acids by transporting them from the cytosol to the mitochondrial matrix for β-oxidation. Carnitine is supplied by the diet from meat, poultry, fish, and some dairy (69) products but is not found in plant foods. Like creatine, serum concentrations of carnitine have been found to be lower in vegetarians (67) despite endogenous synthesis from lysine and methionine in the liver (69). Not surprisingly, carnitine has been targeted as a potential promoter of fat loss and endurance performance. Many well-controlled studies, however, have demonstrated that carnitine supplementation has no effect on fuel utilization at rest or during exercise and does not enhance endurance performance or promote body fat loss (69). Nevertheless, vegetarian athletes may be a target of aggressive marketing and express interest in this supplement.

Nutrition before, during, and after Exercise

Pre-exercise nutrition. Nutritional intake in the meal before a competition or exercise session should increase fuel stores, provide adequate hydration, and prevent both hunger and gastrointestinal distress. Studies have shown that consumption of between 1 and 5 g of carbohydrate/kg body weight 1 to 4 hours before endurance exercise has the potential to improve endurance performance by as much as 14% (18) and is also thought to benefit high-intensity activity lasting several hours. Vegetarian athletes should be encouraged to consume familiar, well-tolerated, high-carbohydrate meals that are low in sodium, simple sugars, and fiber. Vegetarian athletes who are used to eating "gas-producing" foods such as legumes, which are not typically recommended in the pre-event meal, may tolerate these foods without complication. Interestingly, several studies have suggested that consumption of carbohydrate with a low-glycemic index (lentils versus potatoes) 1 hour before exercise may prolong endurance during strenuous exercise by maintaining higher blood glucose concentrations toward the end of exercise (70,71) and may also confer an advantage by providing a slow-release source of glucose without an accompanying insulin surge (70). (The glycemic index of common foods can be found in the Tools section.) As with all athletes, the guidelines for fluid consumption should be followed. These include consuming at least 2 cups of fluid about 2 hours before exercise, followed with another 2 cups approximately 15 to 20 minutes before endurance exercise (17).

Supplementation during exercise. Carbohydrate ingestion at levels between 45 and 75 g per hour have been shown to benefit prolonged, moderate-intensity exercise (≥2 hours) and variable intensity exercise of shorter duration (10) presumably by maintaining blood glucose levels as endogenous glycogen stores become depleted. Ingestion of fluid replacement beverages, at the recommended concentration of 6% to 8% (72), easily provides carbohydrate requirements while simultaneously meeting fluid needs. Interestingly, both fluids and carbohydrate are shown to have an accumulative effect on performance (73). While commercial sports drinks work well, vegetarian athletes may prefer diluted fruit juice (4 oz juice in 4 oz water = 6% solution) or low-sodium vegetable juices such as carrot juice (7% solution). A pinch of table salt can also be added which may be beneficial for events lasting longer than 3 to 4 hours (72). On the other hand, vegetarians may prefer solid foods which work equally well provided they are ingested with water (74) and are easily digestible. In this case athletes should be instructed to consume approximately 8 oz (240 mL) of water with every 15 g of carbohydrate ingested (6% solution).

Postexercise nutrition. Glycogen and fluid replacement are the immediate concern after prolonged or strenuous exercise. Vegetarian athletes in heavy training should make an effort to consume carbohydrate immediately and at frequent intervals following exercise (75). Foods with a high glycemic index (76), or those containing both carbohydrate and protein (~1 g protein: 3 g CHO) may increase the rate of muscle glycogen storage after exercise by stimulating greater insulin secretion. Consumption of carbohydrate (1 g/kg body weight) or a carbohydrate protein combination after resistance training is also found to stimulate glycogen resynthesis (77) and reduce muscle protein degradation (ie, resulting in a more positive body protein balance) (78). Current recommendations for postexercise fluid requirements are to consume at least a pint of fluid for every pound of body weight deficit (79). Athletes participating in heavy, prolonged workouts should also make an effort to include sodium and potassium in the recovery meal(s). While vegetarians are likely to choose foods containing ample potassium (eg, fruits, vegetables), they may intentionally or unintentionally avoid sodium-containing foods. Sodium intake can be of concern during periods of heavy training (ie, the typical sweat loss is ~30 mEq/L or 690 mg of sodium per hour) (72) in athletes consuming diets containing limited processed food. Sodium replenishment is needed to help restore fluid and electrolyte balance. Thus, more liberal intakes of sodium are often appropriate in the athletic population.

SPECIAL CONCERNS FOR THE FEMALE ATHLETE

The prevalence of amenorrhea among exercising women is reported to be between 3.4% and 66% (80) with higher prevalence in runners as opposed to cyclists and swimmers (81). The cause of this secondary hypothalamic amenorrhea is unknown but may be related to training level, nutritional status, body composition changes, stress, and hormone changes with exercise (80). While some studies have noted higher prevalence of secondary amenorrhea among "vegetarians" (82,83), others have not (84). By definition, however, "vegetarians" in the former studies consumed "low-meat" diets and not necessarily vegetarian diets. In nonathletic females, Goldin et al (85) found lower circulating estrogen levels in vegetarians compared to nonvegetarians which were associated with higher fiber and lower fat intakes, higher fecal outputs, and two to three times more estrogens in feces. Among athletes several studies have generally found lower intakes of energy (83,86), protein (83,86), fat (83,87), and zinc (87), and higher intakes of fiber (87,88) and vitamin A (87) in amenorrheic compared to eumenorrheic athletes. These findings suggest that the nutrient composition of some vegetarian diets could be predisposing to amenorrhea.

Given the high prevalence of amenorrhea among athletic women, nutritionists should take a menstrual cycle history as part of the screening procedure and, if appropriate, refer the athlete for medical evaluation and treatment. Nutrition evaluation and education of vegetarian athletes should focus on adequacy of energy, protein, fat, zinc, and fiber intakes. If appropriate, amenorrheic athletes can increase energy intake and decrease fiber by consuming one-third to one-half of their cereal/grain servings from refined rather than whole-grain sources and by replacing some high-fiber fruit/vegetable servings with juice servings.

COUNSELING AND WORKING WITH VEGETARIAN ATHLETES

Assessment

Vegetarian athletes come in all sizes and shapes and have different reasons for being vegetarian. In the counseling session a dietary assessment is necessary to determine which foods are eliminated from the diets and what foods are acceptable. This will help in the evaluation of nutrient adequacy to ensure that nutrients in foods that are not consumed can be met with foods that are acceptable. Although definitions including "lacto-ovo-vegetarian," "lacto-vegetarian," "vegan," or "strict vegetarian" are commonly used to describe vegetarians, they are not always realistic. Vegetarians do not fall into distinct categories based on food selection or philosophies on vegetarianism. For example, two "lacto-ovo-vegetarians" may have very different eating philosophies concerning dairy products, which would require different types of nutrition education. One may consume several servings of dairy products a day, while the other may eat only cheese and the small amounts of dairy found in processed foods. Similarly, some "vegans" may be extremely strict, eliminating all commercially available foods that contain any ingredient that is animal derived or processed with an animal derivative (eg, commercial bread), while another will simply avoid foods of obvious animal origin. Also, some individuals claim to follow vegetarian diets when they mean that they avoid red meat or eat only fish.

A thorough diet history followed by an analysis of kilocalories and key nutrients such as fat, calcium, iron, zinc, riboflavin, and vitamin B-12 is the best way to get a reliable assessment of the vegetarian athlete's diet. Computer nutrient databases may be helpful, but many do not contain an adequate selection of vegetarian foods. In many cases it is useful to have the athlete keep food records and bring in food labels from any or all vegetarian products. In addition to the dietary assessment, it is often valuable to discuss why the active vegetarian has chosen a vegetarian diet. While health, ecology, animal welfare, and religion are admirable reasons, weight loss or lack of time is not. In fact, individuals who "don't eat meat" because it is the socially acceptable way to lose weight or because of shrinking time or food budgets have been labeled "new wave" vegetarians (89). These individuals may be health and nutrition risks because of their haphazard eating patterns and lack of the solid philosophy that drives many vegetarians in their desire to eat well. The focus in "new wave" vegetarians should be on improving the diet with healthier plant-based but not necessarily vegetarian foods. A final concern is that vegetarianism may be used as a convenient and socially acceptable way for individuals with eating disorders to reduce fat and energy intakes and thus mask their disordered eating behaviors. Clinical studies have found that a large number of anorexia nervosa patients profess to be vegetarian (90,91). A recent population-based survey has also noted that adolescents who report being "vegetarian" were more likely to engage in disordered eating behaviors (frequent dieting, binge eating, and self-induced vomiting) (92). Again, the motivation for following a vegetarian diet and the adequacy of energy intake may be valuable when screening for potential eating disorders.

Guidelines have been developed for counseling pregnant vegetarians (93) which are quite useful in working with any vegetarian (94). These have been adapted for vegetarian athletes and are listed in the *Box 26.3*. It is also important to remember that nutritional requirements are for essential nutrients not for specific foods.

BOX 26.3   Guidelines for Counseling Vegetarian Athletes

- Establish rapport.
- Reinforce positive nutrition practices.
- Prioritize nutrition concerns to help athlete choose appropriate dietary changes.
- Individualized counseling.

Adapted from: Johnston P. Counseling the pregnant vegetarian. *Am J Clin Nutr*. 1988;48:901-905.

RESOURCES FOR IMPROVING THE DIET

Some athletes or active persons, vegetarian or omnivorous, find selection of a varied diet to be difficult (94). Factors such as lack of knowledge of food preparation, lack of time, and economic constraints may lead to a monotonous diet. This pattern is very common in college athletes. Basic vegetarian cookbooks and videos can be used to provide ideas for increased dietary variety (see *Box 26.4*). A tour of the supermarket or natural food store will help identify products that are suitable for use by vegetarians. Vegetarian cooking classes for teams or individual athletes are also a great way to provide hands-on education and introduce new vegetarian foods and recipes.

BOX 26.4   Recommended Resources for Vegetarians

General Vegetarian

Being Vegetarian, by The American Dietetic Association. John Wiley Publishers, 1996. ISBN 0-471-34661-6

The Vegetarian Way: Total Health for You and Your Family, by Virginia Messina, MPH, RD and Mark Messina. Crown Trade Paperbacks, 1997. ISBN 0-157-88275-2

Vegetarian Journal. Bi-monthly publication by The Vegetarian Resource Group, PO Box 1463, Baltimore, MD 21203. ISSN 0885-7636. www.vrg.org

Vegetarian Cookbooks

Low-Fat Ways to Cook Vegetarian, edited by Susan M. McIntosh, MS, RD. Oxmoor House, 1996. ISBN 0-8487-2206-x

The Be Healthier Feel Stronger Vegetarian Cookbook, by Susan M. Kleiner, PhD, RD and Karen Friedman-Kester, MS, RD. A Simon & Schuster Macmillan Company, 1997. ISBN 0-02-861014-8

The Essential Vegetarian Cookbook, by Diana Shaw. Clarkson Potter/Publishers, 1997. ISBN 0-517-88268-x

Vegetarian Express: Easy, Tasty, and Healthy Menus in 28 Minutes (or Less), by Nava Atlas and Lillian Kayte. Little, Brown and Company, 1995. ISBN 0-316-05740-1

Vegetarian Professional

The Dietitian's Guide to Vegetarian Diets. Issues and Applications, by Mark Messina, PhD and Virginia Messina, MPH, RD. Aspen Publishers, Inc, 1996. ISBN 0-8342-0635-8

---

continued

> **BOX 26.4** Recommended Resources for Vegetarians (continued)
>
> **Vegetarian Quantity Recipes**
>
> *Campus Favorites: Quantity Vegetarian Recipes*, 2nd ed. Dietitians in College and University Food Service subgroup of Management in Healthcare Systems Dietetic Practice Group, 1995
>
> *Vegetarian Quantity Recipes*, by Debra Wasserman. The Vegetarian Resource Group. ISBN 0-931411-0804
>
> *Vegetarian Journal's Foodservice Update*, by The Vegetarian Resource Group, PO Box 1463, Baltimore, MD 21203. ISSN 1072-0820
>
> **Vegetarian Resources**
>
> The Vegetarian Resource Group, PO Box 1463, Baltimore, MD 21203. www.vrg.org
>
> Vegetarian Nutrition. A dietetic practice group of the American Dietetic Association.
>
> **Vegetarian Travel**
>
> *Vegetarian Journal's Guide to Natural Foods Restaurants in the US & Canada*, 3rd ed. Avery Publishing Group, Garden City Park, NY, 1998

CONCLUSION

Nutritionists can play an essential role in optimizing the health and performance of athletes and active persons following vegetarian diets. However, nutritionists who work with vegetarian athletes and their coaches and trainers need to be sensitive to and knowledgeable about vegetarian issues. In this setting the role of the nutritionist is to work with the athlete to ensure adequate nutritional status given his or her vegetarian beliefs, income, and lifestyle. While athletes should be encouraged to eat a wide variety of plant foods, they should not be told that they need poultry, fish, or dairy products to obtain adequate nutrition. The American Dietetic Association's position on vegetarian diets states that "appropriately planned vegetarian diets are healthful, are nutritionally adequate, and provide health benefits in the prevention and treatment of certain diseases" (95).

REFERENCES

1. Goran M. Variation in total energy expenditure in humans. *Obes Res*. 1995;3:59-66.
2. Poehlman E, Melby C, Goran M. The impact of exercise and diet restriction on daily energy expenditure. *Sports Med*. 1991;11:78-101.
3. Toth MJ, Poehlman ET. Sympathetic nervous system activity and resting metabolic rate in vegetarians. *Metabolism*. 1994;43:621-625.
4. Grandjean A. The vegetarian athlete. *Phys Sports Med*. 1987;15:191-194.
5. Houtkooper L. Food selection for endurance sports. *Med Sci Sports Exerc*. 1992;24:S349-S359.
6. Messina M, Messina V. *The Dietitian's Guide to Vegetarian Diets*. Gaithersburg, Md: Aspen Publishers Inc; 1996.
7. Bergstrom J, Hermansen L, Hultman E, Saltin B. Diet, muscle glycogen, and physical performance. *Acta Physiol Scand*. 1967;71:140-150.
8. Nilsson L, Hultman E. Liver glycogen in man—the effect of total starvation or a carbohydrate-poor diet followed by carbohydrate refeeding. *Scand J Clin Lab Invest*. 1973;32:325-330.

9. O'Keeffe K, Keith R, Wilson G, Blessing D. Dietary carbohydrate intake and endurance exercise performance of trained female cyclists. *Nutrition Research*. 1989;9:819-830.

10. Brewer J, Williams C, Patton A. The influence of high carbohydrate diets on endurance running performance. *Eur J Appl Phys*. 1988;57:698-706.

11. Coggan AR, Swanson SC. Nutritional manipulations before and during endurance exercise: effects on performance. *Med Sci Sports Exerc*. 1992;24:S331-S335.

12. Spencer M, Yan Z, Katz A. Carbohydrate supplementation attenuates IMP accumulation in human muscle during prolonged exercise. *Am J Physiol*. 1991;261:C71-C76.

13. Maughan R, Poole D. The effects of a glycogen-loading regimen on the capacity to perform anaerobic exercise. *Eur J Appl Phys*. 1981;46:211-219.

14. Pizza F, Flynn M, Duscha B, Holden J, Kubitz E. A carbohydrate loading regimen improves high intensity, short duration exercise performance. *Int J Sport Nutr*. 1995;5:110-116.

15. Larson DE, Hesslink RL, Hrovat MI, Fishman RS, Systrom DM. Dietary effects on exercising muscle metabolism and performance. *J Appl Physiol*. 1994;77:1108-1115.

16. Hargreaves M, Costill D, Coggan A, Fink W, Nishibata I. Effect of carbohydrate feedings on muscle glycogen utilization and exercise performance. *Med Sci Sports Exerc*. 1984;16:219-222.

17. Position of The American Dietetic Association and The Canadian Dietetic Association: Nutrition for physical fitness and athletic performance for adults. *J Am Diet Assoc*. 1993;93:691-696.

18. Coyle E, Coggan A, Davis J, Sherman W. Current thoughts and practical considerations concerning substrate utilization during exercise. *Sports Sci Exch*. 1992;Spring:1-4.

19. Lemon P. Do athletes need more dietary protein and amino acids? *Int J Sport Nutr*. 1995;5:S39-S61.

20. Lemon P, Mullin J. Effect of initial muscle glycogen levels on protein metabolism during exercise. *J Appl Physiol*. 1980;48:624-629.

21. Young V, Pellett P. Plant proteins in relation to human protein and amino acid nutrition. *Am J Clin Nutr*. 1994;59:1203S-1212S.

22. Martin W. Effect of endurance training on fatty acid metabolism during whole body exercise. *Med Sci Sports Exerc*. 1997;29:635-639.

23. Muoio D, Leddy J, Horvath P, Awad A, Pendergast D. Effect of dietary fat on metabolic adjustments to maximal VO_2 and endurance in runners. *Med Sci Sports Exerc*. 1994;26:81-88.

24. Jones N, Heigenhauser G, Kuksis A, Matsos C, Sutton J, Toews C. Fat metabolism in heavy exercise. *Clin Sci*. 1980;59:469-478.

25. Ornish D, Brown S, Scherwitz L, et al. Can lifestyle changes reverse coronary heart disease? The Lifestyle Heart Trial. *Lancet*. 1990;336:129-133.

26. Kiens B, Essen-Gustavsson B, Gad P, Lithell H. Lipoprotein lipase activity and intramuscular triglyceride stores after long-term high fat and high carbohydrate diets in physically trained men. *Clin Physiol*. 1987;7:1-9.

27. Klesges R, Ward K, Shelton M, et al. Changes in bone mineral content in male athletes. *JAMA*. 1996;276:226-230.

28. Barr SI. Changes in bone mineral density in male athletes [letter]. *JAMA*. 1997;227:22-23.

29. Schneider P, Reiners C. Changes in bone mineral density in male athletes [letter]. *JAMA*. 1997;277:23-24.

30. Heaney R, Recker R, Saville P. Menopausal changes in calcium balance performance. *J Lab Clin Med*. 1978;92:953-962.

31. Linkseiler H, Zemel M, Hegsted M, Schuette S. Protein-induced hypercalciuria. *Federation Proc*. 1981;40:2429-2433.

32. Myburgh K, Hutchins J, Fataar A, Hough S, Noakes T. Low bone density is an etiologic factor for stress fractures in athletes. *Ann Intern Med*. 1990;113:754-759.

33. Wolman R, Clark P, McNally E, Harries M, Reeve J. Dietary calcium as a statistical determinant of trabecular bone density in amenorrhoeic and oestrogen-replete athletes. *Bone Mineral.* 1992;17:415-423.

34. Weaver C, Plawecki K. Dietary calcium: adequacy of a vegetarian diet. *Am J Clin Nutr.* 1994;59:1238S-1241S.

35. Minihane A, Fairweather-Tait S. Effect of calcium supplmentation on daily non-heme-iron absorption and long-term iron status. *Am J Clin Nutr.* 1998;68:96-102.

36. Hallberg L. Does calcium interfere with iron absorption [editorial]? *Am J Clin Nutr.* 1998;68:3-4.

37. Robertson J, Maughan R, Davidson R. Faecal blood loss in response to exercise. *BMJ.* 1987;295:303-305.

38. Waller M, Haymes E. The effects of heat and exercise on sweat iron loss. *Med Sci Sports Exerc.* 1996;28:197-203.

39. Eichner E. Runner's macrocytosis: a clue to footstrike hemolysis. *Am J Med.* 1985;78:321-325.

40. Snyder A, Dvorak L, Roepke J. Influence of dietary iron source on measures of iron status among female runners. *Med Sci Sports Exerc.* 1989;21:7-10.

41. Craig W. Iron status of vegetarians. *Am J Clin Nutr.* 1994;59:1233S-1237S.

42. Lamanca J, Haymes E. Effects of low ferritin concentrations on endurance performance. *Int J Sports Med.* 1992;2:376-385.

43. Zhu Y, Haas J. Iron depletion without anemia and physical performance. *Am J Clin Nutr.* 1997;66:334-341.

44. Herbert V. Everyone should be tested for iron disorders. *J Am Diet Assoc.* 1992;92:1502-1509.

45. Lukaski H. Micronutrients (magnesium, zinc, and copper): are mineral supplements needed for athletes? *Int J Sport Nutr.* 1995;5:S74-S73.

46. Manore M, Helleksen J, Merkel J, Skinner J. Longitudinal changes in zinc status in untrained men: effects of two different 12-week exercise training programs and zinc supplementation. *J Am Diet Assoc.* 1993;93:1165-1168.

47. Singh A, Moses F, Deuster P. Chronic multivitamin-mineral supplementation does not enhance physical performance. *Med Sci Sports Exerc.* 1992;24:726-732.

48. Gibson R. Content and bioavailability of trace elements in vegetarian diets. *Am J Clin Nutr.* 1994;59:1223S-1232S.

49. Hunt J, Matthys L, Hohnson L. Zinc absorption, mineral balance, and blood lipids in women consuming controlled lacto-ovo-vegetarian and omnivorous diets for 8 weeks. *Am J Clin Nutr.* 1998;67:421-430.

50. Belko A. Vitamins and exercise—an update. *Med Sci Sports Exerc.* 1987;19:S191-S196.

51. Soares M, Satyanarayana K, Bamji M, Jacob C, Ramana Y, Rao S. The effect of exercise on the riboflavin status of adult men. *Br J Nutr.* 1993;69:541-551.

52. Than T-M, May M-W, Aug K-S, Mya-Tu M. The effect of vitamin B-12 on physical performance capacity. *Br J Nutr.* 1978;40:269-273.

53. Herbert V. Vitamin B-12: plant sources, requirements, and assay. *Am J Clin Nutr.* 1988;48:852-858.

54. Rauma A, Torronen R, Hanninen O, Mykkanen H. Vitamin B-12 status of long-term adherents of a strict uncooked vegan diet ("living food diet") is compromised. *J Nutr.* 1995;125:2511-2515.

55. Kreider R, Miriel V, Bertun E. Amino acid supplementation and exercise performance. Analysis of the proposed ergogenic value. *Sports Med.* 1993;16:190-209.

56. Clarkson P. Antioxidants and physical performance. *Crit Rev Food Sci Nutr.* 1995;35:131-141.

57. Kanter M. Free radicals and exercise: effects of nutritional antioxidant supplementation. *Exerc Sports Sci Rev.* 1995;12:375-397.

58. Krajcovicova-Kudlackova M, Simoncic R, Bederova A, Klvanova J, Brtkova A, Grancicova E. Lipid and antioxidant blood levels in vegetarians. *Nahrung.* 1996;40:17-20.

59. Harris RC, Soderlund K, Hultman E. Elevation of creatine in resting and exercised muscle of normal subjects by creatine supplementation. *Clin Sci.* 1992;83:367-374.

60. Birch R, Noble D, Greenhaff P. The influence of dietary creatine supplementation on performance during repeated bouts of maximal isokinetic cycling in man. *Eur J Appl Phys.* 1994;69:268-270.

61. Balsom P, Soderlund K, Sjodin B, Ekblom E. Skeletal muscle metabolism during short duration high-intensity exercise: influence of creatine supplementation. *Acta Physiol Scand.* 1995;154:303-310.

62. Grindstaff P, Krieder R, Bishop R, et al. Effects of creatine supplementation on repetitive sprint performance and body composition in competitive swimmers. *Int J Sport Nutr.* 1997;7:330-346.

63. Rossiter H, Cannell E, Jakeman P. The effect of oral creatine supplementation on the 1,000-m performance of competitive rowers. *J Sports Sci.* 1996;14:175-179.

64. Earnest C, Snell P, Rodriguez R, Almada A, Mitchell T. The effect of creatine monohydrate ingestion on anaerobic power indices, muscular strength and body composition. *Acta Physiol Scand.* 1995;153:207-209.

65. Volek J, Kraemer W, Bush J, et al. Creatine supplementation enhances muscular performance during high-intensity resistance exercise. *J Am Diet Assoc.* 1997;97:765-770.

66. Balsom P, Soderlund K, Ekblom B. Creatine in humans with special reference to creatine supplementation. *Sports Med.* 1994;18:268-280.

67. Delanghe J, De Slypere J-P, De Buyzere M, Robbrecht J, Wieme R, Vermeulen A. Normal reference values for creatine, creatinine, and carnitine are lower in vegetarians. *Clin Chem.* 1989;35:1802-1803.

68. Clarys P, Zinzen E, Hebbelinck M. The effect of oral creatine supplementation on torque production in a vegetarian and nonvegetarian population: a double blind study. *Vegetarian Nutrition: An International Journal.* 1997;1:100-105.

69. Sharma D, Mathur R. Correction of anemia and iron deficiency in vegetarians by administration of ascorbic acid. *Indian J Physiol Pharmacol.* 1995;39:403-406.

70. Thomas D, Brotherhood J, Brand J. Carbohydrate feeding before exercise: effect of glycemic index. *Int J Sports Med.* 1991;12:180-186.

71. Thomas D, Brotherhood J, Miller J. Plasma glucose levels after prolonged strenuous exercise correlate inversely with glycemic response to food consumed before exercise. *Int J Sport Nutr.* 1994;4:361-373.

72. Gisolfi C, Duchman S. Guidelines for optimal replacement beverages for different athletic events. *Med Sci Sports Exerc.* 1992;24:679-687.

73. Below P, Mora-Rodriguez R, Gonzalez A, Coyle E. Fluid and carbohydrate ingestion independently improve performance during 1 hour of intense exercise. *Med Sci Sports Exerc.* 1995;27:200-210.

74. Yaspelkis B, Patterson J, Anderla P, Ding Z, Ivy J. Carbohydrate supplementation spares muscle glycogen during variable-intensity exercise. *J Appl Physiol.* 1993;75:1477-1485.

75. Sherman W. Recovery from endurance exercise. *Med Sci Sports Exerc.* 1992;24:S336-S339.

76. Burke L, Collier G, Hargreaves M. Muscle glycogen storage after prolonged exercise: effect of the glycemic index of carbohydrate feedings. *J Appl Physiol.* 1993;75:1019-1023.

77. Roy B, Tarnopolsky M. Influence of differing macronutrient intakes on muscle glycogen resynthesis after resistance exercise. *J Appl Physiol.* 1998;72:890-896.

78. Roy B, Tarnopolsky M, MacDougall J, Fowles J, Yarasheski K. Effect of glucose supplement after resistance training on protein metabolism. *Clin J Sport Med.* 1997;8:70.

79. Maughan R. Rehydration and recovery after exercise. *Sports Sci Exch.* 1996;9:1-5.

80. Otis CL. Exercise-associated amenorrhea. *Clin Sports Med.* 1992;11:351-362.

81. Sanborn C, Martin B, Wagner W. Is athletic amenorrhea specific to runners? *Am J Obs Gyn.* 1982;143:859-861.

82. Brooks S, Sanborn C, Albrecht B, Wagner W. Diet in athletic amenorrhoea [letter]. *Lancet*. 1984;2:559-560.

83. Kaiserauer S, Snyder A, Sleeper M, Zierath J. Nutritional, physiological, and menstrual status of distance runners. *Med Sci Sports Exerc*. 1989;21:120-125.

84. Slavin J, Lutter J, Cushman S. Amenorrhea in vegetarian athletes [letter]. *Lancet*. 1984;1:1474-1475.

85. Goldin B, Adlercreutz H, Gorbach S, et al. Estrogen excretion patterns and plasma levels in vegetarian and omnivorous women. *N Engl J Med*. 1982;307:1542-1547.

86. Nelson M, Fisher E, Catsos P, Meredith C, Turksoy R, Evans W. Diet and bone status in amenorrheic runners. *Am J Clin Nutr*. 1986;43:910-916.

87. Deuster PA, Kyle SB, Moser PB, Vigersky RA, Singh A, Schoomaker EB. Nutritional intakes and status of highly trained amenorrheic and eumenorrheic women runners. *Fertil Steril*. 1886;46:636-643.

88. Lloyd T, Buchanen J, Bitzer S, Waldman C, Myers C, Ford B. Interrelationship of diet, athletic activity, menstrual status, and bone density in collegiate women. *Am J Clin Nutr*. 1987;46:681-684.

89. Szabo L. The health risks of new-wave vegetarianism. *Can Med Assoc J*. 1997;156:1454-1455.

90. Huse DM, Lucas AR. Dietary patterns in anorexia nervosa. *Am J Clin Nutr*. 1984;40:251-254.

91. O'Connor MA, Touyz SW, Dunn SM, Beumont JV. Vegetarianism in anorexia nervosa? A review of 116 consecutive cases. *Med J Aust*. 1987;147:540-542.

92. Neumark-Sztainer D, Story M, Resnick MD, Blum RW. Adolescent vegetarians. A behavioral profile of a school-based population in Minnesota. *Arch Pediatr Adolesc Med*. 1997;151:833-838.

93. Johnston P. Counseling the pregnant vegetarian. *Am J Clin Nutr*. 1988;48:901-905.

94. Mangels A. Working with vegetarian clients. *Issues in Vegetarian Dietetics*. 1995;5:1,4-5.

95. Position of The American Dietetic Association. Vegetarian diets. *J Am Diet Assoc*. 1997;97:1317-1321.

27

MANAGING BODY WEIGHT

Brenda Davy, MS, RD

Athletes' primary nutrition concern is body weight (1). In many sports the percentage of body fat as well as body weight correlates inversely with performance (2). This relationship is largely limited to sports where performance involves movement of the body either vertically (eg, high jumping) or horizontally (eg, running) (3-5). Additional body fat may be detrimental to performance in these types of activities because of the nonforce-producing mass added to the body (6). Excessive fatness and body weight also increase the metabolic cost of physical activity (6). Swimmers, however, may benefit from somewhat higher levels of body fat because of its effect on buoyancy (7). In general, physical activity involving movement of body mass would be predicted to be more efficient mechanically or metabolically at lower levels of body fat and body mass.

High levels of body mass may be advantageous in certain sporting events (eg, sumo wrestlers and weightlifters). Athletes participating in sports involving the movement of an external load may benefit from both an increased body weight and lean body mass. For example, a heavy individual with a large amount of lean tissue will be more successful in overcoming the inertia of stationary (eg, barbells) or moving (eg, other competitors) objects.

Many athletic performances are judged on aesthetic qualities as well as the completion of specific physical tasks (eg, gymnastics, figure skating, bodybuilding, ballet dancing). Physical appearance may be as important a factor in a particular athlete's weight goals as is minimizing the amount of nonforce-producing body mass.

This chapter reviewes three aspects of weight management that pertain to the athlete: weight maintenance, weight reduction, and weight gain. More specifically, the use of body composition, rather than body weight, will be emphasized by discussing approaches for increasing or maintaining lean body mass while decreasing fat mass. The general approach for helping the athlete achieve his or her weight goals will rely on the energy balance concept. In simplistic terms body weight remains stable when the amount of energy consumed is equal to the amount of energy expended. When energy intake exceeds energy expenditure a state of positive energy balance is achieved and body weight will increase. Conversely, when energy expenditure exceeds energy intake a state of negative energy balance is achieved and body weight is lost. For further information on this topic, its relationship to macronutrient balance, and physical activity, a recent review is suggested (8). The role of the sports nutritionist is to assist the athlete in achieving his or her body weight and composition goals by modifying energy intake and/or expenditure in a way that does not negatively impact health.

ESTABLISHING APPROPRIATE GOALS

The athletic individual will likely have a higher lean body mass than a sedentary individual. For this reason using traditional height/weight tables to assess the athlete's current weight may result in categorizing the athlete as overweight, even when he or she is not overfat. Since the athlete generally strives to minimize body fatness while achieving an appropriate weight, body composition rather than body weight should be the focus in determining weight goals. It is important to note that these guidelines apply to adults only; using adult body composition guidelines in prepubescent athletes may adversely affect normal growth and development (9).

While acceptable body fat ranges for the general population may be 15% to 18% fat for men and 20% to 25% fat for women, optimal ranges for the athlete may be 5% to 12% for men and 10% to 20% for women (10). Ranges indicating potential risk for eating disorders are <4% in men and <10% in women (10). Optimal body composition will vary by gender, sport, and even position within a sport. For example, ideal percent body fat ranges may differ for a female swimmer versus a male marathon runner. See *Table 27.1* for ranges of actual body fat values for athletes in various sports.

TABLE 27.1   Ranges of Relative Body Fat Values for Men and Women Athletes* in Various Sports

	% Fat	
Sport	Men	Women
Baseball/Softball	8-14	12-18
Basketball	6-12	10-16
Bodybuilding	5-8	6-12
Canoe/Kayak	6-12	10-16
Cycling	5-11	8-15
Fencing	8-12	10-16
Football	6-18	—
Golf	10-16	12-20
Gymnastics	5-12	8-16
Horse Racing	6-12	10-16
Ice/Field Hockey	8-16	12-18
Orienteering	5-12	8-16
Pentathlon	—	8-15
Racquetball	6-14	10-18
Rowing	6-14	8-16
Rugby	6-16	—
Skating	5-12	8-16
Skiing	7-15	10-18
Ski Jumping	7-15	10-18
Soccer	6-14	10-18
Swimming	6-12	10-18
Synchronized Swimming	—	10-18
Tennis	6-14	10-20
Track and Field, running events	5-12	8-15
Track and Field, field events	8-18	12-20

continued

TABLE 27.1   Ranges of Relative Body Fat Values for Men and Women Athletes* in Various Sports (continued)

Sport	% Fat Men	% Fat Women
Triathlon	5-12	8-15
Volleyball	7-15	10-18
Weightlifting	5-12	10-18
Wrestling	5-16	—

Source: Wilmore J, Costill D. *Physiology of Sport and Exercise*. Champaign, Ill: Human Kinetics; 1994:394. Reprinted by permission.

*The values in this table are for elite athletes. A combination of laboratory techniques was used to estimate body composition. The ranges reflect variations within a sport and different studies from which the data were collected. (Personal communication, J. Wilmore)

Other considerations in establishing an appropriate body weight goal may include an individual's personal weight history (eg, lowest adult body weight) and errors in measurement techniques used to estimate body composition. Assessing body composition allows the athlete and the nutritionist to determine appropriate and realistic weight goals that can help to optimize performance without compromising health.

Case Study 1 gives an example of how to calculate an appropriate body weight goal based upon optimal body composition. For examples involving weight loss, it has been assumed that the vast majority of weight lost will be from fat tissue. A meta-analysis by Ballor et al (11) examined the effects of energy restriction with and without exercise training on losses of fat versus fat-free weight. Energy restriction alone resulted in approximately 25% of total weight lost as fat-free mass, while energy restriction in combination with exercise training resulted in an average of 12% of weight lost as fat-free mass. However, a great deal of variability exists due to factors such as the type and volume of activity, the degree of energy deficit, the macronutrient composition of the diet, and even individual differences. The ideal strategy is to revise further calculations and adjustments based on repeated body composition measurements.

CASE STUDY 1

Calculating Body Weight Based on Optimal Body Composition

Lori is a 25-year-old competitive endurance cyclist. She feels she would perform better in the upcoming season if she lost some weight. She is currently 5'4" and 135 lb. She underwent a hydrostatic weighing procedure which estimated her body fat at 23%. Since high school she has never weighed less than 120 lb.

Current Weight	= 135 lbs (61.4 kg)
Body Fat	= 23%
Fat Mass	= 135 x 0.23 = 31 lbs
Fat-free Mass	= 135 – 31 = 104 lbs
Body Fat Goal	= 15% (85% lean weight)
Goal Weight	= 104 ÷ 0.85 = 122 lbs

Lori's estimated intake from her food record is 2,655 kcal per day, with a macronutrient distribution of 18% protein, 32% fat, 48% carbohydrate, and 2% alcohol. Her needs based on the World Health Organization equation multiplied by an activity factor of 2.0 (for "planned vigorous activities") are 2,798 calories. These two estimates are reasonably close, with a difference of about 143 calories.

DETERMINING ENERGY REQUIREMENTS

Once an appropriate weight goal is determined, energy needs should then be assessed. Factors such as age, gender, body composition, sport, and training schedules may influence energy requirements. While a sedentary individual might require 25 to 35 kcal/kg per body weight per day, an active individual engaging in 90 minutes of daily exercise might require 45 to 50 kcal/kg per body weight per day. Estimates are not always guaranteed to be extremely accurate, but there is a scientific basis for estimated energy requirements. A simple method is to use an equation to predict resting energy expenditure (REE) at the athlete's current body weight, then apply an appropriate activity factor. Several such equations are presented in *Tables 27.2 to 27.5*.

TABLE 27.2   Equations for Predicting Resting Energy Expenditure from the World Health Organization (12)

	Age Range (years)	REE in kcal/day
Males		
	10-18	(17.5 x wt (kg)) + 651
	18-30	(15.3 x wt (kg)) + 679
	30-60	(11.6 x wt (kg)) + 879
	>60	(13.5 x wt (kg)) + 487
Females		
	10-18	(12.2 x wt (kg)) + 746
	18-30	(14.7 x wt (kg)) + 496
	30-60	(8.7 x wt (kg)) + 829
	>60	(10.5 x wt (kg)) + 596

TABLE 27.3   Revised Harris-Benedict Equations for Estimating Resting Energy Requirements (13)

Males:	88.362 + (4.799 x ht) + (13.397 x wt) – (5.677 x age)
Females:	447.593 + (3.098 x ht) + (9.247 x wt) – (4.330 x age)

wt = weight in kg   ht = height in cm   age = age in years

TABLE 27.4   General Estimate of Resting Metabolic Rate (RMR) and Activity Factors

Estimating RMR:	1 kcal/kg body weight/hour x 24 hours	
Activity Factors		
Very light	(extremely sedentary, largely bedrest)	1.2 - 1.3
Light	(no planned activity, mostly officework)	1.5 - 1.6
Moderate	(walking, stairclimbing during the day)	1.6 - 1.7
Heavy	(planned vigorous activities)	1.9 - 2.1

TABLE 27.5   Estimates of Energy Expended in Physical Activity Using METs

1 MET = 3.5 mL O_2/kg body weight/minute or about 1 kcal/kg body weight/hour

Multiply kg of body weight x MET value of activity x duration of activity (hours)

Example: Lori cycles for 1.5 hours fairly vigorously (about 15 mph), at an intensity of about 10 METs. (See the Tools section for the MET values of various activities.)

61 kg x 10 METs x 1.5 = 915 kcal

A comprehensive list of MET values has been published by Ainsworth BE, Haskell WL, Leon AS, et al. Compendium of physical activities: classifications of energy costs of human physical activities. *Med Sci Sports Exer*. 1993;25:71-80.

Usual dietary intake should also be assessed. A variety of tools may be used including 24-hour recalls, food intake records, and food frequency questionnaires. Such tools are described in the *Dietary Assessment Resource Manual* (14). Combining multiple assessment tools may provide a more accurate assessment of usual habits (eg, a spontaneous 24-hour recall plus a 3- or 4-day food intake record). In addition to helping determine energy requirements, these tools may identify eating patterns and food preferences and can be used for menu planning. For more information on dietary assessment, see Chapter 9, Dietary Assessment.

An assessment of energy expenditure is also needed. An activity log kept with a food intake record will allow the dietitian to examine the athlete's exercise schedule and how it relates to his or her diet and intake patterns (see *Figure 27.1*). Over- and under-reporting can be potential problems with using intake and activity records to estimate requirements. Under-reporting food intake may be a greater problem in heavier athletes or in athletes who have greater concerns about their weight (7). For this reason self-reports should be considered together with several other pieces of information. For example, how does the athlete's estimated intake from the food record compare with needs estimated using an equation with an appropriate activity factor?

FIGURE 27.1   Sample Food and Activity Record

Food and Activity Record

Name _____

Date _____

Day (circle):   1   2   3   4   Other _____

Time	Place	Description of Food Item (Include brand names and cooking methods, if known.)	Portion Size (such as cups, ounces)	Office Use

Time	Description of Activity	Intensity	Duration

DETERMINING MACRONUTRIENT NEEDS

Compared to sedentary individuals, athletes have increased carbohydrate and protein needs (10). The optimal macronutrient composition for the diet will vary by sport. Some athletes have a very high energy intake while others consume a low amount of energy. Therefore, for diet prescription it is best to calculate macronutrient needs relative to current body weight rather than as a percentage of total calories. As indicated in *Table 27.6*, the athlete should consume adequate amounts of carbohydrate and protein, with the balance of calories coming primarily from dietary fat. In the case of weight reduction, this approach should allow the athlete to maintain his or her activity level and help to conserve lean tissue.

TABLE 27.6   Macronutrient Needs of Athletes (8,15,16)

Carbohydrates

General Guideline	60% to 65% of total energy
Endurance Athletes	65% to 70% of total energy, or 7 to 10 g/kg body weight

Protein

General Guideline	0.8 g/kg body weight, or 12% to 15% of total energy
Endurance Athletes	1.2 to 1.4 g/kg body weight
Strength Athletes	1.6 to 1.7 g/kg body weight

Dietary Fats

The balance of calories following the calculation of carbohydrate and protein needs, to a maximum of 30% of total energy

COUNSELING THE ATHLETE

Weight Maintenance

The goal with weight maintenance is maintaining a state of energy balance. Case Study 2 illustrates these steps in helping athletes maintain weight.

1. **Assess current eating and activity habits.** Have the athlete keep a food intake record and activity log for 3 or more days. Provide instructions on the level of detail needed on the record such as portion sizes, brand names of products, names of restaurants, and mealtimes. Have the athlete provide product labels to assist you in accurately analyzing intake and ask that he or she record activity habits including his or her training schedule. The athlete will likely be motivated and want to have an accurate assessment of intake and expenditure. For clarity and completeness review the record with the athlete when it is returned. Attention to detail will result in a better assessment of needs.

2. **Establish current energy requirements and analyze the intake record.** Many software programs are available for this. Be aware that under- and over-reporting are often a problem with assessing intake,

but food intake records are still useful in providing an estimate of needs and establishing current habits. Consider his or her workout routine as well as usual daily activities. Evaluate the reported intake versus a calculated estimate of requirements.

3. **Determine the appropriate macronutrient composition for the diet.** Consider the athlete's sport and training regimen.

4. **Devise practical, individualized strategies for meeting the athlete's goal of weight maintenance.** Suggestions include the following:
   - Sample menus may be helpful to provide usable examples of how to meet calorie and macronutrient needs.
   - Suggestions for snacks to keep on hand, in the workout bag, and in the desk at work are helpful. Try trail mixes, dried fruits, fig bars and cookies, or dry ready-to-eat cereals.
   - "Sports" products such as energy bars and drinks may be good postworkout snacks.
   - If the athlete has a limited amount of time for meal preparation, suggest meal options that can be prepared in 10 minutes or less. Convenience items such as microwave burritos, instant soup, pasta cups, and frozen entrees may be helpful items to keep on hand.

5. **Follow up. Monitor weight for stability on a weekly basis.** For individuals who have a difficult time maintaining their weight, suggest that they regularly monitor their weight if they do not already do so. This can help prevent major fluctuations that could impact performance. If further troubleshooting is needed, repeated records of food intake may be helpful.

CASE STUDY 2

Weight Maintenance

Tracy is a 31-year-old distance runner who is about to begin training for a marathon. She is 5'5" and weighs 115 lb (52 kg). Her body fat, estimated using skin fold measurements, is approximately 12%. She reports difficulty maintaining her weight when she increases her mileage. She has a busy work schedule and often skips meals. She would like some help with maintaining her present weight during her marathon training, which she plans to begin soon.

Steps 1 and 2: Tracy's 4-day food and activity records indicate that she consumes an average of approximately 2,600 kcal, with a macronutrient distribution of 15% protein, 20% fat, and 65% carbohydrate. She generally eats two meals per day with an occasional postworkout snack. She eats a lot of bagels, yogurt, and fruit and tries to avoid "high-fat things" like fried foods and red meat. Her typical day at work is very sedentary, mostly seated at a computer. Her activity records indicate that she runs an average of about 8 to 10 miles per day at a "moderate" pace; about 7 minutes per mile (14 METS). She typically performs one or two "intense" interval workouts per week, at five to six 1-mile intervals. She feels that she does not really eat that much more when she begins to increase her running mileage due to a lack of time.

Estimated intake from food record   = 2,600 kcal

Estimated REE = 52 kg x 1 kcal/kg body wt/hour x 24   = 1,248

Daily energy needs (without running):

REE x "light" activity factor of 1.5 for seated work   = 1,248 x 1.5 = 1,872

Estimated expenditure for running (noninterval days):

52 kg x 14 METS x approximately 1 hour   = 728

Estimated daily needs with current schedule (1,872 + 728) = 2,600 kcal

Step 3: Tracy is an endurance athlete, so a recommended macronutrient distribution is:

Carbohydrate: 65% to 70% of total energy, or 7 to 10 g/kg body weight

(2,600 x .65) ÷ 4 kcal/g = 423 g

Protein: 1.2 to 1.4 g/kg body weight

52 kg x 1.2 = 62 g

52 kg x 1.4 = 73 g

= 62 – 73 g

Fat: 20% to 30% of total energy, or the balance after calculating carbohydrate and protein needs

(423 x 4 kcal/g) + (73 x 4 kcal/g)   = 1984

2,600 – 1,984 = 616 ÷ 9 kcal/g   = 68 g (24%)

Step 4: Since Tracy's current fat intake is 20% of total calories, she could add extra energy by using some higher-fat spreads such as cream cheese and peanut butter on her bagels. When she prepares meals at home, she can use items such as olive oil, nuts, and cheeses more freely. She will keep energy-dense snacks such as raisins, dried apricots, and whole-wheat fig bars in her desk at work. Since Tracy tends to get busy at work and lose track of time, she will try scheduling her meals into her work day. She is going to wake up 10 minutes earlier in the morning to allow extra time for breakfast at home. Tracy was also given information on nutritious options at fast-food establishments. A week's worth of sample menus at her recommended calorie level will assist her in meal planning so that she can more easily meet her energy needs.

Step 5: Tracy is going to weigh herself once a week on her bathroom scale and return in 2 weeks for a follow-up session with her sports nutritionist.

Weight Reduction

If weight reduction is desired, a state of negative energy balance must be achieved. Energy restriction may impair performance due to factors including a reduction in energy stores, impairment of immune function, alterations in mood, changes in enzyme activity, and structural alterations in the muscle (7). For this reason weight reduction is best accomplished in the off-season so as to not interfere with the athlete's training regimen. An eating plan that is high in carbohydrates (eg, 60% to 70%) and adequate in protein (eg, 1.4 to 1.7 g/kg body weight) may help to minimize some of the effects of energy restriction, such as maintaining nitrogen balance (7). If the sport is year-round, weight loss should be accomplished very gradually. Focus on decreasing levels of body fat, except for some endurance and weight-category sports where the primary goal may be to decrease overall weight (although weight loss goals should still be based upon decreasing fat mass). For endurance athletes who must move their entire body weight for a prolonged period of time (eg, cyclists, long-distance runners), a larger total body mass may be detrimental to performance.

The recommended rate for safe, gradual loss is 0.5 to 1.0 lb (0.2 to 0.5 kg) per week (8). If the commonly accepted figure of 3,500 calories per pound of body fat is used, this would correspond to a caloric deficit of approximately 250 to 500 calories per day. A goal of small weekly decrements in body weight should be emphasized with the athlete as larger and more rapid losses can result in greater losses of muscle glycogen and lean tissue, thereby decreasing strength and performance. Additionally, recent evidence suggests that rapid weight loss, such as the case of wrestlers trying to "make weight," may result in a temporary impairment of cognitive function (17). Other negative consequences of rapid weight loss, largely due to fluid losses, include compromised cardiac function, altered ability to maintain body temperature, and muscle cramping due to electrolyte disturbances (9). Large changes in scale weight within a short period of time (eg, 1 or 2 days) most likely reflect changes in fluid balance or glycogen stores rather than changes in body fatness. If an athlete must reduce his or her body weight below the "natural" weight, such as in weight category sports, "quick" losses should be accomplished over a 6- to 8-week period, and weekly losses should not exceed 2 to 3 lb (18). Following these athletes after such a loss is important to help them safely return to their precompetition weight.

Progress during weight reduction should ideally be monitored by tracking changes in body composition rather than body weight. Using a graph or chart to monitor changes may reinforce the goals of the athlete, while serving as a quick reference for the nutritionist. Case Study 3 illustrates these steps.

1. **Assess current weight and body composition.** Devise an appropriate goal weight, considering the athlete's gender, sport, and personal weight history.
2. **Evaluate current diet and activity habits.** Have the athlete keep a food intake record and activity log for 3 or more days. Provide instructions on the level of detail needed on the record such as portion sizes, brand names of products, names of restaurants, and mealtimes. Have the athlete provide product labels to assist in accurately analyzing his or her intake, and ask that he or she record activity habits including training schedule. Encourage athletes to be as accurate as possible so that you may better evaluate their current intake. For clarity and completeness, review the record with the athlete when it is returned.

    When reviewing the record, consider some of the following points:
    • Does the athlete eat three regular meals, or does he or she often "skip" meals?
    • Does he or she eat one to two large meals per day?

- Does the athlete tend to snack frequently?
- Does he or she get many "empty" calories, for example from soft drinks or alcohol?
- Does he or she consume some "obviously" high-fat foods, which could easily be eliminated to create a caloric deficit?
- Does the athlete use large quantities of sports-type products, such as energy bars and drinks?
- Does his or her diet appear to be lacking in one or more areas? Is the athlete eating according to the Food Guide Pyramid guidelines?

3. **Estimate current energy requirements.** Analyze the intake record. What is the athlete's activity level? Consider his or her workout routine as well as usual daily activities. Consider the reported intake and an estimate of his or her requirements.

4. **Devise an individualized approach for achieving negative energy balance.** This is best accomplished by decreasing intake modestly while increasing aerobic exercise. For example, for a loss of 1 lb per week, decrease daily intake by 250 kcal and increase expenditure by 250 kcal. The inclusion of exercise may serve to prevent a decrease in metabolic rate and loss of lean tissue due to excessive caloric restriction (11). Encouraging increased aerobic exercise for athletes who do not expend a large number of calories in their typical workouts, for example strength or power athletes, can create a greater caloric deficit and promote a greater loss of body fat.

Dietary Strategies:
- Limit fat to 20% to 25% total calories.
- Maintain high carbohydrate intake (60% to 70%) to help maintain energy level for workouts.
- Ensure that protein intake is adequate (1.4 to 1.7g/kg/body weight).
- Encourage a regular meal schedule, with snacks as needed.

Exercise Strategies:
- Increase exercise (primarily aerobic, endurance) to 30 to 60 minutes on most days of the week.
- Resistance training may help to increase/preserve muscle mass and prevent a decline in resting metabolic rate (19).

5. **Follow the athlete's progress.** Monitor changes in body weight on a weekly basis. For females, monitor menstrual cycles for irregularities. Consult recent reviews on this topic (20) for information on the adverse consequences of, and interventions for, menstrual dysfunction. Body composition should be reassessed after 2 or more weeks of intervention. Periodic records of food intake may help to monitor the athlete's dietary practices.

Be attentive to the athlete's "motivation" or psychological state surrounding weight and weight changes. The sports nutritionist should be aware that many athletes they counsel may be at risk for the development of eating disorders and a preoccupation with their body weight. Be aware of sudden or excessive losses of body weight. Compulsive eating behaviors and large fluctuations in body weight may indicate an eating disorder (10). Follow up on warning signs of excessive negative energy balance (fatigue, poor training, frequent illness, menstrual irregularities). Are they able to complete their workouts? What do they report about their "energy level"?

CASE STUDY 3

Weight Reduction

Step 1: Jenny is a 16-year-old gymnast who states that she has "slacked off" with her workout schedule over the summer. She wants to get "in shape" for the upcoming gymnastic season and would like to "lose a few pounds." She is 4'10" and weighs approximately 120 lb (54.5 kg). She thinks she usually weighs about 110 lb during gymnastics season. A recommended body fat level for Jenny would be in the range of 8% to 16% according to *Table 27.1*. Her current body fat level was estimated to be at 24% using skinfold calipers.

Step 2: Establishing Jenny's goal weight range
Current Weight	= 120 lb (54.5 kg)
Body Fat	= 24%
Fat Mass	= 120 x 0.24 = 29 lb
Fat-free Mass	= 120 – 29 = 91 lb
Body Fat Goal	= 8 - 16%
Goal Weight Range	= 99 - 108 lb

Step 3: Jenny's food intake record indicates that she consumes about 2,350 kcal, with fat and protein comprising 34% and 11% of total energy, respectively. She indicates that recently she has been eating a vegetarian diet, something a lot of her friends are also doing. She has not been eating regular meals at home but has been stopping for quick snacks (french fries, soft drinks) with her friends at fast-food restaurants.

According to her activity record, she has been working out at the gym (mostly strength-type workouts using weights) for 1 to 1 1/2 hours, 3 to 4 days per week. As part of her workout, she rides an exercise bicycle at the gym for 20 to 30 minutes.

Estimated intake from food record	= 2,350 kcal
Estimated REE	= 1,411 kcal
Estimated daily needs (without workout), assuming "light" activity factor of 1.5	= 2,117 kcal
Energy expended in activity:	
Cycling: 54.5 kg x 7 METs x 0.5 hours	= 191 kcal
Weights: 54.5 kg x 6 METs x 0.5 hours	= 164 kcal
Estimated expenditure on workout days	= 2,472 kcal
Estimated average daily expenditure	= 2,270 kcal

Step 4: Jenny needs an estimated daily intake of 2,270 kcal to maintain her present weight. To lose 1 lb per week, she could reduce her intake to a level of around 2,000 kcal (estimated needs less 250 kcal) and add more aerobic exercise to her present workout routine. To expend an additional 250 kcal per day (1,750 additional kcal per week), Jenny could add 1 hour of cycling exercise three times per week (1,145 kcal) and cycle for an additional 15 to 30 minutes on her strength workout days (287 to 573 kcal).

To limit her fat intake to 20% to 25% of total energy (44 to 56 g per day), Jenny could be more careful about her choices at fast-food restaurants. Low-fat protein sources, such as reduced-fat cheeses, vegetarian-style beans, and nonfat yogurt, may be used. She should try to eat regular meals and consume high-carbohydrate snacks in moderate amounts, such as fruit, graham crackers, and pretzels (rather than soft drinks or french fries).

Maintaining her muscle mass during weight loss is of particular importance. Her strength training workouts should help to prevent loss of lean tissue, but an adequate protein intake is also crucial. At her current weight she should consume at least 76 g of protein per day. Vegetarian protein sources were discussed and Jenny's mom was provided with suggestions for nonmeat entrees to try at home for the whole family. Both Jenny and her mom were given sample vegetarian menus at her recommended calorie intake level.

Step 5: Jenny will return in 1 week to follow up on her progress. She will complete another 3-day food intake record before she returns. Her skinfold measurements will be repeated in 2 weeks.

Weight Gain

To gain weight an individual must be in a state of positive energy balance. As with weight reduction, efforts to increase body weight are best accomplished during the off-season so as not to interfere with training. The focus is usually on increasing lean body mass, although some athletes may need to increase their overall body mass. Caution should be exercised in this instance, as large increases in body fatness may have adverse effects on the immune system (21). An emphasis on strength training rather than aerobic exercise will help to stimulate muscle growth, while not creating such a substantial energy deficit. The optimal protein intake for muscle protein deposition is 1.5 g/kg body weight (10). However, the limiting factor for muscle protein deposition is energy intake, not protein intake (10). This deserves reinforcement and is a common misconception among many athletes. Many athletes attempting to increase their body or muscle mass will try nutritional supplements purported to enhance weight gain. Several of these, such as chromium, creatine, beta-hydroxy-beta-methylbutyrate (HMB), and amino acids, were recently reviewed by Clarkson (22). (See Chapter 7, Egrogenic Aids for information on dietary supplements.) However, increased muscular work combined with an adequate energy and protein intake is the only proven safe and effective means to increase muscle size and strength (10,22). Case Study 4 gives an example of counseling an athlete who wants to gain weight using these steps.

1. **Assess current body weight and composition.** Devise an appropriate goal weight and a realistic weekly weight increment. A general guideline is 0.5 to 1.0 lb per week. Greater than this will be extremely difficult given the large amount of daily energy required to create a sufficient positive energy balance.

2. **Evaluate current diet and activity habits.** Have the athlete keep a food intake record and activity log for 3 or more days. Provide instructions on the level of detail needed on the record, such as portion sizes, brand names of products, names of restaurants, and mealtimes. Have the athlete provide product labels to assist in accurately analyzing intake, and ask that he or she records activity habits including training schedule. Encourage athletes to be as accurate as possible so that you may better evaluate their current intake. For clarity and completeness, review the record with the athlete when it is returned. Consider the following points:

   - Is his or her current energy intake adequate to maintain present weight?
   - Is his or her current protein intake within the recommended range at his or her present weight?

3. **Estimate the additional energy needed to create the positive energy balance.** For an increase of 0.5 to 1.0 lb per week, an additional 400 to 500 calories per day will be required. Devise an individualized food and activity plan to accomplish the caloric excess. Encourage the athlete to choose his or her additional calories wisely from foods with nutritional value (eg, foods that will provide additional nutrients as well as calories), rather than "empty" calorie foods.

   Dietary Strategies:
   - Encourage regular meals with frequent snacks.
   - Increase portion sizes at mealtimes, particularly of high energy-dense foods.
   - Include sports products, such as bars and drinks.
   - Include a "meal replacement" beverage each day to be used between meals, not with meals.
   - Include the use of more nutrient- and energy-dense foods in meal preparation. These include olive and canola oil, nuts, cheese, and dried fruits.
   - Include one extra meal each day.

   Exercise Strategies:
   - Add resistance-training workouts

   Box 27.1 gives more suggestions for increasing calorie intake.

4. **Follow the athlete's progress on a weekly basis.** Reassess body composition after 2 or more weeks of intervention or after a substantial increase in weight. Periodic records of food intake may be kept to monitor the athlete's dietary habits.

CASE STUDY 4

Weight Gain

Richard is a 23-year-old competitive bodybuilder who thinks his performance would improve if he could "bulk up." He states he has been drinking high-protein shakes to increase his muscle mass. He has gained only 1 lb since starting to drink the shakes 3 weeks ago. Richard is 5'8" and weighs 195 lbs. His body fat, using the bioelectrical impedance machine at the gym, was estimated to be around 5%. He works at a restaurant during the day and spends a lot of time walking. He currently lifts weights 5 days per week, 2 hours per session. He also works out on the stair climber two times per week, 30 minutes per session. His goal is to accomplish this weight gain over an 8-week period.

Step 1: Richard's coach would like to see him put on 10 to 15 lb of muscle mass. Since the impedance test may have been inaccurate, his body composition was reassessed using Dual Energy X-ray Absorptiometry (DXA). This test estimated his body fat at 9%. He would like his body fat to be in the range of 5% to 6%.

Current Weight	= 195 lb (88.6 kg)
Body Fat	= 9%
Fat Mass	= 195 x 0.09 = 17.6 lb
Fat-free Mass	= 195 – 17.6 = 177.4 lb
Desired Fat-free Mass	= 177 + 10 = 187 lb
Body Fat Goal	= 6% (94% lean weight)
Goal Weight	= 187 ÷ 0.94 = 199 lb

Step 2: Richard's 3-day food intake record indicated that he consumed an average of 3,900 calories, with a fat and protein intake of 32% and 21%, respectively.

Estimated intake from food intake record	= 3,900 kcal
Estimated REE (Harris-Benedict)	= 1,974 kcal
Daily energy needs (without workouts):	
REE x "moderate" activity factor of 1.7 (walking)	= 1974 x 1.7 = 3,356 kcal
Estimated expenditure for aerobic activity:	
88.6 kg x 6 METs x 0.5 hours	= 266 kcal per session
Estimated needs (with aerobic session)	= 3,622 kcal per day
Estimated expenditure for strength workouts:	
88.6 kg x 6 METs x 2 hours	= 1,063 kcal per session
Estimated needs (with strength workout)	= 4,419 kcal per day
Estimated average daily needs	= 4,191 kcal per day

Step 3: For Richard to gain 1 lb per week, he should consume an additional 500 calories per day, for a total recommended energy intake of 4,691 kcal. Since he has 8 weeks to accomplish this goal, adjustments in his intake may be required depending on his progress after several weeks of intervention. He and his coach do not plan to change his training schedule at this time.

Richard is still concerned about getting enough protein. At his present weight he requires about 133 g protein per day (88.6 kg x 1.5 g/kg/body weight) and 136 g per day at this goal weight. According to his food intake record, he consumes about 205 g per day (3,900 kcal x 0.21 = 819 kcal (4 kcal/g = 205 g) which is more than adequate. At his recommended intake level, this amount of protein would comprise approximately 11% of total energy.

Richard would benefit from a reduction in fat intake from 32% to 25%. Many of the high-protein foods he has been including in his diet are high in fat. This reduction could easily be accomplished by choosing leaner meats and lower fat nonmeat proteins such as legumes. A lower fat intake would allow him to consume a greater amount of carbohydrate (64%), for an overall macronutrient profile that should facilitate the desired changes in body composition.

Richard was provided with a week's worth of sample meal plans. His plan is to eat three regular meals and three substantial mini-meals throughout the day. He will continue to make protein shakes but will use 1% milk rather than whole milk and will add berries or a banana. He was provided with a list of nutritious foods to try that will help "boost" his overall intake, as well as the tips in *Box 27.1*.

Step 4: Richard will return after 1 week of following his new eating plan. He will have a DXA repeated in 4 weeks to see if he has had any changes in body composition.

BOX 27.1   Suggestions for Increasing Calorie Intake (23)

- Choose nutrient-dense cereals such as granola, muesli, and Grape-Nuts. Top with nuts, sunflower seeds, bananas, or dried fruits.
- Cook hot cereals with milk rather than water. Mix in powdered milk, margarine, peanut butter, nuts, wheat germ, or dried fruit.
- Drink juices such as apple, cranberry, grape, pineapple, and apricot. To increase the caloric content of frozen juices, add less water than the directions indicate.
- Use fruits such as bananas, pineapple, raisins, dates, dried apricots, and other dried fruits rather than fruits with a high water content such as grapefruit, plums, and peaches.
- To increase the calories in milk, add 1/4 cup powdered milk to 1 cup of 2% milk, or add powdered beverage mixes such as Carnation Instant Breakfast, Ovaltine, and Nestle's Quik.
- Make homemade blender drinks such as milkshakes and fruit smoothies.
- Spread toast with generous amounts of peanut butter, margarine, jam, jelly, fruit preserves, or honey.
- Choose hearty, dense breads such as sprouted wheat and honey bran. Use thick slices for sandwiches. Stuff with tuna salad, chicken, or other fillings.
- Make canned soups more substantial by adding evaporated milk in place of water or regular milk, or add extra powdered milk. Garnish with parmesan cheese or croutons.
- Try bean dishes such as lentils, split pea soup, chili with beans, hummus, and limas.
- Sauté chicken or fish in canola or olive oil. Add sauces and breadcrumb toppings.
- Include higher-calorie vegetables such as peas, corn, carrots, winter squash, and beets. Top with margarine, slivered almonds, grated cheeses, or sauces. Try stir-frying vegetables in olive oil.
- Add cottage cheese, garbanzo beans, sunflower seeds, chopped nuts, raisins, croutons, and dressings made with olive oil to salads.
- Add extra margarine and powdered milk to mashed potatoes.
- Enjoy desserts such as oatmeal raisin cookies, fig bars, puddings, stewed fruit compotes, frozen yogurt, cornbread with honey, muffins, and fruit breads.
- Try healthful snacks such as fruit yogurt, low-fat cheese and crackers, peanuts, sunflower seeds, granola, pretzels, bagels with low-fat cream cheese and jelly, and peanut butter crackers.

Adapted by permission. Clark N. *Nancy Clark's Sports Nutrition Guidebook*, 2nd ed. Champaign, Ill: Human Kinetics; 1997:292-294.

SUMMARY

Successful management of body weight is of critical importance for competitive athletes. Having an excessive amount of body fat or an inadequate amount of lean or total body mass may negatively impact physical performance. The sports nutritionist can best assist the athlete in achieving body weight and composition goals through an individualized approach using the energy balance concept. Once a realistic weight or body composition goal has been determined, needs and expenditure can be assessed. A personalized food and activity plan can be designed, taking into account the athlete's specific needs and preferences. Follow-up should occur on a weekly basis to monitor progress and troubleshoot problems. This process should help to ensure that the desired outcome is achieved, while not negatively affecting present and future overall health.

REFERENCES

1. Parr RB, Porter MA, Hodgson SC. Nutrition knowledge and practices of coaches, trainers, and athletes. *Phys Sports Med*. 1984;12:127-138.
2. Optimal body weight for performance. In: Wilmore JH, Costill DL. *Physiology of Sport and Exercise*. Champaign, Ill: Human Kinetics; 1994:389-398.
3. Boileau RA, Lohman TG. The measurement of human physique and its effect on physical performance. *Orthop Clin North Am*. 1977;8:563-581.
4. Malina RM. Physique and body composition: effects on performance and effects on training, semistarvation, and overtraining. In: Brownell KD, Rodin J, Wilmore JH, eds. *Eating, Body Weight, and Performance in Athletes*. Philadelphia, Penn: Lea & Febinger; 1992:94-114.
5. Pate RR, Slentz CA, Katz DP. Relationship between skinfold thickness and performance of health related fitness test items. *Res Q Exerc Sport*. 1989;60:183-189.
6. Houtkooper LB. Body composition assessment and its relationship to athletic performance. In: Berning JR, Steen SN, eds. *Nutrition for Sport & Exercise*. Gaithersburg, Md: Aspen Publishers; 1998:155-166.
7. Walberg-Rankin J. Changing body weights and composition in athletes. In: Lamb DR, Murray R, eds. *Perspectives in Exercise Science and Sports Medicine, Vol 11: Exercise, Nutrition and Weight Control*. Carmel, Ind: Cooper Publishing; 1998:199-236.
8. Melby CL, Commerford SR, Hill JO. Exercise, macronutrient balance, and weight control. In: Lamb DR, Murray R, eds. *Perspectives in Exercise Science and Sports Medicine, Vol. 11: Exercise, Nutrition and Weight Control*. Carmel, Ind: Cooper Publishing; 1998:1-60.
9. Clarkson P, Manore M, Opplinger B, Steen S, Walberg-Rankin J. Methods and strategies for weight loss in athletes. *Sports Sci Exch*. 1998;9(1).
10. Position of The American Dietetic Association and The Canadian Dietetic Association. Nutrition for physical fitness and athletic performance for adults. *J Am Diet Assoc*. 1993;93:691-696.
11. Ballor DL, Poehlman ET. Exercise-training enhances fat-free mass preservation during diet-induced weight loss: a meta-analytical finding. *Int J Obes*. 1994;18:35-40.
12. Food and Nutrition Board. *Recommended Dietary Allowances*. 10th ed. Washington, DC: National Academy Press; 1989.
13. Roza AM, Shizgal HM. The Harris-Benedict equation reevaluated: resting energy requirements and body cell mass. *Am J Clin Nutr*. 1984;40:168-182.

14. Thompson FE, Byers T, Kohlmeier L. Dietary assessment resource manual. *J Nutr.* 1994;124(11S):2245S-2315S.

15. Lemon PW. Dietary protein requirements in athletes. *J Nutr Biochem.* 1997;8:52-60.

16. Lemon PW. Influence of dietary protein and total energy intake on strength improvement. *Sports Sci Exch.* 1989;2(4).

17. Choma CW, Sforzo GA, Keller BA. Impact of rapid weight loss on cognitive function in collegiate wrestlers. *Med Sci Sports Exerc.* 1998;30:746-749.

18. Smith NJ. Weight control in the athlete. *Clin Sports Med.* 1984;3(3):693-704.

19. Bryner RW, Ullrich IH, Sauers J, et al. Effects of resistance vs. aerobic training combined with an 800 calorie liquid diet on lean body mass and resting metabolic rate. *J Am Coll Nutr.* 1999;18:115-121.

20. Dueck CA, Manore MM, Matt KS. Role of energy balance in athletic menstrual dysfunction. *Int J Sport Nutr.* 1996;6:165-190.

21. Shephard RJ, Shek PN. Immunological hazards from nutritional imbalance in athletes. *Exerc Immunol Rev.* 1998;4:22-48.

22. Clarkson PM. Nutritional supplements for weight gain. *Sports Sci Exch.* 1998;11(1).

23. Clark N. *Nancy Clark's Sports Nutrition Guidebook*, 2nd ed. Champaign, Ill: Human Kinetics; 1998:292-294.

The author would like to thank Kevin Davy, PhD, Tracy Horton, PhD, Susie Parker, MEd, and Christopher Melby, DrPH for their helpful comments during the preparation of this chapter.

28
EATING DISORDERS IN ATHLETES

Jaime S. Ruud, MS, RD; Monika M. Woolsey, MS, RD; and Lisa Dorfman, MS, RD

The importance of physical activity as a component of wellness and disease prevention is well documented and is a cornerstone of the philosophy that led to the founding of Sports, Cardiovascular, and Wellness Nutritionists (SCAN). Sports nutritionists are an important part of the physical fitness movement, as their knowledge of the impact of diet and exercise on physical training can help the novice, collegiate, or professional athlete develop a program that maximizes the physical and mental benefits of exercise. As positive as the fitness movement is for the majority of those who exercise, when taken to an extreme, sports participation can be dangerous and even deadly.

The sports nutritionist is often the person in an athlete's life with the ability to identify and intervene in an eating disorder. Since the behaviors accompanying eating-disordered pathology create an energy deficit, they impact sports performance in a number of ways. Athletes are likely to arrive at a consultation with complaints of fatigue, poor performance, slower competition times, inability to sleep, inability to gain weight with strength training, and inability to lose body fat, with the hopes that a nutrition supplement or "special diet" will provide a simple, concrete answer to the problem. While nutrition supplements can be a solution for some athletes, for others they may divert attention away from a much more serious condition.

While education is a vital role of the sports nutritionist, the recent increase in the incidence of eating disorders has also produced a need for understanding when to recommend a supplement and when to engage in a multidisciplinary intervention. The sports nutritionist may be the first (or only) professional the athlete consults about the problem. The line between appropriate, high-level training and pathological behavior is so fine that only one who has the athlete's confidence will have the opportunity to obtain the information necessary to make such decisions.

DEFINITION AND DIAGNOSTIC CRITERIA

According to the fourth edition of the *Diagnostic and Statistical Manual of Mental Disorders* (DSM-IV), eating disorders are characterized by severe disturbances in eating behavior (1). The term "eating disorder" commonly refers to anorexia nervosa or bulimia nervosa. However, eating disorders can also be applied to eating disorders not otherwise specified (NOS), a category for disturbances in eating behavior that do not meet the criteria for anorexia or bulimia. Compulsive overeating, obesity, and anorexia athletica fall into this classification. Binge eating disorder is currently classified as a research category in the DSM-IV.

Anorexia Nervosa

Anorexia nervosa is characterized by four distinct criteria (1):

1. A refusal to maintain a normal weight for age and height (see *Box 28.1*)
2. An intense fear of gaining weight or getting fat, although underweight
3. A distorted body image
4. Amenorrhea (the absence of three consecutive menstrual cycles)

BOX 28.1   *Calculating Minimum Ideal Body Weight*

When possible, perform this assessment in a fully hydrated condition.

1. Estimate body composition. (Note: As many eating-disordered behaviors are dehydrating in nature, any body composition method that relies on total body water measurement is likely to overestimate body fat and underestimate goal weight. Calipers are the preferred method in this population.)

2. Estimate midarm circumference (MAC) and midarm muscle circumference (MAMC). (*Note:* The technique of measuring MAMC can be found in Chapter 11, Assessment of Body Size and Composition.)

3. Determine what percentage of minimum recommended MAMC (21 cm in adults) the athlete has.

4. If the athlete is hydrated and does not have an adequate MAMC, calculate how much muscle mass needs to be gained to achieve this MAMC.

5. From this adjusted Lean Body Mass (LBM), calculate an ideal weight based on a desired body fat percentage.

6. Always give goal weight in a range. A range of ±5% is usually more acceptable with eating-disordered thinking than is the usual ±10% range. The diagnostic threshold for an eating disorder is based on 85% of desired weight.

Example:

The client is a distance runner: 5' 6", 103 lb, MAMC 18 cm, 13% body fat.
The nutrition therapist and the athlete agreed on a goal body fat percentage range of 13% to 16%.

18 cm ÷ 21 cm = 85.7% desired MAMC

103 lb x 0.13 = 13.4 lb fat, 89.6 lb lean

Since the athlete is 85.7% of minimum MAMC, 90.6 lb lean is used in the subsequent equations; 89.6 lb LBM is 85.7%; therefore 90.6 lb is 100%.

90.6 ÷ 0.857 = 105.7 lb desired LBM

Desired weight at 13% body fat	**Desired weight at 16% body fat**
x lb fat + x lb lean = desired weight	x lb fat + x lb lean = desired weight
13.4 + 90.6 = 104 lb	16.6 + 90.6 = 107 lb
Range: 99-109 lb (104 lb ± 5%)	Range: 102-112 lb
Diagnostic threshold = 88 lb (104 x 85%)	Diagnostic threshold = 91 lb

---

It is important to point out that there can be more than one kind of anorexic. Two subtypes have been identified by the DSM-IV (1). They are either the restricting type or the binge-eating/purging type. The first subtype loses weight by severely restricting calories. The second subtype engages in bingeing or purging behaviors such as self-induced vomiting, laxative abuse, and enemas to keep weight down.

The classic anorexic is intelligent, high achieving, and well organized. As a child she may have been nondemanding, quiet, well-behaved, and willing to please. She or he may have been slightly overweight initially, and on the subtle suggestion of family, a friend, or coach went on a diet. She or he achieves a very low body weight by severely reducing food intake. In the process she or he becomes enmeshed in daily rituals, including frequent weigh-ins, conscious denial of hunger, avoiding foods with fat, skipping meals, counting calories, and excessive exercise.

Although the most obvious physical consequence of anorexia is extreme weight loss, there are other distinguishing features including lanugo (a fine, downy hair on arms, legs, and face), cold intolerance, and complaints of bloating or constipation. Common symptoms of anorexia nervosa are amenorrhea, compulsive exercising, sleep disturbance, and anxiety at mealtime.

Bulimia Nervosa

Bulimics often eat a normal diet but binge and purge to cope with emotional stress and low self-esteem. Vomiting, laxative abuse, and excessive exercise are purging methods used to control weight. To qualify for this diagnosis, bingeing and purging must occur, on average, at least twice a week for 3 months. Bulimics by their very nature are secretive, which makes this disorder very difficult to diagnose. They also have a tendency to abuse legal and illegal substances including alcohol, amphetamines, and cocaine and present themselves with a dual diagnosis of depression, bipolar, or other mood disorders which can also mask their eating disorder.

Bulimia nervosa is characterized by the following criteria (1):

1. Recurrent episodes of binge eating
2. Recurrent, inappropriate, compensatory behavior to prevent weight gain (such as self-induced vomiting; misuse of laxatives, diuretics, enemas or other medications; fasting; or excessive exercise)
3. The binge eating and compensatory behaviors both occur at least twice a week for 3 months.
4. Self-evaluation is influenced by body shape and weight.
5. The bingeing and purging are not accompanied by anorexia nervosa.

As with anorexics there can be more than one kind of bulimic: the purging type, who engages in self-induced vomiting or abusing laxatives, diuretics, or enemas; and the nonpurging type who compensates by fasting or using excessive exercise. Excessive exercise is defined as more than 1 hour of exercise a day for the "sole purpose of controlling weight."

There is a very fine line between dieting/exercise and bulimia nervosa. *Box 28.2* lists some questions that the sports nutritionist can ask to ascertain exercise behaviors.

BOX 28.2	Five Questions to Ask Your Client about Exercise
1.	Do you skip a meal because you missed a workout?
2.	Do you consciously tailor workouts to burn the calories you intend to eat?
3.	Are you a compulsive record-keeper when it comes to your workout?
4.	Do you exercise more if you have eaten more than you wanted to?
5.	Do you sacrifice many other opportunities to socialize in order to workout?

The typical bulimic is an 18- to 25-year-old female who is overly concerned about her appearance, although she is usually within 85% of a normal weight range. To maintain and preserve her perceived body image, she becomes entrapped in a vicious cycle: diet, starve, binge, guilt and shame, purge, relief, and diet. Purging is the coping mechanism that alleviates the shame and guilt of the binge.

Unlike anorexia nervosa many physical signs of bulimia do not appear until late in the course of the illness. Although bingeing can be harmful to the body, purging is usually the more dangerous of the two behaviors. Methods of purging include vomiting and the use of laxatives, diuretics, diet pills, and ipecac. Excessive exercise can also be considered a form of purging; what distinguishes this as part of the disease is the relative compulsivity of the physical activity. An inability to take a day off without experiencing guilt, adjusting exercise based on caloric intake, and doing exercise over and above regular team workouts are all signs and symptoms that the physical activity is not productive. Common signs of binge-purge behavior include dental erosion, cavities, swollen cheeks (swollen parotid glands), calluses on the back of hands, and orthostatic blood pressure changes due to dehydration.

EATING DISORDERS NOT OTHERWISE SPECIFIED

The eating disorders not otherwise specified category is for eating disorders that meet several but not all of the criteria for anorexia nervosa and bulimia nervosa. Examples include obesity, compulsive overeating, body weight less than 85% of minimal ideal weight without amenorrhea, and binge eating disorder.

Binge Eating Disorder

Binge eating disorder (BED), where large amounts of food are eaten within a relatively short time, is not officially recognized as an eating disorder. Yet it is much more common than either anorexia nervosa or bulimia nervosa. Binge eating disorder is different from bulimia nervosa because people with binge eating disorder usually do not purge after eating by vomiting or using laxatives. Binge eating disorder is characterized by the following criteria (1):

1. Recurrent episodes of binge eating (within any 2-hour period, eating a large amount of food and a lack of control over eating during the episode)
2. Eating until uncomfortably full
3. Eating large amounts of food, even when not physically hungry
4. Eating alone out of embarrassment
5. Feelings of disgust, depression, low self-esteem, and lack of willpower
6. Binge eating occurs at least 2 days a week for at least 6 months.
7. Binge eating disorder is not associated with the regular use of inappropriate compensatory behaviors (ie, purging, fasting, excessive exercise).

Binge eating disorder's specific criteria do not include all cases of overweight or "compulsive overeating"; however, as nutrition therapists become more fluent with the use of the DSM-IV and psychosocial assessment, it is likely that improvement in the ability to diagnose binge eating disorder will increase the incidence of this disorder in the population. (See *Box 28.3.*) Binge eating disorder is usually not an issue with the elite athlete but is likely to manifest in the case of a debilitating injury. If sports participation is the major or only form of emotional outlet, prolonged inactivity may bring this dysfunction to the surface. A serious injury that eliminates the ability to exercise may bring the athlete face-to-face with the degree of communication and coping physical activity provides. Weight gain during this time should always be monitored for the possibility that an eating disorder may be surfacing.

BOX 28.3   How to Differentiate BED from Other Weight-related Disorders

"I was too embarrassed to buy everything I wanted to eat at one place. So I would drive through 10 fast-food restaurants on the way home and collect everything I wanted to eat in bits and pieces."

Such a scenario is not uncommon to binge eating disorder. Unlike anorexics and bulimics, who can receive praise for their weight and exercise prowess, the binge eater is looked at by society with disdain. Weight is one of the few characteristics that is still culturally appropriate to tease, reject, mock, taunt, and label. This vulnerability to judgement creates a tremendous amount of shame for the BED individual. One client shared, "Even drug addicts can hide their issues to a point. When you're fat, it's like you're wearing your problems for the whole world to see, and everyone thinks they have the answer and the right to give me advice."

The sense of shame, rejection, and low self-esteem can be what drives BED individuals to seek help, often in the form of nutrition counseling. Given the negative cultural attitude toward obesity, it is natural for someone with BED to believe that losing weight will create a sense of well-being and erase the negative. It is important for the sports nutritionist to be able to identify and differentiate BED from other weight-related disorders, as BED often requires multidisciplinary intervention (including antidepressant medication) before lasting relief can be achieved.

Binge eating and the shame it creates can impair client disclosure about eating habits. It is crucial to work toward a relationship of unconditional acceptance to foster trust on the part of the client. Even when such acceptance is provided by the practitioner, it may take months, even years, for the client to share what is truly happening with food. Because of this secrecy, a true BED diagnosis is often not possible in the first few visits of a counseling relationship.

In addition to conscious denial of binge eating, a significant percentage of binges occur during dissociation, or eating during a "zoning out" period. If a client is dissociating, it is important to refer him or her for a mental health evaluation, as this emotionally protective mechanism may hint at issues not appropriate to address in nutrition therapy.

Anorexia Athletica

This term is used to describe a subclinical eating disorder frequently found among athletes. In general, a person with a subclinical eating disorder shows signs of disordered eating and distorted body image but fails to meet the criteria for anorexia nervosa or bulimia. (See *Box 28.4.*) The classic features of anorexia athletica include (2,3):

1. An intense fear of gaining weight or becoming fat even though an individual is already underweight (< 5% of expected body weight)
2. Restriction of food (< 1,200 kcal per day)
3. Compulsive exercise
4. Amenorrhea
5. Occasional bingeing or purging (once a week or once every 3 months)

BOX 28.4   What is disordered eating?

The terms "disordered eating" and "eating disorders" are often used interchangeably. Are they the same? Anorexia nervosa and bulimia nervosa have specific diagnostic criteria, and binge eating disorder is currently classified as a "research" category in the DSM-IV. In contrast, disordered eating is not a specific diagnosis.

Current thinking tends to view disordered eating and eating disorders as a continuum of behaviors, rather than distinct diseases or diagnoses. Individuals with eating disorders often describe periods of their life in terms of what their food behaviors were (eg, "That was my anorexic phase," or "I was a compulsive overeater until I went to school. That's when I got into bulimia.") These disorders almost never have a distinct starting point, but tend to be behavior patterns that gradually encroach on one's life until they completely control it.

Although not every dietetics practitioner is an eating disorder specialist, every dietitian who counsels encounters disordered eating. Because dietitians are in the unique position of meeting clients at the less severe end of the spectrum, they can coordinate an intervention before a life-threatening eating disorder develops. For all of us, regardless of our area of focus, the basic concepts of treatment for eating disorders have application in our counseling work.

Source: Sports, Cardiovascular, and Wellness Nutritionists. What is disordered eating? *SCAN'S Pulse*. 1997;16(1):8-10.

HOW COMMON ARE EATING DISORDERS IN ATHLETES?

Eating disorders have been widely studied in the general population, but only in the last decade have researchers examined the risk in athletes. The DSM-IV (1) reports that 0.5% to 1% of adolescent and young women meet the full criteria for anorexia nervosa. The prevalence of bulimia nervosa is approximately 1% to 3% of the female population. Both disorders have a female to male ratio of 10:1. Binge eating disorder reportedly affects 2% of all adults and is the most common eating disorder.

In the last 10 years, eating disorders have become very visible in the sports world. Research figures show that the prevalence of eating disorders in female athletes ranges from 1% to 62% depending on the sport and the diagnostic tool used to measure eating attitudes and behaviors (3,4). Sundgot-Borgen (6) studied elite female athletes representing 35 different sports and reported a greater incidence of eating disorders among athletes in aesthetic (34%) and weight-dependent sports (27%) compared to endurance (20%), technical (13%), and team sports (11%). The prevalence of eating disorders also varied within sports groups. For example, among endurance athletes, the prevalence was higher in runners and cross-country skiers than in cyclists, swimmers, and orienteers. These findings clearly support the theory that athletes participating in sports where leanness or a specific weight are important are at greater risk of developing an eating disorder. The number of athletes who develop subclinical eating disorders is not known; however, it appears to be more prevalent than previously thought and may lead to the development of a clinical eating disorder. According to Beals and Manore (2):

> "Severe food restriction may cause an increase in energy conservation or energy efficiency, which may undermine further attempts at weight loss or weight maintenance. This in turn may cause the athlete to resort to more extreme dietary measures and perhaps eventually develop a clinical eating disorder."

While most athletes diagnosed with anorexia or bulimia are women, male athletes who participate in low-weight sports such as wrestling, running, and crew are also at risk. Oppliger et al (7) reported that 1.7% of high school wrestlers meet the criteria for bulimia nervosa, a rate higher than expected for adolescent males. Eating and weight disturbances have also been reported in lightweight rowers (8,9). Lightweight rowers and wrestlers often develop distorted beliefs similar to female athletes about food, weight, and performance. In an effort to achieve a certain weight classification, they use a variety of weight-loss methods. Restricting food intake rapidly and severely is one of the most common weight control practices, followed by restricting fluids, increased exercise, and the use of a sauna. The psychological effects of "making weight" can lead to depression, low self-esteem, and preoccupation with food—personality features frequently seen in eating disordered persons.

Athletes who deliberately diet and overtrain may also be at risk for "muscle dysmorphia," a psychiatric disorder recently identified by Pope et al (10). Muscle dysmorphia is an excessive preoccupation with being musclar and fit. It is a form of body dysmorphic disorder (BDD) which is an obsession with a defect in visual appearance, specifically the face, hair, nose, and skin (1). Those suffering from muscle dysmorphia have a severely distorted body image. Despite being large and muscular, they see themselves as small and weak and some go to great lengths to improve their appearance. The classic symptoms of this condition include abuse of anabolic steroids and other substances, excessive exercise, withdrawal from social activities and relationships, depression, low self-esteem, and obsessive compulsive disorder (OCD) (10).

The number of athletes afflicted with muscle dysmorphia is not known. Bodybuilders are likely the most common suffers of the disorder because they already possess a certain amount of obsessiveness. Bodybuilders typically follow rigid diets and workout several hours a day in an effort to get more muscular and leaner.

Treatment for muscle or body dysmorphia is often difficult and there are no guarantees. Some success has been shown with drugs used to treat OCD, such as the selective serotonin reuptake inhibitors. Cognitive behavioral therapy may also be beneficial.

WHAT CAUSES AN ATHLETE TO DEVELOP AN EATING DISORDER?

Eating disorders result from a combination of biological, psychological, behavioral, social-environmental, and cultural factors (11). (See *Table 28.1.*) Females generally are at greater risk because our society places demands on women to achieve and maintain an ideal body shape. Even young girls who are underweight for their height are dieting to combat the fear of being overweight (12). Factors associated with weight concerns in adolescent girls include peer pressure, trying to look like girls/women on TV and in magazines, and being teased about their weight (11). Female athletes are also under pressure to perform and meet specific requirements for their sport (13).

TABLE 28.1   Risk Factors for Eating Disorders

Biological factors	Body weight
	Early maturation
	Pubertal development
Psychological factors	Body dissatisfaction
	Low self-esteem
Behavioral factors	Excess dieting
	Bingeing
Socio-environmental factors	Peer pressure to be thin
	Negative parental attitudes toward weight control
Cultural norms	Society's glamorization of thinness

Adapted from: Taylor et al. Factors associated with weight concerns in adolescent girls. *Int J Eat Disord.* 1998;24:31-42.

The close relationship between body image and performance makes athletes very vulnerable to an overemphasis on weight. Sundgot-Borgen (14) has identified several risk factors that may be responsible for precipitating the onset of eating disorders in athletes.

1. Dieting at an early age or to make a certain weight class
2. Personality factors—high self-expectation, perfectionism, persistence
3. Traumatic experiences with weigh-ins or comments from a coach or teammate about weight
4. Sudden increase in training
5. Emotional circumstances—an injury or loss of a coach
6. Sports emphasizing leanness—dance, figure skating, long-distance running
7. Sports requiring weight classifications—rowing, wrestling, weight-lifting

It has been suggested that female athletes most at risk for eating disorders are those who are experiencing considerable distress achieving a separate and adequate sense of self, who are conflictually dependent on their parents, and who engage in harsh, destructive forms of self-restraint (15). While athletics alone does not cause an eating disorder, social pressure for thinness from coaches and peers combined with anxiety about athletic performance and negative self-appraisal can set the stage (16). The very personality that promotes excellence in athletic participation is the personality that predisposes one to compulsions. It is often a way to get parental attention, and in emotionally blunted families sports can become a form of emotional expression.

EARLY CLUES TO AN EATING DISORDER

There is a distinct difference between restricting food to stay thin and having anorexia, and between vomiting to reach a desired weight and having bulimia (17). Preoccupations with weight and dieting do not always indicate an eating disorder is at bay. Some athletes may show signs of disordered eating during training but resume normal eating habits and gain weight during the off-season (18). A few telltale signs to look for include menstrual irregularity, gastrointestinal complaints, injuries, low self-esteem, and dieting or restrictive eating habits.

Menstrual Irregularities

Menstrual irregularities include amenorrhea (the absence of three to six consecutive menstrual cycles) and oligomenorrhea (three to six menstrual cycles a year at intervals greater than 36 days) (19). In the general population the prevalence of amenorrhea is between 2% and 5%. Among female athletes, however, the prevalence of amenorrhea is reported to be as high as 44% (20). A number of factors have been implicated in the cause of amenorrhea, including low body weight, excessive exercise training, insufficient calorie intake, and inadequate vegetarian diets (21).

There is a tendency to think of amenorrhea as always directly related to percent body fat and that restoring body fat will reverse the menstrual irregularity. While much of athletic amenorrhea is related to the low estrogen levels found when body fat is decreased, it is important not to discount the impact that chronically elevated stress hormones (ie, cortisol) have on menstrual function. Cortisol elevation tends to suppress reproductive function. In some studies amenorrheic athletes regained their cycles within days of being sidelined for an injury or taking a vacation. It is important to address low body fat if it exists, but to be aware that the symptom may result from hypothalamic dysfunction and not dietary deficiency.

Gastrointestinal Complaints

Complaints of constipation and bloating should also raise suspicions of an eating disorder. Constipation is caused by decreased gastric motility due to starvation, irregular eating habits, and/or laxative abuse (22). Constipation is a common side effect after bulimic clients eliminate laxatives and diuretics from their daily routine. Because there is a tendency for psychosomatic complaints in eating disorders, it is important to ascertain whether the client is constipated (experiencing bowel function that varies from normal) or overly focused on physical symptoms. A thorough history of the actual complaint, frequency of bowel movement, hydration, and dietary intake are vital to making this assessment. Until a gastrointestinal workup rules out any physical explanation for the complaints, they should be considered as real.

Response to Injury

Another important clue to the presence of an eating disorder may be the athlete's response to injury. Athletes often use extreme exercise as a method of controlling weight and become very anxious when an injury prevents them from participating in their regular routine. Christy Henrich, a world-class gymnast who died after a long battle with eating disorders, exercised to exhaustion in an effort to lose weight. Athletic trainers and physical therapists need to be educated about eating disorders since they are in long-term contact with the injured athlete and can be the person who develops the trust that results in referral.

Low Self-esteem

Low self-esteem is also a well-known trait of athletes with eating disorders and may be a motivating factor in the development of anorexia and bulimia (23). Persons with eating disorders generally have a history of low self-esteem and difficulty coping with stress. Performing as an athlete may be a focus that helps to build self-esteem.

Dieting or Restrictive Eating Habits

What often begins as a casual diet in an effort to shed a few pounds or decrease body fat often ends in a lifetime battle with food. It has been shown time and again that many cases of anorexia nervosa and bulimia nervosa develop following a period of restrictive dieting (24). Restrictive eating behaviors can range from inadequate nutrition to voluntary starvation coupled with extreme exercise regimens (25). Many athletes cautiously watch the amount of fat they consume, striving for intakes less than 10% of total calories. Dairy products, meats, and sweets are often omitted from the diet because these foods are believed to cause weight gain. The more restrictive the behavior, the more obsessive and controlling the athlete becomes about what foods she or he can and cannot eat. Two studies have examined the nutritional status of female athletes with eating disorders (26,27). Sundgot-Borgen (26) reported that a significant number of the athletes' diets were low in energy and carbohydrate. Additionally, there were low intakes of several micronutrients (ie, calcium, vitamin D, and iron). Beals and Manore (27) also reported low-energy intakes as well as low intakes of protein, carbohydrate, and fat due to food restriction and avoidance of red meat and dairy products.

Restrictive eating behaviors, bingeing and purging, and prolonged severe energy restriction can result in decreased performance, serious medication complications, and even death. Health professionals working with athletes should become more aware of the health problems associated with eating disorders, most notably amenorrhea and osteoporosis. (See *Box 28.5*.)

BOX 28.5   The Female Athlete Triad: A New Position Statement

In 1997, the American College of Sports Medicine published its position statement on the female athlete triad. The triad consists of disordered eating, amenorrhea, and osteoporosis. It occurs in physically active girls and women as well as elite athletes. The components of the triad are interrelated in cause, progression, and outcome. Alone or in combination, triad disorders can reduce physical performance and have serious medical and psychological consequences.

Women and girls are subject to inner and societal pressure to reach and maintain unrealistically low levels of body weight and/or body fat. These forces contribute to the development of disordered eating behaviors that help to initiate the triad. Other factors that are specific to athletes include sport-related emphasis on body weight and body fat, perfectionism, lack of nutrition knowledge, drive to excel at any cost, impact of injury, and pressure to lose weight from parents, coaches, judges, and others.

Obtaining accurate prevalence data for athletic populations is difficult because athletes often deny disordered eating behaviors. Furthermore, those who chronically engage in disordered eating practices generally do not meet the strict DSM-IV diagnostic criteria for anorexia nervosa or bulimia nervosa. Many athletes erroneously believe that losing weight by any method enhances performance and that disordered eating behaviors are harmless. Inadequate caloric intake and disordered eating practices jeopardize health and performance due to muscle glycogen depletion, dehydration, loss of muscle mass, hypoglycemia, electrolyte disturbances, anemia, amenorrhea, and osteoporosis.

The amenorrhea component of the triad is believed to be hypothalamic in origin and caused by decreased ovarian hormone production and a hypoestrogenemia similar to menopause. The hypothesis is that low-energy availability disrupts the hypothalamic gonadotrophic-releasing hormone pulse generator. Thus, menstrual disorders are caused by a failure to consume enough energy to compensate for the energy cost of exercise, rather than by exercise itself. To avoid alterations in their reproductive hormones and menstrual function, active women should consume enough calories to match their calorie expenditure.

Amenorrhea is the most discernible symptom of the triad. Unfortunately, many women welcome the convenience of not menstruating and do not report the amenorrhea because they consider it to be benign. However, the low concentration of ovarian hormones in amenorrheic athletes is associated with reduced bone mass and an increased rate of bone loss. Clinicians should exclude all other causes of amenorrhea and encourage amenorrheic women to consume at least 1,500 mg of elemental calcium per day. Although reduced training, increased intake, weight gain, and hormone replacement therapy may restore menses, bone mineral density may not return to normal levels. Poor nutrition and amenorrhea may reduce skeletal accretion during the critical years of bone formation in the adolescent athlete, placing the athlete at risk for stress fractures and premature osteoporosis.

Sport medicine professionals should be aware of the interrelated development and the varied presentation of triad components because the triad is often not recognized, denied, and under-reported. They should be able to recognize, diagnose, treat, or refer women who present with any triad component. Athletes who have one triad component should be checked for others. Screening can occur during the preparticipation examination and/or clinical evaluation for menstrual change, weight change, disordered eating patterns, cardiac arrhythmia (including bradycardia), depression, or stress fracture.

All sports medicine professionals, trainers, coaches, and officials of sports-governing bodies should learn how to prevent and recognize the symptoms and risks of the triad. Those who work with active girls and women, including parents, should promote a training environment that is medically and psychologically sound. There should not be pressure to lose weight. Sports medicine professionals should have a fundamental knowledge of nutrition and be able to recommend resources for nutrition, medical and psychological evaluation, and counseling. Active girls and women should learn about proper nutrition, safe training practices, and the warning signs and risks of the triad.

IDENTIFICATION

If you suspect an athlete has an eating disorder, it is important to intervene. Many colleges and universities have developed policies and procedures for the prevention, treatment, and intervention regarding eating disorders in athletes. A multidisciplinary team of professionals who have knowledge in the different aspects of recovery offers the best therapeutic approach. The team includes a physician, psychologist, psychiatrist, nutrition therapist, and coach or trainer. Each member of the team works together on problems related to the eating disorder. For instance, the physician monitors the athlete's medical condition, the psychiatrist manages the use of medication, the nutrition therapist addresses food and weight-related behaviors, and the psychologist focuses on family and peer issues. The coach and/or trainer provides support and works with the athlete on performance-related issues. (See *Box 28.6*.)

BOX 28.6   The Initial Intervention: What to Do, What Not to Do

WHAT TO DO

- The coach or trainer who has the best rapport with the person should arrange a private meeting.
- Express support for the person and concern for his or her best interests. Stress that health and happiness transcend the athletic arena. Be empathic and caring.
- In an objective and nonpunitive way, list what you have seen and what you have heard that have led you to be concerned. Let the athlete respond fully. Expect denial and rationalization.
- Emphasize that the person's place on the team or in the program will not be endangered by an admission that he or she has an eating disorder.
- Add that athletic participation will be curtailed only if the eating disorder has compromised the person's health or put him or her at risk for injury.
- If the athlete admits having an eating disorder, try to determine if he or she can voluntarily abstain from the behaviors.
- If, in the face of compelling evidence, the athlete refuses to admit that a problem exists, or if it seems that the problem has either been long-standing or cannot be corrected readily, consult a clinician with expertise in eating disorders.
- Remember that most people with eating disorders have tried repeatedly, and failed, to correct the problem on their own. Failure is especially demoralizing to athletes who are constantly oriented toward success.
- Let the person know that eating disorders are treatable, and people do recover from them. Almost always, though, professional help is necessary. Needing help should not be regarded as a sign of weakness, inadequacy, or lack of effort.
- Arrange for regular, private, follow-up meetings apart from practice times.
- If the athlete is working with a physician or counselor, ask that resource person how you can best help and then do it.
- Remember that many athletes who develop eating disorders have been told in the past that they need to lose weight. Realize that past or present coaches or trainers may have contributed to the eating disorder. Let the athlete know that you know that the demands of the sport may have played a role in the development of the problem.

---

continued

BOX 28.6   The Initial Intervention: What to Do, What Not to Do (continued)

WHAT NOT TO DO

- Don't question teammates or talk to them about the athlete. Talk directly to him or her.

- If you have evidence that a problem exists, intervene. Don't hope it will go away if you ignore it. It won't.

- Don't tell the person that you know he or she has a problem without giving him or her your reasons and the evidence. He or she will only become defensive.

- Don't tell the athlete to straighten up. Don't threaten to keep checking on him or her.

- Never conclude that if the athlete really wanted to stop the behaviors, he or she would make it happen. Don't make the mistake of believing that failure to improve shows a lack of effort. Even the fastest recoveries, facilitated by mental health professionals, take several months to years.

- Don't refuse to admit that you, and the demands of the sport, may have contributed to the eating disorder.

- Don't try to keep the problem hidden by attempting to deal with it yourself when professional intervention and treatment are clearly appropriate.

- Don't nag, bribe, threaten, or manipulate. These tactics don't work; they only make matters worse.

Reproduced with permission. Anorexia Nervosa and Related Eating Disorders (ANRED). Identifying the athlete with an eating disorder and the initial intervention. http://www.anred.com/ath-id.html. Accessed October 25, 1998.

It is essential that members of the eating disorder team work closely together so the messages communicated to the athlete are consistent (17). Grandjean et al (17) note that "most guidelines for the treatment of eating disorders have been developed based on clinical experience with nonathletes. There may be inherent differences in the treatment of athletes." The treatment team should also have experience working with athletes and an appreciation for the sport environment. Athletes can be afraid to talk about eating disorders because they are afraid of losing a financial scholarship. For an athlete, losing their sport means losing their identity.

The treatment team should determine who will dispense advice on weight and body fat. An athlete who is given different advice from different team members will tend to listen to the advice that best fits his or her disordered thinking. Agreeing as a team to relegate this authority to the team physician and/or nutrition therapist and encouraging coaches and trainers to refrain from comments about losing weight to improve performance are in the best interest of the athlete. Each athlete's recovery process is unique and, therefore, treatment plans and goals should be individualized (28). One of the issues likely to arise in treatment is whether or not the athlete should continue to train and compete. According to Sundgot-Borgen (29), "Suspension from sports is a good solution only for a few cases." Harris and Nattiv (30) believe if the athlete is not willing to comply with treatment, he or she should not be allowed to stay on the team. In most cases the decision is based on the severity of the eating disorder. Short-term restrictive eating habits or excessive exercise may not be severe enough to cause serious health risk to the athlete. However, prolonged starvation, laxative abuse, and self-induced vomiting place the athlete at great health risk and can jeopardize performance. If an athlete's eating disorder puts him or her in physical danger, a written contract signed by the coach, treatment team, and the athlete may be necessary. The contract mandates that the athlete show up for counseling and medical appointments in order to stay on the team.

THE ROLE OF THE SPORTS NUTRITIONIST

The goal in nutrition therapy for eating disorders (ED) is to develop awareness of emotions and a battery of communication and coping skills that address the issues to which these emotions relate. It is important to develop a supportive relationship that will keep the athlete returning for appointments. This can be achieved by developing and frequently referring to a list of nonweight-related recovery goals and providing assignments that encourage awareness of behaviors. ED individuals also need to learn how to have a healthy relationship with food. They have often used food almost exclusively as a means of emotional expression; nutrition therapy can introduce these athletes to the joys of tasting, smelling, moving, playing, nourishing oneself—all of which are virtually impossible under the constraints of a rigid diet and exercise plan.

The responsibilities of the nutrition therapist include (24):

1. Evaluating the athlete's food intake
2. Sharing with the psychologist and physician any behavior changes and/or dietary information
3. Educating the athlete about normal and abnormal food intake patterns
4. Helping the athlete understand weight and performance-related issues
5. Dispelling myths and misconceptions about diet, exercise, and health
6. Teaching the principles of good nutrition and meal planning

The Initial Interview

A 3-day food intake record is likely to reveal only a small part of the whole nutrition picture. While the anorexic client's intake may be monotonously regular, he or she may overexaggerate the portions consumed by describing the amount served instead of the amount actually eaten. The bulimic client may have difficulty recalling all the foods eaten or the number of times purging occurred. Do not assume portion sizes; ask specifically. To obtain a more complete evaluation of nutritional status, ask about alcohol or caffeine intake, supplements, laxatives, diuretics, and other medications (what kind, how much, how often, and when taken). These may represent cross-addictions, and the therapist should be aware of them.

Inquire about the client's attitudes toward eating, the eating environment (eg, companions), where food is eaten (eg, car, bathroom, kitchen, basement), how quickly food is eaten, and how soon purging is induced. Obtain the details of physical exercise (type, frequency, duration, and intensity). Intensity can be described in terms of heart rate, ability to talk, and heavy or light breathing.

The measurement of body composition via skinfold thickness may be perceived as too invasive during the initial interview, but when attained, this information will certainly complement the nutrition report.

For the underweight client, the most important goals are to establish 95% of normal body weight and to overcome the medical complications of malnutrition. Although these disorders typically take several months or years to develop and generally as long to correct, the medical consequences require immediate attention and care through an adequate nutrition program.

The nutrition plan should consist of approximately 20% to 30% of total calories as fat, and provide about 1.5 to 2.0 g protein per kg body weight. The meal plan should include five to six small meals. A word of caution: In the athlete who needs 4,000 calories per day to support his or her physical activity, 133 g of fat equals 30% of calories. It is important to ascertain the athlete's comfort level with this amount of fat, provide a meal plan that illustrates its incorporation, and emphasize that adding fat will decrease hunger, bloating, and the volume of food needed to reach this goal. Many athletes are struggling to eat 10 or fewer grams of fat; a jump to 133 g, if not provided with supportive nutrition education, will never be achieved.

Specific meal guidelines can be provided to avoid the anxiety of selecting foods. It is important to take into consideration the food preferences of clients and to provide support for their self-selected individualized diet plans (eg, vegetarianism), as long as their choices are generally healthful in nature. High-calorie supplements should be used only when the client has an extremely low body weight or is extremely anxious about eating six meals daily. Support should be given regarding fear-of-fatness issues, and clients should be reassured that the program will help them achieve their personal health and performance goals.

After the initial visit increments of 200 kcal each week can be added in conjunction with a supervised exercise program to achieve a weight gain of 0.5 to 2.0 lb per week. Bizarre food practices previously followed may be discussed at this time. It is important to express to clients that they will not feel any better about themselves, nor will they benefit from their newly adopted eating habits, if they continue abusing their bodies with laxatives, diuretics, diet pills, or recreational substances such as alcohol, marijuana, and cocaine to avoid feelings and food issues.

A food, mood, and activity diary may help clients with eating disorders feel like active participants in their treatment. Tools such as the computerized dietary analysis and blood examinations can give clients additional feedback on their progress. Positive support and education from the nutritionist strengthen the recovery process.

Nutrition treatment for the bulimic who is of normal weight is similar to that for the low body weight anorexic; the principal exception is that withdrawal from laxatives, diuretics, and other bulimic behaviors can create significant physical distress. In addition, there is a strong correlation between bulimia and physical and/or sexual abuse. Therefore, achieving dietary goals may require more gradual steps and psychotherapy to address the issues that drive the behavior. Avoidance of binge foods is suggested initially; the client can gradually progress to eating these foods in a controlled environment. For clients with bulimia, behavioral changes in eating habits are as important as restoring normal metabolism. Encourage bulimic clients to avoid excessive hunger by eating at least three meals per day. These clients should be encouraged to eat in the presence of others, because more often than not these individuals tend to eat most of their meals alone.

Exercise can be a healthy tool for achieving a better body image, fitness, and ideal body size, but it can be detrimental if it becomes another compulsion to replace the vomiting and other purgative agents. The food, mood, and activity diary may help to open conversations regarding this potential problem.

When counseling eating-disordered clients, it is important to remember that anorexics and bulimics are experts in deception and manipulation. If they sense the dietitian or therapist is vulnerable or inexperienced, they might attempt to exploit a perceived weakness by lying, creating a feeling of inadequacy in the dietitian, or trying to arouse conflict among professional consultants. A confident attitude on the part of the dietitian can be helpful in the treatment of the client. The goal is to reverse the client's distorted thinking about food, weight, and body image while promoting self-esteem and positive feelings about body weight.

PREVENTION

Athletes, coaches, trainers, parents, and physicians need to be educated about eating disorders—what they are, warning signs, who is most at risk, what to do if a problem arises, and what treatment options are available. Eating disorders are serious and complex problems. Being prepared to intervene when an athlete is identified as having an eating disorder reduces anxiety and fear and assures that the athlete will receive the proper support and treatment. The American College of Sports Medicine and the American Academy of Pediatrics have issued position statements warning against the dangers of unhealthy weight control practices in athletes (20,31).

Educational programs aimed at reducing our cultural obsession with thinness and society's distorted meaning of both femininity and masculinity are needed (32). Eating Disorders Awareness and Prevention, Inc. (EDAP) is a national, nonprofit organization dedicated to the prevention of eating disorders. It provides information to health care professionals, K-12 and college educators, families, friends, and sufferers. One of the programs established by EDAP is Eating Disorders Awareness Week (EDAW). During this week (every February) and throughout the year, volunteer coordinators, health professionals, and educators organize educational outreach programs and presentations in schools and communities. EDAP provides these coordinators with educational and promotional materials.

HUGS, International is an organization whose vision is to "challenge the myths of the diet industry by shifting the attitudes and beliefs of the public from the preoccupation with weight and size to an acceptance and appreciation of healthier living" (33). Programs and materials for teens and adults emphasize eating for energy, physical activity for fun, and size acceptance. HUGS, International sponsors the annual public awareness campaign, "International NoDiet Day" (33). The goal of NoDiet Day is to debunk diet myths and embrace healthier alternatives.

Girls on the Run is another innovative program that combats the cultural and social pressures facing adolescents today (34). This 12-week program is designed exclusively for preteen girls. It uses physical activity and experimental learning to teach social and personal skills. According to Molly Barker, founder and director of the Girls on the Run program, "It is the development of these skills that can prevent future at-risk behaviors for eating disorders" (34).

Girls on the Run provides girls with an opportunity to enhance self-esteem and develop physically, emotionally, and spiritually. *Box 28.7* lists helpful websites.

BOX 28.7   Web sites about Eating Disorders

• After the Diet Disordered Eating Resources	http://www.afterthediet.com
• Anorexia Nervosa and Related Eating Disorders, Inc. (ANRED)	http://www.anred.com
• Gurze Books	http://www.gurze.com
• Something Fishy	http://www.somethingfishy.com
• Sportfuel Sports Nutrition Resources	http://www.sportfuel.com
• HUGS International, Inc.	http://www.hugs.com
• Eating Disorders Awareness and Prevention, Inc.	http://www.edapinc.com
• The Renfrew Center	http://www.renfrew.org
• National Eating Disorders Organization	http://www.aureate.com

---

REFERENCES

1. American Psychiatric Association. *Diagnostic and Statistical Manual of Mental Disorders.* 4th ed. Washington, DC: American Psychiatric Association; 1994.
2. Beals KA, Manore MM. The prevalence and consequences of subclinical eating disorders in female athletes. *Int J Sport Nutr.* 1994;4:175-195.
3. Sundgot-Borgen J. Prevalence of eating disorders in elite female athletes. *Int J Sport Nutr.* 1993;3:29-40.
4. Burckes-Miller ME, Black DR. Male and female college athletes. Prevalence of anorexia nervosa and bulimia nervosa. *Athletic Training.* 1988;2:137-140.
5. Sports, Cardiovascular, and Wellness Nutritionists. What is disordered eating? *SCAN's Pulse.* 1997;16(1):8-10.
6. Sundgot-Borgen J. Risk and trigger factors for the development of eating disorders in female elite athletes. *Med Sci Sports Exerc.* 1994;26:414-419.
7. Oppliger RA, Landry GL, Foster SW, Lambrecht AC. Bulimic behaviors among interscholastic wrestlers: a statewide survey. *Pediatrics.* 1993;91:826-831.
8. Thiel A, Gottfried H, Hesse FW. Subclinical eating disorders in male athletes. A study of the low weight category in rowers and wrestlers. *Acta Psychiatr Scand.* 1993;88:259-265.
9. Sykora C, Grillo CM, Wilfley DE, Brownell KD. Eating, weight, and dieting disturbances in male and female lightweight and heavyweight rowers. *Int J Eat Disord.* 1993;14:203-211.

10. Pope HG, Gruber AJ, Choi P, Olivardia R, Phillips KA. Muscle dysmorphia. An underrecognized form of body dysmorphic disorder. *Psychosomatics*. 1997;38:548-557.

11. Taylor CB, Sharpe T, Shisslak C, et al. Factors associated with weight concerns in adolescent girls. *Int J Eat Disord*. 1998;24:31-42.

12. Koff E, Rierdan J. Perceptions of weight and attitudes toward eating in early adolescent girls. *J Adolesc Health*. 1991;12:307-312.

13. Wilmore JH. Eating and weight disorders in the female athlete. *Int J Sport Nutr*. 1991;1:104-117.

14. Sundgot-Borgen J. Eating disorders, energy intake, training volume, and menstrual function in high-level modern rhythmic gymnasts. *Int J Sport Nutr*. 1996;6:100-109.

15. Skowron EA, Friedlander ML. Psychological separation, self-control, and weight preoccupation among elite women athletes. *J Counseling Devel*. 1994;72:310-315.

16. Williamson DA, Netemeyer RG, Jackman LP, Anderson DA, Funsch CL, Rabalais JY. Structural equation modeling of risk factors for the development of eating disorder symptoms in female athletes. *Int J Eat Disord*. 1995;17:387-393.

17. Grandjean AC, Woscyna GR, Ruud JS. Eating disorders in athletes. In: Mellion MB, ed. *Office Sports Medicine*. 2nd ed. Philadelphia, Penn: Hanley & Belfus; 1996:113-119.

18. Leon GR. Eating disorders in female athletes. *Sports Med*. 1991;12:219-227.

19. Putukian M. The female triad: eating disorders, amenorrhea, and osteoporosis. *Med Clin North Am*. 1994;78:345-356.

20. American College of Sports Medicine. The female athlete triad. *Med Sci Sports Exerc*. 1997;29:i-ix.

21. Benson JE, Engelbert-Fenton KA, Eisenman PA. Nutritional aspects of amenorrhea in the female athlete triad. *Int J Sport Nutr*. 1996;6:134-145.

22. McClain CJ, Humphries LL, Hill KK, Nicki NJ. Gastrointestinal and nutritional aspects of eating disorders. *J Am Coll Nutr*. 1993;12:466-474.

23. Lindeman AK. Self-esteem: its application to eating disorders and athletes. *Int J Sport Nutr*. 1994;4:237-252.

24. Reiff DW, Reiff KKL. *Eating Disorders: Nutrition Therapy in the Recovery Process*. Mercer Island, Wash: Life Enterprise; 1997.

25. Johnson MD. Disordered eating in active and athletic women. *Clin Sports Med*. 1994;13:355-369.

26. Sundgot-Borgen J. Nutrient intake of female elite athletes suffering from eating disorders. *Int J Sport Nutr*. 1993;3:431-442.

27. Beals KA, Manore MM. Nutritional status of female athletes with subclinical eating disorders. *J Am Diet Assoc*. 1998;98:419-425.

28. Position of The American Dietetic Association. Nutrition intervention in the treatment of anorexia nervosa, bulimia nervosa, and binge eating. *J Am Diet Assoc*. 1994;94:902-907.

29. Sundgot-Borgen J. Eating disorder. In: Berning JR, Steen SN, eds. *Nutrition for Sports & Exercise*. Gaithersburg, Md: Aspen Publishers; 1998:199.

30. Harris SS, Nattiv A. Controversies in sports medicine: should women with eating disorders be allowed to participate in athletics? *Sports Med Digest*. 1995;17:1-4.

31. Committee on Sports Medicine and Fitness. Promotion of healthy weight-control practices in young athletes. *Pediatrics*. 1996;97:752-753.

32. Eating Disorders Awareness and Prevention, Inc. http://www.edapinc.com. Accessed April 1, 1999.

33. Hugs International, Inc. http://www.hugs.com. Accessed April 1, 1999.

34. Barker M. Girls on the Run: coping with the crisis of cultural pressure. *Healthy Weight*. 1997;12:89-91.

29

EXERCISE AND PREGNANCY

Kelly Kullick, RD, ACE-certified personal trainer and Lynn Dugan, MS, RD

Physical fitness and activity are important in the lives of many women. Women are staying more active during pregnancy and are looking for guidance on safety and the appropriate exercise duration and intensity. Historically, exercise during pregnancy has not been widely studied. This is attributed to concern about putting pregnant women at risk during clinical trials (1). As a result, health care providers are cautious in recommending exercise during pregnancy. Despite sanctioned guidelines, questions remain regarding the extent to which a pregnant woman can exercise without compromising the growth and development of the fetus. Recently, research has begun to provide answers and is leading to a more liberal, often more practical, school of thought on exercise for active women during pregnancy (2). The most recent guidelines for exercise during pregnancy from the American College of Obstetricians and Gynecologists (ACOG) were published in February 1994 (3). They can be obtained by requesting Technical Bulletin No. 189 in writing to ACOG, 409 12th Street SW, Washington, DC 20024.

Available data suggest that beginning or maintaining an exercise program is suitable for most healthy women during pregnancy, especially in the second and third trimester. Although no level of exercise has been conclusively demonstrated to improve perinatal outcome, exercise can enhance maternal fitness and sense of well-being (3). Exercise is also associated with fewer discomforts during pregnancy (4).

In contrast to the lack of knowledge on the effects of exercise on pregnancy and perinatal outcomes, there is a more comprehensive understanding of the effect of pregnancy on exercise. Specifically, physiologic changes during pregnancy, such as blood volume expansion and the change in the center of gravity, can significantly affect exercise performance.

Whether a pregnant woman has been sedentary or athletic, all should share common goals during pregnancy. The emphasis shifts from athletic performance, body sculpting, and weight loss to health goals that protect the mother and the fetus and provide enhancements to muscular strength, cardiovascular fitness, flexibility, and posture.

In fact, for many pregnant women, the breadth of exercise expands beyond aerobic and strength training. In addition to pelvic floor strengthening exercises, pregnant women benefit from relaxation techniques and flexibility exercises. Furthermore, the maximum benefit of exercise for the pregnant women is achieved by expanding the workout routine to incorporate total body exercises. For instance, adding head and neck exercises to a program already focusing on abdominal muscles, arms, legs, and back will round out the program for the pregnant woman.

Helping a pregnant client identify the physiologic changes that occur in pregnancy related to nutrition and exercise will allow her to attain the benefits available from exercise. In addition, as research advances in the area of exercise and pregnancy, it is critical that the sports nutritionist stay abreast of developments to continue to contribute to the health care team.

WEIGHT GAIN

The role of the dietetics professional is valuable to ensure adequate weight gain during pregnancy. The food choices a client makes are critical for the growth and development of the fetus. This is especially true for an athletic pregnant client, since she has increased energy expenditure during exercise. As a result, caloric needs to gain the appropriate amount of weight are greater than those for a sedentary woman of equal weight for height.

While the daily energy needs for the athletic pregnant woman increase, the individual needs may not increase based on exercise changes. For example, if the pregnant woman was a competitive athlete, or a very strenuous exerciser, and decides to cut back on exercise intensity and/or duration during pregnancy, daily caloric needs will likely decrease. Therefore, even with the increased energy needs to support the growth of the fetus and to move the heavier pregnant body, the less active pregnant woman may not have energy needs that were as high as during prepregnancy. The dietetics professional should evaluate the caloric needs of the pregnant woman throughout pregnancy, since needs will likely change to accommodate activity level. Further, the pregnant woman should be encouraged to listen to her body for hunger signals.

"How much weight should I gain?" This is one of the first questions asked by a new mother. Weight gain guidelines differ depending on prepregnancy weight. A 25- to 35-lb weight gain is appropriate for women within the normal weight-for-height guidelines based on body mass index (BMI). Underweight women should strive for a 28- to 40-lb weight gain, and overweight women should keep their weight gain to 15 to 25 lb. Women expecting multiple births, however, should strive for additional weight gain. For example, a 35- to 45-lb weight gain is appropriate for women of "normal" weight-for-height expecting twins. Because the metabolic needs of the pregnant athlete are often higher than a sedentary woman, one of the roles for a dietetics professional is to monitor weight gain and recommend an appropriate calorie intake (5).

Studies show a high correlation between inadequate maternal weight gain and high-risk, low-birth-weight babies (5-7). If a client is exercising excessively, or intentionally keeping her weight down, consult her physician. Unfortunately, many women with a history of eating disorders insist on maintaining an excessive exercise routine and restrictive eating habits during pregnancy. Encourage the weight-conscious woman to think of her child and the risks associated with low birth-weight.

"Normal" weight gain for women is based on individual needs. Generally, a 3- to 5-lb weight gain during the first trimester is adequate. During the second and third trimesters, however, a weight gain goal of just under 1 lb per week is an acceptable guideline. An additional 300 kcal per day is recommended during the second and third trimesters to reach this goal. Encourage a client to monitor her weight weekly when adequately hydrated. If she is not gaining approximately 1 lb per week, increase calorie needs appropriately. She may be expending more than 300 kcal per day in exercise that may negate weight gain.

NUTRITION NEEDS

The additional 300 kcal needed for pregnancy should come from adding one protein and one dairy serving (5). However, an exercising client may need extra calories given her increased metabolism and higher energy expenditure. Because carbohydrate and protein are the two major fuel sources of energy for the fetus, additional calories needed for exercise should come from added servings of carbohydrate (8). Carbohydrate intake meets the growth needs of the fetus and provides energy for the physiological changes of pregnancy.

Soultanakis et al (8) found that during periods of exercise greater than 20 minutes, both extracellular glucose and hepatic glycogen stores are depleted and free fatty acids become the major source of energy. Free fatty acids are elevated to spare glucose for the growing fetus as well as for maternal brain needs. Because blood glucose levels in pregnant women decrease more quickly during exercise and remain lower postexercise, hypoglycemia is more likely to occur during and after exercise in pregnancy (8). Therefore, women who exercise should eat a small (15-g carbohydrate) snack approximately 1 hour prior to their workout (9). *Box 29.1* lists examples of snacks that contain 15 g of carbohydrate.

BOX 29.1 Examples of 15-g Carbohydrate Snacks

- 1 slice of bread
- 2 graham crackers
- 10 saltines
- 1/2 English muffin
- 1/2 bagel
- 1 cup milk
- 1 medium piece of fruit
- 4 oz fruit juice
- 1/2 cup canned fruit
- 7 pretzels
- 7 wheat crackers
- 1/2 cereal bar
- 1/4 cup pudding prepared with milk
- 1 toaster pastry

Sports drinks are recommended to replete carbohydrate, fluid, and electrolyte losses for pregnant women who exercise more than 30 to 45 minutes per session. Sports drinks should contain 6% to 8% carbohydrate. Sports drinks containing less than 5% do not provide enough carbohydrate, whereas those containing 10% or more tend to cause nausea, diarrhea, and intestinal cramping (10).

Due to increased blood supply, water is a critical nutrient for a healthy pregnancy. Expectant women should be encouraged to drink 8 to 12 cups of water or other hydrating fluids per day. Water is the preferred source of hydration; however, other fluids may include decaffeinated beverages, soups, milk, juice, or sports drinks for strenuous exercisers. Strenuous exercise induces significant water loss and puts women at greater risk for dehydration. Exercising women should allow for additional fluid intake to keep well hydrated and keep body temperature within normal limits. Specifically, encourage the client to consume 16 oz at least 1 to 2 hours prior to exercise and 4 to 8 oz during exercise at 15- to 20-minute intervals, and to replenish fluids after exercise (10).

Pregnant women should consume two to three servings, or 6 to 7 oz, of protein per day. For fetal development, protein is an essential building block for cellular growth as well as for the development of hair, skin, muscles, nerves, and brain tissue.

Eating three to four servings of high-calcium foods per day, such as dairy products, calcium-set tofu, salmon with bones, or calcium-fortified beverages, will help pregnant women reach the prenatal calcium requirement of 1,000 to 1,300 mg per day. Soy and dairy products also provide significant amounts of protein. Calcium-fortified food products can be used to add variety to food choices.

Societal attitudes often discourage a diet with a reasonable amount of fat. However, dietary fat has a vital function in utilizing fat-soluble vitamins. In addition, body fat has many vital functions including regulating body temperature and supplying fuel, and as a precursor for hormones, bile, and vitamin D. Remind the exercising client that fat is a needed nutrient. Fat intake should be limited to 30% of daily caloric intake (11).

Prescribed routinely, the prenatal multivitamin provides a source of iron, folic acid, and additional vitamins and minerals. However, the prenatal vitamin is a supplement not a replacement for a nutritious, healthy diet. Encourage the client to eat a variety of foods to meet daily nutrition needs.

Because pregnancy and exercise put a greater demand on the body for oxygen, women who exercise during pregnancy should have adequate iron intake. Iron is essential to build the fetal blood supply as well as to support maternal erythropoiesis during pregnancy (5). Symptoms of iron deficiency anemia include fatigue, anorexia, pagophagia, immunocompetence, and impaired muscle function (12). If anemia is suspected, ask the physician to evaluate iron status.

Progesterone is released during pregnancy to relax the smooth muscles of the uterus to accommodate fetal growth; however, it also relaxes other smooth muscles such as the muscles of the gastrointestinal tract. As a result, motility in the gut is prolonged allowing for greater nutrient absorption. Along with this benefit comes one side effect. Slowed motility is often the cause of constipation in pregnancy (5). Fiber decreases intestinal transit time and increases fecal volume so an adequate supply of fiber (25 to 35 g per day) is critical to maintain consistent gastrointestinal function. Fiber can also help to alleviate another common occurrence of pregnancy—hemorrhoids. To ensure consistent bowel function, the woman should be encouraged to exercise regularly, choose 6 to 11 servings of complex carbohydrates, at least five servings of fruits and vegetables, and at least eight 8-oz glasses of water and hydrating beverages daily.

EFFECTS OF PREGNANCY ON EXERCISE

Pregnancy has specific effects on exercise. Physiological changes require a client to modify her exercise routine. Educating pregnant women about what changes to expect will help them to maintain a safe and healthy exercise routine. Safety is a high priority for prenatal exercise. The recommendations for exercise in pregnancy are designed to protect the health of the fetus as well as to assist maternal adaptation to physiological and hormonal changes.

Traditionally, exercise in the supine position (ie, exercises that include abdominal and leg exercises while lying on the back) has not been recommended after the first trimester. The additional weight of the enlarging uterus puts pressure on the inferior vena cava that can cause hypotension with resulting dizziness, nausea, and shortness of breath (9).

Clapp (2), however, has not found any objective information to indicate that exercise in the supine position should be avoided. He contends that as long as the legs and torso are moving, blood flow back to the heart should not be hindered. If a woman begins to feel dizzy, she should roll to her left side to allow the blood flow to freely move through the inferior vena cava (2).

Given the controversial information on exercising in the supine position after the first trimester, it is best to advise women to monitor the effects of the fetus on blood flow. As always, a pregnant woman should listen to her body and make adjustments when necessary. If she begins to feel dizzy while lying on her back, she should roll to the left to maximize blood flow back to the heart. She may recognize this as a signal that the weight of her uterus is now too heavy to continue exercising in this position.

Women should subjectively monitor intensity using a perceived exertion scale (6 = no exertion, 20 = maximal exertion) rather than target heart rate or body temperature. A safe exertion rate is defined as "somewhat hard" (13) on the Rating of Perceived Exertion scale (RPE) (9). However, depending on prepregnancy RPE, a safe exertion rate during pregnancy may range from 11 to 15.

Animal studies indicate that body temperature of 102°F or higher can lead to abnormalities of the fetal central nervous system including spina bifida or hydroencephalopathy. While most women do not exercise to this level of exertion, the increased demands of any exercise routine present a greater risk of hyperthermia. Because this risk is highest in hot, humid weather, exercise should be limited or avoided in such conditions. *Box 29.2* offers suggestions on preventing dehydration and hyperthermia. Pregnant women should monitor body temperature immediately after exercise to make sure it does not rise to 102°F (10,13).

BOX 29.2 Prevent Dehydration and Hyperthermia

- Drink plenty of fluids—water, milk, fruit juice, vegetable juice, sports drinks, broths and soups, caffeine-free soft drinks, sparkling water.
- Drink enough liquid to keep the urine dilute and almost colorless.
- If getting up to urinate during the night, drink water in preparation for morning exercises.
- Avoid exercising during midday heat.
- Avoid exercising indoors without air conditioning.
- Wear cotton or the newer "wicking" fabrics to keep cool.

Because maximum heart rate decreases during pregnancy and resting heart rate increases, especially in late gestation, the usefulness of target heart rates for determining exercise intensity is questionable (14). However, target heart rate monitoring is still the most commonly used method to measure exercise intensity. The American College of Obstetricians and Gynecologists recommends maintaining heart rate <150 beats per minute (15).

To compensate for the changes in breathing and to avoid breathlessness and hyperventilation, exercise intensity should be closely monitored. Caution must be advised to avoid breath holding and instead to focus on inhaling and exhaling deeply, evenly, and slowly. To adjust for the diminished cardiac reserve that causes women to tire more easily, the pregnant woman should adjust her workout. She may stop or slow down when fatigued, or she may lower the intensity of her entire workout so she may exercise for the length of time she desires. Exhaustive exercise, however, should be avoided (4,9).

Peripheral joint laxity increases in pregnancy to allow joints to stretch and ligaments to relax, thereby allowing the body to accommodate the size of the baby as it grows. To protect the body, caution clients to avoid stretching to the maximum. The exercising pregnant woman may be particularly prone to injury because her body can stretch beyond her comfort zone, resulting in injury (9).

Because the growing uterus presses against the bladder, the pregnant woman urinates more frequently. Although frequent visits to the bathroom are inconvenient, adequate fluid intake is necessary for hydration and increased blood flow, especially while exercising.

As the pelvic floor muscles weaken during the last trimester, incontinence may become a problem. Therefore, it is recommended that Kegel exercises to strengthen muscles and control the bladder be performed. Kegels are performed by repetitively contracting and releasing the pelvic floor muscles. These exercises produce the same feeling as stopping the flow of urine while urinating. Encourage clients to incorporate Kegels into their daily exercise routine (9). Clients should not, however, perform these exercises while urinating because it increases the risk of urinary tract infections.

A pregnant woman's center of gravity changes as the baby grows. Balance may be affected, especially in the third trimester. Therefore, consider the necessary modifications for physical activity in which balance is important.

Mild abdominal muscle separation, known as diastasis recti, is a common problem among pregnant and postpartum women; it is caused by a stretching of the linea alba, the long ligament separating the abdominal muscles. While this problem is common, it is not serious. Encourage your client to check for diastasis recti before each workout. Instruct her to lay on her back and place two of her fingers just above or below the navel. She should then lift her head and shoulders off the ground and press down with her fingers. If a separation greater than the width of the fingers is felt, she should modify abdominal exercise (9).

If diastasis recti is present, exercises may be modified from a full crunch to a supported crunch and an omission of the oblique exercises. To modify a crunch, the woman should wrap her arms across one another across the abdominal area. As she crunches up, she should tighten her arms to support her separated muscles (9). Another suggested abdominal exercise is the pelvic tilt. The woman lays on her back, feet on the ground, hip distance apart, and lifts the gluteus maximus muscle off the floor; she then gently contracts and releases the abdominal muscles. It is important to include a good abdominal routine to provide extra support and stability for the back.

Encourage daily abdominal exercises to take pressure off of the back, thereby minimizing lower back pain. Weak abdominal muscles commonly cause lower back pain, a condition which is typical during pregnancy due to the increased frontal weight load and tense back muscles (9).

Common sense should dictate never to exercise in sickness or pain, or in very hot or humid weather. Heat dissipation should be assisted with proper clothing and adequate hydration. Regular exercise is preferred to sporadic bouts of physical activity. Activities to be avoided include those that may involve risk of abdominal trauma such as snow skiing and water skiing, or activities that may result in a fall.

EFFECTS OF EXERCISE ON PREGNANCY

There are many benefits to exercising during pregnancy. Exercise increases energy level and overall sense of well-being. The endorphins released during a workout create an additional psychological boost. Exercise may also help to maintain self-esteem. Furthermore, an exercise routine gives the pregnant woman an opportunity to take some time for herself (1,9). Many physical benefits accompany an exercise routine as well. These include improved circulation, reduced swelling and leg cramps, strengthened abdominal muscles, reduced backaches, and increased muscular balance. Exercise also increases the rate of digestion, absorption, and utilization of nutrients (1,9).

The benefits of exercise are different in early versus late pregnancy. Early pregnancy exercise improves placental growth and functional capacity. Later pregnancy exercise maintains maternal fitness and limits weight gain (2).

EFFECTS OF EXERCISE ON CONCEPTION, LABOR, AND FETAL OUTCOME

Results from several studies (14,16) indicate that pregnant women who have been exercising prior to pregnancy may continue to exercise at the same intensity without putting themselves or their unborn child at risk. Clapp (14,16) found that women who exercised at least 3 days per week for 30 minutes per session did not decrease their rate of conception, nor did they increase the incidence of spontaneous abortion. Therefore, exercising at this level does not decrease a woman's chances of conceiving, nor does it increase her risk of miscarriage. Clapp also found that exercising women did not have greater incidences of ectopic pregnancy or placental weakness.

Exercise during pregnancy has little or no effect on labor and fetal outcome. The primary benefit is the maternal comfort and well-being during labor, pregnancy, and prior to conception. Maternal comfort, however, is a significant factor that should not be discounted. In addition, exercising women tend to gain less weight than their less active counterparts (16).

Clapp (16) found that offspring of women who continued to exercise throughout their pregnancy had lower body-fat percentages and weighed approximately 14 oz less than offspring of less active women. Clapp concluded that infants born to exercising women, although lighter and leaner, were just as healthy as their heavier, fatter counterparts. Interestingly, offspring of women who exercised preconceptually and had stopped exercising during pregnancy weighed approximately 8 oz more than offspring of the control group (17).

Clapp (17) also found that offspring of exercising women have normal growth and development during the first year of life. Specifically, head circumference and length were similar in both groups of offspring, as were motor, integrative, and academic-readiness skills. Children of active and nonactive women were followed at both 1 and 5 years of age and found to have similar growth and development of head circumference, length, weight, and fat measurements. And, at both 1 and 5 years of age, they had similar morphometric and neurodevelopmental outcomes (18). These data suggest that offspring born to exercising women had less subcutaneous fat, yet no developmental or growth impairments compared to the offspring of the less active women (17).

DEVELOPING AN EXERCISE PROGRAM

Women who do not have additional risk factors for adverse maternal or perinatal outcome can engage in exercise safely without compromising fetal growth and development or complicating pregnancy, labor, or delivery (3,14). Regardless of the exercise history of a pregnant client, considerations in developing an exercise program are universal; yet, the prescription must be individualized. The goal of exercise during pregnancy is to safely reach or maintain fitness while avoiding dehydration, hyperthermia, hypoglycemia, and physical injury. For this, caution is emphasized although there are no data in humans to indicate that pregnant women should limit exercise intensity and lower target heart rates because of potential adverse effects (3). Secondary goals include improving or maintaining cardiovascular fitness, maintaining muscular strength, improving flexibility, and improving posture.

Most healthy, active women with normal pregnancies do not require special exercise prescriptions. However, women at the extremes of performance, beginners and serious athletes, as well as those with goals to increase their exercise program will benefit from a detailed exercise prescription (2). The specific exercise prescription needs to be formulated with the complete understanding of the changes imposed by pregnancy. Exercise prescriptions should include a health assessment. Decisions about exercise type, frequency, duration, and intensity must be individualized and guided by a client's health status and athletic experience and interest, as well as common sense (3).

The approach to developing an exercise plan for the previously sedentary individual is to start slowly and preferably at the beginning of the second trimester because increase in body temperature is more serious in the first trimester. It is also important to get an exercise program approved by the medical caregiver. Pregnancy tends to be a period in a woman's life when she is prone to make positive health changes (14). Pregnancy could be a good time to establish routine physical activity.

Women who are recreational athletes whose well established exercise regimens are at low to moderate intensity (about three times a week for at least 20 minutes) can usually continue to exercise without changing their program. For example, women who walk or jog two or three times weekly or who participate in weekend sports (hiking, swimming, golf, or tennis) can continue their activities without change (2).

A 50-minute exercise session recommended by the YMCA of the USA (9) provides structure for both the beginner exerciser and the recreational athlete who desires adding diversity to her exercise program. This program is detailed in *Box 29.3*.

BOX 29.3 Suggested Exercise Session (9)

- Warm-up (5 minutes) — As in a traditional exercise prescription, the warm-up is necessary to prepare the muscles for exertion and stretching.
- Aerobic (20 minutes) — The aerobic phase is another component of a traditional workout. Intensity must be monitored with Borg's Rating of Perceived Exertion (19).
- Strengthening (10 minutes) — All major muscle groups should be included in the strengthening phase: abdominals, shoulders and arms, back, legs, and pelvic floor muscles. All strengthening exercises should be performed in a slow and controlled manner.
- Cool down (5 minutes) — Five minutes of the aerobic phase should be used for cool down. These additional 5 minutes should follow the strengthening phase.
- Stretching (5 minutes) — To lengthen muscles and increase their flexibility, stretching is essential. Joints may be loosened by the increase in the hormones progesterone and relaxin. Therefore, it should be advised not to stretch to the maximum point of resistance or to use jerky, bouncy movements. All stretches should be performed by supporting joints to avoid injury.
- Relaxation (5 minutes) — A phase of the workout that is most likely a new addition for the pregnant woman is relaxation. It fits well at the end of a workout when the muscles are slightly fatigued. Relaxation techniques are valuable to a pregnant woman because of the resulting release of muscular and mental tension, reduced fatigue, and lessened stress. These can also be employed during childbirth and labor to help control the pain. Relaxation exercises include progressive relaxation, massage, and visualization.

Some women who participated in weight-bearing exercise prior to pregnancy may begin to notice a decline in performance early in pregnancy. Several factors may contribute to the decline: pregnancy fatigue, nausea, vomiting, and morphological changes (3). Recreational athletes should be guided to limit abrupt changes in the endurance component of their exercise regimen in early pregnancy and focus attention on four areas: environmental conditions, eating habits, hydration status, and balance of rest time with exercise (16). Clapp (16) recommends matching time spent exercising with time at restful, nonphysical activity.

The competitive athlete may need to decrease exercise intensity because perception of exertion may be the same as the prepregnant level. Serious competition as an "all-out" effort is strongly discouraged until more is known about the effect on fetal growth and development (4). Equally significant, the competitive athlete may need support shifting the focus from improving athletic performance to optimizing health benefits. Clapp (16) recommends that this be done early in the reproductive process, ideally before conception.

Exercise for the pregnant, competitive athlete must be monitored closely. Special laboratory analysis and equipment are necessary. Clapp (2) recommends twice monthly assessments to include:

- Continuously monitored maternal core temperature before, during, and for 10 minutes after exercise

- Measurement of maternal weight before and after the exercise session
- Hematocrit or plasma protein concentration to assess fluid shifts
- Measurement of maternal blood glucose levels before and after exercise
- Measurement of workload, oxygen consumption, perceived level of exertion, and blood lactate levels
- Measurement of fetal heart rate and behavioral responses to exercise

A change in well-being or abnormal physiological response indicates that the training regimen needs modification. As the athlete will soon discover, specific symptoms associated with pregnancy will likely indicate the modifications necessary during pregnancy related to intensity, frequency, or duration. It is critical that the athlete and health care providers work together.

SPECIFIC-SPORT RECOMMENDATIONS

Weight-bearing exercise is most beneficial for obtaining the additive effects of pregnancy and exercise (2). However, physical adjustments to the physiologic and morphologic changes of pregnancy appear to favor nonweight-bearing exercise, especially during the later months of pregnancy.

Swimming is a nonweight-bearing exercise and an excellent activity for pregnancy. Swimmers should warm up by walking in the water or swimming slowly. Remind clients to avoid holding their breath while swimming and not to swim alone. Diving is not recommended.

Cycling is another good exercise because it is nonweight-bearing. Cycling in a racing position may cause back pain and should be avoided in the later stages of pregnancy due to the protruding abdomen. Switching to a stationary bike may be practical once the center of gravity is altered. Remind clients to avoid cycling on wet pavement or winding paths due to a risk of falling.

Aquatic exercise offers another nonweight-bearing option. Water enhances the workout by providing a natural resistance as well as lessening the impact of body movements. Aquatic shoes may add stability during water exercise and prevent slipping on the pool deck.

Walking is an excellent exercise and a good start-up exercise, especially for women who have not been previously active or who may have taken a break in their exercise routine due to first trimester fatigue and morning sickness. Remind clients who walk or jog to wear a supportive bra (often two are necessary) and walking shoes.

Jogging is safe for those who have previously jogged. Many women find jogging increasingly uncomfortable as gestation progresses due to tension on the round ligaments, uterine mobility, or pelvic instability. In addition, the sensation of needing to urinate in the later stages of pregnancy may prohibit this activity. Lower abdominal support belts (found at maternity stores) are often helpful (4). It is important to prevent overheating and dehydration while jogging. Therefore, remind clients to wear comfortable clothing (cotton or "wicking" fabrics in warm weather), to drink plenty of water, and to monitor exertion.

Lower impact aerobic classes are acceptable for women familiar with the routines. Clients should be cautioned to avoid twists and turns that can strain the knees and back. Special attention needs to be placed on changes in balance to prevent falling. Some women can safely participate in high-impact aerobics with proper monitoring if they engaged in this activity prepregnancy.

Racquet sports are acceptable for those familiar with them—tennis, badminton, and racquetball. Caution is advised for the third trimester when balance and lateral movements may become unsafe. During participation, the player should focus on making directional changes slowly.

Strength training—using proper technique with light weights—is recommended for women familiar with weight training. It can help to improve upper body strength. Women should be advised to avoid increasing weight loads, repetitions, or sets until after the first trimester. Weight training programs should be designed to increase strength (with multiple repetitions and sets) rather than muscle mass (maximal weight and limited repetitions) (2). Remind clients to avoid breath-holding and to use a spotter.

Other forms of exercise generally considered safe for the pregnant woman include the use of rowing machines, stair climbers, and treadmills.

Certain activities are to be avoided due to a risk of abdominal trauma or extreme environmental conditions. These include board diving, Scuba diving, water skiing, horseback riding, hang gliding, and contact sports (14).

There are circumstances when pregnant women should not exercise. *Box 29.4* identifies the contraindications to physical activity in pregnancy.

BOX 29.4   Contraindications to Exercise during Pregnancy (3)

The ACOG recommendations are intended for women who do not have any additional risk factors for adverse maternal or perinatal outcome. ACOG recommends that the following conditions are contraindications to exercise during pregnancy:

- Pregnancy-induced hypertension
- History of preterm rupture of membranes
- Preterm labor during the prior or current pregnancy, or both
- Incompetent cervix
- Persistent second- or third-trimester bleeding
- Intrauterine growth retardation

In addition, the following medical conditions will further impact the recommendations of whether an exercise program is appropriate:

- Chronic hypertension
- Active thyroid disease
- Cardiac, vascular, or pulmonary disease

BED REST

Best rest is recommended for a variety of conditions associated with pregnancy. As a result, even the most active women may find themselves unable to carry out daily routines much less a regular workout schedule. Although total bed rest throughout pregnancy is rare, many women may be partially restricted to bed rest. This rest keeps the body's physical stress level at a minimum and helps to prevent miscarriage or early delivery (20).

With the permission of her physician, many women will be able to perform very light exercises at this time. Whether in the form of stretching, toning, or deep breathing, some exercise is important to maintain proper circulation. The physician may recommend simple exercises such as deep breathing routines or wiggling the fingers and toes every 20 to 30 minutes. These help promote circulation and relaxation. The physician may even recommend toning exercises. Proper breathing technique is important to prevent a rise in blood pressure. The client should inhale during the release and exhale during the contraction. For example, exhale during a bicep curl up and inhale on the curl back down. Remind clients to exhale when the movement is hardest to prevent breath-holding.

Pelvic tilts keep the abdominal muscles strong and prevent lower back pain and stiffness. Bicep curls with soda cans strengthen the arms for picking up the baby. Inner thigh and pelvic floor muscles may be strengthened as the woman squeezes a large pillow between her knees while laying on her back. Finally, Kegel exercises are important in maintaining pelvic floor strength and bladder control. It is essential that the woman seek physician approval for any exercise while on bed rest (20).

The importance of a healthy diet must be emphasized during bed rest. The activity level of women on bed rest is, obviously, very low. Therefore, it is important to emphasize the importance of increased water and fiber intake to prevent constipation. Encourage women to eat plenty of fruits and vegetables and drink plenty of fluids.

Energy needs for the pregnant woman on bed rest differ from those of active pregnant women. Caloric needs decrease as activity decreases. Therefore, the recommended increase in calories for pregnancy may not be needed. The client's pace of weight gain (discounting fluid retention) dictates energy requirements. The dietetics professional should help the client adjust daily needs based on rate of weight gain.

THE SPORT NUTRITIONIST'S ROLE

Dietetics professionals have many opportunities to become involved with women during their pregnancy and many resources are available. *Box 29.5* shows what one dietitian has achieved with this population. *Box 29.6* identifies useful resources.

BOX 29.5   Exercise, Pregnancy, and the Registered Dietitian

Kelly Kullick RD/LD, ACE-certified personal trainer, and coauthor of this chapter, founded HealthyMoms, a home-based personal training and weight management company specializing in prenatal and postpartum care for women. HealthyMoms brings exercise equipment and nutrition expertise to women in the comfort of their own homes. This is just one example of a "custom designed" career for the dietetics professional.

BOX 29.6   Resources for Dietetics Professionals

Web Sites:

- All-inclusive pregnancy and parenting web station (www.storknet.com)
- Exercise and pregnancy (www.fitfor2.com)
- The American Dietetic Association (www.eatright.org)

Books:

- *Essential Exercises for the Childbearing Year* by Elizabeth Noble
- *Exercising Through Your Pregnancy* by James Clapp, MD
- *Fit for Two: The Official YMCA Prenatal Exercise Guide*, YMCA of the USA with Thomas W. Hanlon
- *Maternal Fitness* by Julie Tupler and Andrea Thompson
- *Nutrition in Pregnancy and Lactation* by Bonnie Worthington-Roberts and Sue Rodwell Williams
- *Positive Pregnancy Fitness* by Sylvia Klein Olkin
- *Taking Charge of Your Fertility: The Definitive Guide to Natural Birth Control and Pregnancy Achievement* by Toni Weschler, MPH
- *The Complete Prenatal Water Workout Book* by Helga Hughes

Videos:

- "Before Your Pregnancy: Prepare Your Body for a Healthy Pregnancy. Expert Advice on Nutrition and Exercise." Amy Ogle, MS, RD. Ordering information: 1-800-955-5115

REFERENCES

1. Aerobics and Fitness Association of America. *Fitness Theory & Practice.* Sherman Oaks, Calif: Aerobics and Fitness Association of America; 1993.
2. Clapp JF. *Exercising Through Your Pregnancy.* Champaign, Ill: Human Kinetics; 1998.
3. The American College of Obstetricians and Gynecologists. Exercise during pregnancy and the postpartum period. *Technical Bulletin No. 189.* Washington, DC: American College of Obstetricians and Gynecologists; 1994.
4. Clapp JF. A clinical approach to exercise during pregnancy. *Clin Sports Med.* 1994;13:443-458.
5. Worthington-Roberts B, Williams SR. *Nutrition in Pregnancy and Lactation.* 6th ed. Dubuque, Iowa: Brown & Benchmark Publishers; 1997.
6. Brown JE: Improving pregnancy outcome in the United States: the importance of preventive nutrition services. *J Am Diet Assoc.* 1989:89:631.
7. Food and Nutrition Board. *Nutrition During Pregnancy.* Washington, DC: National Academy Press; 1990.
8. Soultanakis HN, Artal R, Wiswell RA. Prolonged exercise in pregnancy: glucose homeostasis, ventilatory and cardiovascular responses. *Seminars in Perinatology.* 1996;20:315-327.
9. YMCA of the USA with Thomas W. Hanlon. *Fit for Two: The Official YMCA Prenatal Exercise Guide.* Champaign, Ill: Human Kinetics; 1995.
10. American Council on Exercise. *Personal Trainer Manual.* San Diego, Calif: American Council on Exercise; 1996.
11. Whitney EN, Cataldo CB, Rolfes SR. *Understanding Normal and Clinical Nutrition.* 4th ed. St. Paul, Minn: West Publishing Company; 1994.

12. Mahan LK, Escott-Stump S. *Krause's Food, Nutrition, and Diet Therapy*. 9th ed. Philadelphia, Penn: W B Saunders Co; 1996.

13. McMurray RG, Katz VL. Thermoregulation in pregnancy. Implications for exercise. *Sports Med*. 1990;10:146-158.

14. Sternfeld B. Physical activity and pregnancy outcome. Review and recommendations. *Sports Med*. 1997;23:33-47.

15. Bailey DM. Safety guidelines for exercise during pregnancy. *Lancet*. 1998;351:1889-1890.

16. Clapp JF. The effect of continuing regular endurance exercise on the physiologic adaptations to pregnancy and pregnancy outcome. *Am J Sports Med*. 1996;24:S28-S29.

17. Clapp JF, Simonian S, Lopez B, Appleby-Wineberg S, Harcar-Sevcik R. The one-year morphometric and neurodevelopmental outcome of the offspring of women who continued to exercise regularly throughout pregnancy. *Am J Obstet Gynecol*. 1998;178:594-599.

18. Clapp JF. Morphometric and neurodevelopmental outcome at age five years of the offspring of women who continued to exercise regularly throughout pregnancy. *J Pediatr*. 1996;129:856-863.

19. Borg GAV. *Borg's Perceived Exertion and Pain Scales*. Champaign, Ill: Human Kinetics; 1998.

20. The American College of Obstetricians and Gynecologists. *Planning for Pregnancy, Birth & Beyond*. 2nd ed. New York, NY: The Signet Group; 1995.

EXERCISE IN EXTREME TEMPERATURES

Charlene Harkins, MEd, RD, FADA

Temperature is a key factor in exercise, training and athletic performance, and outdoor activities. Many athletic events and training regimes occur in either very cold or very hot temperatures. Also, the young and the old have responses to ambient temperatures that differ from the population at large. Sports nutritionists need to consider the nutritional implications of extreme temperatures on the body when working with athletes.

The body's metabolic response to heat and cold can be impaired by inadequate nutrition. Appetite and thirst responses are frequently inappropriate in environmental extremes, leading to inadequate energy or fluid intakes. The availability of food and water is often limited due to logistical constraints. Backpackers, mountaineers, and explorers are usually limited to the food they can carry in their packs. The weight of the pack is critical; often food and water are sacrificed to make room for essential equipment, clothing, and gear. Inadequate dietary energy can result in glycogen depletion and loss of lean body mass. Inadequate fluid intake coupled with increased sweating, loss of lung-humidified air to an arid environment or altitude, or cold-induced diuresis can lead to dehydration and compromised thermoregulation and endurance. Persistent negative energy and fluid balances can combine to cause substantial decreases in physical performance capacity.

Expeditionary or recreational outdoor activities are frequently conducted in hot, cold, high-altitude, or rugged-terrain environments. Mountaineering, cross-country skiing, snowshoeing, sledding, and backpacking can be as physically demanding as more conventional sporting events, plus there is an added element of danger. The wilderness is much less forgiving of mistakes than an urban environment where medical care is nearby. A miscalculation of physical ability or inadequate preparation can be life-threatening in environmental extremes. Proper education, planning, preparation, equipment, and training are essential for work in the heat, cold, and high altitudes. Proper nutrition is an often-overlooked but critical component of planning to support effective work under these conditions.

PHYSIOLOGICAL RESPONSES IN HOT ENVIRONMENTS

The young and the old may have problems exercising in the heat. The Academy of Pediatrics noted that when compared to adults, young children may produce more metabolic heat during exercise in comparison to their body size, do not have as great a sweating capacity, and have a reduced capacity to convey heat from the core to the skin. These factors increase the chances of heat injury for children (1). At high levels of heat stress, tolerance to the heat is decreased in older individuals, possibly because they sweat less. Reduced ability to tolerate heat in the elderly may also be related to fitness levels. As more people become physically active throughout middle age and remain physically active into advanced years, the older person may tolerate exercise in the heat as well as younger adults (2).

Another subset of the population, obese persons, may also have difficulty exercising in hot environments. Obese individuals generally have high amounts of body fat that deter heat loss; they also tend to generate more heat during exercise due to low levels of fitness (1).

A fourth group, individuals who have previously experienced a heat injury, may also be less tolerant to exercise in the heat. Current thinking is that heat sensitivity caused by a previous injury is due to damage to the temperature-regulating centers in the brain. This causes the transfer of heat from the core to the skin to be impaired and thus allows the body temperature to rise faster. This particular type of heat injury is of concern for competitive athletes (1).

ATHLETES IN A HOT ENVIRONMENT

From a physiological standpoint the most severe stress an athlete can encounter is exercise in the heat (3). About 75% of the energy turnover during exercise is wasted as heat, causing the body's core temperature to rise. In cool environments most of the body's heat is transferred to the air (4); however, when the environmental temperature exceeds skin temperature, heat is gained and body temperature can rise to dangerous levels. At high ambient temperatures when it is not excessively humid, the only effective means of heat loss is by the evaporation of sweat secreted onto the skin. The evaporation of sweat is effective in dissipating large amounts of heat and will limit the rise in core temperature to no more than 3° to 4°C in all but the most extreme conditions of heat and humidity (3).

To minimize the adverse impact of hot, humid conditions, the training staff must address three issues:

1. An acclimatization strategy
2. A rehydration strategy
3. Lifestyle issues

Heat Acclimatization

Regular exposure to hot, humid conditions causes a number of physiological adaptations that serve to reduce the adverse effects on exercise performance and lessen the risk of heat injury. Such responses include an increase in blood volume and an enhanced ability to sweat. The increase in blood volume helps assure that the body can meet the demand for blood supply by both muscles and skin. Acclimatization also results in a faster onset of sweating, a greater distribution of sweat over the body, and an increase in the sweat rate. In addition, the sodium content of sweat tends to be reduced with acclimatization as the body attempts to retain sodium to help conserve extracellular fluid volume.

The rate of adaptation to physical activity in the heat depends on the intensity and duration of exercise and the environmental conditions. Some physiological adaptations can occur within the first few days of training in the heat so that even a few session of exercise in the heat may be beneficial (5).

The process of heat acclimation, or the physiologic adjustments that improve an athlete's heat tolerance, can be achieved best when the athlete trains in a warm environment (6). Consistent training in heat produces physiologic adjustments that make athletes more tolerant of hot-weather exercise. It is possible for an athlete to become fully acclimatized with as little as 30 minutes per day of exercise over an 8- to 12-day period while working out at a relatively intense level (ie, 70% VO_2max) (7).

The physiologic adjustments that accompany acclimatization are critical to enhance an athlete's performance in the heat. With acclimatization, blood volume increases allowing for greater transport of metabolic heat from deep tissues to the body's shell and cooling the inner core more effectively. The threshold for the onset of sweating is lowered, allowing the cooling process to begin earlier in exercise. After 10 days of heat exposure, the sweating capacity is nearly doubled; the sweat is more evenly distributed over the entire body and becomes more dilute, preserving the body's electrolytes in the extracellular fluid. Extracellular fluid increases in volume by 8% to 20% (5). Unfortunately, the benefits of the acclimatization process can be lost quickly if the individual is not well hydrated, or for an athlete, if training in the heat is postponed for 2 or 3 weeks (6).

Although an acclimatized athlete would undoubtedly perform better in high heat than someone not acclimatized to heat, neither athlete would perform at his or her maximal ability. Exercise in heat increases the rate of muscle glycogen use, contributing to earlier fatigue and exhaustion than in a cooler climate. Athletes who must train in the heat for repeated days without being acclimatized experience a rapid depletion of energy reserves and may feel the onset of chronic fatigue-type symptoms. Acclimatization can reduce the rate of glycogen usage by as much as 50%, thereby enhancing hot-weather training capacity and performance (6).

Hydration Concerns

Exercising in hot weather puts special emphasis on the importance of adequate hydration and the replacement of glucose during exercise. In hot conditions water loss through sweat can exceed 2 L per hour and may peak around 3 L per hour in an acclimatized athlete (1). Without adequate replacement of lost fluids, circulating blood volume decreases, stoke volume decreases, and heart rate increases causing an overall deterioration in circulatory efficiency.

Adequate hydration is essential to meet the metabolic and thermic needs of exercise in the heat. The American College of Sports Medicine Position Stand on Exercise and Fluid Replacement (6) recommends that active people maintain a hydrated state before, during, and after exercise. Cool, flavored sports drinks are encouraged. Solutions containing 6% to 8% carbohydrate in the form of sugars (glucose or sucrose) or starch (maltodextrin) have been shown to effectively provide substrate for immediate energy use and fluid for hydration. The inclusion of sodium may help to enhance the palatability, promote fluid retention, and possibly prevent hyponatremia in individuals drinking excessively large quantities of fluids.

Considerations for Exercise in the Heat

Monitoring individual responses to heat stress and the rate and extent of adaptation are an essential part of preparation for competition in the heat. When exposed to the heat, athletes often become dehydrated despite the availability of fluids. Regular monitoring of body mass can give useful information on the athlete's hydration status, provided some precautions are observed. Body mass measurements should always be made at the same time of day, under the same conditions. Measurement of weight loss during training sessions should also be monitored so these measurements can be combined and compared with the normal daily pattern. A progressive decrease in body mass over the course of a few days is a likely indication of dehydration. Alternatively, longer-term weight loss could also be due to a loss of appetite and decreased food intake, a common response to hot conditions.

Athletes should be encouraged to keep a record of subjective symptoms associated with travel, training, and competition to make note of the patterns that may emerge. The record should include daily body weight and some information on urine output (eg, the time of day urine is passed, an estimate of the urine volume via a measurable cylinder, and the urine color). This information has value if it is collected in hot conditions and can be compared with the normal pattern established over a period of at least a few weeks of training in a cool environment.

Heat implications for children. Children's physiologic responses to exercise are generally similar to those of adults, but there are several age- and maturation-related differences in their responses. For example, children respond differently to the combined stresses of exercise and climatic heat than adults do (8). Children's responses to exercise in the heat include low sweating rates per gland, high concentrations of lactic acid in sweat, lower cardiac output, high metabolic heat of locomotion, shorter exercise tolerance time, slower acclimatization rate, and rapid increase in core temperature during dehydration (9).

During exertion metabolic heat created during muscle contraction increases, thus increasing the need for the body to dissipate heat faster. In addition, children's metabolic heat production per kilogram of body mass is greater than in adults, thus adding an extra load to their thermoregulatory systems (10). The smaller the child, the greater is the excess in heat production.

Another issue for children is the difference in sweat capacity as compared to adults. During activities in hot climates, evaporation of sweat is the main avenue for heat dissipation. It is the only means for cooling the body when ambient temperature exceeds skin temperature. Children, with a lower sweating rate per sweat gland (8), are at greater risk for heat injury than adults in similar environments. In addition, children's exercise tolerance is reduced in climactic heat.

Children, like adults, do not drink enough when offered fluids ad libitum during exercise in the heat (9). However, one important difference is that for any given level of hypohydration, children's core temperatures rise faster than those of adults. Thus, supervising adults need to prevent "voluntary dehydration" in children. Instructing and encouraging children to drink above and beyond their thirst at frequent intervals should be a rule of thumb in hot and humid environments. To enhance a child's willingness to drink, beverages should be palatable and stimulate further thirst. Carbonated soft drinks should be avoided as should beverages with caffeine.

Recommendations for Activities in Hot Environments

Participation in activities in hot environments creates a need for awareness of signs and symptoms of exhaustion and heat stroke. Chills, goose pimples, dizziness, weakness, fatigue, mental disorientation, nausea, and headaches are some symptoms that may signify the onset of heat illness. If this occurs, the participant should stop the activity, sit or lay in a cool place, and consume cool fluids.

Heat-related stress can be minimized by taking precautions:

- Exercise in the cooler parts of the day—early morning or evening.
- Wear lightweight and light-colored clothing.
- Exercise in shady environments away from pavement that may add to radiative heat.
- Modify training to reduce intensity and duration.
- Drink cold fluids periodically and plan for adequate water stops.
- Take frequent breaks to restore hydration and energy stores.
- Avoid caffeinated, alcoholic, and carbonated beverages.
- Replenish lost electrolytes.
- Plan ahead and acclimatize to the environment over a period of days.

ATHLETES IN A COLD ENVIRONMENT

Cold-temperature activities also create concerns for athletes, the very young, and the old. This section will investigate issues created by cold weather and provide guidelines for the sports nutritionist in dealing with the nutrition concerns of persons pursuing activities in cold environments.

Exercising in Cold Weather

The greatest problem posed by outdoor activities in cold weather is hypothermia—the body's inability to keep a core temperature at or close to 98.6°F. In cold weather activities the body must convert stored food (usually fat) to heat in order to maintain the core temperature. If heat is being pulled out of the body faster than it can be replaced, the body begins to cool. As the body cools, it automatically begins restricting blood flow to the extremities.

Physiological adaptations that accompany exercising in the cold allow most athletes to continue their training programs during the winter months. Cold acclimatization, fitness level, and body fat all play a role in the physiological factors that affect performance for cold-weather athletes.

The process of cold-weather acclimatization is less understood and less documented than warm-weather acclimatization, but it is known that cold-weather acclimatization is more difficult to attain (11). Athletes who have become acclimatized to cold-weather training typically demonstrate increased blood flow to peripheral areas, increased skinfold thickness for greater insulation, and elevated metabolic rate for greater heat production (12). This greater metabolic rate translates into a greater caloric requirement for weight maintenance, regardless of the intensity and duration of exercise (13).

Maintaining body temperature requires a high level of fitness (11). Ongoing intensive exercise training appears to improve an athlete's tolerance to cold (14); therefore, it is beneficial to develop the highest possible level of fitness to perform effectively in cold-weather sports.

Athletes with slightly higher body-fat levels can usually tolerate cold-weather exercise better than leaner athletes. This appears to be due to the peripheral blood temperature tending to remain more stable in individuals with a higher percentage of body fat, allowing their core temperature to remain stable for longer periods of time than persons with less body fat (11).

Ambient Temperature and Wind

Air temperature alone is not an adequate measure of the true temperature felt on the exposed portions of the body (ie, hands, face, and neck). An additional measure, the wind chill factor, is a necessary consideration. On a windy day blowing air magnifies heat loss via convection because the warm layer of air surrounding the body is constantly being replaced by cooler air (15).

Considerations for Exercise in the Cold

- Check the weather. If it is raining and cold, wear outer garments that repel water. For wind chill temperatures below -15ºF, consider a scarf or a mask to warm the air breathed. Wind chills below -20ºF threaten exposed skin and it may be wise to avoid outdoor activities at these temperature levels.
- Wear a hat. Wind chills below freezing can result in up to 50% of body heat loss coming from the head.
- Wear gloves or mittens. Mittens are better than gloves; gloves are better than nothing. In aggressive physical activities, the participant may be unaware that his or her hands are getting too cold.
- Keep feet warm and dry. Wear woolen socks. Light cotton socks underneath thick woolen socks may be more tolerable if the participant is bothered by wool fabric.
- Dress in layers. With several layers of clothing, athletes can adjust to conditions as they warm or cool and the weather and exercise intensity change.
- Pick warm materials. Wool is still the best natural fiber choice since it absorbs moisture without losing insulation value. Polyester fleece fabrics are improving as a choice, while polypropylene is excellent in drawing moisture away from the skin. Cotton is a poor choice because it has very little insulation value and it retains moisture when wet. Moisture against the body tends to draw heat away quickly.
- Attempt cold-weather activities during daylight hours. This may be difficult depending on the time of year and the latitude.

While most research efforts are aimed at protection against cold exposure, some research is investigating ways to improve cold tolerance by modifying the thermoregulatory response to cold (16). The main strategies are oriented toward thermal acclimation, physical exercise, dietary enhancement of thermogenesis, pharmacological enhancement of thermogenesis, and manipulation of the thermoregulatory set point. While none of these strategies has concrete results that routinely improve cold tolerance, pharmacological enhancement of cold thermogenesis using ephedrine in combination with methylxanthine represents the most promising method for delaying the onset of hypothermia in humans (16).

Diets for Cold-weather Activities

While there is no consensus about the most appropriate diet for activity in the cold, evidence is strong that adequate amounts of carbohydrate are necessary (17). Doubt (17) analyzed the dietary needs of cold-weather exercise and suggested that carbohydrate-loading appears to be efficacious, as it is for other athletic endeavors. Contrary to conventional wisdom, the combination of exercise and cold exposure does not act synergistically to enhance the metabolism of fats. Free fatty acid levels are not higher, and may even be lower, when exercising in cold air or cold water compared to exercising in warmer conditions. Glycerol, a good indicator of lipid mobilization, is likewise reduced in the cold, suggesting impaired mobilization of fat from adipose tissue. Catecholamines, which promote lipolysis, are higher during exercise in cold air and cold water, indicating that the reduced lipid metabolism is not due to a lack of adequate hormonal stimulation. It is proposed that cold-induced vasoconstriction of peripheral adipose tissue may account, in part, for the decrease in lipid mobilization. Venous glucose is not substantially altered during exercise in the cold, but lactate levels are generally higher than with activity performed in milder conditions. The time lag between production of lactate within the muscle and its release into the venous circulation may be increased by cold exposure. Exercise VO_2max is generally higher in the cold, but the difference between warm and cold environments becomes less as workload increases. Increases in oxygen uptake may be due to shivering during exercise, an increase in muscle tone in the absence of overshivering, or nonshivering thermogenesis. Heart rate is often, but not always, lower during exercise in the cold (17).

Water requirements for work in cold environments are similar to those for temperate environments (18). Although water requirements are not as high in the cold as in the heat, the consequences of dehydration are still important. Exposure to cold can cause a reduction in the sense of thirst and consequently reduced water consumption.

Hypohydration in the cold can reduce food consumption, efficiency of physical and mental performance, and resistance to cold exposure (19). While adequate fluid intake is paramount in preventing hypohydration in the cold, it is also prudent to consider the temperature of the fluid and food provided for work in the cold. Whenever possible, warm fluid and heated foods are generally recommended in the cold to impart a feeling of warmth and well-being. The warming effect of a hot beverage in the cold is probably related to its effect on subsequent vasodilatation and increased blood flow to cold extremities rather than the actual quantities of heat contained in the ingested fluid.

Weight loss is common during cold-weather field expeditions, often due to the monotony of the diet and difficulty in preparing food, coupled with increased energy expenditures. Water requirements are not increased in cold-weather operations, but intakes may be decreased due to the difficulty of melting snow and ice and the tendency of cold-weather travelers to utilize dry foods that will not freeze and can be eaten without thawing. Inadequate hydration may decrease the body's ability to adjust to cold stress (19).

Nutrition needs vary with activity in extreme conditions. Consideration needs to be given to changes in energy needs with changes in environmental conditions, temperature, and clothing needs. Hydration is of utmost importance whether the temperature is hot or cold. Nutrition is a cornerstone in the completion of tasks done in varying temperatures and conditions (20).

REFERENCES

1. Williams MH. *Nutrition for Health, Fitness and Sport.* 5th ed. Boston, Mass: WCB McGraw-Hill; 1999.
2. Guccione AA. *Geriatric Physical Therapy.* St Louis, Mo: Mosby; 1993.
3. Maughan RJ, Shirreffs SM. Preparing athletes for competition in the heat: developing an effective acclimatization strategy. *Sports Sci Exch.* 1997;10(2).
4. Nadel J. Temperature regulation in cold environments. *Sports Sci Exch.* 1988;2(3):73-76.
5. Lind AR, Bass DE. Optimal exposure time for development of heat acclimation. *Federal Proceedings.* 1963;22:704-708.
6. American College of Sports Medicine. Position stand on exercise and fluid replacement. *Med Sci Sports Exerc.* 1996;28:i-vii.
7. Dawson B. Exercise training in sweat clothing in cool conditions to improve heat tolerance. *Sports Med.* 1994;17:233-244.
8. Bar-Or O. Children's responses to exercise in hot climates: implications for performance and health. *Sports Sci Exch.* 1994;7:2-8.
9. Bar-Or O. Climate and the exercising child. *Int J Sports Med.* 1980;1:53-65.
10. MacDougall JD, Bar-Or O, Roche O, Moroz JR. Maximal aerobic capacity of Canadian school children: prediction based on age-related oxygen cost of running. *Int J Sports Med.* 1983;4:194-198.
11. Askew EW. Environmental and physical stress and nutrient requirements. *Am J Clin Nutr.* 1995;61(suppl):S631-S637.
12. Vallerand AL, Jacobs I. Energy metabolism during cold exposure. *J Sports Med.* 1992;13:191-193.
13. Lickteig JA, Foster C. Nutrition for winter sports. In: Casey MJ, ed. *Winter Sports Medicine.* Philadelphia, Penn: Davis; 1990:22-23.
14. Edwards JSA, Askew EW, King N, Fulco CS. Nutritional intake and carbohydrate supplementation at high altitude. *J Wilderness Med.* 1994;5:20-33.
15. Horvath SM. Exercise in cold environment. *Exerc Sport Sci Rev.* 1982;8:28-30.
16. Mercer JB. Enhancing tolerance to cold exposure—how successful have we been? *Arctic Med Rev.* 1995;54 (suppl):70-75.
17. Doubt TJ. Physiology of exercise in the cold. *Sports Med.* 1991;11:367-381.
18. Welch BE, Buskirk ER, Iampietro PF. Relation of climate and temperature to food and water intake in man. *Metabolism.* 1958;7:141-144.
19. Freund BJ, Sawka MN. Influence of cold stress on human fluid responses. In: Marriot BM, ed. *Nutritional Needs in Cold and in High-altitude Environments.* Washington, DC: National Academy Press; 1996:161-164.
20. Murray R. Fluid needs in hot and cold environments. *Int J Sport Nutr.* 1995;5(suppl):S62-S73.

31

EXERCISE AT HIGH ALTITUDES

Julie Ann Lickteig, MS, RD, FADA

Athletes traveling abruptly to altitudes above 8,000 feet (2,400 meters) may experience symptoms representative of low levels of available oxygen. Each person adjusts at his or her own pace, and every trip to altitude presents a new situation for each individual. The inability to adapt results in one of three forms of altitude illness. The three forms and their symptoms are:

1. **Acute Mountain Sickness (AMS)**
   Persons experience headaches, mild nausea, vomiting, anorexia, broken sleep patterns, lethargy, and some weakness. Generally symptoms will disappear in 3 days (1-3). If not, descend and try a staged ascent.

2. **High Altitude Pulmonary Edema (HAPE)**
   Noticeable symptoms are dyspnea, a distinctive dry cough, gurgling sounds from the chest indicating water has replaced air, watery sputum, a staggered gait, and sometimes irrational behavior patterns. Limited time remains, usually just hours for such persons, until unconsciousness and possible death occur. An immediate trip to lower altitudes is advised.

3. **High Altitude Cerebral Edema (HACE)**
   The traveler with HACE experiences extremely severe headaches combined with diminished judgment, confusion, difficulty in coordinating muscular activity and balance, and hallucinations leading to coma and death. No time should be lost in evacuating this person to lower altitude, regardless of the time of day or night.

Gradual acclimatization of even the most physically fit individuals will reduce the percentage and the degree of altitude illness. Affecting one out of four individuals, AMS is the mildest of the three forms of altitude illness (4). The causes of altitude illness are less known than the effects. As scientists search for the answers relating to hypoxia and the retention of fluid leading to edema, some progress is being made. Recent photos of cerebral edema by magnetic resonance imaging (MRI) show some transfer of plasma through the blood-brain barrier (5). In all cases of altitude illness, descent of 1,000 to 2,000 feet (300 to 600 meters) is the preferred treatment; this is usually followed by a quick recovery. A slower reentry to altitude is advised when the athlete contemplates a return to a higher environment.

NUTRITION GUIDELINES

Without previous altitude experience, athletes do not know how their body will react, especially when training and competing. The following approaches will not eliminate illness, or even death, but are highly recommended.

- With increased breathing due to altitude and physical exertion, the body responds by humifying the inspired dry air, resulting in great loss of body fluids. It is recommended that the athlete increase sea-level consumption of nonalcoholic fluids to 2 L if at moderate altitude and up to 4 L at high altitude. The ability to replace fluid loss can be judged by a copious flow of light-colored urine. When flying, begin an increased fluid regimen at sea-level, avoiding any alcoholic drink that enhances dehydration since flying suddenly puts the athlete at altitude. If additional calories are needed, beverages of 6% to 8% carbohydrate will increase the total caloric and fluid intake.

- Anorexia in the initial 72 hours at altitude may drop caloric intake 40% to 60% compared to that at sea-level (6). Training and performance levels also decrease as the body adapts. The ability to maintain nutritional balance and physical performance corresponds to the body's adaptation to each successively higher elevation. Dietary intake will parallel that success or failure, especially if the anorexia continues. Unflavored glucose polymers used as a calorie enhancer in mashed potatoes and hot cereals, as well as other simple liquid and solid foods, are often an acceptable alternative to larger meals that go unconsumed (7). Liquid-type foods such as gelatins, puddings, instant breakfast drinks, and light soups may meet a double need for fluids and some calories. No dietary measures can prevent altitude symptoms, but small frequent feedings of beverages and transition foods can assist the body in adjusting to unfamiliar altitudes. Examples of transition foods for acclimatization include mashed potatoes, cooked cereals, rice, noodles, pasta, breads, crackers, pudding, gelatin, sherbet, canned fruit, dried fruit, cooked vegetables, yogurt, cottage cheese, vanilla wafers, oatmeal cookies, hot cocoa, eggs, baked or broiled chicken, turkey or fish, stewed meats, processed cheese slices, instant breakfast drinks, light soups, fruit nectars, and juices.

Examples of menus for the casual traveler and for an aggressive sportsperson are given in *Tables 31.1* and *31.2* (8).

TABLE 31.1   Altitude Adjustment Menus for the Aggressive Sportsperson (8)

Food	Serving Size	Calories	Carbohydrate (g)	Protein (g)	Fat (g)
Breakfast					
Applesauce	1/2 cup	52	13.8	0.2	0.1
Oatmeal	1 package	104	18.1	4.4	1.8
Sugar	2 t	31	8.0	0	0
Skim milk	1 cup	86	11.9	8.4	0.4
Cracked-wheat bread	1 slice	66	13.0	2.2	0.6
Margarine	1 t	4	tr*	tr	3.8
Jelly	1 t	13	3.3	tr	0
Fluids (ad lib):					
• Milk cocoa	2 cups	227	49.4	6.8	2.7
• Sweetened tea	1 cup	88	22.0	0.3	0
• Water	2 cups	0	0	0	0
Lunch					
Granola bars	2 bars	594	67.3	15.0	33.2
Banana chips	1 cup	346	88.3	3.9	1.8
Raisins	1/2 cup	217	57.4	2.3	0.3
Fluids (ad lib):					
• Eggnog	1 cup	261	38.9	8.2	8.4
• Lemonade	2 cups	223	57.5	0	0
• Sweetened tea	1 cup	88	22.0	0	0
• Water	2 cups	0	0	0	0
Dinner					
Vegetable soup	1 cup	122	19.0	3.5	3.7
Macaroni & cheese	1 cup	430	40.2	16.8	22.2
Pita bread	1	203	38.8	6.4	2.1
Fruit cocktail	1/2 cup	57	14.7	0.6	tr
Fluids (ad lib):					
• Apple juice	1 1/2 cups	175	43.5	0.2	0.4
• Drinking gelatin	2 cups	267	41.9	24.5	1.1
• Water	2 cups	0	0	0	0

continued

TABLE 31.1 Altitude Adjustment Menus for the Aggressive Sportsperson (8) (continued)

Food	Serving Size	Calories	Carbohydrate (g)	Protein (g)	Fat (g)
Snacks					
Fig bars	8	401	84.5	4.4	6.3
Dried apricots	1/2 cup	155	4.1	2.4	0.3
Hard candy	1 oz	108	27.2	0	0.3
Totals		4,348	820.7	110.6	89.5
			(75% of calories)	(10% of calories)	(19% of calories)

General hints

- Gradually increase calories as activity increases.
- Plan one-pot meals that cook in 15 minutes.
- Drink 3 to 5 L water per day. Drink frequently.
- Know that it takes 15 to 20 minutes to melt snow to water; it takes 10 to 15 minutes to boil water.
- Increase carbohydrate intake drastically.

Moderate climbing: 3,500 kcal

- 4.4 kg (2 lb) dry food per person
- 75% kcal from carbohydrate
- 15% kcal from fat
- 10% kcal from protein
- 4 L fluid

Heavy climbing: 5,000 kcal

- 5 kg (2 1/4 lb) of dry food per person
- 5 L fluid

*tr = trace, <0.05 g

TABLE 31.2 Altitude Adjustment Menus for the Casual Sportsperson (8)

Food	Serving Size	Calories	Carbohydrate (g)	Protein (g)	Fat (g)
Breakfast					
Orange juice	1/2 cup	56	13.4	0.9	0.1
Cornflakes	3/4 oz	83	18.3	1.7	0.1
Sugar	2 t	31	8.0	0	0
Skim milk	1 cup	86	11.9	8.4	0.4
Cracked-wheat bread	1 slice	66	13.0	2.2	0.6
Margarine	1 t	34	tr*	tr	3.8
Jelly	1 t	13	3.3	tr	0
Fluids (ad lib):					
• Sweetened tea	1 cup	88	22.0	0.3	0
• Water	2 cups	0	0	0	0

continued

TABLE 31.2   Altitude Adjustment Menus for the Casual Sportsperson (8) (continued)

Food	Serving Size	Calories	Carbohydrate (g)	Protein (g)	Fat (g)
Lunch					
Chicken noodle soup	1/2 cup	26	3.7	1.5	0.6
Saltine crackers	6	74	12.2	1.5	2.0
Low-fat cottage cheese	1/2 cup	82	3.1	14.0	1.2
Gelatin salad	1/2 cup	80	19.7	1.6	0.1
Canned peaches	1/2 cup	55	14.3	0.8	tr
Fluids (ad lib):					
• Lemonade	2 cups	223	57.5	0	0
• Water	1 cup	0	0	0	0
Dinner					
Broiled salmon	3 oz	184	0	23.2	9.3
Baked potato	1 small	124	28.6	2.6	0.1
Mixed vegetables	1/2 cup	54	11.9	2.6	0.1
Sherbet	1/2 cup	135	29.4	1.1	1.9
Fluids (ad lib):					
• Sweetened tea	1 cup	88	22.0	0	0
• Water	2 cups	0	0	0	0
Snacks					
Banana	1/2	52	13.4	0.6	0.3
Apple	1 medium	81	21.1	0.3	0.5
Totals		1,750	326.8	63.4	21.1
			(75% of calories)	(15% of calories)	(11% of calories)

General hints:

- Resume normal patterns after 36 to 48 hours.
- Keep exercise to a minimum.
- Avoid alcohol; increase other fluids.
- Drink 3 to 4 L water per day. Drink frequently.

*tr = trace, <0.05 g

- Unless an athlete works diligently to meet daily energy requirements, prolonged visits to altitude, such as expedition climbing, can result in loss of body mass, body fat, and eventually muscle mass. To compensate, athletes should think in terms of a performance diet with carbohydrate (CHO) representing about 60% of total calories. For climbers using available packaged foods, the percentages suggested are 57% CHO (500 to 600 g), 14% protein, and 29% fat (9). Previously, it was believed that the body favored CHO at altitude. However, after acclimatization, some foods with up to 40% of their calories from fat, such as sausage and processed cheese slices, can be included. This provides caloric density in a smaller space due to the physical limitations of a backpack, sled, animal pack, and other needs.

- Total calories should replace those expended, but the active athlete who is enduring a long visit at higher altitudes is rarely able to meet those requirements, even with supplements (9-11). Depending on the type of physical performance, 3,800 to 6,000 kcal may be required; careful manipulation of intake over shorter periods of time has resulted in caloric/activity equilibrium up to 14,000 feet (4,666 meters) (12). Gender differences are now being studied relative to intake and basic metabolic rate during acute exposure to altitude. Results show that women tend to cope with the differences more quickly than men (13). Up to 18,000 feet (5,500 meters) absorption is not impaired, but the ability to eat is compromised (14). Due to the intricacies of the sodium and fluid balance at the cellular level, there is still uncertainty about the body's ability to retain sodium leading to peripheral edema. One way to counter this imbalance is to consider a moderate to low sodium intake along with a continued high consumption of fluids from a safe water source (15). The sodium content of processed foods and sports drinks tends to generally meet or sometimes exceed the normal athlete's needs.

- Knowing one's hemoglobin level is helpful. The athlete does not want to compromise his or her potential to carry additional oxygen, since diminished atmospheric pressure may lessen the iron content of the individual red blood cells (11,15).

- Sleeping one or two nights at an intermediary elevation enroute to the higher elevations often minimizes the altitude symptoms and allows for a better normalization of dietary intake. For example, to acclimate for a ski trip to the Colorado Rockies, schedule an overnight stay in Denver (5,280 feet or 1,600 meters) on the way to ski at Breckenridge (base of 10,000 feet or 3,030 meters). Climbers, hikers, snowshoers, or hunters going over 8,000 feet (2,400 meters) should ascend by 1,000- to 2,000-foot (300- to 600-meter) increments on a daily basis. If possible, a routine of working and climbing higher but sleeping at a lower altitude is preferred. For example, hunt at 11,000 feet (3,333 meters) but sleep at 9,000 feet (2,727 meters).

- The success of an athlete's adaptation and correlated performance are related to the speed of the ascent from lower to higher elevations, the intensity and duration of exercise expended especially during the initial days at a new elevation, the actual altitude achieved, and the length of time that the athlete will spend at that altitude.

- One of the realities of altitude, especially higher elevations, is that it takes longer to perform normal functions. Melting snow for water, cooking, and ultimately eating and digesting food take longer than most people realize. Cooking time doubles for each 5,000-foot (1,515-meter) increase in elevation. Spacing and timing of activities should be adjusted accordingly. Production of work at 18,000 feet (6,000 meters) is one-half of sea-level efficiency.

- For competing athletes, shorter distance events such as sprints may be handled quite well, or even at slightly improved performance. However, endurance events like triathlons challenge the athlete the most. For example, a 100-mile foot-race over irregular terrain with changing altitudes of 8,000 to 12,000 feet (2,424 to 3,636 meters) requires good acclimatization and a consistent monitoring of small quantities of appropriate foods and fluids (see *Box 31.1*). Lower performance levels and higher training times are the result of a 1.5% to 3.5 % reduction in VO$_2$max for every 1,000 feet (305 meters) above 5,000 feet (1,524 meters) (6). Up to 8,000 feet (2,666 meters) athletes should reserve 2 weeks for adjustment but attempt to train with the best intensity possible; this enables the body to minimize some of the effects of the initial "detraining period." An additional week is needed for each 2,000-foot (610 meters) increment up to 15,000 feet (4,545 meters). One must accept the fact that maximum sea-level aerobic capacity is impaired at altitude, even after many months. The athlete's diet should reflect a decrease in intensity, but it also needs to compensate for an increase in basal metabolic rate (6,10,13,16). The trained sports professional can help athletes achieve this balance.

BOX 31.1   Foods for Athletes on the Move at Altitude

Skim milk mozzarella string cheese, bread sticks, bagels, dried sweetened cranberries, honey bars and straws, whole-wheat tortillas, fruited newtons, grain bars, toaster pastries, yogurt-covered raisins, flavored corn nuts, Rice Krispie/marshmallow bars, honey-nut Cheerios, popcorn, dried banana slices, dried apricots

By knowing the altitudes to which one will travel and the type of activity to be pursued, appropriate plans can be made for adaptation and the related dietary needs. The information presented in *Box 31.2* and *Table 31.3* enables the athlete to make decisions appropriate to the sport.

BOX 31.2   Sports Often Performed at Altitude

Skiing—alpine, cross-country, and telemark; hockey; snowshoeing; mountain climbing; hiking; backpacking; ice climbing; gliding; hang gliding, hot-air ballooning; parapenting; bicycling; distance running; marathons; roller blading; ice skating; swimming; hunting; fishing; bouldering; back-country skiing; ice climbing; biathlon; speed skating; trekking

TABLE 31.3   Altitudes of Popular Sporting Areas

Low Altitudes	Feet	Meters
Mt. Katahdin, Maine	5,267	1,596
Sun Valley, Idaho	5,750	1,742
Park City, Utah	6,900	2,300
Moderate Altitudes		
Pressurized plane cabin	7,500	2,273
Ski resorts, Rocky Mountains	7,500–9,500	2,121–2,879
Zugspitze, Germany	9,738	2,951
Leadville, Colorado	10,000	3,030

continued

TABLE 31.3   Altitudes of Popular Sporting Areas (continued)

High Altitudes	Feet	Meters
Ski summits, Rocky Mountains	11,000–12,000	3,333–3,636
Bugaboo Spires, Canada	11,150	3,379
Grand Teton, Wyoming	13,767	4,173
Pikes Peak, Colorado	14,110	4,276
Mt. Ranier, Washington	14,410	4,366
Mt. Blanc, France	15,782	4,782
Extremely High Altitudes		
Mt. McKinley, Alaska	20,320	6,157
Aconcagua, Peru	22,900	6,939
Cho Oyo, Nepal	26,750	8,106
Mt. Everest, Nepal	29,028	8,796

REFERENCES

1. Bezruchka S. *Altitude Illness*. Seattle, Wash: The Mountaineers; 1994.
2. Houston CS. *Going Higher*. Rev ed. Boston, Mass: Little Brown and Co; 1987.
3. Forgey WW, ed. *Wilderness Medical Society Practice Guidelines for Wilderness Emergency Care*. Merrillville, Ind: ICS Books; 1995:22-24.
4. Honigman F, Theis MK, Koziol-McLain J, et al. Acute mountain sickness in a general tourist population at moderate altitudes. *Ann Intern Med*. 1993;118:587-592.
5. Hackett PH, Yarnell PR, Hill R, Reynard K, Heit J, McCormick J. High-altitude cerebral edema evaluated with magnetic resonance imaging. *JAMA*. 1998;280:1920-1925.
6. McArdle WD, Katch FI, Katch VL. *Exercise Physiology, Energy, Nutrition, and Human Performance*. Philadelphia, Penn: Lea & Febiger; 1986.
7. Lickteig JA. Nutrition for winter sports. In: Casey MJ, Foster C, Hixson EG, eds. *Winter Sports Medicine*. Philadelphia, Penn: FA Davis Co; 1990:22-33.
8. Lickteig JA. Nutrition for high altitudes and mountain sports. In: Casey MJ, Foster C, Hixson EG, eds. *Winter Sports Medicine*. Philadelphia, Penn: FA Davis Co; 1990:383-392.
9. Reynolds RD, Lickteig JA, Howard MP, Deuster P. Intakes of high fat and high carbohydrate foods by humans increased with exposure to increasing altitude during an expedition to Mt. Everest. *J Nutr*. 1998;128:50-55.
10. Reynolds RD, Lickteig JA, Deuster P, et al. Energy metabolism increases and regional body fat decreases while regional muscle mass is spared in humans climbing Mt. Everest. *J Nutr*. 1999;129:1307-1314.
11. Jones TE, Hoyt RW, Baker CJ, et al. Voluntary consumption of a liquid carbohydrate supplement by special operations forces during a high altitude cold weather field training exercise. *USARIEM Technical Report T20-90*. Natick, Mass: US Army Research Institute of Environmental Medicine; September 1990:1-113.
12. Butterfield GE, Gates J, Fleming S, Brooks GA, Sutton JR, Reeves JT. Increased energy intake minimizes weight loss in men at high altitude. *J Appl Physiol*. 1992;72:1741-1748.
13. Butterfield GE, Mawson JT. Energy requirements of women at altitude. In: Houston CS, Coates G, eds. *Hypoxia: Women at Altitude*. Burlington, Va: Queen City Printers; 1997:8-19.
14. Kayser B. *Factors Limiting Exercise Performance in Man at High Altitude* [dissertation]. Geneva, Switzerland: University of Geneva; 1994.
15. Houston C. *High Altitude: Illness and Wellness*. Merrillville, Ind: ICS Books; 1993:1-72.
16. Reynolds R. Effects of cold and altitude on vitamin and mineral requirements. In: Marriott BM, Carlson SJ, eds. *Nutritional Needs in Cold and in High-Altitude Environments*. Washington, DC: National Academy Press; 1996:215-244.

SECTION 4 SPORTS-SPECIFIC NUTRITION GUIDELINES

More and more, sports nutrition professionals are being asked to address the unique needs of athletes involved in specific sports. They must be able to provide practical solutions to real-world, real-time food and nutrition issues which today's athletes are facing. Various sources are available, but many do not address the issues specific to individual sports. This section offers the unique perspectives of sports nutrition professionals who provide nutrition consultation to athletes in specific sports or, in some cases, the authors are (or were) participants themselves in the sport. Because there are many gaps in the literature on the nutrition needs and considerations of athletes participating in specific sports, much of the following information about the nutrition needs and concerns of athletes is based on the authors' unique experiences and expert opinions. Insightful comments and useful tips are offered to help practitioners address the unique nutrition needs and concerns of athletes in many different sports.

SECTION 4 CONTENTS

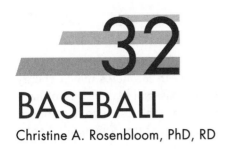

32

BASEBALL

Christine A. Rosenbloom, PhD, RD

Many credit Abner Doubleday of Cooperstown, New York, with the invention of the game of baseball in 1839, even though similar games with bases, such as rounders in England, were played earlier. While the exact origin of baseball is not certain, Alexander J. Cartwright set down many of the rules for the game in 1845. Baseball became popular among Civil War soldiers and when the war ended, they spread the game throughout the country (1). Baseball, dubbed "The Great American Pastime," is played professionally by 31 teams (29 United States teams and 2 Canadian teams). It is also played by minor league professional clubs; semi-professional teams; amateur clubs; women's leagues; college, high school, middle school, and elementary school teams; and little league teams. It became an Olympic sport in 1992 (2).

ENERGY AND MACRONUTRIENT NEEDS

Energy

Baseball is considered a "skill" sport requiring fine motor control, coordination, and reaction time (3). Baseball is not a game of continuous activity. While there are elements of the game that require aerobic fitness (general conditioning for the players) and anaerobic power (pitching a fastball, batting, running the bases, throwing a baseball from the outfield to the infield, or throwing a baseball from the catcher to an infielder), baseball players do not have increased demands for energy, protein, carbohydrate, or fat as compared to athletes in other sports. Katch and McArdle (4) suggest that pitchers have higher energy needs than fielders. A 183-lb pitcher burns 7.5 kcal per minute of activity (900 kcal in 2 hours), whereas a 183-lb fielder burns 5.1 kcal per minute of activity (612 kcal in 2 hours). These are relatively low states of energy expenditure, considering 5.1 kcal per minute of activity is burned during food shopping. By comparison, a 183-lb competitive tennis player burns 11.9 kcal per minute of activity or 1,428 kcal in 2 hours (4).

Carbohydrate

Baseball players should strive to achieve at least 60% of energy intake as carbohydrates. This recommendation is consistent with advice offered by many health organizations to sustain good health (5). Carbohydrate is the preferred fuel for athletes, as reviewed elsewhere in this manual. For the baseball player, a diet rich in complex carbohydrate provides fuel to maintain muscle and liver glycogen stores and, because complex carbohydrates are low in fat, helps match energy intake and expenditure to control body weight (5). Baseball players do not have the high-energy demands of competitive endurance athletes, such as runners, cyclists, or soccer players, so carbohydrate intake approaching 70% of total energy intake is not necessary.

While the need for total carbohydrate does not differ from that of the general population, baseball players should adhere to the same general guidelines for the timing of carbohydrate ingestion as other athletes. A precompetition meal containing ample carbohydrate and containing 500 to 600 kcal should be eaten 3 to 4 hours before games. Meals that are high in carbohydrate-containing foods are more easily and quickly digested and absorbed than a high-protein or high-fat meal (6).

Protein

Although the protein needs of baseball players have not been determined, it is reasonable to assume that a diet of 12% to 15% of total kcal from protein will meet the needs of baseball players. This recommendation is consistent with recommendations for good health (5). Lemon (7) points out that the Recommended Dietary Allowance (RDA) for protein was established on sedentary individuals, and current research indicates an increased need for protein in active people. Dietary protein for the endurance athlete is estimated to be 1.2 to 1.4 g per day and may be as high as 1.6 to 1.7 g/kg per day for those who regularly strength train (7). These protein recommendations are 150% to 212% greater than the current RDA of 0.8 g/kg per day. Many high school, college, and professional baseball players engage in strength training and their protein needs could be higher than those athletes not involved in strength training. To determine protein needs of an individual baseball player, total energy intake, carbohydrate intake, degree of strength training, and amount of aerobic exercise should all be considered. Athletes who restrict energy intake for weight loss or those who strength train may need to consume protein intakes at the high end of the range (7).

Fat

For many athletes, baseball players included, the problem is too much fat in the diet rather than too little (5). A high-fat diet leaves little room for carbohydrates—the preferred fuel for exercise. Athletes should restrict total fat intake to <30% of total calories, with saturated fats contributing no more than 10% of total calories to help reduce the incidence of cardiovascular disease. Baseball players frequently must eat out due to travel schedules, pick up fast food after a game, or eat late at night after games, thereby easily exceeding the recommended intake of fat.

MICRONUTRIENT NEEDS

The vitamin and mineral needs of baseball players have not been determined. Baseball players should aim to meet the RDA for vitamins and minerals through wise food selection and use supplements only if dietary intake is lacking in nutrients.

Some baseball players ask about supplements of vitamin A and beta-carotene because of their role in night and peripheral vision. Retinol is the biologically active form of vitamin A and beta-carotene can be converted to retinol in the body. Retinol is important in night vision and peripheral vision (8). The RDA for vitamin A is 1,000 Retinol Equivalents (RE) or 5,000 International Units (IU) for adult men and 800 RE or 4,000 IU for adult women. Children need slightly less (8). There is no RDA for beta-carotene. Since vitamin A is toxic when taken in excess (>7,500 RE or 37,500 IU) and can accumulate in the liver, a single-dose supplement of vitamin A is not recommended (4). There is no known toxicity from beta-carotene supplements. It is clear that a deficiency of retinol adversely affects vision, but there is no research supporting the notion that extra vitamin A or beta-carotene will improve a baseball player's vision. Baseball players can get ample vitamin A and beta-carotene in their diets by eating sweet potatoes, carrots, mangoes, turnip and collard greens, spinach, papaya, red and green bell peppers, apricots, cantaloupe, romaine lettuce, eggs, tomatoes, broccoli, oranges, and milk. Many fortified foods, such as breakfast cereals and energy bars, are also good sources of retinol (9).

FLUID NEEDS

Fluid may be the most important need for a baseball player. Traditionally, baseball is played in the summer when heat and humidity are high, plus it is one of the few sports that has no time limit. While most baseball games are played in nine innings (less in little league) which last less than 4 hours, longer games are possible. The longest major league baseball game on record was played on May 1, 1920 between the Brooklyn Robins and the Boston Braves. The game was called after 26 innings and a 1-1 tie (2).

Fluid replacement helps maintain hydration, which in turn promotes the health, safety, and optimal physical performance of an athlete (10). Exercise in the heat can limit physical performance by leading to dehydration, hyperthermia, and glycogen depletion (11). Consuming sports drinks at appropriate intervals can eliminate the danger from dehydration; yet, despite the recognition that athletes should consume adequate fluids during exercise, they often do not.

Yoshida et al (12) measured the aerobic capacity, sweat rate, and fluid intake of nine college baseball players to assess their thermoregulatory response at high temperatures. The subjects participated in baseball practice without drinking fluids for 2 hours. After 30 minutes of rest, they played a 2 1/2-hour baseball game and were allowed free access to a sports drink. The rate of sweat loss during the practice was 56.53 mL/kg, while the mean fluid consumption during the game was 44.78 mL/kg, with recovery of sweat loss at 76%. Athletes with free access to fluids did not consume enough to replace sweat losses (12).

Broad et al (13) studied body weight changes and voluntary fluid intakes during training and competition in team sports in both indoor and outdoor conditions. Although baseball was not among the team sports included in this study (soccer, basketball, and netball teams were studied), the authors found that athletes did not respond predictably to environmental conditions to meet their fluid needs and that fluid consumption should be considered a learned behavior (13).

Horswill (14) notes that the effect of dehydration on performance varies depending on the degree of dehydration and the type of performance; however, "dehydration doesn't enhance absolute performance and largely diminishes performance." Horwill offers several behavioral strategies to help athletes meet their fluid needs. These are summarized in *Box 32.1*. More suggestions for increasing fluid intake are found later in this chapter.

BOX 32.1 Fluid Guidelines for a Typical Baseball Game Schedule (10,14,20,26)

Guidelines for a 7 PM Baseball Game

Time	Drink
5 PM	2 cups (16 oz) of sports drink
7 PM-10 PM	1/2 to 1 cup (4 to 8 oz) every 15 to 20 minutes
After the game	Enough to at least replace lost body weight (Drinking 50% more than needed to restore lost body weight is even better.)

Strategies to Increase Fluid Intake:

- Practice scheduled drinking—drink during warm-ups and between innings.
- Give each player a sports bottle.
- Drink a sports drink that tastes good while exercising.
- Offer cool fluids which are usually preferred over warm fluids.
- Avoid carbonated beverages, as athletes tend to drink less when the beverage is carbonated.

ERGOGENIC AIDS

Baseball players are getting taller and heavier. Today's player is 5.1% taller than 100 years ago and 2.4% taller than 50 years ago (15). Average weights of major league baseball rookies have increased by 17.5 lb from the 1800s to the decade of the 1980s (15). Greg Lozinski finished his career with the Chicago White Sox at 279 lb (15). In addition, today's baseball players are interested in increasing muscle mass to achieve the "power swing." Mark McGwire's and Sammy Sosa's much publicized use of legal (by Major League Baseball rules) ergogenic aids during the record home run-setting season of 1998 shined a spotlight on creatine and androstenedione.

Creatine

Baseball players use creatine for the "power swing," although no research studies to date have examined the effect of creatine on a baseball player's swing. In theory creatine could be ergogenic to a baseball player by increasing the amount of creatine and phosphocreatine in resting muscle cells, increasing the rate of phosphocreatine resynthesis between activities, and enhancing the training ability so that more lean body mass can be accrued (16).

The most well-documented side effect of supplemental creatine use is weight gain. Two- to 7 lb-weight gains have been observed with creatine use, depending on the length of supplementation (17). Currently three leading theories explain the weight gain: fluid retention, protein synthesis, and improved quality of training which provides a potent adaptive stimulus to the development of lean mass (17).

Although there are anecdotal reports of muscle pulls, cramps, strains, or prolonged recovery from injury while using creatine, these effects have not been documented in published studies (16,17). However, since long-term safety is unknown, teams should adopt an official policy about creatine use. Creatine is a legal substance and is not banned by any sport-governing bodies. More information about creatine is found in Chapter 7, Ergogenic Aids.

Baseball players who choose to use creatine should use only recommended amounts (ie, 20 g per day for 5 to 7 days for loading and 5 g per day for maintenance) and consume extra water to avoid the potential dehydrating effects of extra protein (16,17).

Androstenedione

Androstenedione is a weakly androgenic hormone that has been touted as a "natural" way to boost testosterone levels without the harmful effects of anabolic steroids (18). It is classified as a dietary supplement, not a Schedule III substance like anabolic steroids (18). Androstenedione is reported to have its roots in the training of East German athletes who were advised to inhale it through a nasal spray immediately before competition to increase aggression (19). While proponents of androstenedione claim that it can increase lean mass, strength, and performance, no studies to date have shown this to be true. Presently, the science is not available to advise athletes if androstenedione use is safe or unsafe, helpful or harmful (18,19). Androstenedione is not banned by Major League Baseball, but it is banned by other organizations governing baseball players. College and Olympic baseball players should be aware that both the National Collegiate Athletic Association (NCAA) and the International Olympic Committee (IOC) ban its use.

The Endocrine Society has issued cautions about androstenedione use and has called for more research (20). The Endocrine Society, representing specialists who conduct and study hormone research and who treat endocrine disorders, recommends that androstenedione not be classified as a dietary supplement because it is not part of a normal diet. The use of androgens can be especially dangerous for adolescents because too much exogenous androgen can shut off the body's own natural production of testosterone, which can stunt growth (20). It is not known if androstenedione has the same side effects as anabolic steroids, but caution is warranted (18).

The National Federation of State High School Association's Medicine Advisory Committee issued a position statement about the use of dietary supplements in light of the publicity surrounding creatine and androstenedione use by major league baseball players (21). The position states that high school personnel and coaches should never supply, recommend, or permit the use of any drug, medication, or food supplement (including creatine and androstenedione) solely for performance-enhancing purposes (21).

PRECOMPETITION MEALS

Collegiate and professional baseball players frequently play night games. Since players report to the clubhouse about 4 to 5 hours before an evening game and a pregame meal should be consumed 3 to 4 hours before a game, food should be available in the clubhouse. Eating 3 to 4 hours before a game allows enough time for food to leave the stomach but yet avoids sensations of hunger (8). The pregame meal should contain foods rich in carbohydrate, moderate in protein, and low in fat and fiber, but the professional baseball player's clubhouse usually contains a wide range of foods—from high-carbohydrate to high-fat foods. Helping players identify the most appropriate pregame food choices can minimize fat while increasing carbohydrate intake. If an athlete has gastrointestinal discomfort from eating foods before a game, the following options can be suggested (22).

- Before competition, try eating small amounts of food more frequently.
- Four hours before competition, eat low to moderate glycemic index foods. (A list of foods with their glycemic index can be found in the Tools section.)
- Consume a sports drink that contains 6% to 8% carbohydrate (14 to 19 g per 8 oz).

Precompetition meals should also include foods that are familiar to the baseball player. Sammy Sosa, who hails from the Dominican Republic, helped to focus attention on the increasing number of Latino players in major league baseball; 30% of all major league baseball players are Latino, up from 14% in 1990 (23). Team managers should be sensitive to the ethnic food preferences of their players. *Box 32.2* identifies some Hispanic food preferences that would be appropriate to include in clubhouse meals.

BOX 32.2   Food Choices for Latino Players

Food Group	Common Foods
Grains	Short-grain rice
	Short-grain rice served with legumes
	Legumes (black beans preferred by Cubans; red and kidney beans by Puerto Ricans)
	Wheat flour breads
	Corn tamales and tortillas
	Cassava bread
	Cornmeal
Vegetables	Cabbage
	Chilies
	Corn
	Cucumber
	Eggplant
	Green beans
	Lettuce
	Onions

---

continued

BOX 32.2   Food Choices for Latino Players (continued)

Food Group	Common Foods
Vegetables (continued)	Spinach
	Plantains
	Potatoes
	Tomatillos
	Tomatoes
	Yams
Fruits	Bananas
	Breadfruit
	Coconut
	Grapes
	Guava
	Mangoes
	Oranges
	Papayas
	Passion fruit
	Pineapple
	Sapodilla (a member of the persimmon family)
	Raisins
Protein Foods	Beef
	Chicken
	Turkey
	Chicken eggs
	Mackerel
	Snapper
	Tarpon
	Aged cheeses
Seasonings	Cilantro
	Chili peppers
	Cinnamon
	Garlic
	Nutmeg
	Thyme
Beverages	Hot chocolate
	Coffee
	Soft drinks
	Refrescas (cold drinks made with tropical fruit flavors)

Source: Kittler PG, Sucher KP. *Food and Culture in America: A Nutrition Handbook*. 2nd ed. Belmont, Calif: West/Wadsworth; 1998.

TOP NUTRITION CONCERNS

Eating on the Road

Major league, minor league, collegiate, and Olympic baseball players travel often. Choosing high-carbohydrate foods is possible while dining out—even at fast-food restaurants—but some athletes have to make the conscious choice to eat more healthfully and, therefore, might have to retrain their taste buds. Clark (24) points out that a typical big burger, fries, and shake can provide 1,165 calories with 45% carbohydrate and 42% fat—missing the mark for a performance diet of <30% fat and at least 60% carbohydrate (24). The following suggestions can improve a baseball player's diet while eating out.

Breakfast:
- Choose blueberry pancakes, waffles, or French toast with syrup and request the butter or margarine on the side.
- Opt for cooked or dry cereal with low-fat milk and sliced bananas, strawberries, raspberries, blackberries, or blueberries.
- Order a large glass of juice.
- Choose English muffins, wheat toast, or muffins with jelly or jam instead of margarine or butter. Biscuits, croissants, pastries, and doughnuts are all high-fat items.
- Order an egg omelette with one whole egg and two egg whites and fill it with vegetables instead of cheese or high-fat breakfast meats like bacon or sausage.
- If breakfast meat is desired, ham or Canadian bacon is a leaner choice than bacon or sausage.

Lunch:
- Order a triple decker sandwich (three slices of bread) to increase carbohydrate intake. Opt for turkey, chicken, or tuna over high-fat luncheon meats like bologna or salami.
- If peanut butter and jelly are available, go heavy on the jelly and lighter on the peanut butter.
- Order the regular burger or cheeseburger over the specialty sandwiches (ie, triple meat patties with bacon and cheese). Two regular hamburgers contain more carbohydrate and less fat than one specialty sandwich.
- Choose regular size fries over the super-sized order.
- Survey the menu for items like chili, baked potatoes, grilled chicken, salads with grilled chicken, three-bean salad, coleslaw, or barbecued chicken.
- Turkey sub sandwiches loaded with lettuce, tomato, onion, and peppers are good alternatives to burgers and fries.

Dinner:
- Start with soup—vegetable, minestrone, chicken, or bean soups with crackers are high-carbohydrate choices to start the meal.
- Opt for a house salad instead of a higher-fat Caesar salad. Ask for the dressing on the side.

- Choose meat, fish, or poultry that is broiled, grilled, baked, or blackened. Leaner cuts of meat contain the words "loin" or "round" in the cut.
- Ask for an extra portion of the carbohydrate-rich rice, mashed potatoes, noodles, or beans.
- Eat plenty of bread or rolls—just skip the butter or margarine.
- Look for fruit-based desserts instead of higher-fat pies or cakes.

Late-night Eating after Games

Many baseball games are played under the lights and when the game ends, the eating begins. Eating foods rich in carbohydrate can help replenish muscle glycogen, and studies have shown that the glycogen resynthesis rate is greater during the first few hours after exercise than it is several hours later (22). Eating carbohydrate-rich foods immediately after a game can help a baseball player recover more quickly, which can be important in a long baseball season. Strategies to fuel the body yet feed the hunger after late night baseball games include:

- Drink sports drinks that contain carbohydrate. This will help replace carbohydrates and fluids lost through sweat.
- Opt for foods with a high glycemic index. These are more effective in replenishing muscle glycogen stores. Bagels with honey, crackers, raisins, bananas, bread (both white and whole wheat), and sports drinks with sugar or glucose polymers are all high glycemic index foods (8).
- Thick crust pizza (especially if the crust is eaten) with vegetable toppings or leaner meat options (ie, ham or Canadian bacon) can be an appropriate late night snack to boost carbohydrate intake.
- Be aware that consuming caffeinated drinks (ie, coffee, tea, some soft drinks) may lead to insomnia. Some over-the-counter pain remedies (Vanquish, Anacin) and some prescription pain drugs (Cafergot, Fiornal, Darvon) contain caffeine and can also lead to insomnia (25).

Increasing Fluid Consumption

As mentioned earlier in this chapter, fluid could arguably be the most important substance for baseball players of all ages. The following strategies will help increase fluid consumption.

- Players should include "fluid training" during spring training or preseason practice. While players always think about training their muscles or training their minds to learn new strategies and game plans, they rarely think about training their bodies to tolerate greater fluid intake during games.
- Players should drink fluids during the warm-up period (13).
- Players should drink fluids in the dugout between innings.
- Alcohol is not a good fluid replacement and can exaggerate the dehydrating effect of exercise in warm weather and impede rehydration after exercise (25).

TIPS FOR WORKING WITH COACHES AND TRAINERS

- Set up a meeting with the athletic trainer during the off-season and offer to provide a nutrition seminar or workshop during the preseason. A nutrition seminar for players will be more meaningful if both the coach and athletic trainer share their concerns about nutrition and the eating behaviors of their players.
- Encourage coaches and trainers to help players stay hydrated and choose more healthful foods. For example, providing scheduled fluid breaks and ensuring all players have water bottles will help increase fluid intake.
- Encourage coaches and trainers to model behavior by making healthful food choices when dining with players.
- Inform coaches about the most current dietary supplements and ergogenic aids that players might be using. Let coaches know which dietary supplements contain substances banned by their governing bodies.
- Offer to plan pregame meals or clubhouse food choices.

CASE STUDY

Mickey is an 18-year-old college freshman playing second base for a Division I NCAA team. In high school Mickey played football (fullback) as well as baseball. He is 5'10" with a stocky, compact build. He weighed 240 lb when he reported for his physical. Body plethysmography revealed a body fat percentage of 23%. Mickey's high school playing weight was 215 lb. Although that appeared to be heavy for his height, he ran the 40-yd dash in 4.6 seconds and was recruited for his quickness and strength. Blood chemistry taken at freshman physicals showed a total cholesterol level of 273 mg/dL with LDL-cholesterol of 164 mg/dL. His blood pressure was elevated on three different occasions, averaging 134/93. He has a positive family history of heart disease.

After Mickey completed a 3-day food diary, analysis showed the following:

Average calorie intake:	4,830 kcal
Carbohydrate intake:	495 g (41% of total kcal)
Protein intake:	253 g (21% of total kcal)
Fat intake:	204 g (38% of total kcal)
Cholesterol intake:	625 mg

Vitamin A, folate, and calcium intakes were <67% of RDAs.

Mickey usually skipped breakfast; his first meal of the day was around 11 AM. He would go back to his dorm room and cook two packages of Ramen noodles and make two egg salad and cheese sandwiches. His beverage choice was 24 oz of Kool-Aid or a soft drink. Before baseball practice, he would eat a 20-piece chicken nugget "snack." Dinner was eaten after baseball practice and was usually a large pepperoni, sausage, and extra cheese pizza with 1 L of cola. Favorite desserts included ice cream and cookies.

Mickey told the sports nutritionist that after high school graduation he was very sedentary and for 3 months did little other than "watch television." He knew he had gained weight, but was surprised at the 25-lb weight gain. While aware of his family history for high blood pressure and heart disease, he said he was never told his blood pressure was high and he had never had his cholesterol level measured.

Assessment

Mickey's energy needs were calculated as follows:

- He requires ~2, 900 kcal based on a desired body weight of 215 lb at 30 kcal/kg. That is almost 2,000 kcal less than his current intake.
- Carbohydrate needs were estimated to be 435 g per day (60% of energy needs).
- Protein needs were estimated to be 110 g per day (15% of energy needs and ~1.2 g/kg per body weight of 215 lb).
- Fat intake was calculated as 80 g per day, or 25% of energy needs.

These recommendations were realistic goals for Mickey based on his current intake and his goal to reach 215 lb. During his initial meeting with the sports nutritionist, both short-range and long-range goals were agreed upon. Mickey signed a performance contract with the sports nutritionist. (See the Tools section for an example of a performance contract.)

Short-range goals (2 months):
- Alter eating habits to achieve a weight loss of 10 lb during the preseason.
- Eat breakfast every day, consisting of banana, 1/2 bagel with jelly, and orange juice.
- Buy a meal ticket for lunch and dinner so that these meals can be consumed at the training table instead of in the dorm room. The sports nutritionist will show Mickey how to make appropriate selections for lunch and dinner.
- Eat at least five servings of fruits and vegetables every day.
- Limit fast-food meals and pizza to two times per week.
- Meet with the sports nutritionist at least once a week to monitor progress.

Long-range goals (12 months):

- Reduce body weight by 25 lb to high school weight of 215 lb.
- Reduce body fat percentage to 15% to 18%. Body fat percentage will be remeasured in 6 months.
- Learn to make more heart-healthy, performance-enhancing food choices when eating out.
- Reduce blood pressure without use of medication.
- Reduce blood cholesterol to < 200 mg/dL and reduce LDL-cholesterol to < 130 mg/dL.
- Institute an aerobic exercise program (established by the strength and conditioning coach) to help with weight loss and body fat loss.
- Remeasure blood lipids at the end of the season.

REFERENCES

1. Baseball: The great American game. http://www.adventure.com/encyclopedia/general/rfibaseb.html. Accessed May 28, 1998.
2. Major League Baseball. http://www.majorleaguebaseball.com.html. Accessed May 3, 1998.
3. Bucci L. Dietary supplements as ergogenic aids. In: Wolinsky I, ed. *Nutrition in Exercise and Sport.* 3rd ed. Boca Raton, Fl: CRC Press; 1998:315-368.
4. Katch FI, McArdle WD. *Introduction to Nutrition, Exercise, and Health.* 4th ed. Philadelphia, Penn: Lea & Febiger; 1993.
5. Williams C. Macronutrients and performance. *J Sports Sci.* 1995;13:S1-S10.
6. Williams C, Chryssanthopoulos C. Pre-exercise food intake and performance. In: Simopoulos AP, Pavlou KN, eds. *Nutrition and Fitness: Metabolic and Behavioral Aspects in Health and Disease.* Basel, Switzerland: Karger; 1997:33-45.
7. Lemon PWR. Effects of exercise on dietary protein requirements. *Int J Sport Nutr.* 1998;8:426-447.
8. Williams MH. *Nutrition for Health, Fitness, and Sport.* 5th ed. Boston, Mass: WCB McGraw Hill; 1999.
9. Duyff RL. *The American Dietetic Association's Complete Food and Nutrition Guide.* New York, NY: Wiley Publishers; 1998.
10. American College of Sports Medicine. Position stand on exercise and fluid replacement. *Med Sci Sports Exerc.* 1996;28:i-vii.
11. Millard-Stafford M. Fluid replacement during exercise in the heat. *Sports Med.* 1992;13:223-233.
12. Yoshida T, Nakai S, Yorimoto A, Kawabata T, Morimoto T. Effect of aerobic capacity on sweat rate and fluid intake during outdoor exercise in the heat. *Eur J Appl Physiol.* 1995;71:235-239.
13. Broad EM, Burke LM, Cox R, Heeley P, Riley M. Body weight changes and voluntary fluid intakes during training and competition sessions in team sports. *Int J Sport Nutr.* 1996;6:307-320.
14. Horswill CA. Effective fluid replacement. *Int J Sport Nutr.* 1998;8:175-195.
15. Topp R. Demographics. http://www.totalbaseball.com.html. Accessed October 1, 1998.
16. Volek JS, Kraemer WJ. Creatine supplementation: its effect on human muscular performance and body composition. *J Strength Cond Res.* 1996;10:200-210.
17. Plisk SS, Kreider RB. Creatine controversy? *Strength Cond J.* 1999;21:14-23.

18. Rosenbloom C. Androstenedione: its potential safety concerns. *SCAN's Pulse*. 1999;18:4-6.

19. Gwartney DL, Stout JR. Androstenedione: physical and ethical considerations relative to its use as an ergogenic aid. *Strength Cond J*. 1999;21:65-66.

20. Hunt, V. Endocrine Society, NSCA urge caution with androstenedione. *NATA News*. December, 1998:14.

21. NFHS takes position on androstenedione. http://www.nfsha.org/PR-position.htm. Accessed April 19, 1999.

22. Williams C, Nicholas CW. Nutrition needs for team sports. *Sports Sci Exch*. 1998;11:1-7.

23. Emerson T, Zarembo A. Sosa's streak. *Newsweek*. October 5, 1998:66-68.

24. Clark N. Eating nutritiously on the road. *Phys Sports Med*. 1985;13:133-139.

25. McArdle WD, Katch FI, Katch VL. *Sports and Exercise Nutrition*. Philadelphia, Penn: Lippincott Williams and Wilkins; 1999.

26. *Fluids 2000*. Chicago, Ill: The Gatorade Company; 1998.

33

BASKETBALL

Julie H. Burns, MS, RD and Kathy Engelbert-Fenton, MPH, RD

The fast-paced nature of basketball makes the game one of the most exciting in sports. Players must possess the unique combination of speed, agility, and power. They also need an endurance base to maintain high-intensity effort and allow for the execution of intricate and skillful maneuvers throughout the game.

A basketball player's nutritional training practices can have a significant impact on the overall development of a first-class athlete. Without the proper fuel and fluid intake, athletes may fall short of reaching their potential. Like other sports, maintaining appropriate levels of energy, fluid, and carbohydrate is an important contribution to peak performance.

ENERGY SYSTEMS

Basketball players utilize all three energy systems (ATP-CP or phosphagen system, lactic acid or anaerobic glycolysis, and oxidative or aerobic system) to generate power during training and games. Basketball action is intermittent. Quick bursts of power required for fast breaks, steals, and jump shots are fueled by the ATP-CP and lactic acid systems. Slower-paced play, longer sustained actions, and brief recovery periods are fueled by oxidative energy production. All three energy systems are active all the time, continually varying in their use for energy production. Each system is tapped according to the physiologic demands placed on the player at any given time. The primary determinants of fuel use during basketball play are intensity and duration of movement, and fuel availability and access (1,2). Both anaerobic and aerobic training are integral parts of most basketball players' conditioning programs. In particular, aerobic training and fitness improve heat tolerance and increase the capacity of trained skeletal muscles to store muscle glycogen, the only fuel that can be used to generate ATP anaerobically (3).

MACRONUTRIENT NEEDS

The general nutrient needs of basketball players do not differ from athletes of other sports. Consumption of a well-balanced and varied diet based on foods in the Food Guide Pyramid that meet daily energy expenditure will satisfy macronutrient and micronutrient requirements. A diet rich in carbohydrate (60%), moderate in protein (15% to 20%) and low in fat (25%) is the recommended sports diet for health and optimal performance (4-6). Carbohydrate requirements should be individualized and expressed based on body weight (g/kg BW)

509

instead of a percentage of total calories. Most basketball players require approximately 7 to 10 g/kg per day of carbohydrate (5,7). For basketball players who do exhaustive glycogen-depleting exercise on a daily basis, the goal for muscle repletion is to consume 7 to 9 g/kg BW in a 24-hour period or up to an upper level of 500 to 600 g carbohydrate per day (7). Because the capacity to store carbohydrate is limited, there appears to be no additional benefit to consuming more than 600 to 700 g of carbohydrate daily. When discussing carbohydrate needs with athletes, it may be helpful to begin with a quick and simple discussion about which fuels are utilized during the sport, with an emphasis on dietary carbohydrate, and follow with a list of foods and amounts (based on g/kg BW) that will supply carbohydrate (grains, cereals, fruits, starchy vegetables, fruit juices, dried peas and beans, lean milk and yogurt, sports drinks, high-carbohydrate beverages, etc).

The current recommendation for protein intake for athletes is 1.2 to 1.4 g/kg BW for endurance athletes and 1.4 to 1.7 g/kg BW for strength athletes (8). Based on these recommendations basketball players who engage in cross-training would likely have maximum protein needs of 1.7 g/kg BW for adults and about 2.0 g/kg BW for adolescents. Some athletes incorrectly believe that protein is the primary fuel burned during physical activity. Often, these athletes are surprised to learn that protein is not burned for fuel under circumstances where total energy intake and carbohydrate are adequate.

Basketball players have fat requirements of at least 1.0 to 1.2 g/kg BW (15% to 20% of total calories) based on the World Health Organization recommendations for fat intake for good health for sedentary or lightly active adults (9). Basketball players who have high-caloric needs may require even higher fat intakes (25% to 30% of total calories) to meet their energy needs. Sports nutritionists can provide guidance to basketball players on practical ways to include more healthful sources of fat in their diet (eg, olives, olive oil, avocado, flaxseed, fatty fish, nuts, seeds, etc) and limiting excessive saturated fat.

MICRONUTRIENT NEEDS

Minerals

The minerals sodium, potassium, chloride, calcium, magnesium, and phosphorus serve a variety of critical physiological functions key to athletic performance, including the maintenance of fluid balance and bone mass, nerve impulse propagation, force generation, and muscle contraction (10). Most men participating in team sports such as basketball tend to consume a diet adequate in calories and, thus, micronutrients and minerals (10). With heavy sweat losses, however, additional intakes of sodium, chloride, and possibly potassium may be warranted and can be obtained from foods and sports drinks after exercise and at subsequent meals (10). In contrast to men, female athletes need to pay special attention to the minerals calcium, iron, and possibly zinc in their diets (5), and supplementation may be indicated when dietary changes are pursued but found to be unsuccessful in remedying a situation. Providing samples of meal plans that meet the Recommended Dietary Allowances (RDAs) for vitamins, minerals, and energy will help shift the athlete's focus away from a heavy reliance on supplements to meet nutrient needs and toward the use of nutrient-dense whole foods that provide abundant essential nutrients for performance and health.

Vitamins

Research is not available to firmly support an increased need for vitamins beyond the RDAs for athletes, except for thiamin, which is required in proportion to the number of calories consumed. Athletes require more thiamin because of their increased energy needs. Thiamin is easily obtained from whole-grain and enriched grain products. Some athletes may benefit from a multiple vitamin and mineral supplement because of particular food habits, such as a high consumption of processed foods and frequent meals on the road, food intolerances or allergies, exclusion of an entire food group, or other dietary practices. According to Dr. William Evans (11), supplementation of antioxidant vitamins in particular should not exceed the levels established by the Task Force on Guidelines for Dietary Supplementation, United States Olympic Committee. (See *Table 33.1*.) As always, the ideal sports performance diet should be customized to meet the unique dietary patterns and needs of each athlete.

TABLE 33.1   USOC Guidelines for Dietary Supplementation with Antioxidant Vitamins (11)

Nutrient	Maximum Dosage
Beta-Carotene	3,000-20,000 µg or 5,000-33,340 IU
Vitamin C	250-1,000 mg
Vitamin E (as alpha-tocopherol)	100-400 IU

ENERGY NEEDS

The energy needs of basketball players vary considerably from individual to individual and are dependent on many factors, notably body size and activity level (12). For example, a young, small, female basketball player training for 60 minutes per day may require only 2,000 kcal per day while a male professional player may need three times this amount or approximately 6,000 kcal. Sports nutritionists can get an idea of whether an athlete is meeting energy requirements by looking at the amount of calories normally consumed versus those expended daily and tracking body mass and body composition fluctuations for a period of time. Assuming these two indices stay fairly consistent and the health and performance of the athlete are maintained, caloric intake is most likely adequate (10).

Total daily energy expenditure includes three components: resting energy expenditure (REE), activity calories for daily living, and activity calories for purposeful exercise (basketball or other exercise training). To provide an estimate of energy needs for a basketball player desiring weight maintenance, determine REE that is proportional to lean body mass (9) and assign an appropriate activity factor for daily living and purposeful exercise ranging from 1.6 to 2.4 for light training through very heavy training, respectively. (See *Table 33.2.*) Specific caloric expenditures for each activity may also be used in place of an activity factor. The estimated amount of calories per minute expended during basketball is shown in *Table 33.3.* Basketball players tend to engage in other physical activities including aerobic conditioning and resistance training, both of which contribute significantly to energy expenditure. Energy expenditure fluctuates on a daily basis due to changes in the intensity and duration of physical activity and will affect energy intake and needs.

TABLE 33.2   Resting Energy Expenditure (9)

Age (years)	Males	Females
10-18	(17.5 x BW) + 651	(12.2 x BW) + 746
18-30	(15.3 x BW) + 679	(14.7 x BW) + 496
30-60	(11.6 x BW) + 879	(8.7 x BW) + 829

BW is body weight in kilograms.

TABLE 33.3   Energy Expenditure for Competitive Basketball (2)

kg	lb	Calories/minute
55	120	7.8
59	130	8.5
64	140	9.2
68	150	9.9
77	170	11.2
82	180	11.9
86	190	12.5
91	200	13.2
95	210	13.8

Caloric requirements can also be estimated in a general way for those athletes who train for 90 or more minutes per day. Economos et al (13) recommend that male athletes consume >50 kcal/kg per day (23 kcal/lb) and females consume 45 to 50 kcal/kg per day (20 to 23 kcal/lb).

FLUID NEEDS

Like energy needs, fluid requirements vary widely among basketball players and are dependent on many variables, such as the athlete's genetic make-up for sweating, level of fitness and acclimation, playing temperature and environment, amount and type of clothing worn, and intensity of training or competition (14). Ideally, individual sweat rates for each athlete can be calculated by recording changes in pre- and postexercise body weight and adjusting for fluid intake during a typical training session (15). (See Chapter 6, Fluid and Electrolytes.)

The most common cause of early fatigue during exercise is not lack of fuel, but dehydration. Fortunately, preventing dehydration is easily achievable. Basketball players need to be taught that even slight losses in body weight can impair performance (as little as a 1% loss or less than 2 lb in a 175-lb player). An aggressive approach taken by the coaching staff during practice and competition to prevent dehydration by promoting the liberal intake of fluids before, during, and after exercise will lead to increased stamina and stronger play on the court.

The following steps for promoting fluid intake can help maximize performance and prevent heat-related illness (15).

- Make certain that fluid is always nearby and easily accessible to the athlete.
- Provide sports drinks, sports gels (follow with at least 8 oz of fluid), and foods with a high liquid content, such as orange slices, during time-outs, half-time, and rest breaks when feasible.
- Encourage players to drink on a schedule (5 to 10 oz every 15 to 20 minutes) instead of waiting until thirsty.
- Serve cool, flavored fluids that contain sodium (like sports drinks) to encourage adequate drinking so fluid requirements are more likely to be met.
- Assign individual squeeze bottles to each player. By providing players with their own sport bottles, the importance of staying hydrated is emphasized and the quantity of fluid ingested by each player can be monitored. Individual bottles also decrease the chance of spreading viral infections. For school-aged players, a sports bottle filled with fluids can be frozen and sent to school to keep the fluid cool for after-school practice.
- "Train" athletes to drink. Most players are unaccustomed to drinking the recommended volume of fluid to fully replace sweat losses. They need to incorporate hydration strategies into practice sessions. Refer to *Table 33.4* for the specific amounts of fluid to consume before, during, and after exercise (15,16).

TABLE 33.4   Fluid and Carbohydrate Needs for Basketball Players (5,15,16,20)

	Rationale	Carbohydrate	Fluid
High-intensity Training	For basketball players who train hard daily and need to maximize daily muscle glycogen recovery	7-10 g/kg BW per day or 500-600 g per day	10-12 cups per day (~2.5-3 L) plus fluids before, during, and after exercise
Moderate-intensity Training	For basketball players who train less than 1 hour daily at a moderate intensity	5-7 g/kg BW per day	10-12 cups per day (~2.5-3 L) plus fluids before, during, and after exercise
Pre-exercise	To enhance fuel availability and prehydrate for a practice or game	1 g/kg BW 1 hour prior 2 g/kg BW 2 hours prior 3 g/kg BW 3 hours prior 4 g/kg BW 4 hours prior	17 oz or ~2 cups (~1/2 L) 2 hours prior (noncaffeinated, nonalcoholic)
During Exercise	To provide an additional source of carbohydrate fuel during moderate- and high-intensity basketball practice and games	30-60 g per hour	5-10 oz every 15 minutes for hydration purposes

continued

TABLE 33.4   Fluid and Carbohydrate Needs for Basketball Players (5,15,16,20) (continued)

	Rationale	Carbohydrate	Fluid
Recovery	To speed early recovery and rehydration after hard training or a game, especially during the season when there are back-to-back games and daily practices	1.0-1.5 g/kg BW high-glycemic carbohydrate beverages and foods immediately following exercise and every 2 hours. Total carbohydrate intake over the next 24 hours at 7-9 g/kg or approximately 500-600 g in 24 hours	~20 oz (~3 cups) per lb lost during exercise

- Teach athletes to monitor their hydration status by checking urine color. (Even very young athletes think that this a fun way of tracking their fluids.) A clear, odorless, light-colored urine indicates good hydration status, whereas dark urine suggests an athlete may be dehydrated.
- Encourage athletes to weigh-in before and after training sessions to assess individual fluid losses.

ERGOGENIC AIDS

Professional basketball players are most interested in supplements that claim to enhance power output, muscle mass, and quickness, and maintain energy levels throughout the long season. Younger basketball players may have some of these same concerns. Sports nutritionists can be a reliable source of information on the safety and efficacy of supplements—input that is especially needed and important for the young athlete. (Refer to Chapter 7, Ergogenic Aids for review of dietary supplements commonly used by athletes.)

To date, no studies have been conducted on the effects of specific nonnutritive nutritional supplements on basketball performance. One study (17) showed an improvement in jumping height after creatine ingestion, which may have some application to basketball. In general, about half of the studies have found that creatine ingestion improved short-term exercise performance while the other half showed no effect. The greatest concerns regarding creatine supplementation include quality assurance and the lack of long-term safety data. Since the FDA does not regulate dietary supplements for quality, purity, safety, or effectiveness, the buyer must assume the responsibility for obtaining quality assurance information from individual manufacturers. At present, many trainers are not recommending creatine use because of possible adverse effects on hydration status, recently reported cases of renal problems (18,19), anecdotal reports of muscle strains and pulls, and the lack of long-term safety studies.

Other dietary supplements, such as Chinese herbs and herbal remedies (especially those with ginseng and ginkgo biloba), are of great interest to adult basketball players because of their potential role in enhancing mental acuity and feelings of well-being. Sports nutritionists need to acquire additional knowledge and training in herbal medicine so that they can provide credible input on the proper and safe use of these therapies.

NUTRITIONAL CONSIDERATIONS FOR TRAINING AND COMPETITION

The primary fuel used during basketball is carbohydrate. A challenge for the sports nutritionist is assisting basketball players in understanding their carbohydrate needs and practically applying this information to food choices. For many players this will mean more emphasis on carbohydrate and less on protein. See *Table 33.4* for specific carbohydrate and fluid needs during training (15,16,20).

Providing practical tools to educate the athlete on ways to obtain foods that contain adequate carbohydrate, fluids, energy, and other nutrients is useful. Taking the basketball player (and/or spouse/significant other/parent) to the grocery store teaches and shows the athlete, or the person responsible for food preparation, how to buy appropriate training foods. Some basketball players, in particular the professional athlete, may wish to hire a personal chef to take the pressure off of meal preparation. Sports nutritionists can work with personal chefs to devise delicious gourmet meal plans that satisfy both the nutrient and energy requirements of a sports performance diet.

Eating on the road is a challenge for basketball players, especially those who travel out of town for extended periods of time. Providing mini-seminars and handouts on healthful meal selection when dining out is helpful. Traveling basketball players, especially high-profile athletes who must spend a lot of time in their rooms, may also need guidance in selecting meals and snacks from hotel room service menus. Sports nutritionists may also be involved in selecting the foods and fluids that are served during in-flight meals on team airline charters.

Pregame Meal and Fluid Recommendations

Many basketball players need guidance on what to eat before they train or compete. The pre-exercise meal prevents the athlete from feeling hungry and fatigued and may also help prepare him or her mentally for competition. Some professional players who must report to play 90 minutes before tip-off have their pregame meal at midday, rest for a few hours in the afternoon, and follow with a substantial snack, including fluids, about 3 hours before game time. They then eat a light snack (like an energy bar) and drink fluids once they arrive at the sports arena. Others (probably those with faster gastric-emptying rates) may opt to have their pregame meal about 3 to 3.5 hours before tip-off. For those athletes eating 3 to 4 hours or more before play, including a small amount of lean protein as part of a high-carbohydrate pregame meal may enhance satiety and alleviate hunger during the game. Each athlete needs to experiment with what foods feel best both physiologically and psychologically. After determining what works well, many athletes choose to eat the exact same foods at the same time as part of their pregame ritual. See *Table 33.5* for a sample meal plan and *Table 33.6* for pregame fuel and meal-timing recommendations.

TABLE 33.5   Sample 3,200 kcal Meal Plan Menu (65% of total kcal from carbohydrate or ~7 g/kg BW) for Meeting Carbohydrate Needs for an 80-kg (175-lb) Male Basketball Player (age range 10 to 17 years)

Breakfast	CHO (g)	Lunch	CHO (g)	Postexercise Snack	CHO (g)	Dinner	CHO (g)
1 cup orange juice	30	2 slices whole-wheat bread	30	1 can Gatorlode	71	2 cups pasta	80
1 large banana	30	4 oz turkey breast meat	0	1 cup vanilla yogurt	36	1 cup marinara sauce	20
1 cup Raisin Bran	42	1 T light mayonnaise	0	4 graham crackers	22	2 T parmesan cheese	0
12 oz 1% milk	16	2 lettuce leaves	0	Water	0	1 cup broccoli	8
1 slice whole-wheat toast	15	2 tomato slices	2			2 cups green salad	3
2 t margarine or olive oil	0	1 small pear	15			3 T Italian dressing	0
Water	0	2 oz pretzels	45			1 slice French bread	15
		8 oz apple juice	30			2 t margarine or olive oil	0
		Water	0			12 oz 1% milk	16
						Water	0
						Total g CHO	526

This diet meets minimum daily carbohydrate needs of ~7 g/kg BW: 526 g CHO.

Note: Sports drink carbohydrate and energy consumed prior to and during practice were not accounted for in meal plan calculation.

CHO = carbohydrate

TABLE 33.6   Pre-exercise Carbohydrate Needs for 80-kg (175-lb) Player (5,7)

Time Before Exercise	Calculation for CHO (g)	Sample Snacks and Meals Meeting Selected Needs
1 hour	1.0 g/kg BW = 80 g	1 bagel (30 g), 4 t jam (20 g), 8 oz 1% milk (12 g), 1 large banana (30 g) provide 92 g carbohydrate. Add additional fluids if tolerated.
2 hours	2.0 g/kg BW = 160 g	
3 hours	3.0 g/kg BW = 240 g	
4 hours	4.0 g/kg BW = 318 g	2 cups pasta (80 g), 1.5 cups lean meat sauce (20 g), 1 cup cooked vegetables (10 g), 2 slices bread and spread or oil (30 g), 2 T honey (30 g), 2 cups 1% milk (24 g), 1 cup applesauce (30 g), 8 vanilla wafers (20 g), 1 cup fruit yogurt (43 g), and 2 cups orange juice (60 g) provide 347 g carbohydrate.

Many athletes practice or train in the morning without eating breakfast. This should be discouraged. High-carbohydrate liquid meals (homemade or commercial) work well for the player who is not hungry or does not wish to eat a meal in the morning. Athletes who eat a high-carbohydrate light meal before practice can avoid feelings of fatigue and lightheadedness caused by low blood-sugar levels. Young athletes who practice after school may have had lunch several hours before and should be sent to school with a high-carbohydrate snack and beverage to eat after school to raise blood-sugar levels and provide energy.

TOP NUTRITION CONCERNS

Basketball players want to maximize speed, agility, and power. To accomplish these goals from a nutrition standpoint, players need a training diet that has enough energy and key nutrients, most notably carbohydrate and fluids. Mental sharpness and stamina during play, especially during the fourth quarter when the game may be on the line, are also top concerns of basketball players. Fluids, like sports drinks and water, ingested during play will help delay the deterioration in play that occurs during prolonged exercise. Carbohydrate gels taken with at least 8 oz of fluid may also be helpful. A recent study (21) examined the performance effects (both physical and mental) of a 6% carbohydrate-electrolyte beverage during intermittent, high-intensity exercise. The study was designed to closely mimic the demands of an actual competitive sporting event such as a basketball game by using a "shuttle run" course. Subjects (5 males, 5 females) were experienced in sports such as soccer and basketball. The exercise periods consisted of four, 15-minute quarters of intermittent shuttle running at various percentages of VO_2max (walking, jogging, running, sprinting, and jumping) accompanied by a 20-minute half-time rest period, followed by a shuttle run to fatigue. Carbohydrate or placebo (artificially flavored water) drinks were consumed prior to exercise (5 mL/kg, 6% solution), at half-time (18% solution), and during the four, 15-minute quarters (3 mL/kg, 6% solution). Subjects then underwent physical function tests (shuttle run to fatigue, 20-meter maximal sprint, and 10 repetition maximal vertical jumping) and mental function tests (a whole-body motor skills test, a profile of "mood states," and a concentration test). Subjects who consumed the sports drink ran 37% longer before becoming fatigued and completed the 20-meter sprint during the fourth quarter faster than the placebo group. In addition, whole-body motor skill test performance and the perception of fatigue were improved in the carbohydrate-supplemented subjects. These preliminary results suggest a beneficial role of carbohydrate supplementation on physical as well as mental performance tasks that are similar to the demands of many intermittent, high-intensity sports including basketball.

Basketball players are also often concerned about fatigue and staleness, especially during the latter part of the regular season and in the postseason. Effective recovery practices are key to preventing a plateau or dip in performance, and require specific fluid and carbohydrate intakes for prevention. When there is limited time for recovery (as occurs with back-to-back games and daily training sessions and practices), 150% of the fluid lost during exercise should be replaced before the next game or practice to speed recovery (~20 to 24 oz for every lb of weight lost during exercise) (22). To replenish glycogen stores, 1.0 to 1.5 g/kg BW of high-glycemic carbohydrate beverages and foods should be consumed immediately following exercise and every 2 hours at a carbohydrate level of ~1 g/kg per 2 hours in snacks or meals. The total carbohydrate intake over the next 24 hours should be about 7 to 9 g/kg or approximately 500 to 600 g in 24 hours (7,23). A sports drink is a good choice when rehydration is a goal, whereas a high-carbohydrate energy drink is acceptable when hydration status is adequate and additional energy is desired during recovery. A 200-lb basketball player could replete his carbohydrate stores by consuming approximately 600 g carbohydrate per day or 7 g/kg BW. See *Boxes 33.1* and *33.2* for sample recovery foods handouts.

BOX 33.1   Sample Recovery Foods Handout for Athletes

MAXIMIZE YOUR RECOVERY WITH CARBOHYDRATES!

Here are some items that you can mix and match to reach your individual recovery carbohydrates. Remember that you should try to eat or drink about 0.5 g/lb of carbohydrate (for example, about 85 g for a 175-lb player) **within 15 minutes after playing and again every 2 hours for the next 6 to 8 hours.**

10-15 g CHO	25-30 g CHO
1 fruit roll-up	1 banana
1 oz pretzels	1 cup mashed potatoes
2 cups cottage cheese (2%)	1 bagel
1 medium piece of fruit (orange, apple)	1 large fruit or bran muffin
6 saltine crackers	3/4 cup cereal
2 T reduced-fat peanut butter	16 oz 1% milk
3 cups popcorn	3 Mrs. T's Pierogies
1/3 cup rice	1 cup instant soup
1/2 cup stuffing	2 frozen pancakes
12 oz Gatorade	1 1/2 oz box raisins
1 frozen fruit juice bar	2 tortillas (6 in)
3 T wheat germ	1/2 cup low-fat refried beans
	6 oz yogurt
	1 cup frozen yogurt

40-45 g CHO	50-60 g CHO
4 graham cracker squares	11 oz Gatorpro
4 Fig Newtons	2 cups apple or orange juice
1 Powerbar	8 oz sherbet
12 oz can soda	2 cups applesauce
1 cup cranberry juice cocktail	1 cup chocolate pudding
1 baked potato with skin	1 Met-Rx bar

Source: Burns JH. Western Springs, IL: SportFuel, Inc.

BOX 33.2   Sample Recovery Foods Handout for Basketball Team
of Higher Body Weight

YOUR GUIDE TO QUICK RECOVERY

Your recovery carbohydrate needs have been calculated based on your body weight. Because of your heavy training schedule and long season, your requirements have been determined at the high end of the recommendations (range: 0.3 to 0.7 g carbohydrate/lb of body weight). You can put back more carbohydrate into your muscles (and speed recovery) by taking in high-carbohydrate foods and drinks within 15 to 30 minutes of completing exercise and again every 2 hours for the next 6 to 8 hours.

Usually, it's easier to replace the 15- to 30-minute carbohydrate requirement with fluids since they can be consumed quickly, help you rehydrate, and can provide carbohydrate. You can then complete your carbohydrate recovery with your postgame meal, eaten within 2 hours of a game or practice. Of course, this meal should be rich in carbohydrate-containing foods, low in fat, moderate in protein, and loaded with noncaffeinated, nonalcoholic fluids. If you have lost more than 2% of your body weight during exercise, continue drinking fluids such as sport drinks and add a few salty items (such as soup or pretzels) to speed up the rehydration and recovery process. The following table gives you several options for meeting your carbohydrate recovery requirements.

120 g	150 g	180 g
2 cups applesauce	2 cans Gatorlode	1 cup ready-to-eat cereal
4 Fig Newtons	1 orange	1 cup skim milk
8 oz sports drink	*or*	1 banana
or	10 cups sports drink	2 cups cran-grape juice
1 cup raisins or dried cherries	*or*	*or*
or	2 cups apple-cranberry juice	1 can Gatorlode
1 cup fruit yogurt	1 large bagel	1 Met-Rx bar
1 pear		1 cup ready-to-eat pudding
4 graham cracker squares		

Source: Burns JH. Western Springs, IL: SportFuel, Inc.

WORKING WITH COACHES AND TRAINERS

Many coaches and trainers are aware of the impact that good nutrition practices have on performance and health. Often the difficulty lies in finding the time for nutrition education because of other priorities and demands made on the team's, the trainer's, and the coaching staff's time. At the professional level, the athletic trainer is usually the sports nutritionist's main and best contact and knows the most about the athletes' nutrition habits and needs. The best time to contact the trainer or coach is well before training camp begins (~2 months) when plans for training camp are just being drawn. Preventing injuries is one of the trainers' and coaches' top concerns. Approaching the trainer and/or the coach with specifics on how sound nutrition practices can help keep the team healthy will more than likely be of interest. The services that the sports nutritionist can provide during the preseason to help maximize the health and conditioning of the team can be compiled and sent to the trainer, with additional copies to the strength and conditioning coaches, head coach, and other coaching staff. Once the season begins, it becomes increasingly difficult to meet with the team as a group, although playoffs may be an opportunity for a nutrition refresher session.

Some strategies that have worked to spur interest in nutrition and have lead to individual counseling sessions at the professional level include mini-seminars (15 to 20 minutes) on various nutrition topics accompanied by user-friendly handouts and food samples. Other materials sent during the season via the trainer have included a quarterly sports nutrition newsletter and other nutrition items of interest such as a play-off preparation memo, various nutrition suggestions for injured players, etc.

CASE STUDY

Danny is a single, 22-year-old professional basketball player who plays back-up center. His team is in the process of rebuilding after losing an all-star to retirement and several other players to free agency. With a less experienced line up, Danny believes that the coaches will likely adopt an up-tempo game plan. He asked to meet with the sports nutritionist for help in increasing his quickness on fast breaks and on building his strength for low-post (under the basket) play.

Baseline Information

- Current Weight: 262 lb (stable)
- Height: 6'9"
- Best Playing Weight Range: 252-257 lb
- Baseline Body Fat: 17% (calipers)
- Current intake based on 4-day diet record: 5,900 kcal (26% protein, 35% carbohydrate, and 39% fat)

Recommendations

- General recommendation: Identify higher-fat foods that are routinely consumed and reduce consumption and/or substitute with healthful choices to reduce both total fat and calories in the diet. In this case, bacon and sausage were eaten daily, 2% and whole milk were used regularly, and meat portions were very large, high-fat cuts.
- Calculate caloric needs.
  — Caloric needs based on current training of 90 minutes or more at high intensity are approximately 5,950 kcals daily (based on 23 kcals per median goal body weight of 255 lb or REE x 2.4).
  — Subtract 500 kcals per day for desired fat loss and arrive at estimated 5,450-kcal meal plan.
  — Devise a meal plan using 1.7 g/kg BW protein totaling 196 g protein, 1.3 g/kg fat totaling 151 g, and about 7.0 g/kg BW carbohydrate/lb totaling 815 g. The percentage of calories translates into approximately 15% protein, 25% fat, and 60% carbohydrate.

(Please note that when developing meal plans, particularly very-high-calorie diets, the g/kg and the total g carbohydrate daily are more useful measures than percentages of total calories.)

— Note that the meal plan was provided as a guide for intake only; caloric and macronutrient adjustments can easily be made by substituting lean meat and dairy for high-fat meats and dairy selections, and by reducing meat portions and increasing fruit, vegetable, and whole-grain intake.

- Increase dietary carbohydrate.
  — Add additional fruits, vegetables, whole grains, fruit juices, sports drinks, and high-energy carbohydrate drinks based on individual food preferences to increase carbohydrate intake. Initial carbohydrate intake was 516 g or about 100 g less than the recommended 600 g per day for adequate carbohydrate repletion.
  — Address a strong family history of prostate cancer (his father and uncle) with tomatoes, guava, watermelon, red grapefruit, cantaloupe, winter and summer squash, and pumpkin (seed). Recommend these as good choices for daily fruit and vegetable consumption. Other foods which may be important in the prevention of prostate cancer include fish, flax, olive and canola oils, sesame, avocado, and soy.
  — Provide recipes for fruit blender drinks (smoothies) for use in the morning and for quick high-carbohydrate snacks.
- Attend a grocery shopping tour.
  — Identify high-carbohydrate foods and fluids needed for performance enhancement during a tour with the sports nutritionist. Danny also learned how to select lean protein foods and received recipes for leaner grilling.
- Increase fluid intake.
  — Provide a handout with specific requirements, including amount and timing suggestions for intake because fluid intake was inadequate.
- Exercise.
  — Increase aerobic exercise to five times per week to reduce body fat (to an approximate range of 13% to 15% which corresponds to a weight range of 250 to 256 lb, or to where Danny feels his performance goals are reached). Continue the resistance program set up by the strength and conditioning coach to build muscle mass.
- Educate about recovery foods and fluids.
  — Provide a handout on recovery foods to give suggestions for rehydrating and refueling with high-glycemic index foods postexercise. Danny was never hungry after training and tended to drink only water after exercise. He felt that his recovery from hard training was slow. He needs between 81 to 174 g of carbohydrate postexercise (0.7 to 1.5 g/kg BW x range of 252 to 257 lb BW) and 20 to 24 oz of fluid for every 1 lb of weight lost during exercise (usually about 3 lb).

- Discuss tips for dining out.
  —Obtain menus from restaurants that Danny frequented and review them together so that he could learn to make the best choices when dining away from home.
- Check plan regularly.
  —Recheck diet intake, performance effects, ability to recover between sessions, exercise tolerance, feeling of well-being, and body-fat measurement in 3 to 4 weeks and make adjustments as needed.

REFERENCES

1. McArdle WD, Katch FI, Katch VI. *Exercise Physiology: Energy, Nutrition, and Human Performance*. 4th ed. Baltimore, Md: Williams and Wilkens; 1996.
2. Williams MH. *Nutrition for Health, Fitness and Sport*. 5th ed. Boston: McGraw-Hill; 1999.
3. Gollnick P, Hermansen L. Biochemical adaptation to exercise: anaerobic metabolism. In: Wilmore J, ed. *Exercise and Sports Sciences Reviews*. Vol. 1. New York, NY: Academic Press; 1973:1-43.
4. Coleman E. Carbohydrate—the master fuel. In: Berning JR, Steen SN, eds. *Nutrition for Sport and Exercise*. 2nd ed. Gaithersburg, Md: Aspen Publishers; 1998:29,21-44.
5. Hawley J, Burke L. *Peak Performance: Training and Nutritional Strategies for Sport*. Sydney, Aus: Allen & Unwin; 1998.
6. Berning JR, Steen SN. *Nutrition for Sport and Exercise*. 2nd ed. Gaithersburg, Md: Aspen Publishers; 1998.
7. Coyle E. Substrate utilization during exercise in active people. *Am J Clin Nutr*. 1995;61(suppl):968S-979S.
8. Lemon PWR. Effects of exercise on dietary protein requirements. *Int J Sports Nutr*. 1998;8:426-447.
9. World Health Organization. *Energy and Protein Requirements. Report of a Joint FAO/WHO/UNO Experts Consultation*. Technical report series 724. Geneva, Switzerland: WHO; 1985.
10. Murray R, Horswill CA. Nutrient requirements for competitive sports. In: Wolinsky I, ed. *Nutrition in Exercise and Sport*. 3rd ed. Boca Raton, Fla: CRC Press; 1998:521-556.
11. Evans W. The Protective Role of Antioxidants on Exercise-induced Oxidative Stress. Paper presented at: 1996 Sports, Cardiovascular, and Wellness Nutritionists (SCAN) Symposium; 1996; Scottsdale, Ariz.
12. Brotherhood J. Nutrition and sports performance. *Sports Med*. 1984;1:350-389.
13. Economos CD, Bortz SS, Nelson ME. Nutritional practices of elite athletes. *Sports Med*. 1993;16:381-399.
14. Sawka MN, Wenger CB. Physiological responses to acute exercise-heat stress. In: Pandolf KB, Sawka MN, Gonzalez RR, eds. *Human Performance Physiology and Environmental Medicine at Terrestrial Extremes*. Indianapolis, Ind: Benchmark Press; 1988:153-197.
15. Horswill CA. Effective fluid replacement. *Int J Sport Nutr*. 1998;8:175-195.
16. American College of Sports Medicine. Position stand: exercise and fluid replacement. *Med Sci Sports Exerc*. 1996;28:i-vii.
17. Bosco C, Tihanyi J, Pucspk J, et al. Effect of oral creatine supplementation on jumping and running performance. *Int J Sports Med*. 1997;18:369-372.

18. Pritchard NR, Kalra PA. Renal dysfunction accompanying oral creatine supplements. *Lancet*. 1998;351:1252-1253.
19. Kuehl K, Goldberg L, Elliot D. Renal insufficiency after creatine supplementation in a college football athlete. *Med Sci Sports Exerc*. 1998;30:S235.
20. Coyle EF. Fuels for sport performance. In: Lamb DR, Murray R, eds. *Perspectives in Exercise Science and Sports Medicine, Vol 10. Optimizing Sport Performance*. Carmel, Ind: Cooper Publishing Group; 1997:95-138.
21. Welsh RS, Byam S, Bartoli W, Burke JM, Williams H, Davis JM. Influence of carbohydrate ingestion on physical and mental function during intermittent high-intensity exercise to fatigue. *Med Sci Sports Exerc*. 1999;31:S123.
22. Shirreffs SM, Taylor AJ, Leiper KB, Maughan RJ. Post-exercise rehydration in man: effects of volume consumed and drink sodium content. *Med Sci Sports Exerc*. 1996;28:1260-1271.
23. Williams C, Nicholas CW. Nutrition needs for team sports. *Sports Sci Exch*. 1998;11(3).

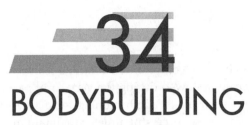

BODYBUILDING

Susan M. Kleiner, PhD, RD

Historically, a controversy has continued among nutritionists, exercise scientists, and practitioners about whether bodybuilders should be considered athletes. The goals of their sport are relatively subjective, since they are judged on the size, definition, symmetry, and vascularization of their muscular development, rather than objective measures of time, distance, or accuracy. But step into a gym where serious bodybuilders are training and talk to them about their exercise regimens, and there is little doubt that these individuals are elite athletes, equally dedicated to their sport as any cyclist, long jumper, or marksman.

Due in part to this controversy, the scientific study of nutrition for strength training and bodybuilding has lagged behind the study of nutrition for aerobic and endurance training. Nutritionists and dietitians have been left in the dark as to the best dietary advice for bodybuilders. And bodybuilders have had no choice but to go to more popular sources like magazines, trade books, and other successful bodybuilders to find nutrition information relevant to their sport. However, the last decade has seen an increase in the research community's interest in studying the nutritional requirements of strength training and bodybuilding. Today the science of nutrition for strength training is in its infancy, but there is a body of evidence to support nutritional recommendations that will help bodybuilding athletes achieve their goals of gaining muscle, losing fat, and becoming physically prepared for bodybuilding competitions.

GOALS AND STRATEGIES

Muscle cells generate adenosine triphosphate (ATP) through three energy systems: the phosphagen system, the glycolytic system, and the oxidative system. The phosphagen and glycolytic systems dominate during strength training, and the oxidative system is predominant during aerobic and endurance activity. Because bodybuilders participate heavily in strength training and aerobic activity (more or less depending on the timing of competition), they must be well fueled to support all energy systems.

There are four training and diet strategies that all competitive bodybuilders follow. Each has different goals and slightly different nutritional requirements.

1. Maintain muscle.
2. Build muscle.
3. Taper the body.
4. Cut weight.

The goal of maintenance is to maintain body composition, avoiding lean tissue loss or fat gain. This strategy is typically followed during the very early part of the off-season, just after the competitive season. Strength training for maintenance is the predominant exercise, but the most successful athletes maintain an aerobic exercise routine as well. Workouts are usually once a day, four to six times per week.

The muscle-building strategy is begun once the bodybuilder feels rested from the previous season and ready to begin training for the next season of competition. The goal is to build lean tissue and minimize fat gain. Strength training is still the predominant exercise, with some aerobic exercise included. Workouts are often twice a day, 5 to 6 days per week.

Tapering is begun approximately 12 weeks prior to competition. The goal of the tapering strategy is to maintain or continue to slightly build muscle, lose fat, and gain muscular definition. The style of strength training changes to support the goals, and the amount of aerobic exercise is significantly increased to incur larger kilocalorie deficits.

The cutting strategy is used only if tapering has not been completely successful. It is a way of giving the diet a final tweak to chisel away the last bits of unwanted body fat. Kilocalories are cut to a minimum while strength training and aerobic exercise remains high. This diet should be followed for only 1 week prior to competition.

ENERGY AND NUTRIENT NEEDS

Energy and macronutrient needs change depending on the diet strategy and the athlete's goals (see *Table 34.1*). It is recommended that energy intakes start at the low end and then gradually increase so that weight gain is slow, maximizing muscle gain and minimizing fat gain.

Protein recommendations should be increased by 10% during all of the above diet strategies for athletes who avoid animal protein. During the tapering and cutting phases, dietary protein is increased to cover the needs of a hypocaloric diet. Carbohydrate recommendations are decreased during these same phases to enhance lipolysis. However, carbohydrate intake should remain high enough to allow for muscle glycogen replenishment. After protein and carbohydrate amounts are calculated, fat gram recommendations are based upon the remaining total calories.

TABLE 34.1   Energy and Nutrient Recommendations for Strength Trainers and Bodybuilders*

	Maintenance Diet**	Building Diet**	Tapering Diet**	Cutting Diet**
Men	g/kg/day	g/kg/day	g/kg/day	g/kg/day
Protein	1.2	1.4	1.8	1.8
Carbohydrate	8	9	6	5
Fat	remaining kcals	remaining kcals	remaining kcals	remaining kcals
Calories	*44/kg/day*	*52-60/kg/day*	*38/kg/day*	*33/kg/day*
Women	g/kg/day	g/kg/day	g/kg/day	g/kg/day
Protein	1.2	1.4	1.8	1.8
Carbohydrate	8	9	6	5
Fat	remaining kcals	remaining kcals	remaining kcals	remaining kcals
Calories	*38-40/kg/day*	*44/kg/day*	*35/kg/day*	*30/kg/day*

*Recommendations are based on personal experience and references 1-13.

**Definitions:

    Maintenance diet: Maintaining body weight, fat-free and fat mass

    Building diet: Increasing fat-free mass and body weight

    Tapering diet: Decreasing fat mass, increasing fat-free mass

    Cutting diet: Further decreasing body weight and fat mass

DIETARY SUPPLEMENTS

A multitude of dietary supplements are used by bodybuilders, only a few of which have a sound scientific basis for positively influencing their goals. Many supplements are under study, yet have not been adequately shown to enhance strength or tissue growth. This section will discuss only those supplements that have been shown to be effective.

Liquid energy supplements and sports beverages are important additions to the bodybuilder's high kilocalorie diet. They are an alternative to solid food because they are easily digested and allow for rapid stomach emptying.

Fluid and electrolyte beverages are especially beneficial during long, intense, strength-training workouts. High-carbohydrate beverage supplements are an easy way to boost carbohydrate intake. Meal replacement beverages serve several purposes: They are easy to carry snacks that supplement calories on the road; the carbohydrate-protein complex assists with glycogen replenishment after exercise (14); and theoretically, the carbohydrate-protein complex may also enhance the anabolic hormonal environment after exercise to promote muscle building (14,15).

Since intensive strength-training exercise increases the production of free radicals, supplementation of antioxidants, particularly vitamin E which is only marginally available in a low-fat diet, may help reduce muscle soreness (16). Dosages of 100 to 400 mg per day are recommended.

Once diet and training are maximized, creatine supplementation may enhance muscle growth and strength (17). Loading dosages of 5 g, four times a day for 5 to 7 days are effective. This can be followed by a maintenance dose of 2 g to 5 g per day. See Chapter 7, Ergogenic Aids for a further discussion of creatine.

NUTRITION CONCERNS

The fiber intakes of bodybuilders are low due to poor fruit, vegetable, and whole-grain consumption (8,9,18,19). Since one major concern of these athletes is the flatness of their abdomens, they avoid foods that cause bloating or fullness of the stomach and intestines. In order to increase the fiber content of the diet, as well as the intake of micronutrients and phytochemicals from these important foods, recommend foods that do not cause gaseous reactions (see *Box 34.1*). The antigas-forming product Beano is also an important addition to the dietary supplement arsenal of serious bodybuilders.

BOX 34.1   Recommended High-fiber Foods for Bodybuilders

- Fresh fruits with skin
- Dried fruits
- Fruit juices with pulp
- Potatoes, sweet potatoes, and yams with skin
- Peas
- Carrots
- Winter squash
- Tomatoes
- Romaine, leaf, Boston, and bibb lettuce
- Whole grains and cereals

Since the precompetition tapering and cutting phases can last at least 12 weeks, their diets can have a significant impact on nutritional health. Bodybuilders, especially female bodybuilders, eliminate dairy and red meat from the diet during this time due to misconceptions about these foods and their impact on leanness and muscular definition (8,9,18,19). Dietary calcium and zinc intakes are generally inadequate during the precompetition season for all bodybuilders and may be inadequate year round for females. Since these dietary inadequacies may negatively impact the health and performance of the athletes, increasing intakes of fat-free dairy products and lean red meats should be recommended.

Bodybuilders partake in the notorious "making-weight" practices often associated with wrestlers. When too much fat is gained during the training season, if dieting was not appropriate during the precompetition tapering phase, or if the weight category entered is unrealistically low, many bodybuilders will severely dehydrate themselves to make their weight category for competition. This practice is both unhealthy and unnecessary. A dehydrated athlete looks poor on stage and has a diminished sense of balance, making poses wobbly and unattractive. By choosing a realistic weight category and following an appropriate diet and training strategy, dehydrating practices become unnecessary.

WORKING WITH BODYBUILDERS

Historically, little credible nutrition information has been available to bodybuilders and strength trainers. Madison Avenue played the major role in influencing the diets of these athletes, and promotional product advertising was poorly refuted. Today, nutrition and exercise scientists have better information regarding the nutrition needs of bodybuilders. There are useful supplements to replace ineffective ones. As with all athletes, gaining their trust and working with their goals in mind are essential to developing a good client-counselor relationship.

Since the use of anabolic steroids and other drugs to enhance training and performance is still pervasive in this sport, it is essential that the counselor be well-informed on the topic. Often questions will reflect drug use and its potential impact on nutritional requirements. Answers must be truthful and, if appropriate, a referral to a sports medicine physician can be recommended.

Website addresses useful for the dietetics professional working with bodybuilders can be found in *Box 34.2*

BOX 34.2   Useful Web sites for the Sports Nutritionist Working with Bodybuilders

http://www.sportsci.org/
The peer-reviewed journal and site of Internet Society for Sport Science

http://www.wheatfoods.org/strs/
Wheat Foods Council. Set the record straight on fad diets.

http://www.sportfuel.com/
A sports nutrition company, SportFuel, Inc, founded by Julie Burns, MS, RD

http://www.NutriFit.org/
Sports, Cardiovascular, and Wellness Nutritionists, a dietetic practice group of The American Dietetic Association

http://www.gssiweb.com
Gatorade Sports Science Institute

http://www.powereating.com/
Susan M. Kleiner's website on Power Eating

CASE STUDY

Mitch is a 24-year-old bodybuilder who has competed successfully in several regional competitions but would like to move up into the national arena. He knows that this will take some work, and he has really been dieting but does not seem to be having any success. He is 5'8" tall, weighs 192 lb, and has 11% body fat. He needs to drop closer to 6% body fat to compete at the national level. He feels like he does not have enough energy to complete his full workouts, and he is exhausted at the end of the workout. His workouts consist of :

- Boxing 1.5 hours, three times per week
- Alternating upper and lower body strength-training workouts plus abdominals and stretching, six times per week
- Running 5 miles (10-minute mile, three times per week)
- Jumping rope for an hour, three times per week

Assessment

His present diet consists of 2,100 calories: 114 g protein, 315 g carbohydrate, and 41 g fat. He drinks about 3 qt of deionized water every day. According to the exchange system, Mitch is eating the following diet:

7.5	Bread
2.5	Fruit
4.0	Other carbs
0.5	Vegetable
6.0	Very lean meat/protein
3.5	Lean meat
1.0	Skim milk
2.5	Fat

Mitch takes the following supplements:

Creatine phosphate	10 g, once per day
L-ornithine	35 g, once per day
L-carnitine	500 mg, once per day
Vanadyl sulfate	15 mg, twice per day
Bee pollen	45 oz, twice per day
Selenium	200 µg, once per day
Coenzyme Q	100 mg, once per day
Chromium picolinate	200 µg, once per day
Vitamin E	1,000 IU, once per day
Vitamin C	2,000 mg, once per day
Thermadrene (ephedra)	300 mg, once per day

Recommendations

The following adjustments can be made to Mitch's diet and supplements to enhance his training program and his fat loss.

- Calorie intake is too low. Increase to 38 kcal/kg per day for a total of 3,316 kcal.
- Increase protein intake to 1.8 g/kg per day for a total of 157 g.
- Increase carbohydrate intake to 6 g/kg per day for a total of 524 g.
- Fat intake will increase according to calorie increase.
- Adjust milk, fruit, and vegetable intake to healthy levels.
- Educate regarding supplements, focusing on adding liquid supplements when useful and eliminating any harmful supplements as soon as possible.

Suggestions:
- Eliminate the following supplements based on the scientific evidence that they do not enhance performance, muscle building, or fat loss: L-ornithine, L-carnitine, vanadyl sulfate, bee pollen, coenzyme Q, chromium picolinate.
- Eliminate thermadrene (ephedra) because it can be a health hazard.
- Decrease vitamin E supplementation to 100 to 400 mg per day.
- Slowly taper vitamin C supplementation to a maximum of 500 mg per day.
- Continue 200 μg selenium per day since it is not taken in any other form.
- Continue creatine once the diet is appropriate but suggest changing to a creatine monohydrate supplement, which may work better.
- Discuss timing of meals and supplements to enhance exercise performance, glycogen replenishment, and muscle growth.
- Discuss the benefits of fluids and the differences between various waters available on the market.

Bodybuilders are uniquely aware of the influence of diet on their performance. Many seek nutrition information from a variety of sources, not all of which are credible. The diet to support strength training and muscle-building is not the same as diets to support endurance training. It is essential that when counseling these athletes dietitians use state-of-the-science information so that the athlete can gain confidence through successful outcomes. Staying current on the latest nutritional supplements, diet fads, and drug use is also essential so that the dietitian can fully answer athletes' questions in an informed way, thereby gaining their trust and confidence.

REFERENCES

1. Coyle EF. Fuels for sport performance. In: Lamb D, Murray R, eds. *Perspectives in Exercise Science and Sports Medicine. Vol 10. Optimizing Sport Performance.* Carmel, Ind: Cooper Publishing Group; 1997:95-125.

2. Coyle EF. Fat metabolism during exercise. *Sports Sci Exch.* 1995;8:1-7.

3. Frentsos JA, Gaer JR. Increased energy and nutrient intake during training and competition improve elite triathletes' endurance performance. *Int J Sport Nutr.* 1997;7:61-71.

4. Gornall J, Villani RG. Short-term changes in body composition and metabolism with severe dieting and resistance exercise. *Int J Sport Nutr.* 1996;6:285-294.

5. Harberson DA. Weight gain and body composition of weightlifters: effect of high-calorie supplementation vs anabolic steroids. In: Garrett WE Jr, Malone TE, eds. *Report of the Ross Laboratories Symposium on Muscle Development: Nutritional Alternatives to Anabolic Steroids.* Columbus, Ohio: Ross Laboratories; 1988:72-78.

6. Keim NL, Belko AZ, Barbieri TF. Body fat percentage and gender: associations with exercise energy expenditure, substrate utilization, and mechanical work efficiency. *Int J Sport Nutr.* 1996;6:356-369.

7. Kleiner SM, Calabrese LH, Fiedler KM, Naito HK, Skibinski CI. Dietary influences on cardiovascular disease risk in anabolic steroid-using and non-using body-builders. *J Am College Nutr.* 1989;8:109-119.

8. Kleiner SM, Bazzarre TL, Litchford MD. Metabolic profiles, diet, and health practices of championship male and female bodybuilders. *J Am Diet Assoc.* 1990;90:962-967.

9. Kleiner SM, Bazzarre TL, Ainsworth B. Nutritional status of nationally ranked elite bodybuilders. *Int J Sport Nutr.* 1994;4:54-69.

10. Lemon PW, Tarnopolsky MA, MacDougall JD, Atkinson SA. Protein requirements and muscle mass/strength changes during intensive training in novice body-builders. *J Appl Physiol.* 1992;73:767-775.

11. Lemon PW. Do athletes need more dietary protein and amino acids? *Int J Sport Nutr.* 1995;5(suppl):S39-S61.

12. Walberg-Rankin J. Dietary carbohydrate as an ergogenic aid for prolonged and brief competitions in sport. *Int J Sport Nutr.* 1995;5(suppl):S13-S28.

13. Walberg JL, Leidy MK, Sturgill DJ, Hinkle DE, Ritchey SJ, Sebolt DR. Macronutrient content of a hypoenergy diet affects nitrogen retention and muscle function in weight lifters. *Int J Sports Med.* 1988;9:261-266.

14. Zawadzki KM, Yaselkis BB, Ivy JL. Carbohydrate-protein complex increases the rate of muscle glycogen storage after exercise. *J Appl Physiol.* 1992;72:1854-1859.

15. Chandler RM, Byrne HK, Patterson JG, Ivy JL. Dietary supplements affect the ana-bolic hormones after weight training exercise. *J Appl Physiol.* 1994;76:839-845.

16. Kanter MM, Nolte LA, Holloszy JO. Effects of an antioxidant vitamin mixture on lipid peroxidation at rest and postexercise. *J Appl Physiol.* 1993;74:965-969.

17. Kreider RB, Ferreira M, Wilson M, et al. Effects of creatine supplementation on body composition, strength, and sprint performance. *Med Sci Sports Exerc.* 1998;30:73-82.

18. Sandoval WM, Heyward VH. Food selection patterns of bodybuilders. *Int J Sport Nutr.* 1991;1:61-68.

19. Walberg-Rankin J, Edmonds CE, Gwasdauskas FC. Diet and weight changes of female bodybuilders before and after competition. *Int J Sport Nutr.* 1993;3:87-102.

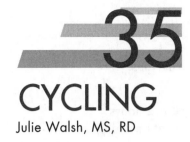

CYCLING

Julie Walsh, MS, RD

Cycling is one of the most popular activities in the United States. While individuals of all ages and abilities ride for pleasure or fitness, there are three main competitive forms of bicycle racing: road, mountain, and track. Road racers ride events on paved roads; mountain bikers ride off-road in either cross-country or downhill events; and track riders race sprint competitions on tracks. Both road and cross-country mountain bikers are considered endurance athletes, while downhill mountain bikers and track riders are power athletes.

The type of energy systems utilized when cycling depends on the type of event in which the cyclist competes. Cross-country and road racing require primarily aerobic metabolism because these are endurance events lasting anywhere from over an hour to up to 5 hours or more. During these races cyclists must sprint or use extra power up hills, so they also utilize anaerobic pathways. However, the nutritional requirements of cyclists who compete in track events or downhill mountain bike races are not the same because their events last only a few seconds to a few minutes, which requires anaerobic power rather than endurance. The nutrition needs of these riders are more similar to athletes competing in power events such as weightlifting or sprinting.

Because cross-country road cycling and cross-country mountain biking are the most popular cycling events, this chapter will discuss the demands of competitive cross-country riding.

CROSS-COUNTRY CYCLING

The cycling racing season begins in early April and extends into October. During the off-season, November through March, riders usually adhere to a weightlifting program to gain muscle. When the season begins riders log 250 to 400 miles a week at slow to moderate paces to build endurance and help lose excess body fat that they may have gained during the off-season. Once the racing season begins, training rides are reduced in duration and intensity in order to race on weekends. Competitive cyclists typically train 15 to 24 hours per week. Due to this amount of training and racing, nutritionists need to help these athletes ensure an adequate food and fluid intake.

A typical rider's week during the racing season looks like this:

- Sunday: Race 2 to 4 hours
- Monday: Easy spin (50% to 60% VO$_2$max) for 1 to 2 hours
- Tuesday: 2- to 4-hour moderate ride; 1 hour weight training
- Wednesday: 2- to 5-hour endurance ride
- Thursday: 2- to 4-hour moderate ride; 1 hour weight training
- Friday: Off or easy spin for an hour
- Saturday: Race 2 to 4 hours

Energy Requirements

It has been estimated that cycling at speeds of 14 to 16 mph requires 10 metabolic equivalents (METs) (one MET equals 1 kcal/kg/hour); 16 to 19 mph requires 12 METs; and racing at speeds over 20 mph requires 16 METs (1). Based on limited data, mountain biking has been estimated to require 8.5 METs (1). However, experts in the field contend that mountain bikers expend 12 to 16 METs during a race, similar to the estimates for road cyclists, due to the intensity of mountain biking compared to road cycling. In fact, because mountain biking does not have drafting, the energy expenditure may actually be higher than road cycling.

A 73-kg rider riding at 18 mph for 3 hours would expend about 2,628 kcal (73 kg x 12.0 x 3 hours). Because cyclists ride in packs and their energy needs are constantly changing throughout the course, some experts contend that while racing cyclists burn anywhere from 600 to 900 kcal per hour (2).

Several studies have examined the nutritional intake of competitive cyclists (3-6). A study of competitive male cyclists found that their mean caloric intake is 4,162 kcal during training days and 4,460 kcal on race days (3). Another study found that elite male cyclists racing in Spain consumed 5,600 kcal during a 24-hour period (4). One study revealed that female road racers consumed, on average, 2,900 to 3,000 kcal/day when training and 2,100 to 2,200 kcal on noncycling days (5). The recommended macronutrient distribution for cyclists is the same for most other endurance athletes: 65% to 70% of calories from carbohydrate or 8 to 10 g carbohydrate/kg body weight; 15% of calories from protein or 1.2 to 1.4 g protein/kg body weight; and the remainder of calories from fat.

CYCLING-SPECIFIC NUTRITION CONCERNS

The key nutritional issues for cyclists include hydration and energy consumption during training and racing, maintaining body weight and an optimal percent body fat, and nutrition needs to hasten recovery from injury.

Hydration

Most cyclists know fluids are important, but few meet their fluid requirements during exercise. One study found that during a 100-mile stage of a 3-week race, elite road racers consumed only 1.26 L fluid during a 170-km race at high altitudes (4). Lack of fluid intake during training and racing is a result of many factors. First, cyclists can only carry two water bottles at a time and they cannot refill them whenever they wish. While racing they must wait until they reach a designated "feed zone" until they can be handed additional fluids and/or food. In addition, when cyclists are riding technical sections or trying to "break away" from the pack, they are usually unable to drink because they are unable to take one hand off the handlebars in order to do so. Since it is harder for mountain bikers to drink than it is for road riders, many off-road riders choose to wear back-mounted hydration systems that allow for hands-free drinking.

Working with cyclists to help them develop appropriate hydration strategies can lead to improved performance. Fluid needs are based on a rider's sweat rate and intensity of the ride, but a starting point is to recommend drinking a standard cyclist's water bottle (20 oz) before riding, 1/4 of a bottle every 15 minutes of riding, and 1 1/2 to 2 water bottles after riding. Although many riders eschew sports drinks for plain water, sports drinks should be recommended because fluid requirements can be met, as well as the recommended 30 to 60 g carbohydrate per hour of exercise. Helping a rider estimate his or her sweat rate by weighing before and after cycling can help determine how much fluid he or she needs to drink during exercise. (See Chapter 6, Fluid and Electrolytes for calculating sweat rate and more recommendations for fluid consumption.)

Nutritionists should give fluid guidelines in terms of the number of standard water bottles (20 oz) the rider should consume per hour of riding. Developing a set drinking schedule (ie, drink every 10 minutes) will help cyclists meet fluid needs. Cyclists may also want to experiment with back-mounted hydration systems that hold a liter or more of fluids or use larger water bottles that hold 28 oz of fluid.

Carbohydrate Consumption

To obtain adequate carbohydrate calories during long rides and races, solid foods are essential. This is a concern for competitive cyclists because they may not have any appetite during a race, they cannot use their hands for extended periods of time, and they need to be ready to react to an attack at any moment. Foods handed to cyclists should be unwrapped so they can grab and eat as they please. In long races there are feed zones where riders are handed bags that include food and beverages. Each cyclist has his or her own preference for foods, but nutritionists should encourage high-carbohydrate, easy-to-digest, and easy-to-eat options. *Box 35.1* offers suggestions for convenient sources of carbohydrates.

BOX 35.1   Convenient Sources of Carbohydrates

- Energy bars
- Energy gels
- Dried fruit
- Bagels
- Fig bars
- Low-fat toaster pastries
- Crackers
- Candy

Weight and Body Fat

Cyclists must propel their own mass, so the lighter they are the faster they can ride. Excess body fat is a major disadvantage for cyclists, especially when riding uphill. Most cyclists try to lose as much body fat as possible while maintaining or gaining lean muscle mass. Elite male cyclists have body fat levels between 8% to 12% and elite female cyclists fall between 10% to 15% body fat (2). Because cycling is an endurance sport where weight matters, both male and female riders are often at risk for disordered eating. Nutritionists need to be aware that cyclists may try to adhere to a diet lacking in energy to try to achieve a lower body weight or body fat percentage.

In addition, during the preseason cyclists may cut calories drastically to take off excess weight gained during the off-season. Nutritionists can monitor cyclists' body composition throughout the year, especially during the racing season, helping them reduce calories as energy expenditure declines so weight gain is limited during the off-season. When weight loss is necessary, designing eating strategies that enable the rider to lose up to a pound per week is recommended. Riders often want to lose weight rapidly by cutting calories drastically, but they do not understand that this may affect energy levels and decrease muscle mass and metabolic rate.

Recovery

Recovery is an issue for riders because they compete in multiday races or train on consecutive days, and sometimes twice a day. Eating a diet containing 65% to 70% carbohydrate should supply adequate carbohydrate to replenish muscle glycogen stores. A carbohydrate intake of 8 to 10 g/kg body weight is generally recommended to facilitate glycogen resynthesis in competitive cyclists, but elite-level riders in long-stage races such as the Tour de France have consumed as much as 14 g carbohydrate/kg (4).

Cyclists should begin consuming high-carbohydrate foods or fluids immediately after exercise. It has been recommended that 1 g carbohydrate/kg body weight postexercise or 100 g carbohydrate be consumed within the first hour and another 100 g every 2 hours until the next main meal. In addition, a carbohydrate and protein ratio of 3:1 may promote more rapid glycogen resynthesis. Since cyclists may not be hungry following a high-intensity ride, high-carbohydrate recovery drinks are good options. Helping riders choose foods rich in carbohydrates postexercise helps facilitate full recovery.

Ergogenic Aids

Since theirs is an Olympic sport, cyclists must adhere to the rules set forth by the International Olympic Committee (IOC). However, road cycling has a long history of drug use. During the 1998 Tour de France, several riders were expelled because they were caught with banned substances, such as steroid-masking agents and the hematocrit-boosting drug erythropoietin (EPO). In fact, EPO has been used for many years by elite cyclists, and in the past decade nearly 20 cyclists have died from heart attacks linked to EPO. Because cyclists are generally not concerned about building excess muscle mass, anabolic steroids are not as commonly used. (Track and mountain bike downhillers may use steroids.)

In addition to banned substances, many cyclists also experiment with legal substances such as creatine, high-dose vitamins and minerals, amino acids, carnitine, and caffeine. Most cyclists will also use recovery drinks and powders postexercise that may also contain nutrients that athletes believe are performance-enhancing. Chapter 7, Ergogenic Aids covers this topic in detail.

Box 35.2 provides additional information on cycling resources.

BOX 35.2.   Cycling Resources

USA Cycling is the national federation that oversees all cycling disciplines. It is the governing body for all licensed bike racers, including road, track, BMX, and mountain biking. Specific divisions within USA Cycling handle the specific disciplines of cycling. For example, the National Off-Road Bicycle Association is the organization that handles mountain bike racing, and the United States Cycling Federation is the organization in charge of road and track racing.

The phone number for USA Cycling is (719) 635-6212.

CASE STUDY

Mary is a 45-year-old female, lacto-ovo vegetarian. She is a competitive road racer and a Master's National Champion. She is trying to reduce her percent body fat while eating a more balanced and healthful diet.

- Client has no previous medical history; labs all within normal limits. Ht: 5'7"; Wt: 61 kg; Age: 45; Percent body fat: 20%; Desirable body fat percentage: 16% to 16.5%
- Trains 12 to 15 hours per week (12 hours cycling and 3 hours light weightlifting)

Assessment

- Energy requirements = BEE plus Activity Factor plus Cycling and Weightlifting METs
  BEE: $655 + 9.6(61) + 1.8(67) - 4.7(45)$ = Basal Metabolic Rate (BMR) = 1,150 kcal
  (Activity factor, 20% to 25% of BMR)

BMR + 20% = 1,380 kcal (plus sport-specific activity)
12 hours cycling at 10 METs = 7,320 kcal/week spent cycling
3 hours at 6 METs (weightlifting) = 1,098 kcal/week spent lifting
Add 1,200 kcal/day from sport-specific activity = total energy requirements: 2,582 kcal/day

- Diet analysis revealed current diet to contain 2,600 to 3,000 kcal with 77% from carbohydrate, 14% from protein, and 9% from fat. Diet was low in vitamin E, D, iron, zinc, and calcium, and relied on protein supplements rather than food for most protein intake.

Diet recommendation: 2,200 kcal/day to promote gradual fat loss
60% to 70% of calories from carbohydrate or 330 to 385 g carbohydrate
1.2 to 1.6 g protein/kg Ideal Body Weight (59 kg or 130 lb)
88.5 to 94.5 g protein/day
Remainder of calories from fat

Recommendations

- Explain the Food Groups to Mary and plan meals and snacks that meet energy and macronutrient requirements.
- Include three servings of calcium-rich foods daily
- Increase sources of vegetable fats such as olive oil, nuts, and seeds
- Develop strategies to include a wide variety of vegetarian protein sources (ie, lentils, beans, eggs, soy, dairy foods) instead of liquid protein supplements
- Help Mary distinguish between true hunger and external eating cues, such as stress or boredom

Outcome: After 4 months, Mary lost nearly 10 lb and reduced her body fat to 16.5%.

REFERENCES

1. Ainsworth BE, Haskell WL, Leon AS, et al. Compendium of physical activities: classification of energy costs of human physical activities. *Med Sci Sports Exerc.* 1993;25:71-80.
2. Burke ER. *Serious Cycling.* Champaign, Ill: Human Kinetics; 1995.
3. Jensen CD, Zaltas ES, Whittam JH. Dietary intakes of male endurance cyclists during training and racing. *J Am Diet Assoc.* 1992;92:986-988.
4. Garcia-Roves PM, Terrados N, Fernandez SF, Patterson AM. Macronutrient intakes of top level cyclists during continuous competition—change in the feeding pattern. *Int J Sports Med.* 1998;19:61-67.
5. Horton TJ, Drougas HJ, Sharp TA, Martinez LR, Reed GW, Hill JO. Energy balance in endurance-trained female cyclists and untrained controls. *J Appl Physiol.* 1994;76:1936-1945.
6. Clark N, Tobin J, Ellis C. Feeding the ultraendurance athlete: practical tips and a case study. *J Am Diet Assoc.* 1992;92:1258-1262.

36

FIGURE SKATING

Paula J. Ziegler, PhD, RD, CFCS and Satya S. Jonnalagadda, PhD

Figure skating is a competitive sport that involves grace, strength, and endurance. Established in 1921, the United States Figure Skating Association (USFSA) currently has 130,000 members (1). The popularity of the sport has increased tremendously over the past several decades. The United States has won more Olympic medals (38) in the history of this sport than any other country (1).

Competitive figure skating encompasses five major divisions: ladies' singles, men's singles, pairs, ice dancing, and precision team skating. Within each division there are different competition levels such as preliminary, juvenile, intermediate, novice, junior, and senior levels, which although they have similar techniques, get increasingly difficult as the athlete moves up the ladder. Figure skaters are required to develop two main areas: technical merit (ie, difficulty of performance, variety, cleanness, and sureness) and speed, and the presentation of the program (ie, harmonious compositions, variation of speed, ice coverage, carriage and style, ease of movements and sureness in time to the music, originality, and expression of the character of the music). Competition at the higher levels consists of the short program, which has certain required elements that the athlete has to perform, and the long (free) program. In all levels of competition, technique and artistic perfection are prominent features of the skater's performance and significantly influence the judges' scoring. The difficulty of the moves and jumps, how well they are executed, and the overall presentation influence the judging. Therefore, competitive figure skating not only requires athleticism but also artistry.

TRAINING SCHEDULE

On the average figure skaters start training at a very young age (8.1 ± 1.3 years) and typically train throughout the year with no more than a 2-week midwinter break (2). The training schedule includes both on- and off-ice training. It has been reported that figure skaters typically spend 30 to 33 hours per week training, of which approximately 27 hours per week are spent performing on-ice activities, 5.6 hours per week are spent in strength and aerobic activities, and 0.2 hours per week involve preskating warm-up (3,4). Figure skaters need "the balance of a tightrope walker, the endurance of a marathon runner, the aggressiveness of a football player, the agility of a wrestler, the nerves of a golfer, the flexibility of a gymnast, and the grace of a ballet dancer" (5), further emphasizing the uniqueness of the sport and associated training demands.

ENERGY SYSTEMS

Given the short but intense nature of the figure skater's performance, these athletes require a high anaerobic capacity, in addition to good aerobic capacity, to meet the metabolic demands of skating which requires maximal effort for up to 4 minutes in duration (6). Both cardiovascular fitness and upper body strength are essential requirements for the physical performance of the sport. Figure skaters are typically 50% to 60% more cardiovascularly fit (VO$_2$max) than their sedentary counterparts (males: 58.5 mL/kg per minute and females: 48.9 mL/kg per minute) (2,7). During performance, peak oxygen consumption of males was observed to be 80% of their VO$_2$max and for females, 75% of their VO$_2$max (2,7). Because a vast majority of the performance involves jumps, developing higher and harder jumps may contribute to greater technical scores; thus, muscular strength and power are important requirements for the figure skater's performance. Podolsky et al (8) observed a significant positive correlation between strength and jump height. During a performance, generation of speed and its maintenance, especially during the long program, require a high and sustained power output. Therefore, appropriate training programs should be developed to maximize high-power output and increase aerobic power, which will not only delay the onset of metabolic acidosis during performance but also can help delay the onset of fatigue. Additionally, during a performance, the height of the jump may significantly increase the technical and artistic scores of the skater, which to a great part is influenced by the physical abilities of the skater.

BODY COMPOSITION

Studies have shown that the body fat content of elite figure skaters is lower than their nonathletic counterparts (9.1% male skaters, 12.5% female skaters versus 13% nonathletic males, 25% nonathletic females) (7). The percent body fat of figure skaters is similar to that observed in gymnasts and ballet dancers, which may be due to the similar athletic, artistic, and flexibility requirements of these sports (5). Lower body fat composition in these athletes may be related to the requirements of these sports for high aerobic capacity. Ziegler et al (9) observed that heights and weights of both male and female figure skaters are less than the 50th percentile, adjusted for age and gender, which could imply that these athletes are at risk for poor nutritional status. The body composition of these athletes is also influenced by the increased emphasis on leanness, the year-round training program, and the increased demands of growth and development. Additionally, it has been suggested that low body weight is considered a necessary component of performance and appearance, which can partially explain the low percentage of body fat in these athletes (10).

Figure skaters are typically shorter in stature; however, it is unclear if this is a result of the sport or the selective bias associated with the individuals who choose to participate in such sports. For instance, female skaters are smaller, lighter, have less body fat, and are more muscular than inactive females, which may be due to the technical demands and nature of the sport (5,11). Typically, most nonathletic young men and women tend to perceive themselves as overweight and wish to be thinner. Similarly, 72% of the female figure skaters and 39% of the male figure skaters expressed a desire to be thinner with a desired weight loss of 3.6 lb by females and 1.8 lb by males (12). It is of interest to note that during counseling sessions, male skaters typically express the desire to gain muscle weight. In spite of the desire to lose weight, these athletes in general expressed satisfaction with their physical attractiveness and body shape. The low body weight, percent body fat, decreased energy intake, and increased level of physical activity may be one of several factors contributing to the delayed menarche commonly encountered in females participating in sports such as figure skating (13,14).

ENERGY REQUIREMENTS

In spite of the growing popularity of the sport, few studies have carefully examined the dietary intake and nutrient needs of these athletes. Since figure skaters start training at a very early age, their dietary intake and nutritional status will influence their growth and development, training, and performance. Adequate energy intake is required not only to meet the demands of the activity but also to promote optimal development. Their total energy intake is influenced by factors such as age, gender, body size and composition, resting energy expenditure, physical activity level, and physiological status (15).

An examination of reported dietary intake data has identified some potential problems related to inadequate energy intakes and the excessively low-fat content in the diets of these athletes. Delistraty et al (16) observed the mean energy intake of female figure skaters (9 to 17 years) to range from 1,070 to 2,666 kcal per day. Similarly, Ziegler et al (9) observed the energy intake of elite male figure skaters to be 39 kcal/kg of body weight and that of the female figure skaters to be 38 kcal/kg of body weight, which are both below the recommended intakes for active males and females. Although the dietary intakes of these athletes during the week did not vary from that during the weekends, male figure skaters were observed to consume only 75% of their estimated energy needs and female skaters were consuming only 59% of their estimated needs (17). This observed energy restriction could be one of several techniques used by these athletes to achieve weight control. Often figure skaters experience weight loss or gain because they fail to recognize their changing energy needs. This fluctuation in body weight can influence their performance (eg, a weight gain can affect balance, jump, and spin height, whereas a weight loss can result in decreased strength and endurance), resulting in loss of quality training time which otherwise could be spent in learning new skills and techniques. It is therefore important that these athletes maintain energy balance both during the competitive season and during off-season training.

MACRONUTRIENT REQUIREMENTS

To meet the nutrient needs of physical activity and health, the training diet should provide 50% to 55% of total energy as carbohydrate, 12% to 15% from protein, and 25% to 30% from fat (18). However, Delistraty et al (16) observed that the macronutrient contribution to the total energy intake of female figure skaters varied quite substantially, with carbohydrates contributing 38% to 63%, fat contributing 22% to 45%, and protein contributing 11% to 18% of the total energy intake. Similarly, Ziegler et al (9,19) reported that the diets of elite male figure skaters was comprised of 53% carbohydrate, 32% fat, and 16% protein, while that of the female figure skaters was comprised of 58% carbohydrate, 28% fat, and 16% protein. While diets containing less than 30% fat are recommended for the prevention of chronic diseases, they are not necessarily optimal for these young athletes because they can compromise both their macronutrient and micronutrient intake.

MICRONUTRIENT REQUIREMENTS

Micronutrient adequacy of the athlete's diet has come under increased scrutiny because of its influence on growth and performance. Compared to the recommended dietary intakes for the general population, these athletes appeared to be consuming inadequate intakes of all vitamins except vitamin D and vitamin E (9,19). This poor intake of certain vitamins could be due to decreased consumption of certain foods such as skim milk and green leafy vegetables and the increased use of low-fat foods. Likewise, adequate iron, calcium, and zinc intakes were not achieved by elite figure skaters, especially female skaters (9,11,16,19). Zinc is a component of various metalloenzymes, which play a major role in the respiration process and regulate the removal of carbon dioxide from the circulation. Likewise, iron is a major component of hemoglobin and plays an important role in the transport of oxygen to various tissues. Therefore, inadequate intakes of these micronutrients can compromise bone health (calcium) and decrease aerobic capacity (iron and zinc). This can not only influence growth but can also decrease performance capacity and increase risk of stress fractures, osteoporosis, and other health problems such as menstrual dysregulation among these young athletes. Since both the vitamin D and calcium intakes of these athletes are less than adequate and these athletes train mostly indoors with very limited exposure to sunlight, their bone mineral density should be monitored to ensure proper bone health. Possibly the high frequency of multiple, difficult-to-heal stress fractures commonly seen in the lower extremities of figure skaters are due to inadequate intakes of these micronutrients (3,4). Therefore, although there are no sport-specific recommendations for the intake of these micronutrients, it is important that these athletes meet their daily needs through the diet.

FLUID REQUIREMENTS

Prolonged exercise performance can be sustained only with adequate body water and electrolyte balance. Exercise-induced water loss can not only lead to dehydration but can also increase strain on the cardiovascular system which can result in a loss of coordination, impaired performance, and increased risk of injury (20). Typically, male and female figure skaters consume approximately 1 L of fluid per day, with the main sources being carbonated beverages (regular and diet), milk, juice, and water (9). The use of sports drinks by figure skaters is less common, which may be due to the short performance time of this sport compared to other endurance sports such as running where the calories from these sports drinks are needed to maintain performance. Given the nature of the sport and the overall low fluid intake, these athletes need to be educated about the importance of proper hydration and the use of water breaks. It is therefore important to monitor these athletes for symptoms of dehydration on a regular basis and to encourage consumption of adequate fluids during training and competition.

FOOD PREFERENCES

Figure skaters tend to have considerably lower intakes of various food groups compared to the average adolescent in the United States. Female figure skaters expressed preferences for low-calorie foods such as tossed green salads, fruits, and vegetables, while male skaters preferred high-fat, high-salt foods including meat dishes (12). However, they were observed to consume less than the recommended number of servings of the various food groups (12). Increased consumption of nutrient-dense foods from grains, vegetables, fruits, milk products, meat, and meat-alternative groups by these athletes should be encouraged, given that their nutrient intakes are less than adequate.

ERGOGENIC AIDS/SUPPLEMENT USE

Information on supplement use by these athletes is very limited. Available information suggests that the use of ergogenic aids and nutritional supplements by figure skaters is minimal (9). If used, the most common supplements are multivitamins, vitamin C, beta-carotene, iron, and calcium.

INJURIES

Stress and acute fractures, strains, and overuse injuries such as lower back pain are common injuries among figure skaters. This could be due to a combination of factors such as over training, overall dietary intake, physical strength, ice conditions, and equipment (skates). Pecina et al (21) observed that injuries among these competitive athletes occurred anywhere from 6 to 15 years after the initiation of intensive training, with 21% of the athletes suffering from stress fractures which commonly occurred in the take-off leg and were often diagnosed 2 to 10 weeks after the onset of symptoms. Stress fractures could occur as a result of training errors, on-and off-the-ice training regimens, or the continuous repetition of the various jumps that are performed (3,4). Given that some of these athletes have inadequate dietary intake, it is important to regularly monitor their physical well-being to ensure proper and timely medical attention.

MENSTRUAL IRREGULARITIES

A potential consequence of low energy intake by the female skaters may contribute to abnormalities in reproductive endocrinology. Menstrual irregularities are common among female athletes, and the prevalence can range from 1% to 44% compared to 1.8% to 5% in the general population (10). Delayed onset of menarche is commonly observed in these female athletes, with a mean age of 13.2 years (12). This could be a result of increased physical training and a low percent body fat. Amenorrhea may also be associated with alterations in regional fat distribution and the depletion of fat in the femoral area (around hips, thigh, and buttocks) (10).

EATING DISORDERS

There is no doubt that eating disorders are a problem in competitive sports, and typically female athletes are at increased risk for anorexia nervosa and bulimia. (See Chapter 28, Eating Disorders in Athletes.) Elevated scores on the Eating Attitude Test (EAT) have been associated with energy restriction and a greater probability of eating disorder. Rucinski (22) reported that high EAT scores were linked with lower dietary intakes of both macro- and micronutrients among figure skaters. Dieting to lose weight is a common practice among male and female figure skaters (26% and 69%, respectively) (12). Dieting in young females generally follows puberty by approximately 1 year, and the prevalence of dieting increases with age. This may be a result of the increased pressure to remain thin among these athletes who typically seek pathological dieting behaviors, such as starvation, repeated bingeing, and purging, as a way of controlling body weight and deposition of body fat. Additionally, it is unclear whether the risk of eating disorders increases as the skater climbs in rank to the National, World, or Olympic level.

TOP NUTRITION CONCERNS

Adequate Dietary Intake

Figure skaters' poor nutritional status has implications for these athletes at the present time and also has long-term implications since most skaters are at their peak level of growth and development during their training years. It is important that figure skaters consume adequate amounts of calories, macronutrients, and micronutrients. Nutritional status needs to be monitored on a regular basis using a combination of dietary, anthropometric, and biochemical assessments. All figure skaters should be encouraged to consult with dietetic professionals to establish normal eating patterns and attitudes towards food. Additionally, these athletes need to be encouraged to maintain proper hydration status and increase their consumption of water to at least six to eight glasses per day due to the likelihood of dehydration during performance. This is especially a concern when athletes train and perform in cities at high altitudes where dehydration can result due to a shift in fluid balance. Similarly, guardians, coaches, and trainers should also be educated about proper dietary practices to meet the increased needs of these athletes.

Disordered Eating Habits

Since eating disorders are highly probable in a sport such as figure skating where appearance plays a major factor in performance, it is critical that improper eating patterns and behaviors in these athletes be identified early and prevented from developing into serious disorders. These disordered eating patterns not only influence the nutrient intake of the athletes but also can affect the physiological systems of the young athlete, which in the long-term can detrimentally affect the health of these athletes. Additionally, weight cycling, which is a common outcome of poor eating patterns, can result in altered aerobic capacity and decreased performance.

Eating on the Run

Since most figure skaters travel for competition and training either within the country or overseas, it is important that the athletes, trainers, coaches, and parents be educated about making wise food choices while on the road. These athletes should increase their consumption of carbohydrates, especially prior to competition. This can be achieved by increasing their intake of grain products, fruits, and vegetables. When eating out, a high-carbohydrate meal should be chosen over a high-fat meal. If traveling overseas, food-borne illnesses and traveler's diarrhea are commonly encountered either because of food quality, sanitation issues, water safety standards, or the athlete's decreased immunity (23). It is therefore suggested that athletes choose foods with which they are familiar, consume only well-cooked foods, and avoid uncooked foods. Athletes should also consider packing certain nonperishable foods such as breakfast bars, dried foods, pretzels, canned fruit, and sports drinks to be readily available while travelling.

CASE STUDY

Frances is a 14-year-old female figure skater who has been complaining of feeling fat. She achieved menarche when she turned 13 but has not menstruated in the past 6 months. She is 4' 8" in tall and weighs 90 lb. She has become very moody and overly conscious of her appearance. Her performance is suffering, and she is unable to complete her programs successfully. She is exhausted by the end of the short program and has no energy to move. Frances has been skipping meals, especially lunch. She eats only a piece of fruit for breakfast and usually has a very light dinner. She has decreased her fluid intake because she feels bloated.

Recommendations

Frances' daily eating pattern needs to be modified. The importance of proper nutrition and its impact on her performance should be explained to her. Her attitude toward eating should be altered with proper counseling and by providing the appropriate motivation.

- There is a high likelihood that Frances has some form of dysfunctional eating patterns. Conduct an eating attitude test and determine the nature of the disorder. Consider referring Frances to a clinical psychologist or a counselor who specializes in working with disordered eating among athletes to determine the nature of the problem. A nutritionist and psychologist should counsel Frances about the consequences of her poor eating patterns by emphasizing their impact on the short-term (ie, her performance and lack of energy) and long-term (ie, her health, growth, and development). The medical care team, coaches, trainers, and parents should be involved, if needed. Additionally, her feeling of bloating in the absence of adequate fluid intake may be a result of poor eating habits.

- A nutritionist should explain to Frances the role of body fat stores as a source of energy, especially during long training sessions. Additionally, the role of body fat in regulating hormonal status, which in turn can impact menstrual status and bone health, should be explained. Although an actual body fat assessment may make her more self-conscious, it may be worthwhile to discuss in general the percent body fat in sedentary, normal-weight individuals and discuss her particular situation in relation to the role of stored energy.

- Frances should be encouraged not to skip meals and to include appropriate snacks such as fruits, energy bars, and yogurt at regular intervals to provide a source of energy during her performance. Additionally, eating small meals and snacks throughout the day and between training sessions may enable Frances to increase her energy intake and meet her nutrient needs.

- Fluid consumption should be strongly encouraged and monitored. The impact of dehydration on her coordination, stamina, and performance should be explained. Frances should consume water and sports drinks during practice, training, and prior to and after performance to prevent dehydration, to meet her fluid and energy needs during performance, and to restore fluid and electrolyte balance during recovery from exercise training.

- Regular appointments with a nutritionist and psychologist should be encouraged to monitor her eating patterns. Regular communication with Frances, her parents, medical care team, coaches, and trainers should be maintained to monitor her eating behaviors, athletic performance, and social and psychological well-being.

REFERENCES

1. The United States Figure Skating Association. http://www.98.skate.org/usfa.htm. Accessed January 1, 1999.
2. Mannix ET, Healy A, Farber MO. Aerobic power and supramaximal endurance of competitive figure skaters. *J Sports Med Phys Fitness.* 1996;36:161-168.
3. Brock RM, Striowski CC. Injuries in elite figure skaters. *Phys Sports Med.* 1986;14:111-115.
4. Smith AD, Ludington R. Injuries in elite pair skaters and ice dancers. *Am J Sports Med.* 1989;17:482-458.
5. Hawes MR, Sovak D. Morphological prototypes, assessment, and change in elite athletes. *J Sports Sci.* 1994;12:235-242.
6. Aleshinsky SY, Podolsky A, McQueen C, Smith AD, Van Handel P. Strength and conditioning program for figure skating. *Nat Strength Cond Assoc J.* 1988;10:26-30.
7. Niinimaa V. Figure skating: what do we know about it? *Phys Sports Med.* 1982;10:51-56.
8. Podolsky A, Kaufman KR, Cahalan TD, Aleshinsky SY, Chao EYS. The relationship of strength and jump height in figure skaters. *Am J Sports Med.* 1990;18:400-405.
9. Ziegler P, Khoo CS, Kris-Etherton PM, Jonnalagadda SS, Sherr B, Nelson JA. Nutritional status of nationally ranked junior US figure skaters. *J Am Diet Assoc.* 1998;98;809-811.
10. Brownell KD, Neslon-Steen S, Wilmore JH. Weight regulation practices in athletes: analysis of metabolic and health effects. *Med Sci Sports Exerc.* 1987;19:546-556.
11. Rankinen T, Fogelholm M, Kujala U, Rauramaa R, Uusitupa M. Dietary intake and nutritional status of athletic and nonathletic children in early puberty. *Int J Sport Nutr.* 1995;5:136-150.
12. Ziegler P, Khoo CS, Sherr B, Nelson JA, Larson WM, Drewnowski A. Body image and dieting behaviors among elite figure skaters. *Int J Eat Disord.* 1998;24:421-427.
13. Moisan J, Meyer F, Gingras S. A nested case-control study of the correlation of early menarche. *Am J Epidemiol.* 1990;132:953-961.
14. Moisan J, Meyer F, Gingras S. Leisure physical activity and age at menarche. *Med Sci Sports Exerc.* 1991;23:1170-1175.
15. Fogelholm GM, Kukkonen-Harjula TK, Taipale SA, Sievanen HT, Oja P, Vuori IM. Resting metabolic rate and energy intake in female gymnasts, figure-skaters, and soccer players. *Int J Sport Med.* 1995;16:551-556.
16. Delistraty DA, Reisman EJ, Snipes M. A physiological and nutritional profile of young female figure skaters. *J Sports Med Phys Fitness.* 1992;32:149-155.
17. Nevino-Folino NL. Sports nutrition for children and adolescents. In: Queen PM, Lang CE, eds. *Handbook of Pediatric Nutrition.* Gaithersburg, Md: Aspen Publishers; 1993:187-205.
18. Position of The American Dietetic Association: nutrition guidance for adolescent athletes in organized sports. *J Am Diet Assoc.* 1996;96:611-612.
19. Ziegler P, Hensley S, Roepke JB, Whitaker SH, Craig BW, Drewnowski A. Eating attitudes and energy intakes of female skaters. *Med Sci Sports Exerc.* 1998;30:583-586.
20. American College of Sports Medicine Position Stand. Exercise and fluid replacement. *Med Sci Sports Exerc.* 1996;28:i-vii.
21. Pecina M, Bojanic I, Dubravcic S. Stress fractures in figure skaters. *Am J Sports Med.* 1990;18:277-279.
22. Rucinski A. Relationship of body image and dietary intake of competitive ice skaters. *J Am Diet Assoc.* 1989;89:98-100.
23. Nelson-Steen S. Eating on the road: where are the carbohydrates? *Sports Sci Exch.* 1998;11:1-5.

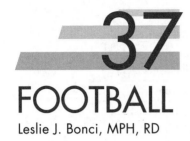

37
FOOTBALL
Leslie J. Bonci, MPH, RD

One of the most astonishing things about working with football players is their size. Football players are large. Today, there are over 200 players in the National Football League (NFL) who weigh over 300 lb. To attain and maintain this size, energy needs must increase dramatically. During twice-daily practice at training camp, a 320-lb player might expend 10,000 kcal a day. Translating this into a realistic eating plan can be a daunting task for a nutrition professional trained in the Food Guide Pyramid portions, which at the maximum accommodate a calorie level of about 3,500 kcal per day.

MACRONUTRIENT REQUIREMENTS

Football is an intermittent activity sport with short bursts of intense effort followed by rest. However, overall calorie needs and specific nutrient requirements may vary depending on the position played. Consequently, counseling strategies for players need to be based on position and the diet adjusted accordingly. Understanding the physiological demands of each position is important. Quarterbacks possess a combination of agility, speed, and strength; running backs, defensive backs, and wide receivers need to be quick; fullbacks, linebackers, and tight ends must be strong and fast; and the linemen need to be strong and are generally larger to effectively block at their position. Therefore, in setting goals with players, it is important to understand their position and formulate a meal plan that will allow for an increase in mass, increase in speed, or decrease in body fat, depending on the athlete. An individualized approach to setting dietary goals is essential when working with football players to ensure that each member of the team is optimally nourished. Adequate carbohydrate stores are critical and yet remain suboptimal in many football players in spite of education about ideal diet composition. Carbohydrate intake averages 43% of daily calories with 40% from fat and 17% from protein (1,2). The use of protein supplements and powders has contributed to misconceptions surrounding the importance of protein as the primary energy source for football. Still, some players have become more nutrition savvy and do try to make an effort to increase carbohydrate in their diets.

Since football players are involved in intensive weight-training programs, their protein needs are higher than other athletes' needs. Protein requirements can be as high as 1.4 to 1.8 g/kg body weight (3,4); however, many players exceed this recommendation by consuming high-protein foods and protein supplements. The recommended diet composition for football players is shown in *Table 37.1*.

TABLE 37.1   Recommended Diet Composition for Football Players (1,2)

Nutrient	Ideal	Current
Carbohydrate	55%	42%
Protein	15%	17%
Fat	30%	40%

To accomplish this goal, education on appropriate carbohydrate choices (including fruits, vegetables, and juices) and education about protein are helpful. Encourage athletes to boost carbohydrate intake through consumption of beverages, or adding a slice of bread, or a serving of pasta to every meal. It is important to educate players on the role of carbohydrates for weight maintenance. Many football players believe that to lose weight they should eat only protein, so it can be challenging to convince a player that carbohydrates are helpful, not harmful.

Decreasing fat in the diet can be especially challenging for football players. Players who have grown up with high-fat foods as regional or ethnic favorites (fried meats, gravy, fatty meats, and/or biscuits) often do not like the taste of the lower fat items. Players who have grown up eating fast food do not always find low-fat foods appealing. Strategies that have been well received for decreasing fat in the diet of football players include:

- Change snacks to include pretzels, light microwave popcorn, reduced-fat chips, or cheese curls in place of regular popcorn or full-fat chips.
- Suggest low-fat granola bars in place of candy bars.
- Recommend fresh fruit on cereal for an evening snack in place of high-fat snack foods.
- Try frozen yogurt in place of ice cream.
- Include a balance of higher and lower fat foods at meals.
- Offer reduced-fat dairy products, mayonnaise, and salad dressings with meals.
- Lower the fat in favorite foods by providing skinless "oven-fried" chicken in place of fried chicken, well-trimmed lean meats in place of heavily marbled cuts of meat, roasted vegetables in place of buttered vegetables, and steamed rice in place of fried rice.

MICRONUTRIENT REQUIREMENTS

Micronutrient needs for football players are not different from the general recommendations for other athletes. Energy needs are higher than for other athletes and, as a result, micronutrient needs are increased; but, since food intake is higher, the need for supplementation is rare. Some teams provide an optional multivitamin-mineral supplement for players. Some players self-supplement, primarily with products they believe will enhance performance or hasten recovery from injury (5).

FLUID REQUIREMENTS

Maintaining adequate hydration can be a challenge for football players, especially the linemen who tend to carry more body fat and may experience more adverse effects of heat illness due to the weight of the uniform and pads during a hot summer practice. Fluid replacement is a key concern, especially to the rookies who may be unfamiliar with the rigors of twice-daily practice in the sweltering sun while wearing pads. In addition, since football players tend to be larger than other athletes, fluid needs are increased based on body size. Gone are the days when water breaks were infrequent if allowed at all during practices. Players are encouraged and even reminded to drink; water bottles and "water boys" are available, as well as sports drinks (6). Fluids are routinely offered in the locker room and large cups are available to encourage players to drink beyond thirst. See Chapter 6, Fluid and Electrolytes for more specific information.

ERGOGENIC AIDS

As in all sports, the goal in football is to win. Since the NFL and the National Collegiate Athletic Association (NCAA) provide routine drug testing, the route to "stronger, bigger, and faster" has to be pursued in a legal but circuitous manner. Many athletes believe that if a supplement is available over-the-counter, it must be safe and legal. A part of every football player's education should be education on dietary supplements that are safe, legal, and effective. The ergogenic aids favored by football players are those that promise increased mass. Most recently, athletes have expressed interest in supplements that may assist with recovery from intense exercise, as well as supplements that increase "energy" and those touted as "fat burners." The most popular supplements are listed in *Box 37.1* (7-11).

BOX 37.1   Ergogenic Aids Most Commonly Used by Football Players (7-11)

- Creatine
- Beta-hydroxy-methylbutyrate (HMB)
- Yohimbine
- Protein powders/amino acids
- Dehydroepiandrosterone (DHEA)
- Androstenedione
- Tribulus terrestris
- Ginseng
- Metabolife 356
- Fat burners (Ripped Fuel, Cutting Edge)
- Melatonin
- Pyruvate
- Glucosamine sulfate/chondroitin
- Gingko biloba
- Enzymes
- Glutamine

Of all the supplements listed in *Box 37.1,* creatine is the most frequently used. A review by Plisk et al (10) discusses the pros and cons of creatine supplementation. The effectiveness of creatine may be position-specific and contingent upon the athlete's underlying nutritional and hydration status. Many football players take creatine and report an increase in mass. Depending on the field position, this may or may not be advantageous. A player who does not have to move as much but is relying more on strength (eg, offensive lineman) will realize more benefit from creatine than the player who adds extra weight that may negatively affect speed (eg, wide receiver). Players are starting to experiment with creatine cycling, as opposed to a continuous high dose, and some players have discontinued use after failing to see any additional increase in mass. It is important to educate players on the proper use of creatine in regard to dosage, frequency of use, and timing of use. Creatine should be taken with simple carbohydrate, not water, for maximum benefit. For further discussion of creatine, see Chapter 7, Ergogenic Aids.

As a consultant to a professional football team, players will often ask questions about supplements and how to use them. Recommended strategies for discussing the effective use of supplements include the following (12):

- Inquire as to what supplement(s) the athlete takes. Ask to see the package or bottle for labeling information.
- Inquire how often and in what dosage the athlete uses the supplement(s).
- Document the name, dose, and frequency of use in the athlete's medical record.
- Determine underlying hydration and nutritional status.
- Discuss the benefits and risk of supplements, especially potential side effects.
- Educate the athlete on the proper use of the supplement.
- Encourage the athlete not to experiment with new products before games.

The player's biggest concern is the legality of a specific substance and whether he will test positive for its use. Players should be told it is better to be safe than sorry when experimenting with dietary supplements. Ask the player if use of a banned or questionable dietary supplement is worth suspension from play. *Box 37.2* contains a list of substances banned by the NFL (13).

BOX 37.2   Substances Banned by the National Football League (13)

Anabolic Agents:

Anabolic/androgenic steroids (DHEA,Testosterone, Androstenedione)

Human or animal growth hormone

Beta-2 agonists

Human chorionic gonadatropin

Masking Agents:

Diuretics (eg, Furosemide, Probenecid, Spironolactone, Hydrochlorthiazide)

Epitestosterone

NUTRITION REQUIREMENTS FOR TRAINING

Football players participate in their most intense workouts during preseason or training camp. During a 5-week training camp for professional players, 4 of 7 days involve twice-daily practices and weight training. During season, a typical day consists of a light morning workout or weightlifting and a more intensive afternoon workout. The player who may require up to 10,000 kcal per day at training camp may need only 5,000 kcal per day during season to maintain weight. The challenge is to meet, but not exceed or fall short of, energy needs. This can be problematic for the player who lives alone and has limited cooking skills. He may be able to eat breakfast and lunch at the stadium but need to provide his own dinner and snacks. As the season winds down, recommendations should be given for weight maintenance in the off-season when activity typically declines, with the goal of preventing excessive weight gain before the start of the next season.

PRECOMPETITION MEALS

For precompetition meals, the football players' personal preferences and superstitions need to be part of the equation. The player who requests a pregame meal of steak and eggs is not going to be happy with pasta but may be willing to have some pancakes or toast to achieve a better balance. Some athletes choose special foods before games. For example, one player ate a whole pie and half a gallon of ice cream the night before a game. Since excess weight was an issue for him, a compromise was reached, settling on half the pie and a pint of ice cream. He eventually learned to like frozen yogurt, did not feel deprived, and lost the extra weight. Offer players a menu of items to choose from for a pregame meal, ranging from breakfast items to grilled chicken to pasta. Many of the players opt for pasta and chicken, but a few request steaks.

Since football is a "stop-start" activity, the fluid of choice during games is water (6). Sports drinks are available to the players, but water is the preferred beverage because energy expenditure is not consistent over a 60-minute game. Providing water as the beverage of choice also prevents taste aversions to particular sports beverages, plus it is the easiest beverage to have available for players. Players are encouraged to drink every time they come to the sidelines. However, in hot, humid game conditions, some players may benefit from a suitable sports drink.

The postgame fluid choice also may be an issue because alcohol is often consumed after games. To encourage a more suitable postgame beverage, the sports nutritionist can stress that alcohol intake can delay muscle glycogen resynthesis (14).

The major nutrition concerns of football players are listed in *Box 37.3*. Football players need practical strategies for achieving body composition and weight goals. Players need and want to know what dietary supplements they can use and how to use them effectively. Since dehydration can occur at summer training camps and playing in indoor stadiums, players should be provided with information on hydration with ample fluid sources and encouraged to take advantage of these fluids.

BOX 37.3 Top Nutrition Concerns of Football Players

- How to achieve weight goals—both weight gain and weight loss
- Legal ways to increase muscle mass
- Maintaining adequate hydration

WORKING WITH COACHES AND TRAINERS

As I enter my seventh year working with a professional football team, the best advice I can give is to be flexible and persistent. My first year of working with the team consisted of menu revisions for training camp and consulting with a few players who were trying to lose weight. I now work with the team year round and am developing a web page devoted to sports nutrition, as well as an educational video to be played on closed-circuit television at training camp. *Box 37.4* provides tips for working with athletic trainers and coaches.

BOX 37.4 Tips for Working with Athletic Trainers and Coaches

- Be available.
- Be creative.
- Be patient but persistent.
- Speak your mind but expect to be challenged.
- Keep it short, simple, and to the point.
- Have fun.

CASE STUDY

Lee is a rookie defensive lineman for an NFL team. Since he had not negotiated his contract, he reported to training camp late. He came into training camp 25 lb above the "desired" weight set for him by the coach. This weight goal was based on achieving a weight that would correlate with a body fat percentage of 18% from standards set by Wilmore et al (15). Having battled weight his entire football career, he resorted to the same weight-loss tactics that had worked for him in high school and college. He would skip breakfast, go to morning practice, eat a piece of fruit for lunch, collapse after lunch, go to afternoon practice, and have a dinner of grilled or broiled skinless chicken and a salad without dressing with water to drink. He went to a local health food store and bought an herbal diet supplement that he was taking daily. After 3 days he was exhausted and passed out on the field at afternoon practice. The athletic trainer and coaches were very concerned and called the sports nutritionist to assess the player's dietary regimen and make recommendations.

Assessment

- Dehydration
- Inadequate calorie intake for energy expenditure
- Lack of variety in diet
- Inadequate knowledge of the proper balance of foods for weight loss
- Inadequate distribution of macronutrients
- Inadequate number of meals per day
- Potential harmful effects of the weight loss supplement:
  — Dehydration
  — Stimulant effect
  — Cathartic
- Unrealistic expectations for weight goals (15,16)

Recommendations

- Dual energy x-ray absorptiometry (DXA) scan to assess actual body composition to set realistic weight goals. Present the results to the strength coach and head coach.
- Guidelines for appropriate fluid requirements regarding:
  — Choices
  — Timing
  — Volume
- Guidelines for appropriate macro- and micronutrient requirements
  — Calorie level and macronutrient composition determined by the sports nutritionist
- Guidelines for number of meals and examples of meals
  — Education regarding meal choices by pointing out acceptable items in the cafeteria
- Guidelines for snacks by developing a list of acceptable snacks which the player likes and accompanying him to the grocery store to stock up on appropriate items
- Education on the role of dietary weight loss supplements on claims made versus reality
- Working closely with the strength coach to increase energy expenditure to facilitate weight loss in conjunction with an appropriate calorie level

REFERENCES

1. Short SH, Short WR. Four year study of university athletes' dietary intake. *J Am Diet Assoc.* 1983;82:632-645.
2. Hickson JF, Wolinsky I, Pivarnik JM, Neuman EA, Itak JF, Stockton JE. Nutritional profile of football athletes eating from a training table. *Nutr Res.* 1987;7:27-34.
3. Lemon PWR. Effects of exercise on dietary protein requirements. *Int J Sport Nutr.* 1998;8:426-447.
4. Paul GL, Gautsch TA, Layman DK. Amino acid and protein metabolism during exercise and recovery. In: Wolinsky I, ed. *Nutrition in Exercise and Sport.* 3rd ed. Boca Raton, Fla: CRC Press; 1998:125-158.

5. Sobal J, Marquart LF. Vitamin/mineral use among athletes: a review of the literature. *Int J Sport Nutr*. 1994;4:320-334.
6. American College of Sports Medicine. Position stand on exercise and fluid replacement. *Med Sci Sports Exerc*. 1996;28:i-vii.
7. Armsey TD, Green GA. Nutrition supplements: science vs hype. *Phys Sports Med*. 1997;25:77-92,116.
8. Eichner ER. Ergogenic aids: what athletes are using and why. *Phys Sports Med*. 1997;25:70-76,79,83.
9. Clarkson PM. Nutritional supplements for weight gain. *Sports Sci Exch*. 1998;11(1).
10. Plisk SS, Kreider RB. Creatine controversy? *Strength Cond J*. 1999;21:14-23.
11. Antonio J, Street C. Glutamine: a potentially useful supplement for athletes. *Can J Appl Physiol*. 1999;24:1-14.
12. Butterfield G. Ergogenic aids: evaluating sports nutrition products. *Int J Sport Nutr*. 1996;6:191-197.
13. National Football League. Policies and Procedures for Anabolic Steroids and Related Substances. June 1997. New York, NY: National Football League.
14. American College of Sports Medicine. Position statement on the use of alcohol in sports. *Med Sci Sports Exerc*. 1982;14:ix-x.
15. Wilmore JH, Parr RB, Haskell WL, Costill DL, Milburn LJ, Kerlan RK. Football pros' strengths and CV weakness—charted. *Phys Sports Med*. 1976;4:45-54.
16. Smith JF, Mansfield ER. Body composition prediction in university athletes. *Med Sci Sports Exerc*. 1984;16:398-405.

38

GYMNASTICS

Kim LaPiana, MS, RD and Kyra Bramble, MS, RD

Gymnastics is a unique sport that requires tremendous strength, coordination, flexibility, intense concentration, motivation, and dedication in order to advance. It has been argued that gymnasts are stronger, pound for pound, than any other type of athlete (1). The sport naturally shapes gymnasts into having very lean, muscular bodies. Nutrition can have a major impact on a gymnast's normal growth, development, training benefit, and athletic performance.

To effectively educate gymnasts, their parents, and coaches, nutrition professionals must understand the sport of gymnastics. The issues and recommendations in this chapter are applicable to all three forms of gymnastics (women's artistic, rhythmic, and men's gymnastics); however, the focus of this chapter is women's artistic gymnastics.

THE SPORT OF GYMNASTICS

USA Gymnastics, the governing body of gymnastics, identified 72,000 registered competing gymnasts during the 1997-1998 season. Of those registered, 87% participated in female artistic, 12% in male artistic, and 1% in rhythmic gymnastics. In addition, there are 87 US colleges with competitive gymnastics teams.

A gymnastics career can begin as early as 3 years of age and continue to about 22 years of age. However, such longevity in the sport is rare. Injuries, sport "burn-out," or other age-related interests cause gymnasts to quit or retire from the sport. In January 1997, the Federation Internationale de Gymnastique (FIG) raised the international competition age eligibility from 15 to 16 years. This measure was taken to encourage athletes to stay in the sport longer and to discourage athletes from peaking at an early age (ie, to prevent "burn-out"). Maintaining a healthy mind and body through adolescence may be rewarded with a college athletic scholarship, which is often the goal of many gymnasts and their parents.

The gymnast who is just beginning in the sport will attend classes 2 to 3 days per week, 1 to 2 hours per session. As skill level improves, he or she advances and begins to complete compulsory routines at various levels between level 1 and the elite level, the highest competitive level. At this point, training increases to 3 to 4 days per week, 3 to 4 hours per session. When the gymnast reaches competition levels 8, 9, and 10, training increases to 4 to 6 days per week, 4 to 5 hours per session. The highest competitive level for women's gymnastics is the elite level. At this level, commitment to training can range from 20 to 36 hours per week, 6 days a week. Some gymnasts have reached the elite level as early as 10 years of age.

The age of the gymnast combined with the time commitment to train presents nutrition-related challenges. Travel time to practice may take up to 1 hour each way in order to train at a particular gym. Often, the gymnast leaves immediately after school and returns home after 9:00 PM. The logistics of transportation and finding time to eat often leave parents and gymnasts confused about the timing of meals and food choices. Because of this time pressure, fast food is often a staple since its convenience far outweighs its nutritional value.

The physical demands of gymnastics are intense, even though it is not a high-calorie-burning sport. Gymnastics is considered an anaerobic sport even though practices may last 3 to 6 hours. Its activities are characterized by short bursts of high-intensity muscular work never lasting longer than 90 seconds. Gymnastics training typically consists of warm ups, flexibility and strength conditioning, and rotations between two to four events (vaulting, uneven parallel bars, balance beam, and floor exercise). These rotations, lasting 30 to 60 minutes each, consist of repetitive skill progressions and/or routines with plenty of recovery time between turns (still using only the anaerobic energy system). Gymnastics is classified predominantly as a speed event that uses nonoxidative glycogenolysis and glycolysis. Vaulting is the exception and is considered a power event that uses the ATP-creatine-phosphate energy system (2). Gymnasts require fast-twitch muscle fibers, which have a limited ability to burn fat in the absence of oxygen. Therefore, gymnasts must maintain optimal liver, muscle glycogen, and muscle creatine stores to fuel their activity.

The sport-specific body type for success in gymnastics is what causes many gymnasts to develop a "diet mentality," often beginning before the onset of puberty. Younger "up-and-coming" gymnasts often emulate the poor dietary practices and beliefs of the older and more advanced athletes at the gym. This diet mentality, coupled with changes in height, weight, and body shape during puberty, presents a challenge to the physical and mental well-being of the gymnast. Gymnasts tend to have personality traits—such as striving for perfection, obsessive behavior, and attention to detail—that are characteristic of adolescents with eating disorders. These behaviors may lead to more significant health problems such as the female athlete triad.

As defined by the American College of Sports Medicine (ACSM), the female athlete triad consists of three interrelated components: disordered eating, amenorrhea, and osteoporosis (3). It is well documented that gymnasts have a high prevalence of disordered eating (4-7), as well as amenorrhea and other types of menstrual dysfunction (8,9). Gymnasts, however, have been shown to have higher bone density than nonathletes and other athletes (eg, runners) despite their prevalence of disordered eating and amenorrhea (9). Sports involving high-impact forces, such as gymnastics, appear to offer some protection against low bone density (10-12). Awareness of the three components of the female athlete triad is essential. An athlete diagnosed with any one component of the triad should be evaluated for the other components. These disorders, alone or in combination, can diminish athletic performance and may result in short- and long-term psychological, medical, and skeletal repercussions.

ENERGY REQUIREMENTS

Few well designed studies of energy balance in young athletes have been published, limiting the current understanding of this topic (13). Energy expenditure and requirements for collegiate gymnasts are not transferable to younger gymnasts, who comprise the majority of the gymnastics population. Predicted energy requirements appear to overestimate what the gymnast needs and, therefore, promote weight gain—the ultimate fear for gymnasts. Additionally, it is difficult to obtain accurate information on dietary intake with gymnasts, as they frequently underreport their energy intake (13). Gymnasts perceive that eating very little is desirable by the researcher because it shows discipline and control outside of the gym environment.

Dietary assessments of elite junior, senior, and college-age gymnasts indicate that most gymnasts consume less than the recommended amount of energy for their age and activity level (4,8,14-16). A recent study of the US national team (n=33) showed that intakes averaged 34.4 kcal/kg and were considered to be 20% less than predicted for age and activity level (16). Other research supports this and indicates that gymnasts between the ages of 9 and 22 years consume anywhere from 20% to 50% below estimated energy requirements (4,8,14,15).

Gymnasts restrict caloric intake to lose weight as a way to obtain the perceived ideal body type. Caloric restriction has a negative effect on training, even though the gymnast may feel lighter. The effects of chronic negative energy balance are well documented in this population. The numerous training and health consequences include nutrient deficiencies, dehydration, fatigue secondary to muscle and liver glycogen depletion, poor concentration, lack of motivation, delayed puberty, short stature, decrease in resting energy expenditure, menstrual irregularities, poor bone health, increased incidence of injuries, and increased risk for developing eating disorders (4,8,13-19).

MACRONUTRIENT RECOMMENDATIONS

According to The American Dietetic Association's position statement for adolescent athletes (20), 55% to 60% of total energy should come from carbohydrate, 12% to 15% from protein, and 25% to 30% from fat. Because the energy demands of gymnastics dictate that carbohydrate is the preferred fuel for high-intensity work (2,21), slightly increasing the carbohydrate contribution in the overall diet is beneficial. Gymnasts should compensate for this change by decreasing overall calories from fat. This promotes better use of fuel for the sport while avoiding weight gain. A diet rich in carbohydrate (60% to 65%), adequate in protein (12% to 15%), and low in fat (20% to 25%) appears to be optimal for the sport of gymnastics.

Carbohydrate

Carbohydrate is the primary fuel for gymnastics activity. Gymnasts training on successive days must consume adequate carbohydrates as well as energy to minimize the threat of chronic fatigue associated with muscle glycogen depletion. Since body storage for this macronutrient is limited, frequent replacement is recommended. The goals for carbohydrate intake include topping off glycogen stores before training and competition, maintaining energy levels during practice, and replenishing glycogen stores after training. Assuming the athlete consumes adequate overall calories, an intake of 6 to 8 g of carbohydrate/kg per day is recommended to ensure adequate glycogen synthesis and replenish muscle glycogen stores (21,22). Consuming amounts greater than this has been suggested; however, a greater level of consumption does not leave room for the balance of protein and fat calories and could promote weight gain.

Optimizing glycogen stores involves the most important meal of the day. Although breakfast may be missed due to time constraints or attempts to limit calories, this is counterproductive to glycogen replenishment and should be discouraged. Quick, easy-to-eat breakfasts (see *Box 38.1*) are available and help to rebuild the breakfast routine as well as replenish glycogen stores.

A carbohydrate snack eaten within 1/2 to 1 hour before practice will "top off" glycogen stores. The snack could be eaten in the car en route to practice or at home while getting ready. The gymnast should be encouraged to choose a snack that contains some protein as it provides greater satiety. *Box 38.2* lists some examples of appropriate snacks.

BOX 38.1   1-minute Breakfast Ideas

- Ready-to-eat cereal topped with blueberries and skim milk
- 6- or 8-oz container of low-fat yogurt
- Small muffin topped with yogurt
- Peanut butter on whole-wheat toast and skim milk
- Small slice of cheese pizza and orange juice
- Instant oatmeal with skim milk
- Breakfast smoothie (skim milk, frozen fruit, and wheat germ whirled in a blender)
- Toasted whole-wheat waffle, topped with fresh fruit
- 1/2 toasted bagel with peanut butter or light cream cheese
- Lean ham on a toasted English muffin and a 6-oz juice box
- Fresh fruit and string cheese
- Packet of instant breakfast mixed with skim milk
- Cottage cheese and fruit

BOX 38.2   High-performance Snacks for Gymnasts

Before Practice	During Practice
(High-carbohydrate foods with some protein)	(Smaller portion of high-carbohydrate foods)
• 1 cup low-fat yogurt	• 1/4 or 1/2 piece of fresh fruit
• 1 cup bean soup and breadsticks	• 3-4 pieces of dried fruit
• 2-3 pieces string cheese and 6 crackers	• 5-6 gingersnaps
• English muffin pizza	• 2-3 graham crackers
• Lean meat sandwich and skim milk	• 10-12 cinnamon "Teddy Grahams"
• Energy bar	• 1/2 energy bar
• Bowl of cereal and skim milk	• 1/4 cup sports drink
	• 5-6 vanilla wafers

After 2 1/2 to 3 hours of gymnastics training, fuel is close to, if not completely, depleted. At this point, the gymnast is usually fatigued and can think only about reaching the end of practice. Concentration levels, motivation, and attitude are dramatically affected, as well as the ability to do muscular work. It is no coincidence that most injuries occur toward the end of practice. Gymnasts often leave the gym feeling discouraged and defeated. The latter part of practice may be physically and mentally counterproductive due to depleted energy stores. Therefore, snack breaks are very beneficial at all levels of training.

Snack breaks are a "win-win" situation for both the gymnast and coach. Including a midpractice snack enables the gymnast to be more productive and positive throughout training. Snack breaks can be taken between rotations and do not need to take up valuable practice time. Snacks should consist of small portions of carbohydrate-rich foods or sports drinks and be convenient and safe to store in a gym bag, and require only moments to eat. USA Gymnastics has promoted snack breaks with great success. This is also a time for coaches to be a role model and reinforce healthy eating that promotes the concept that "food is fuel."

Replenishing glycogen stores after practice is critical. Many times gymnasts are not hungry after practice and skip dinner. If there is a lengthy commute home from the gym, fast food is often the meal of choice. The gymnast should be provided with suggestions for high-carbohydrate, low-fat choices when eating out. It should be emphasized that food is fuel for the body and mind.

Protein

Maintaining the appropriate balance between energy and protein intake is critical for the growth and development of young athletes. If caloric intake is too low, protein will be used for fuel and muscle will be catabolized (23). Furthermore, muscle size and strength will be lost and performance and health will be affected. A diet supplying 12% to 15% of the calories as protein, or 1.2 to 1.7 g/kg, should meet the needs of most young athletes in gymnastics (24). Many gymnasts avoid beef and dairy products (high-protein foods) out of fear that these foods contain too much fat (an observation noted by the authors who participated in the sport for more than 10 years and are currently working with gymnasts). Therefore, it is important that gymnasts be educated and encouraged to include a variety of high-quality, low-fat protein sources in their diets.

Fat

Fat is necessary to provide essential fatty acids, to insulate and protect organs, and to absorb and transport fat-soluble vitamins. Fat also provides satiety and flavor to foods. The latter should not be overlooked when educating adolescent athletes since it promotes normal food consumption. Because gymnastics requires a high strength-to-weight ratio, it is important to keep nonfunctional weight low. Due to the anaerobic nature of gymnastics, fat is not used as a primary fuel source. By reducing fat intake to 20% to 25% of total calories, desirable body composition is easier to maintain.

Many gymnasts think that "fat-free" foods are good choices for snacks. However, most of these snacks are high in sugar and calories with little protein, vitamins, or minerals. Teaching gymnasts to differentiate between fat-free foods and low-calorie, nutrient-dense foods may help them move away from dieting practices and toward making food choices that have positive effects on body composition goals, health, and athletic-training performance.

MICRONUTRIENT RECOMMENDATIONS

A gymnast's intake of calories is usually insufficient to meet 100% of the RDAs/DRIs for most micronutrients (see the Tools section). Calcium and iron are of special concern.

Calcium

Adequate calcium intake is essential to support proper bone growth and development in adolescent gymnasts. Although genetics is the greatest factor in the attainment of peak bone mass, nutrition and physical activity also play important roles (25). Inadequate calcium intake may lead to poorly mineralized bone, placing the gymnast at an increased risk of stress fracture (12,26). Stress fractures are one of the more common injuries in this sport (17). Peak bone density is reached during middle to late adolescence, or just at the age when most gymnasts are reaching their peak competitive years (26,27). Many gymnasts will not drink milk or consume other dairy products. Many claim they are "intolerant" to this food group. However, many of these athletes are simply avoiding these high-calcium foods, as they believe all dairy foods are high in fat. Some have even professed, "Milk products make my skin thick" (ie, difficult to appear lean). The average calcium intake among gymnasts is reported to be as low as 600 mg per day (14), well below the DRI of 1,300 mg per day for 9- to 18-year-olds (8,15,16). Great care should be taken to ensure that gymnasts are obtaining adequate levels of calcium in their diets. Inadequate calcium intake increases the risk of stress fractures, reduces bone density, and contributes to the potential to develop osteoporosis later in life (27).

Iron

The average intake of iron for female gymnasts is 6 to 14 mg per day, which is below the RDA of 15 mg per day (8,14,15). Depletion of iron stores, as indicated by low serum ferritin levels, is a precursor to iron deficiency anemia. Also, iron depletion, in the absence of iron deficiency anemia, may result in impaired endurance performance and slow recovery from exercise. These facts provide a rationale for the routine assessment of iron status in gymnasts, with iron therapy provided when warranted. Many gymnasts forego red meat because it is considered high in fat; thus, they need education on incorporating high-quality iron sources in their diet. Additionally, a multivitamin with minerals taken daily is recommended for gymnasts who consume less than 1,500 kcal per day to ensure overall nutrient adequacy. Encouraging gymnasts to add colorful foods (red, orange, yellow, and green fruits and vegetables) to meals and snacks is a simple and practical way for this age group to improve vitamin, antioxidant, and phytochemical intake (28).

FLUID REQUIREMENTS

Gymnasts do not have special fluid needs compared to general fluid guidelines for other athletes. However, gymnasts may have a harder time with access to fluids. There are only one or two water fountains in a gym and many administrators discourage the practice of bringing sports drinks to the gym because they are concerned that spilled drinks may stain floor mats. Coaches are not always in the habit of encouraging gymnasts to stop for water breaks because this might disrupt practice. In addition, gymnasts do not like to train with a full bladder or take frequent trips to the bathroom.

When dehydrated, gymnasts experience fatigue, lack of concentration, and a high risk of injury. Therefore, it is critical to explain the benefits of fluid intake to both athletes and coaches. Only recently have gymnasts started bringing water bottles to the gym. This is largely due to the increased emphasis on the benefits of proper hydration during training. Fluid guidelines for gymnasts are modified slightly, taking into consideration the age and size of the athlete. Gymnasts should drink 8 oz of fluid 30 minutes before practice, 2 to 3 oz every 15 minutes during practice, and at least 8 oz after practice (29). The change of rotations and waiting in line for a turn are good times for water breaks.

Some gymnasts are concerned with the caloric content of sports drinks and must be reassured that the caloric content is low and the benefits are high. It should be emphasized to the weight-concerned gymnast that the calories from sports drinks are typically used for energy during practice, rather than stored as body fat.

ERGOGENIC AIDS AND SUPPLEMENTS

Scientific research evaluating supplement use has generally not included children and adolescents. Since the majority of the gymnastic population is under 18 years of age, the use of supplements should be discouraged. However, the gymnastics community is close-knit and has been bombarded with supplement claims of improved strength, endurance, and energy, as well as quick weight loss. When high-profile coaches and athletes are paid spokespersons for such products, great interest is generated among other gymnasts, their parents, and coaches. Creatine monohydrate, pyruvate, protein powders, and liquid high-dose multivitamins are currently popular in the gymnastics community. Nutrition professionals have an opportunity to present the facts about such products to those interested; otherwise, the information will be sought from those not qualified. See Chapter 7, Ergogenic Aids for more information.

PRECOMPETITION AND COMPETITION RECOMMENDATIONS

"Nutrition conditioning" should be promoted as an integral component of gymnastics training. The concept of nutrition conditioning includes experimenting with various foods before, during, and after training sessions to determine foods that are satisfying, well-tolerated, and likely to be good choices as competition-day foods. Since the timing of competition may not be the same as for training, some adjustments should be made. In addition, when gymnasts travel to competitions, an overnight stay may offer access only to unfamiliar foods. Due to precompetition jitters, foods and fluids should be familiar to the gymnast. Indigestion and impaired performance may be the result with untested foods or beverages. Planning is the key to success. The sports nutritionist can present a sample meal schedule for the day of competition to the coaches and athletes. It should emphasize nutrition conditioning—the same meals and snacks for training and competition.

DISORDERED EATING AND EATING DISORDERS

Competitive gymnasts are at increased risk of developing disordered eating practices due to their gender, periadolescent age, and the nature of the sport (7,30,31). Disordered eating in female athletes has been reported to range from 15% to 62% (6,7,32-34). Other factors putting gymnasts at risk include psychological traits, self-esteem issues, dieting or restrained eating, and lack of knowledge.

Gymnasts participate in a sport where clothing is scant, perceived ideal body type is thin and very lean, and aesthetics is a component of success. While nothing in the *Code of Points* (35) or other judging regulations relate to body size or appearance, a gymnast often perceives that having a body type similar to her "role model" will improve her chances of success. Gymnasts start to compare their body types, start cutting back on the quantity of food, and begin to focus on how much they weigh. Weight becomes a measure of both self-worth and self-esteem, often lasting for years after participation in the sport has ended. Dieting or restrained eating is a way of life for many gymnasts.

At the completion of their competitive careers, high-level gymnasts often have trouble with weight gain. Former gymnasts report experiencing a decline in self-esteem prior to the development of disordered eating patterns after retiring from the sport (36). This decline in self-esteem has been attributed to the loss of structure, goal-setting, and recognition previously provided by their sport (36). Other gymnasts, surveyed approximately 15 years following the completion of their collegiate gymnastics careers, reported their eating disorder symptoms had abated since college (4). This suggests that these behaviors may have been related to athletic pressure to achieve the ideal body type for gymnastics (4). It also implies that not all gymnasts suffer from disordered eating.

Disordered eating in gymnasts can affect growth, development, and athletic performance and may lead to an eating disorder. There have been several documented cases of elite female gymnasts suffering from anorexia nervosa or bulimia nervosa. However, clear scientific evidence suggesting that eating disorders are more common in gymnastics than in other female competitive sports is lacking (17).

Large-scale, valid research is needed to clearly interpret the prevalence of eating disorders in gymnasts (17).

Public perception has increasingly dictated that gymnastics is a sport that abuses athletes. It has been suggested that participation in gymnastics may cause young athletes to miss out on life, be abused by their coaches, and end up with eating disorders, all having long-term, adverse consequences. It has also been publicized that some coaches are verbally abusive, which contributes to the gymnast's low self-esteem (37,38). These criticisms have been magnified out of proportion. Eating disorders, poor self-esteem, and name-calling by coaches have all happened in the sport of gymnastics, but are not the norm. The number of negative instances in comparison to the number of gymnasts enjoying a healthful and rewarding experience is frequently misrepresented in the media. USA Gymnastics has taken measures to change this public perception as well as to educate all gymnastics participants about proper nutrition practices.

The USA Gymnastics Athlete Wellness Program supports a positive and health-enhancing experience for all involved. Its mission is to insure that gymnasts train in a positive environment and acquire the necessary physical and mental tools needed to pursue their goals, secure their well-being, and enjoy the sport of gymnastics (39). The National Health Care Referral Network, part of the program, consists of health care professionals with an expertise in treating gymnasts and was developed as a resource for gymnasts, coaches, parents, and administrators. Nutritional, psychological, physical, and biomechanical aspects of the sport are covered in the program. In addition, most of the members of this network are former competitive gymnasts to whom other younger gymnasts can relate. Registered dietitians interested in participating in the referral network should contact USA Gymnastics. *Box 38.3* provides information about the referral network.

BOX 38.3   Recommendations for Sports Nutritionists Interested in Working with Gymnasts

USA Gymnastics Health Care Referral Network

For more information regarding the USA Gymnastics Health Care Referral Network, call (317) 237-5050 or visit the web site at http://www.usagymnastics.org/wellness/referralnetwork.html

---

Nutrition professionals have an opportunity to positively affect the young gymnast's life. Strength, training, endurance, motivation, attitude, concentration, and energy levels can be improved by optimizing calorie and nutrient intakes. This, in turn, allows gymnasts to train at a more intense level for a longer time, reduces the risk of injury, and promotes happier and healthier gymnasts. *Box 38.4* offers pointers for effective nutrition messages. *Box 38.5* outlines important "take-home" messages for nutrition education sessions.

BOX 38.4   Pointers for Delivering Effective Nutrition Messages to Gymnasts

---

Gymnasts are strongly influenced by their coaches and peers. It is essential for nutrition professionals to deliver their messages appropriately. Keep these points in mind when working with gymnasts:

1. Teach the coaches, gymnasts, and parents that the information you have can make them better athletes *without spending more time in the gym!*
2. Remember the age group of your audience and tailor your message appropriately.
3. Encourage coaches to use qualified nutrition professionals. This improves the accuracy of information and improves the gymnast-coach relationship.
4. Become involved in a gymnastics organization by offering to write an article for their newsletter or posting monthly bulletin board messages using topics suggested by the coaches, gymnasts, or parents. Schedule weekly or bimonthly visits to the gym and include individual sessions for parents and coaches.
5. Become very familiar with the sport by watching practices and learning the "lingo."
6. Encourage audience participation when speaking to large groups. Ask questions, learn names, and call on people to participate.
7. Picture yourself in a leotard. This will help you understand some of the self-esteem and appearance issues of gymnasts.
8. Use simple, practical, and realistic examples.
9. Use humor and light-heartedness, emphasizing that "food is fuel" and "food is fun."
10. Acknowledge fears associated with puberty and weight gain.
11. Empower coaches and staff to set an example and reinforce positive behavior because their words and actions are taken as gospel. Caution should be taken to avoid negative messages and/or body language.
12. Whenever possible, make sports nutrition recommendations performance-based.

BOX 38.5   Nutrition Take-home Messages

---

1. Nutrition affects strength, power, endurance, perception of energy level, mental concentration and alertness, attitude, mood, flexibility, injury risk, and overall health. Therefore, what a gymnast eats has a direct impact on the level of his or her performance.
2. The main energy-providing nutrient is carbohydrate. Foods high in carbohydrate should comprise the majority the diet.
3. A balanced diet includes a variety of foods.
4. Skipping meals *does not* promote weight control—proper food choices do. Go no longer than 4 hours without eating. Eat healthful snacks between meals.
5. Choose your meals by color. The more orange, yellow, green, and red foods you include in your diet, the more nutrients you will have to be a high-performance gymnast.
6. A multivitamin/mineral supplement is a good idea. Let a dietetics professional determine if you need other supplements.
7. Schedule a refueling snack break after 2 1/2 hours of practice and every hour thereafter.
8. Hydration is critical to athletic performance. Stay hydrated with water for shorter practices and sports drinks for longer practices.
9. Develop a healthy relationship with food. "Food is fuel" and "food is fun."
10. Practice "nutrition conditioning." What you eat before the day of competition needs to be the same as what you eat during the week.

TOP NUTRITION CONCERNS

Achieving the "Ideal" Body Type for Success

Many gymnasts believe their success in gymnastics is largely dependent on their physical appearance. In their eyes the best gymnasts are small, thin, and powerful. Additionally, gymnasts are strongly influenced by their coaches, parents, and peers. If improper dietary practices occur at home or in the gym, a gymnast will most likely adopt similar behaviors. Unfortunately, some coaches and parents are simply misinformed about nutrition and its effect on athletic performance.

Therefore, it is essential that both coaches and parents are educated on proper dietary practices and recognize that achievement of a certain body type is not always realistic. Certain factors, such as genetics and puberty, cannot be changed. In addition, being lighter or smaller does not always equate to better gymnastics performance.

Consuming a High-performance Diet

A high-performance diet for a gymnast is one that provides fuel for the working muscles, quick recovery from exercise training, and adequate energy and nutrients for growth, development, and physical training. Because carbohydrate is the preferred fuel for muscles, a diet rich in complex carbohydrates is ideal. Approximately 65% of total daily calories in a gymnast's diet should be from carbohydrate, 12% to 15% from protein, and 20% to 25% from fat. Caloric intake will vary based on a gymnast's size and activity. A snack break after 2 1/2 hours of practice and every hour thereafter is important for refueling the body and mind for the remainder of practice. Proper hydration is also critical to a gymnast's performance. It is important to emphasize that there are no "good" foods or "bad" foods, but performance foods and fun foods. *Box 38.6* gives an exercise that can be used to educate gymnasts about performance foods.

BOX 38.6   Exercise to Distinguish between "Fun Foods" and "Performance Foods"

This is an exercise to teach gymnasts that all foods can fit into their diet and there are no "good foods" or "bad foods."

1. Tape 2 large sheets of paper to the wall. Label one sheet "Fun Foods" and the other "Performance Foods."
2. Ask the gymnasts to call out their favorite foods while writing them on the appropriate sheet of paper. While doing this, talk about the food's nutritional qualities that make it either "Performance" or "Fun."
3. Encourage gymnasts to eat "Performance Foods" most of the time and "Fun Foods" only some of the time.

This exercise allows the athletes to participate in the nutrition lesson while emphasizing that food is necessary for performance.

Eating the Right Training and Competition Meals

A common question that gymnasts ask is, "What should I eat before a gymnastics meet?" Generally, foods consumed for daily gymnastics training should be similar to those eaten on competition days. "Nutrition conditioning" is recommended to provide consistency for the athletes and also to insure that meals are well-tolerated. Because training is usually a more intense activity over a longer time period, it is essential for gymnasts to consume enough food to maintain adequate energy levels. Foods eaten on a competition day should mimic those eaten on training days. Due to travel schedules and nervousness, gymnasts often forego or forget to eat. Therefore, planning meals, snacks, and fluids in advance of competition helps insure energy needs are met.

CASE STUDY

Mary, a 15-year-old, level 10 gymnast, is not having fun at gymnastics anymore. Since the onset of puberty, she has been overly consumed with her appearance. Her body has been changing over the last year and she "feels fat." She is 5'3" and weighs 115 pounds. Her body fat is 19.5%, as determined at the local health spa. Her ability to perform at her usual level has declined.

Mary is focusing too much on the desire to lose weight. This is contributing to her poor body image and low self-esteem. She occasionally binges and purges to compensate for her feelings of inadequacy. Her coach has recommended a 1,200-calorie, high-protein, low-carbohydrate diet to help Mary "lean out." Mary skips breakfast, eats a very small lunch, and goes to practice having consumed very little food. Following practice, she eats a large dinner and often binges late at night. Mary usually brings a piece of fruit and water to the gym, but chooses not to take snack breaks in an effort to save calories. Mary's mother found weight loss pills in her room and contacted a registered dietitian for nutrition counseling.

Recommendations

1. Determine a realistic goal weight. Although Mary is within clinical guidelines for ideal weight, performance and self-esteem would improve if she weighed less and had less body fat. A competitive gymnast will want to be in the lower 25th percentile (103.5 to 109 lb for Mary) of her normal weight range for height (103.5 to 125.5 lb for Mary). An initial goal reduction of 3 to 4 lb of fat weight will make a noticeable improvement in the way Mary feels about herself and her ability to train. Educate Mary on the components of weight. Evaluate Mary's body composition. Encourage a slow weight loss, no more than 1 to 2 lb per week. Monitor weight on a weekly basis in the privacy of an office (not in the gym). Reevaluate body composition every 2 weeks. Assist Mary with weight loss until her body fat reaches 15% to 17%. For a highly competitive gymnast, the lower quartile weight range for height and 15% to 17% body fat is still considered healthy.

Reevaluate goals every 2 weeks using the following factors: how Mary feels about herself; her energy level during the last half of practice; her ability to concentrate; and her strength and performance gains. An overall weight loss of 5 to 7 lb of fat weight will be ideal for Mary's performance and mental attitude.

2. Educate Mary on the preferred fuel for gymnastics. Gymnasts use carbohydrate for fuel. Her coach recommended a diet that may ultimately harm a gymnast. A low-carbohydrate diet will not adequately fuel her body or replenish her glycogen stores, and may increase her risk of injury. Meet with the coach and explain the importance of a diet comprised of 55% to 60% carbohydrates, 12% to 15% protein, and 20% to 25% fat.

3. Avoid giving specific calorie recommendations to gymnasts. Gymnasts are usually overachievers and are likely to become compulsive with calorie-counting. Initially, work on weight management using improved meal timing, portion sizes, and food selection. If progress is too slow or the athlete is insistent, start with a calorie range of 25 to 30 kcal/kg of actual weight. Monitor intake and adjust calories as weight changes. An intake of 1,200 calories a day for Mary is too low, even when the desired outcome is weight loss. Muscle tissue may be broken down and strength gains compromised. Fat stores will not be utilized for energy due to the anaerobic activity of the sport.

4. Promote realistic and practical weight management techniques. Give Mary a written meal and snack schedule, taking into consideration her school and training schedule and travel time to and from the gym. This will help Mary accept more frequent meals. Review portion sizes and ask Mary to keep a food journal. Review the food journal with Mary every week.

5. Help Mary recognize and respond to true hunger and feelings of fullness. Gymnasts often ignore signs of hunger when focusing on weight loss. When under-fueled, poor athletic performance is inevitable. Fatigue and lack of concentration contribute to increased risk of injury. Mary needs to allow herself to refuel her body for practice and understand the difference between physical hunger and emotional eating.

6. Help Mary to understand there are no "good" or "bad" foods. Mary feels she needs to restrict certain foods because she believes they are fattening. Allowing Mary to eat whatever she wants within the parameters of hunger and fullness will free her from feelings of guilt, which contribute to low self-esteem.

7. Encourage health-enhancing activities. Long-term health means a long-term commitment to an active lifestyle. Mary's weight-for-height is within standard clinical guidelines; however, her perfectionism drives her to believe she is not small enough. She needs to be reminded that the number on the scale is not the ultimate goal; rather, her strength and performance should guide her. Her current actions of bingeing and purging will have long-term health and emotional consequences, which require immediate attention. Proper education and

support will enable Mary to gain confidence and have a more healthful gymnastics experience.

8. Provide positive reinforcement. Each meeting, build upon the positive changes Mary has made, no matter how small. This will motivate her to continue, improve her self-esteem, and boost her self-confidence.

REFERENCES

1. Sands WA. Why gymnastics? *Technique*. 1999;19:5-15.
2. Kendrick ZV. Exercise physiology: implications for sports nutrition. In: Berning JR, Steen SN, eds. *Nutrition for Sports & Fitness*. Gaithersburg, Md: Aspen Publishers; 1998:1-19.
3. ACSM position stand on the female athlete triad. *Med Sci Sports Exerc*. 1997;29:i-ix.
4. O'Connor PJ, Lewis RD, Krichner EM, Cook DB. Eating disorder symptoms in former female college gymnasts. *Am J Clin Nutr*. 1996;64:840-843.
5. Petrie TA. Disordered eating in female collegiate gymnasts: prevalence and personality/attitudinal correlates. *J Sports Exerc Psych*. 1993;15:424-436.
6. Sundgot-Borgen J, Corbin CB. Eating disorders among female athletes. *Phys Sports Med*. 1987;15:89-95.
7. Warren BJ, Stanton AL, Blessing DL. Disordered eating patterns in competitive female athletes. *Int J Eat Disord*. 1990;9:565-569.
8. Krichner EM, Lewis RD, O'Connor PJ. Bone mineral density and dietary intake of female college gymnasts. *Med Sci Sports Exerc*. 1995;27:545-549.
9. Robinson TL, Snow-Harter C, Taaffe DR, Gillis D, Shaw J, Marcus R. Gymnasts exhibit higher bone density mass than runners despite similar prevalance of amenorrhea and oligomenorrhea. *J Bone Mineral Res*. 1995;10:26-35.
10. Cassell C, Benedict M, Specker B. Bone mineral density in elite 7 to 9 yr old female gymnasts and swimmers. *Med Sci Sports Exerc*. 1996;28:1243-1246.
11. Nicholas DL, Sanborn CF, Bonnick SL, Ben-Ezra V, Gench B, DiMarco NM. The effects of gymnastics training on bone mineral density. *Med Sci Sports Exerc*. 1994;26:1220-1225.
12. Taaffe DR, Robinson TL, Snow CM, Marcus R. High-impact exercise promotes bone gain in well-trained athletes. *J Bone Mineral Res*. 1997;12:255-260.
13. Thompson JL. Energy balance in young athletes. *Int J Sport Nutr*. 1998;8:160-174.
14. Benardot D, Schwarz M, Heller DW. Nutrient intake in young highly competitive gymnasts. *J Am Diet Assoc*. 1989;89:401-403.
15. Reggiani E, Arras GB, Trabacca S, Senarega D, Chiodini G. Nutrition status and body composition of adolescent female gymnasts. *J Sports Med Phys Fitness*. 1989;29:285-288.
16. Jonnalagadda SSJ, Benardot D, Nelson M. Energy and nutrient intakes of the United States National Women's Artistic Gymnastics Team. *Int J Sport Nutr*. 1998;8:331-334.
17. O'Connor PJ, Lewis RD, Boyd A. Health concerns of artistic women gymnasts. *Sports Med*. 1996;21:321-325.
18. Theintz GE, Howald H, Weiss N, Syonenke PC. Evidence for a reduction of growth potential in adolescent female gymnasts. *J Pediatr*. 1993;122:306-313.
19. Nattiv A, Mandelbaum BR. Injuries and special concerns in female gymnasts. Detecting, treating and preventing common problems. *Phys Sports Med*. 1998;21:66-81.
20. The American Dietetic Association. Timely statement of The American Dietetic Association: nutrition for adolescent athletes in organized sports. *J Am Diet Assoc*. 1996;96:611-612.

21. Coggan AR, Coyle EF. Effect of carbohydrate feedings during high-intensity exercise. *J Appl Physiol.* 1988;65:1703-1705.

22. Coleman EJ. Carbohydrate—the master fuel. In: Berning JR, Steen SN, eds. *Nutrition for Sports and Fitness.* Gaithersburg, Md: Aspen Publishers; 1998:21-25.

23. Snyder AC, Naik J. Protein requirements of athletes. In: Berning JR, Steen SN, eds. *Nutrition for Sports and Fitness.* Gaithersburg, Md: Aspen Publishers; 1998:45-57.

24. Coleman E, Steen SN. Protein: the great debate. In: Coleman E, Steen SN. *The Ultimate Sports Nutrition Handbook.* Palo Alto, Calif: Bull Publishing Co; 1996:57-64.

25. Nickols-Richardson S, Lewis R, O'Connor P. Gymnastic exercise, dietary intake, and body image: determinants of bone health in prepubescent girls. *SCAN's Pulse.* 1996;15:12-13.

26. O'Connor PJ, Lewis RD, Kirchner EM, Cook DB. Eating disorder symptoms in former female college gymnasts: relations with body composition. *Am J Clin Nutr.* 1996;64:840-843.

27. Heany RP. Calcium intake in the osteoporotic fracture context: introduction. *Am J Clin Nutr.* 1991;54:S242-S244.

28. Craig WJ. Phytochemicals: guardians of our health. *J Am Diet Assoc.* 1997;97(suppl 2):S199-S204.

29. American College of Sports Medicine. Position stand on exercise and fluid replacement. *Med Sci Sports Exerc.* 1996;28:i-vii.

30. American Psychiatric Association. *Diagnostic and Statistical Manual of Mental Disorders: IV.* 4th ed. Washington, DC: American Psychiatric Association; 1994.

31. Johnson MD. Disordered eating in active and athletic women. *Clin Sports Med.* 1994;13:355-369.

32. Nattiv A, Agostini R, Drinkwater B, Yeager KK. The female athlete triad. *Clin Sports Med.* 1994;13:405-418.

33. Rosen LW, Hough DO. Pathogenic weight-control behaviors of female college gymnasts. *Phys Sports Med.* 1988;16:141-145.

34. Rosen LW, McKeag DB, Hough DP, et al. Pathogenic weight-control behavior in female athletes. *Phys Sports Med.* 1986;14:79-86.

35. *Code of Points. Frequently Asked Questions.* http://www.usa-gymnastics.org/faq/019.html. Accessed September 14, 1999.

36. USAG Task Force. USA Gymnastics response to the female athlete triad. *Technique.* 1995;15:16-22.

37. Tofler IR, Stryer BK, Micheli LJ, Herman LR. Physical and emotional problems of elite female gymnasts. *N Engl J Med.* 1996;335:281-283.

38. Ryan J. *Little Girls in Pretty Boxes: The Making and Breaking of Elite Gymnasts and Figure Skaters.* New York, NY: Doubleday; 1995.

39. USA Gymnastics Athlete Wellness Program. In: Theis-Marshall N, ed. *The Athlete Wellness Book.* Indianapolis, Ind: USA Gymnastics Publications; 1998:viii.

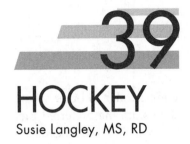

39

HOCKEY

Susie Langley, MS, RD

Ice hockey is a sport of speed, power, stamina, and flexibility. It utilizes both the aerobic and anaerobic pathways, and is played at such high speed that is has been called the fastest team sport ever. It can also be one of the roughest sports, making it very exciting to play and watch—whether at the amateur, collegiate, or professional level (1).

Successful hockey players need muscular strength and conditioning for fast acceleration, quick stopping, and constant physical contact. Sprinting down the ice in 45- to 90-second shifts, shooting the puck at 160 km per hour, checking opponents, and enduring three 20-minute periods of play can be exhausting. Hockey is the only major sport that allows player substitution while a game is in progress. Although each shift can be less than a minute, key players may accumulate 17 to 30 minutes of ice time before the final buzzer (2).

Hockey players can expend 3,000 to 6,000 kcal or more per day. Therefore, a nutrition game plan is crucial in order to survive grueling competitive season and postseason play. Maintaining weight and avoiding injury are difficult to achieve given the physical and psychological stress of consecutive workouts, back-to-back games, and constant travel.

A poorly fueled player is at increased risk of injury. Dehydration and depleted muscle glycogen cause many hockey players to "fade" in the third period or overtime—just when high energy and split-second decisions are needed to make a crucial goal. Today's athletes also need to be made aware that magic bullets like creatine cannot replace the energy from a well-balanced, high-carbohydrate diet throughout a demanding competitive season.

ENERGY NEEDS

A 150-lb (68 kg) hockey player requires about 72 kcal/kg and therefore needs about 5,400 kcal per day (3). (Example: 68 kg x 72 kcal/kg/day = 4,900 kcal + 10% TEF (thermic effect of food) = 4,900 + 490 = 5,390 kcal). Professional hockey players in the weight range of 180 to 210 lb (82 to 95 kg) burn 12 to 14 kcal per minute (4,5). Therefore, in 45 minutes of intense practice, a 180-lb player burns 544 calories (45 x 12.1 kcal/min = 544 kcal). This is in addition to usual daily energy needs.

MACRONUTRIENT NEEDS

The macronutrient recommendations for ice hockey are similar to other sports such as field hockey, soccer, and lacrosse. Carbohydrates are the preferred fuel and are most often underconsumed if energy intake is low (6,7). Protein needs are higher for strength athletes, like hockey players, where there is a significant amount of body checking and wear and tear on muscles, tendons, bones, and teeth. Hockey players have been reported to get more than enough dietary protein (7). However, red-meat restricters or vegetarians with lower intakes of protein may experience delayed growth and maturation and decreased ability to gain or maintain muscle mass. Health-conscious hockey players may choose low-fat products, avoiding red meat, eggs, and dairy foods without good reason. They should be educated about the role of dietary fats and cholesterol for optimum health and disease prevention. *Box 39.1* presents the recommended macronutrient needs and suggested distribution of carbohydrates, protein, and fat for hockey players.

BOX 39.1 Macronutrient Needs and Suggested Distribution for Hockey Players	
60%-65%	Carbohydrate
15%-18%	Protein
20%-30%	Fat

WEIGHT GAIN

Young hockey players who desire to gain more muscle mass are easily lured by advertisements for costly protein and amino acid supplements or the latest ergogenic aids (8). Adolescent athletes need extra protein (1.4 to 1.8 g/kg/body weight (BW)) for growth and building muscle mass (9). They also need a safe program of progressive weight training with appropriate rest days to allow the muscle to hypertrophy. It is recommended that children under the age of 13 not participate in isokinetic exercising or weight training (1).

Sports nutritionists need to assess the athlete's energy input and output before planning meals for weight gain. Consuming regular meals and snacks is essential. Skipping meals and snacks will delay weight gain. Adding an extra 500-kcal minimeal or snack daily should allow for about 1 lb weight gain per week. An expected weight gain of 0.5 to 1.0 lb is considered realistic for young athletes.

WEIGHT LOSS

"Making weight" for training camp may require loss of body fat to ≤12% for professional hockey players. Athletes who try to lose weight rapidly risk losing muscle and will have lower glycogen stores with less energy and stamina to demonstrate their true potential. Gradual weight loss started well in advance of the season (2 to 3 months) is advocated to allow loss of body fat while maintaining muscle mass and high energy levels. High-protein, low-carbohydrate diets are not recommended because of the risk of dehydration and muscle glycogen depletion.

MICRONUTRIENT NEEDS

The micronutrient needs for hockey are not different from general sports nutrition recommendations for vitamins and minerals. However, when complex carbohydrates and enriched grain intakes are low, B vitamins, iron, and fiber intakes may also be low. Iron status should be routinely assessed in hockey players who have low dietary intakes of iron or excessive blood loss through injury or surgery. Low intakes of fruits and vegetables have been reported in hockey players (7). This could result in low intake of antioxidants, fiber, and potassium.

FLUID NEEDS

Hockey players can lose from 3 to 10 lb of fluid in a game (2). Often they are seen spitting out water instead of drinking 4 to 6 oz every shift. Players often say water "sloshes" in their stomach and so avoid drinking fluids. What they may not realize is that dehydration can delay gastric emptying, and the "sloshing" may mean they are already dehydrated (10). Pregame hydration and sipping water or sports drinks throughout play can help prevent dehydration. Drinking fluids on a schedule before, during, and after training and competition should be enforced by the team sport nutritionist and hockey staff. Losing more than 3% body weight in a game is not advisable. Each pound of sweat loss should be replaced with 20 oz (600 mL) of fluid (11). For example, a 180-lb hockey player who loses 3% body weight through sweat is losing 5.4 lb. He would need 5.4 x 20 oz = 108 oz or 13.5 cups of fluid (about 1.5 L) to replace these losses.

Goalies are especially susceptible to dehydration since the weight of heavy equipment causes them to sweat more readily. They need a strategy for keeping water and sports drinks handy to maintain mental alertness and avoid overheating and fatigue. The sport nutritionist should discuss the best possible fluid options with the player, trainer, and medical staff.

Stress can also impact blood sugar levels causing energy slumps, lightheadedness, confusion, and slower reaction time. Encourage athletes to eat ample complex carbohydrates and fewer simple sugars in the pregame meal and in snacks to maintain normal blood sugar.

Drinking an appropriately formulated sports drink before the game and during play may help maintain a constant energy level throughout three 20-minute periods of play (12). Very young athletes do not necessarily need sports drinks and should drink cool water and fruit juice (regular or diluted with equal parts juice to water) as desired. However, it has been shown that elite young athletes will voluntarily drink more fluids and stay better hydrated when drinking a carbohydrate- and sodium-containing beverage in a preferred flavor (13).

Many athletes do not realize that regular soft drinks and fruit juices have almost twice the simple sugar concentration of well-designed sports drinks and during play may cause discomfort or trigger reactive hypoglycemia in sensitive individuals. High-sugar drinks and other foods with a high glycemic index are best consumed postgame when they may promote muscle glycogen repletion (9). *Table 39.1* demonstrates the amount of carbohydrate replacement needed for athletes based on 1 g of carbohydrate per kilogram of body weight. *Table 39.2* lists common carbohydrate-rich food choices for replenishing glycogen stores.

After a practice or a game, hockey players should not leave the locker room until they are hydrated. Cool water is usually preferred after the heat of the game. However, sports drinks, fruit juices, and carbohydrate-rich drinks are recommended to replace glycogen stores within the first 15 to 30 minutes postgame. Often, professional athletes are fatigued or emotionally charged postgame and

TABLE 39.1   Postevent Carbohydrate Replacement

Body Weight	CHO (g)
150 lb (68 kg)	68
160 lb (73 kg)	73
180 lb (82 kg)	82
200 lb (91 kg)	91
220 lb (100 kg)	100
240 lb (109 kg)	109

Example: A 185-lb (84-kg) NHL forward would need 84 g of carbohydrate to replace glycogen stores postgame. That could be fulfilled by drinking a carbohydrate-loading drink (such as GatorLode: 14 oz = 82 g carbohydrate) and 2 hours later eating a meal that provides at least 84 g of carbohydrate-rich foods with moderate protein and fat. Muscles are the most receptive to loading more glycogen in the first 15 to 30 minutes following exhaustive exercise or competition and up to 2 hours later when a balanced meal is frequently eaten.

TABLE 39.2   Common Carbohydrate Foods for Recovery

Food	Amount	CHO (g)	Amount of Food Equal to 100 g CHO
Rice, cooked	1 cup	50	2 cups
Pasta, cooked	1 cup	34	3 cups
Bagel	1	31	3 medium
English muffin	1	30	3
Bran muffin	1 large (4 oz)	49	2
Oatmeal, regular	1 cup	24	4 cups
Raisin bran	1 cup	42	2 1/2 cups
Grapenuts	1 cup	89	1 cup
Muslix	1 cup	60	1 3/4 cups
Low-fat granola cereal	1 cup	85	1 1/4 cups
Whole-wheat bread	1 slice	12	8
Cornbread	4" square	56	2
Bun, hamburger	1	21	4
Pancakes	2 (4" diameter)	18	12
Granola bar	1	16	6
Fig bar	1	10	10
Oatmeal raisin cookie	1	9	10
Date square	1 (60 g)	30	3
Banana bread	1 slice (60 g)	33	3 slices

continued

TABLE 39.2   Common Carbohydrate Foods for Recovery (continued)

Food	Amount	CHO (g)	Amount of Food Equal to 100 g CHO
Fast-food animal cookies	1 serving	39	2¹/2 servings
Pizza (cheese)	1 slice	39	2¹/2 slices
Bean burrito	1	32	3
Raisins, seedless	¹/2 cup	59	³/4 cup
Applesauce	1 cup	60	³/4 cup
Grapes	1 cup	37	2 cups
Fruit cocktail	1 cup	28	3 cups
Banana	1	27	4
Potato, baked	1 large	50	2
Potato, mashed	1 cup	35	3 cups
Sweet potato	1 large	28	3
Corn	1 cup	42	2¹/2 cups
Green peas	1 cup	24	4 cups
Fast-food chili	1 cup	22	5 cups
Lima beans, cooked	1 cup	39	2¹/2 cups
Kidney beans	1 cup	40	2¹/2 cups
Baked beans	1 cup	52	2 cups
Split pea soup	1 cup	28	4 cups
Chunky bean/ham soup	1 cup	27	4 cups
Milk	1 cup	12	8 cups
Frozen yogurt, low-fat	1 cup	34	3 cups
Pudding, chocolate	1 cup	60	1³/4 cups
Low-fat vanilla shake	1 serving	72	1¹/3 serving
Chocolate sundae	1 serving	53	2 servings
Gatorade	8 oz	14	7 cups (56 oz)
AllSport	8 oz	19	5¹/4 cups (42 oz)
PowerAde	8 oz	19	5¹/4 cups (42 oz)
GatorPro	8 oz	58	1³/4 cups (14 oz)
GatorLode	12 oz	70	2 cups (16 oz)
Orange juice	1 cup	26	4 cups
Apple juice	1 cup	28	3¹/2 cups
Cranberry juice	1 cup	36	3 cups
Cola, regular	1 cup	26	4 cups
Soda, fruit flavor	1 cup	28	3¹/2 cups
Power bar	1 (63 g)	41	2¹/2 bars
Crunchy granola bar	1 (46 g)	16	6 bars
Chewy granola bar	1 (28 g)	21	5 bars
Boost chocolate crunch bar	1 (50 g)	30	3¹/3 bars

1 cup = 8 oz (240 mL)

lose their appetite. Carbohydrate-containing drinks and balanced liquid meal replacement drinks should be available to provide fluid, energy, and essential nutrients. Elite hockey players should avoid alcohol during training and competition. If alcohol is consumed socially, postgame fluid loss should be replaced with water and sports drinks prior to consuming alcohol. Alcohol is a diuretic and a central nervous system depressant. The most common symptoms of a hangover are primarily due to dehydration.

ERGOGENIC AIDS

The most common ergogenic aids currently used by hockey players include sports drinks, protein and amino acid supplements, creatine, energy bars, antioxidants, beta-hydroxy beta-methyl butyrate (HMB), and ephedrine (ma huang) (14,15).

Creatine

Creatine is a popular ergogenic aid used by hockey players. Anecdotal reports from hockey trainers suggest it improves anaerobic strength to train longer at a high level of intensity but seems to decrease aerobic performance. The only known side effect of creatine is weight gain. There has been some concern, although not proven, that creatine may increase the risk of muscle tearing and therefore increase the risk of groin injuries (16-19). At the present there are no long-term studies on the effects of creatine in athletes (18). However, there is one report of a soccer player with preexisting kidney disease who suffered kidney dysfunction following creatine supplementation at the level recommended by the manufacturer (19).

Athletes who take creatine supplements should be advised about proper dose loading, maintenance levels, and adequate fluid intakes. However, there is growing concern about the ethics of using ergogenic aids such as creatine, especially in young athletes, due to the potential of its use encouraging more harmful drugs in the future. Young athletes taking creatine anecdotally report some cramping and diarrhea, or loss of gained weight when creatine is stopped. Sport nutritionists should monitor an athlete's diet for adequate high-quality protein intake and emphasize that diets low in energy and carbohydrate intake will have a more negative impact on the ability to train and compete at a high level, than the supposedly positive benefits of creatine.

Protein and Amino Acid Supplements

Use of egg whites, whey protein, and amino acid supplements is popular among rookies to boost power during summer training. The use of raw egg whites is discouraged due to the increased risk of salmonella poisoning and biotin deficiency. Sports nutritionists can educate athletes to choose more tasty and economical protein choices than protein powders or raw egg whites. Many fine educational materials have been developed (ie, materials from Gatorade Sports Science Institute (GSSI) and SCAN) for professionals who are counseling athletes to evaluate the use of protein supplements for gain of lean muscle mass (8,9,14,20).

Sports nutritionists should help athletes understand where they can find protein and amino acids in foods by comparing the content of common foods to amino acid supplement labels. For example, 3 oz of meat, chicken, or fish or 1 1/2 cups of cooked legumes contain 2,000 mg of branched-chain amino acids—more than the amount found in most supplements (21).

Sport drinks are the most common ergogenic aids used successfully in hockey. Sports nutritionists are often asked by hockey trainers to evaluate new sport drinks, energy bars, and vitamin/mineral supplements.

High-protein, high-calorie milkshakes or smoothies, and commercial instant breakfast beverages can be a convenient source of essential amino acids, vitamins, and minerals, and may also be recommended as a tasty and nutritious way to promote healthy weight gain or to prevent weight loss during the hockey season (9,16). Fortified, medical nutritional supplements and meal replacement drinks are also a convenient source of balanced nutrition with high-quality protein that may enhance carbohydrate uptake for glycogen repletion postevent. Many supplements are lactose-free and gluten-free.

PRE- AND POSTGAME MEALS

Hockey players have the same precompetition food or fluid requirements as other athletes, and nutrition recommendations for training are not much different than for competition. The pregame meal should be high in carbohydrate, moderate in protein, and low in fat and fiber. High-fat meals, fried foods, excess simple sugars, and carbonated drinks should be avoided prior to competition. The importance of eating breakfast and making healthy snack and fast-food choices should be part of educating athletes with busy lifestyles. Young rookies living away from home for the first time need advice on shopping and simple strategies for preparing quick and easy meals and snacks.

In professional hockey the pregame meal is often eaten 5 or 6 hours in advance of the evening game. The players usually rest and meet for a pregame snack 2 hours before game time. Individuals who are volume-sensitive (feel full easily) may need to eat more frequently. Use of candy bars and carbonated drinks immediately pregame is discouraged in favor of adequate water and sport drinks (ie, 8 oz of 6% to 8% carbohydrate 15 to 30 minutes before the game). Those who get "pregame jitters" (nervous stomachs) may want to experiment with a chilled liquid meal replacement beverage that can be sipped up to an hour before game time. New products should always be tested during training and never during competition.

Postgame meals are often more important than pregame meals if the athlete is training intensively and playing back-to-back games. Replacing depleted glycogen with a meal high in carbohydrate, moderate in protein, and low in fat is often difficult to achieve due to constant travel, eating on the road, fatigue, lack of appetite, or lack of knowledge. The carbohydrate rule for recovery is 1 g/kg/BW (0.5 g/lb). Athletes should start replacing carbohydrates within the first 15 to 30 minutes after exhaustive exercise and repeat the same every 2 hours for 6 to 8 hours (9). Athletes should be advised to choose a variety of these foods and fluids postgame to replace muscle glycogen based on 1 g/kg/BW. Elite hockey players should be consuming around 600 g of carbohydrates per day during the National

Hockey League (NHL) season. This is based on the need for 7 to 10 g carbohydrates/kg/BW per day.

Consulting with the coaching staff, team chef, and significant others about meal planning can be both challenging and rewarding in helping the athlete achieve optimum fuel and fluid needs.

TOP NUTRITION CONCERNS

1. Gaining or losing weight healthfully
- Add 500 extra kcal per day to build muscle.
- Subtract about 500 kcal per day to lose 1 lb per week.
- Expect about a 0.5 to 1.0 lb per week weight gain or loss.
- Assure adequate energy from a high-carbohydrate, moderate-protein, low-fat diet. Protein needs are higher for growing adolescents building muscle mass.
- Dispel myths about the benefits of high-protein diets or protein and amino acid supplements for muscle-building and weight gain.
- Discuss pros and cons of ergogenic aids such as creatine, HMB, ephedrine, or supplements promoted for weight gain or weight loss, and educate athletes about how to evaluate supplement claims.
- Make practical suggestions for healthy meals, snacks, and fluids.

2. Proper hydration
- Educate athletes on the appropriate use of water, sports drinks, and other fluids, including the negative effects of caffeine-containing beverages and alcohol.
- Determine average fluid loss in athletes through pre- and postgame weight records (see Chapter 6, Fluid and Electrolytes).
- Provide a practical fluid schedule to maintain optimal hydration status on a daily basis throughout training and competition.
- Enforce a fluid schedule before, during, and after practice or games.

3. Adequate carbohydrate intake
- Educate athletes about food sources of carbohydrates to refuel depleted muscle glycogen.
- Encourage a high-carbohydrate diet year round for training and competition.
- Discuss complex versus simple carbohydrates for short versus long-lasting energy sources.
- Educate athletes on the appropriate use of sports drinks before, during, and after exhaustive exercise.
- Offer practical suggestions for postevent replacement of fluids and carbohydrates.
- Help prepare a shopping list for meals and snacks high in carbohydrate.
- Provide a list of portable high carbohydrate snacks to eat at home and on the road.

POINTERS FOR WORKING WITH COACHES AND TRAINERS

- Build a good rapport with the athletic trainer and coaching staff.
- Develop strategies to keep in touch and to reinforce the special expertise of the sports nutritionist.
- Be professional and establish regular contact by phone, fax, e-mail, or letter.
- Suggest establishing a nutrition screening or assessment during team physicals at training camp.
- Propose providing a talk or workshop with the team and staff at training camp or during season breaks.
- Keep the message simple—a difficult task at times. Reinforce and repeat simple concepts on basic fuels and fluids to assure optimum nutrition for the entire team.
- Suggest that rookies and top draft picks keep food records during spring or summer training camp and recommend simple, practical changes that can be monitored easily by the hockey staff.
- Formulate individual high-performance nutrition plans that are simple and practical.
- Be available for last-minute consults with professional athletes who have hectic schedules.
- Realize that follow-up is difficult given busy schedules, travel, and unexpected time demands.
- Translate pre-and postgame meals and snacks for the team using a live food demonstration, or display samples of basic fuels, fluids, and ergogenic aids to stimulate open discussion.
- Suggest a fluid schedule and provide the latest information on sports drinks.
- Stay up-to-date on the latest ergogenic aids and help keep the trainer informed.
- Keep up with the team's progress and attend games when possible.
- Help plan a training table at the home rink and on the road, with ideas for breakfast foods, pregame and postgame meals, airline meals, and restaurant choices during travel.
- Ask to set up a supermarket tour to educate the team and/or their partners.
- When there are language barriers, be prepared to work with a translator.
- Volunteer to do an informal talk or provide a pot luck meal to promote high-performance nutrition with partners or parents of team members.
- Ask the trainer for a referral to work with an NHL farm team.
- Learn all you can about the sport. Resources can be found in *Box 39.2.*

BOX 39.2	Resources on Hockey
The Hockey News	The definitive guide and one of the most popular magazines on hockey
NHL Yearbook	Published by *The Hockey News*. Detailed statistics.
1997-1998 Yearbook	Published by *The Hockey News* for each season. Colorful, entertaining, and a great way to get excited about the season
NHL Hockey	http://www.nhl.com
United States Hockey	http://www.usahockey.com
Canadian Hockey	http://www.canadianhockey.com
Women's Hockey	http://www.usahockey.com/girls.htm
NHL, AHL, CHL, Juniors, Women	http://www.plaidworks.com

CASE STUDY

Scott is a 19-year-old rookie referred during summer training for a high-performance nutrition plan. His goal is to gain about 8 to 10 lb in 2 months and to improve his eating habits before returning to the university on a hockey scholarship. He wants to start taking creatine like some of his teammates and asks about using HMB. The coach thinks he has NHL potential and Scott wants to do all he can to get "the edge." When asked about his fluid intake and pre- and postgame meals, he said he had no particular schedule but usually gets very nervous before each game. He often lacks energy to make it through tough workouts and says he starts to fade by the middle of the third period. He is a serious student and manages to squeeze in other extracurricular activities in addition to hockey.

Height: 71 in (180 cm)	Body fat: 9%
Weight: 167 lb (76 kg)	Goal weight: 176 lb (80 kg)
Frame: medium	Activity level: extremely active
BMI: 23.2	

Boxes 39.3 and *39.4* show Scott's typical diet and energy needs during his summer training period.

BOX 39.3	Typical Summer Training Diet
9:00 AM	8 oz orange juice, 3 scrambled eggs, 1 slice toast
12:30 PM	Slice of double cheese and pepperoni pizza
	12 oz regular cola
4:00 PM	Whey protein supplement shake made with 8 oz pineapple juice
6:30 PM	12 oz steak, 1 baked potato with butter, Caesar salad
	Piece of apple pie and 12 oz 2% milk
11:00 PM	Two chocolate chip cookies and 12 oz diet cola
Analysis: 3,700 kcal, 33% carbohydrate, 24% protein, 44% fat	

BOX 39.4	Summer Training Program
2 hours per day, 5 days per week (10 hours per week)	
Energy output: ~1,000 kcal per session (on average ~700 kcal extra per day)	

Assessment

- Usual intake is low in complex carbohydrates (low in grains, vegetables, and fruit with more simple sugars from cola and cookies). Does not provide enough carbohydrate to sustain heavy workouts for training and competition.
- Excess protein is not needed to build muscle. May contribute to dehydration and place heavier work load on liver and kidneys. Expensive supplements are not necessary.
- High intake of total fat, saturated fat, and cholesterol. May gain undesirable body fat.
- Needs help with timing and planning of meals and snacks.
- Needs education about the pros and cons of whey protein supplements, creatine, and HMB, and the appropriate use of sport drinks.
- Needs information about balanced meal replacement beverages for pregame jitters.
- Needs to set priorities for school and hockey. Too little time for proper meals and rest will affect performance in both areas.

Recommendations

- Eat more whole-grain breads, cereals, and starchy vegetables for adequate energy and optimum muscle and liver glycogen stores.
- Eat more fresh fruits and vegetables for important vitamins, minerals, and fiber.
- Dispel myths about high-protein diets for building muscle. Explain the role of energy and nutrients along with a graduated weight-training program for building muscle.
- Expect about 1/2 lb per week of muscle gain. Start well in advance of the season.
- Educate about protein and amino acid supplements, creatine, and HMB and their relationship to an overall well-balanced diet and adequate carbohydrates.
- Design a meal plan with realistic timing for meals, snacks, and fluids.
- Outline a sensible fluid schedule for training and competition.
- Educate on fast foods, shopping, and quick-and-easy meals and snacks away from home.
- Monitor weight gain and body composition via communication with trainer.
- Stay in touch with the athlete and trainer for continued success. E-mail can be an effective way to communicate with collegiate athletes.

Boxes 39.5 and 39.6 illustrate recommendations for Scott's diet and suggestions for pre- and postgame meal plans.

BOX 39.5   Sample Meal Plan for a Training Diet

7:30 AM	Out of bed
8:00 AM	8 oz orange juice, 2 cups fortified breakfast cereal, 8 oz low-fat milk, banana
	Two slices multigrain toast with soft margarine and jam
	Water
10:00 AM	Training program: strength and conditioning
12:00 PM	Water
1:00 PM	Two turkey sandwiches *or* 12-inch turkey sub with lettuce, tomato, light mayonnaise and raw vegetable sticks
	8 oz low-fat milk or yogurt
	1 apple
	12 oz cranberry-apple juice
3:00 PM	Water
4:00 PM	High-protein fruit smoothie, 2-4 oatmeal cookies *or* 1 energy bar
6:30 PM	4 oz lean beef, 1 large baked potato, 1 pat butter
	1 cup mixed vegetables and garden salad, 2 T vinaigrette
	Fruit cobbler
	Water
10:30 PM	8 oz hot chocolate with 8 oz low-fat milk
	Peanut butter and jam sandwich *or* 6 cups microwave popcorn *or* Cereal, milk, and fruit
	Water

Analysis: 4,500 kcal, 60% to 65% carbohydrate, 15% protein, 20% to 30% fat

---

BOX 39.6   Recommendations for a Pre- and Postgame Meal Plan

1:00 PM	Pregame meal with team:
	4 oz baked chicken breast and 3 cups pasta
	1 cup steamed carrots, small garden salad with 1 T Italian dressing
	1 dinner roll with 1 t soft margarine
	1 cup low-fat frozen yogurt and 2 oatmeal cookies
	10 oz apple juice or low-fat milk
	Water
5:00 PM	Pregame snack with team:
	16 oz water *or* 8 to 10 oz fruit juice *or* sports drink as tolerated
	1 cup applesauce
	1 to 2 slices Italian bread with jam
7:00 PM	8 to 16 oz water (240 to 500 mL)
7:15 PM	8 oz water *or* sports drink
7:30 PM	Game begins:
	4 to 6 oz water *or* sports drink every shift, every time
	At least 2 to 4 cups water *or* sports drink between periods
10:15 PM	Game ends:
	Drink 20 to 24 oz water *or* sports drink for every pound of sweat loss.
	On the road: Carbohydrate-loading sport drink *or* liquid meal replacement
	Beverage may be used by elite players when appropriate.
11:30 PM to 12:00 AM	Postgame meal (home, en route, or hotel):
	4 oz lean meat, poultry, *or* fish
	2 to 3 cups rice, pasta, *or* large potato with margarine
	1 cup cooked vegetables *or* garden salad with dressing
	8 oz low-fat milk *or* low-fat frozen yogurt
	2 to 4 oatmeal raisin and chocolate chip cookies
1:00 AM	Retire

REFERENCES

1. Coles Notes. *Mom's and Dad's Guide to Hockey for Kids*. Toronto, Canada; 1998.
2. Burns J, Dugan L. Working with professional athletes in the rink: the evolution of a nutrition program for an NHL team. *Int J Sport Nutr*. 1994;4:132-134.
3. Paul PH, Snyder A. Predicting energy expenditure. In: Bernardot D, ed. *Sports Nutrition: A Guide for the Professional Working with Active People*. 2nd ed. Chicago, Ill: The American Dietetic Association; 1992:21-25.
4. Coleman E, Nelson-Steen S. *The Ultimate Sports Nutrition Handbook*. Palo Alto, Calif: Bull Publishing Co; 1996.
5. Williams MH. *Nutrition for Health, Fitness and Sport*. 5th ed. Boston, Mass: WCB-McGraw Hill; 1999.
6. Akermark C, Jacobs I, Rasmusson M, Karlson J. Diet and muscle glycogen concentration in relation to physical performance in Swedish elite ice hockey players. *Int J Sport Nutr*. 1996;6:272-284.
7. Houston ME. Nutrition and ice hockey performance. *Can J Appl Sport Sci*. 1979;4:98-99.
8. Roundtable. Methods for weight gain in athletes. *Sports Sci Exch*. 1995;6(3).
9. Clark N. *Nancy Clark's Sport Nutrition*. Champaign, Ill: Human Kinetics; 1997.
10. Maughn R, Rehrer N. Gastric emptying during exercise. *Sports Sci Exch*. 1993;6(5).
11. Gonzalez-Alonso J, Heaps C, Coyle E. Rehydration after exercise with common beverages and water. *Int J Sports Med*. 1992;13:399-406.
12. Davis M, Jackson D, Broadwell M, Queary J, Lambert C. Carbohydrate drinks delay fatigue during intermittent, high intensity cycling in active men and women. *Int J Sport Nutr*. 1997;7:261-173.
13. Rivera-Brown A, Gutierrez R, Gutierrez J, Frontera W, Bar-Or O. Drink composition, voluntary drinking and fluid balance in exercising, trained, heat acclimatized boys. *J Appl Physiol*. 1999;86:78-84.
14. Clarkson P. Nutritional supplements for weight gain. *Sports Sci Exch*. 1998;11(1).
15. Nissen S, Fuller J Jr. HMB (Beta-hydroxy beta-methylglutarate) supplementation and exercise. *SCAN's Pulse*. 1998;17:1-3.
16. Kleiner S, Greenwood-Robinson M. *Power Eating*. Champaign, Ill: Human Kinetics; 1998.
17. Volek J. Creatine monohydrate: is it a performance enhancer? *SCAN's Pulse*. 1996;l:5-6.
18. Kreider R. Creatine supplementation: analysis of ergogenic value, medical safety, and concerns. *J Exerc Physiol*. 1998;1(1). http://www/css.edu/users/tboone2/asep/jan.htlm. Accessed July 14, 1999.
19. Pritchard NR, Kalra PA. Renal dysfunction accompanying oral creatine supplements. *Lancet*. 1998;351:1252-1253.
20. Rosenbloom C, Storlie JA. Nutritionist's guide to evaluating ergogenic aids. *SCAN's Pulse*. 1998;17:1-5.
21. Applegate L. Protein power. *Runner's World*. 1992:22-23.

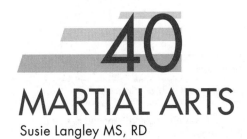

MARTIAL ARTS

Susie Langley MS, RD

The increasing popularity of the martial arts and their current evolution as "sporting" events are opening the door for sport nutritionists (1-5). Movies such as "The Karate Kid" and "Enter the Dragon" with Bruce Lee, and the "Teenage Mutant Ninja Turtles" saga confirm the popularity of the martial arts in all age groups. In 1995 there were an estimated 75 million participants in the martial arts internationally, with 8 million in the United States alone, with women making up the fastest-growing segment (2,3).

The term "martial arts" encompasses those activities concerned with combat and the waging of war (see *Box 40.1*) (1). According to Dr. Jason Su, a sports medicine fellow at the University of Toronto and martial arts expert, there are literally thousands of different styles of martial arts. During the 20th century some developed into organized sports with rules and regulations set forth by official governing bodies. Boxing, wrestling, fencing, and target shooting were historically included among the ancient martial arts. The martial arts that are a part of the Olympic games are judo, taekwondo, and boxing.

BOX 40.1   Martial Arts (1)

Karate	Sumo	Escrima
Judo	Shorinji Kempo	Pentjak Silat
Aikido	Jodo	Taekwondo
Jujitsu	Chinese Kung Fu	Kick Boxing
Kendo	Tai Chi Chuan	Savate
Iaido	H'sing-I Chuan	Indian Martial Arts
Kyudo	Pakua	Hydrids
Ryukyu Kobujutsu	Wushu	
Ninjutsu & Shriken-Do	Wing Chun Kung Fu	

The martial arts represent a true integration of mental and physical skill and demand a high degree of strength, flexibility, speed, agility, explosiveness, and concentration. Participants are attracted to the martial arts for a variety of reasons including self-defense, physical fitness, artistic and spiritual expression, self-discipline, and self-esteem.

For simplicity, the martial arts are subdivided into the categories shown in *Box 40.2*. This chapter will focus on taekwondo with a brief mention of judo and karate since these have become recognized sports in North America.

BOX 40.2   Selected Categories to Classify Martial Arts

1. **Striking arts.** The predominant focus is on hitting an opponent with various parts of one's own body. Includes karate, taekwondo, and kick boxing.
2. **Grappling arts.** The predominant focus is on grappling, throwing, choking, joint controls, and disarticulations. Includes judo, aikido, sumo wrestling, shoot fighting, and jujitsu.
3. **Weapon arts.** These include kendo (fencing), iaido (sword combat), kyudo (archery), target shooting, and jodo (stick or staff).
4. **Hybrid arts.** These have multiple elements of the above and include hapkido, jeet kune do (Bruce Lee system), and certain styles of Phillipino, Indonesian, and Chinese (combat) systems.

TAEKWONDO

Taekwondo ("way of the foot and fist") is fast becoming one of the most popular martial arts and is Korea's national sport (1,3). It is similar to karate and noted for its high kicks and emphasis on breaking or destruction techniques. Taekwondo was previewed as an Olympic sport in 1988 in Seoul, Korea and will become an Olympic event in the year 2000 in Sydney, Australia. The jumping kicks of taekwondo rely on plyometric strength, requiring an explosive muscular action of the legs, driving the body high into the air and thrusting the foot hard into the target with the other foot clear off the floor. Hip joints must be flexible because the leg moves through a wide range of motion. Agility is essential since the kick must be performed without early warning and, with more difficult kicks, the position of the opponent must be visualized at all times (3,4).

During a taekwondo competition the athlete must wear an approved padded jacket as well as head and groin guards. Some female martial artists may also wear a breast guard. Each match consists of three 2-minute bouts (6), with a 1-minute rest between each bout. Competition involves individual bouts held in different weight categories. In 1997 the International Olympic Committee (IOC) set new weight categories for taekwondo (see *Tables 40.1* and *40.2*). The new categories reflect a change in thinking toward healthier weights, especially for women, and may help reduce the risk of dehydration and unhealthy weight-loss practices involved in competing in a lower weight class (6).

TABLE 40.1   Taekwondo: Olympic Weight Divisions (6)

Category	Male (kg)	Female (kg)
1	≤58	≤49
2	58-68	49-57
3	68-80	57-67
4	>80	>67

TABLE 40.2 Taekwondo: Regional and World Class Event Weight Divisions (6)

Category	Male (kg)	Female (kg)
Fin Weight	≤54	≤47
Fly Weight	54-58	47-51
Bantam Weight	58-62	51-55
Feather Weight	62-67	55-59
Light Weight	67-72	59-63
Welter Weight	72-78	63-67
Middle Weight	78-84	67-72
Heavy Weight	>84	>72

Energy Needs

The energy needs for martial arts such as taekwondo, judo, and karate are similar to wrestling and boxing, and a lean, muscular body is desirable. For example, judo and karate athletes at 110 lb (50 kg) expend about 9 kcal per minute versus 9.3 kcal per minute for wrestlers (7,8). Modern martial arts employ both anaerobic energy for explosiveness (eg, executing a flurry of strikes) and aerobic energy for lasting endurance (eg, multiple rounds of fighting and parrying).

Macronutrient Needs

The macronutrient needs for martial arts athletes are similar to other strength-trained athletes such as wrestlers and boxers. General recommendations are 60% to 65% of energy from carbohydrate, 12% to 15% from protein, and 20% to 30% from fat. (Also see Chapter 50, Wrestling.) Carbohydrates are the preferred fuel to supply muscle and liver glycogen and to fuel the brain for split-second decisions and sustain an acute power of concentration. Adequate but not excessive protein (1.2 to 1.7 g/kg) is needed to build and repair muscles, produce blood cells, and maintain a strong immune system. Athletes who consume low-calorie and protein diets, especially those who try to compete in a weight class 10% or more below their usual weight, may risk loss of lean muscle mass, delayed growth, and repair of tissues after injury (9,10). Continued restriction of energy, carbohydrate, protein, and fat, coupled with preoccupation with weight loss, may place both men and women at increased risk for developing an eating disorder (11). For women, overtraining and undereating may slow basal metabolic rate (BMR) and this "energy drain" can lead to menstrual irregularities, risk for overuse injuries, decreased performance, and the female athlete triad (9,12,13). (See Chapter 28, Eating Disorders in Athletes.)

Common symptoms of overtraining and undereating to "make weight" are similar to those of crash dieting—mood swings, fatigue, lethargy, anemia, constipation or diarrhea, decreased libido, and infertility (12,14,15). Very low-fat diets (<10% of energy from fat) and avoidance of animal foods may affect overall health and performance since some fat is needed to help maintain cell membrane integrity, absorb and transport fat-soluble vitamins, synthesize steroid hormones such as estrogen and testosterone, and provide essential fatty acids. A certain amount of body fat is also needed to protect internal organs and insulate nerve fibers.

Micronutrient Needs

The micronutrient needs of martial artists are sparsely reported in the literature. Weight-class martial artists who restrict energy and fluids may be low in thiamin, vitamin B-6, iron, calcium, zinc, magnesium, sodium, potassium, and chloride (9,10,16). Athletes who avoid animal protein and follow low-calorie or strict-vegetarian diets should be monitored for adequate iron, calcium, zinc, and vitamin B-12 (9,10,17).

MAKING WEIGHT

Weight-loss techniques used by weight-class martial artists in taekwondo and judo are similar to those in wrestling where the use of diuretics, laxatives, saunas, rubber suits, and steam rooms, and strict avoidance of food and fluids have become common practice (10,15). Rapid weight loss can adversely affect fluid and electrolyte balance, body composition, thermal regulation, cardiac and renal function, testosterone levels, and strength (18,19). Despite the adverse effects of severe dehydration, Horswill (10) reports that rapid weight loss does not adversely affect high-power exertion lasting less than 30 seconds. In judo competitors, one study (20) showed those who lost weight gradually improved vertical jump height with extra load 6% to 8% compared to no effect for those who lost weight rapidly. However, dehydration does reduce the ability to sustain exercise for longer than 1 or 2 minutes, which means that a dehydrated athlete will not have the endurance to train as hard or last as long in repeated bouts during competition. Glycogen stores may also be depleted by exercise-induced dehydration and food and fluid restriction (10,21). Dehydration can produce the loss of sodium, potassium, chloride, and magnesium (10). It is recommended that safe weight loss (no more than 3 lb per week) should minimize water loss via voluntary dehydration and maximize body-fat loss through a sensible, balanced meal plan. Appropriate cross-training should begin well in advance of the competitive season (10,18,19).

Minimum body fat recommended for martial artists should not fall below 7% for males or 12% for females (9,10). Weight loss ranging from 0.5 to 3.0 lb per week is recommended and should begin at least 3 months ahead of the competitive season. The athlete should be able to focus on optimal training, not on worrying about "making weight" (9,10). Chapter 27, Managing Body Weight discusses weight-loss strategies in detail.

Fluid Needs

Fluid needs for martial artists are the same as for most athletes, except that weight-class athletes need to be carefully monitored to avoid the consequences of severe dehydration including electrolyte imbalance, kidney failure, and death (9,10,22). The use of diuretics, purgatives, and forced sweating techniques to "make weight" before the weigh-in should be discouraged. Many coaches and athletes do not realize that after the weigh-in, at least 48 hours are needed to completely rehydrate (10). During the short time between certification and competition (typically about 4 hours), the consequences of both inadequate hydration and rapid rehydration can have serious consequences to an athlete's health. The risks of rapid rehydration include inappropriate fluid shifts, electrolyte imbalance, and decreased performance (9,10). Water, sports drinks, fruit juice, and other fluids should be recommended before, during, and after competition (23).

PRE- AND POSTEVENT EATING

In weight-class martial arts like judo, karate, and taekwondo, food and fluids are often severely restricted in the days leading up to the event. On the day of the competition, after the early morning weigh-in, martial artists will usually try to consume enough fluids and familiar foods to satisfy their appetite. They are often so hungry and thirsty that they need to be reminded to eat foods high in carbohydrate and low in protein and fat. For some, small amounts of lean protein such as turkey, ham, tuna, or low-fat cheese along with carbohydrate can help settle their stomach and stave off hunger (24). Popular precompetition carbohydrates are bread, bagels, cold cereal, oatmeal, grits, bananas, crackers, rice cakes, rice, boiled potatoes, pasta, low-fat energy bars, oatmeal cookies, fruits, fruit juices, and sports drinks.

In taekwondo, for example, fluids are not consumed during short bouts but should be consumed before and after matches and throughout day-long competitions or weekend tournaments. If the athlete is nervous and unable to eat solid food preevent, a chilled liquid meal replacement beverage can be offered to provide energy and prevent low blood sugar. Postevent, sports drinks, fruit juices, and other carbohydrate-containing fluids are important for replenishing muscle and liver glycogen (23).

ERGOGENIC AIDS

The use of ergogenics in the martial arts is not well documented. Herbal "diet" teas are commonly used as diuretics, and in extreme cases enemas are used in last-minute attempts to make weight. Certain herbal combinations or "stacks," such as ma huang (ephedra), white willow bark (salicylic acid), and kola nut (caffeine), claim to increase metabolic rate and weight loss but can be dangerous (25). Ephedra, the herbal form of ephedrine, acts like an amphetamine and is banned by the IOC (26). Side effects of ephedrine include tremor, nervousness, increased heart rate and blood pressure, myocardial infarction, stroke, seizures, psychoses, and death (9,26,27). Chromium picolinate and polynicotinate have not demonstrated any substantial benefits for losing body fat or gaining muscle (9,10,26,28-30). Whey protein and amino acid supplements may also be popular in the martial arts as with other strength-trained athletes (9,24,26,28,31). The use of creatine among martial artists is unknown, but coaches and athletes should be made aware that long-term studies on its safety are not yet available (26,28,31-34). For more information, see Chapter 7, Ergogenic Aids.

TOP NUTRITION CONCERNS

1. **Making weight safely.**
   - Establish safe weight loss well in advance of the season.
   - Emphasize fat loss versus fluid and muscle loss.
   - Discuss the physiology of starvation and its effect on basal metabolic rate.
   - Discuss the pros and cons of popular ergogenic aids versus a balanced diet.
   - Teach coaches and parents to screen for disordered eating patterns.
   - Communicate with the martial arts team if an individual's weight class seems inappropriate.

2. **Hydrating properly.**
   - Educate coaches and athletes about the consequences of severe dehydration. Athletes, parents, and coaches must know that voluntary dehydration can be life-threatening.
   - Help the coaching staff establish a policy to discourage unsafe dehydration techniques.
   - Establish a fluid schedule for training and competition.
   - Educate athletes about the consequences of rapid rehydration after the weigh-in.
   - Communicate with the sports medicine team if hydration problems exist in athletes.

3. **Choosing healthy meals and snacks for travel and at competitions.**
   - Help athletes plan a list of portable foods and fluids to take when traveling to events.
   - Educate traveling athletes about unfamiliar foods that are safe, accessible, and appropriate sources of carbohydrate.
   - Discuss fluid needs during air travel.
   - Suggest dietary tactics to combat traveler's diarrhea and common gastrointestinal complaints.

WORKING WITH COACHES AND TRAINERS

1. Understand that masters who teach martial arts have not traditionally consulted sports nutritionists. It is essential to understand the coach's philosophy and the background of the sport.
2. Verify realistic weight loss goals within a given timeline with athletes and coaches. Discuss the dangers of voluntary dehydration techniques and rapid weight loss and their effects on health and performance.
3. Demonstrate a successful outcome with a martial artist to show the benefits of good nutrition practices.
4. Volunteer to provide information at an event or practice session.
5. Offer a workshop/seminar for coaches and athletes. Get successful athletes to spread the word about the importance of nutrition to success in their sport.

6. Translate the importance of adequate fluids and electrolytes into a practical fluid schedule for training and competition.
7. Teach coaches and trainers how to recognize signs of eating disorders and how to refer athletes for help.

CASE STUDY

Lori is a 22-year-old elite taekwondo athlete who was referred by her sport physician to "make weight" before a national competition. Returning from an international event, she wanted to qualify for a lower weight class—from bantam weight at 112 lb (50.9 kg) to fly weight at 107 lb (48.6 kg). After several years of "making weight," Lori noted it was harder to drop 5 lb from her slim figure. She occasionally used an herbal diuretic to lose weight and recently tried chromium picolinate without success. Lori's 3-day food record revealed a careful eater, but ethnic foods prepared at home were high in fat. She trained about 12 hours per week and, in addition, worked at a stressful part-time job and maintained high standing at a university. A gold medal winner, Lori expressed her need for sensible nutrition advice. Her body image and eating attitude seemed healthy, but she expressed concern that her recent food obsessions might lead to a full-blown eating disorder.

Factors for Consideration

- Height: 64 in
- Weight: 112 lb (51 kg)
- Frame: small
- BMI: 19
- Body fat: 8%
- Highest adult weight: 118 lb (54 kg at age 20)
- Lowest adult weight: 105 lb (48 kg at age 17)
- Personal weight goal: 107 lb (48.6 kg)

Box 40.3 outlines Lori's training diet.

BOX 40.3	Lori's Training Diet
7:30 AM	Get out of bed
10:30 AM	Banana
1:00 PM	Bagel with light cream cheese, apple juice
7:00 PM	Taekwondo (2 hours)
9:00 PM	Water
9:30 PM	5 oz breaded veal cutlet, fried in olive oil Mixed garden salad dressed with a lot of oil/vinegar dressing Medium potato with olive oil
11:00 PM	1 oz salami 1 oz cheese Apple juice

Menstrual history:

- Menarche: age 14
- Regular menses; taking oral contraceptive pill

Training schedule:

- Taekwondo: 3 to 4 times per week at 90 minutes per session
- Aerobic workout: 4 times per week at 40 minutes per session
- Weight training: 4 times per week at 60 minutes per session
- One rest day per week

Assessment

- While safe weight was below recommendations, the reality of the "win-at-all-costs" attitude makes it sometimes more important to negotiate with elite athletes than risk having them fall victim to more dangerous alternatives in meeting their goal.
- Lori is overtraining and undereating to "make weight" in a lower than usual weight category.
- She risks a potential "energy drain," lowered BMR, disordered eating, and female athlete triad.
- Her pattern is to eat too few calories early in the day with consumption of high-fat foods later in the day.
- The diet is low in calories, protein, iron, B vitamins, calcium, zinc, and other trace minerals.
- Breakfast is too low in calories, complex carbohydrates, and dairy foods.
- Lunch is unbalanced and low in protein, fruit, vegetables, and dairy foods.
- Dinner is high in fat from excess olive oil used in food preparation and low in complex carbohydrates.
- Daily fluid intake is low. Dairy food intake is low. Lori is not meeting calcium needs.
- She allows a large intake of juices high in simple sugar in place of water.
- Diet is low in iron and zinc.

Recommendations

Target: 2,300 kcal, 60% to 65% carbohydrate, 15% to 18% protein, 20% to 25% fat.

Lori's energy needs are greater than 2,300 kcal per day, but this is a sensible compromise since her usual intake is 1,650 kcal per day. A comparison of her target diet versus her actual diet is shown in *Box 40.4*

BOX 40.4 Actual versus Target Intake			
Actual: 1,650 kcal	51% carbohydrate	15% protein	34% fat
Target: 2,300 kcal	60% to 65% carbohydrate	15% to 18% protein	20% to 25% fat

- Eat more enriched complex carbohydrates to meet energy needs and provide B vitamins, iron, and fiber.
- Assure adequate protein, iron, zinc, and calcium from lean meats, low-fat dairy foods, and legumes.
- Space balanced meals and snacks throughout the day to meet energy expenditure for school and for training.
- Build a better breakfast with cereal, fruit, juice, and milk and improve lunch with protein from tuna, and more vegetables and fresh fruit.
- Agree to eat three servings of non-fat milk or yogurt each day.
- Discuss the effects of calorie restriction on fatigue and the risk for eating disorders and female athlete triad.
- Continue eating familiar family foods but minimize olive oil in food preparation.
- Help prepare a shopping list to include lower fat meats, dairy foods, vegetables, fruit, and whole-grain products.
- Suggest portable, healthy snacks and minimeals when on the go.
- Provide education about ergogenic aids and weight-loss products.
- Explain how a negative energy and nutrient balance relates to BMR, fertility, bone health, mood swings, and risk of injury.
- Keep fluid intake at 2 to 3 L per day. Do not restrict fluids.
- Do not weigh-in daily.
- Always work well in advance of the season to "make weight." Discuss realistic weight goals for the off-season.
- Discuss with the master the risks facing young female athletes in "making weight" and how to screen for female athlete triad and eating disorders.

A sample meal plan for Lori is shown in *Box 40.5*.

BOX 40.5   Sample Meal Plan

8:00 AM	1 cup raisin bran cereal, 1 cup skim milk, 4 oz orange juice
10:30 AM	Banana, 1/2 bagel with jam, 8 oz apple juice
1:00 PM	Tuna sandwich: 2 slices multigrain bread, 2 oz water-packed tuna Romain lettuce and tomato, 2 t calorie-reduced mayo 2 plums, water
5:00 PM	Non-fat fruit yogurt, 2 fig bars, water
7:30 PM	Taekwondo training
9:15 PM	Water or 8-oz apple juice
9:30 PM	4 oz grilled, lean veal chop, baked potato, 1 t soft margarine Mixed garden salad with 1 T vinaigrette dressing Steamed spinach, water
11:00 PM	Low-fat French vanilla yogurt, with sliced fresh peach

REFERENCES

1. Crompton P. *The Complete Martial Arts*. Boston, Mass: McGraw-Hill Publishing Co; 1989.
2. Birrer RB. Trauma epidemiology in the martial arts. The result of an eighteen year national survey. *Am J Sports Med*. 1996;24:S72.
3. Mitchell D. *The Complete Book of Martial Arts*. London: Hamlyn Publishing Group Ltd; 1989.
4. Mitchell D. *The New Official Martial Arts Handbook. The Handbook of the Martial Arts Commission of Great Britain*. London: Stanley Paul & Co Ltd; 1989.
5. Corcoran J. *The Martial Arts Sourcebook: The Complete Reference to the Most Frequently Sought Information on the Martial Arts*. New York, NY: Harper Collins Publishers; 1994.
6. World Taekwondo Federation (WTF). *Constitutional Amendments*. Hong Kong: The 13th General Assembly. November 18, 1997.
7. Coleman E, Nelson-Steen S. *The Ultimate Sports Nutrition Handbook*. Palo Alto, Calif: Bull Publishing Co; 1996.
8. Williams M. *Nutrition for Health, Fitness and Sport*. 5th ed. Boston, Mass: WCB-McGraw Hill; 1999.
9. Clarkson P, Manore M, Opplinger B, Steen S, Walberg-Rankin J. Roundtable. Methods and strategies for weight loss in athletes. *Sports Sci Exch*. 1998;9(1).
10. Horswill C. Does rapid weight loss by dehydration adversely affect high-power performance? *Sports Sci Exch.*. 1991;3(30).
11. Benardot D, Engelbert-Fenton K, Freeman K, Hartsought C, Nelson-Steen S. Roundtable. Eating disorders in athletes: the dietician's perspective. *Sports Sci Exch*. 1994;5(4).
12. Dueck C, Manore M, Matt K. Role of energy balance in athletic menstrual dysfunction. *Int J Sport Nutr*. 1996;6:165-190.
13. Nattiv A, Lynch L. The female athlete triad. Managing an acute risk to long-term health. *Phys Sports Med*. 1994;22:60-68.
14. Whitney E, Rolfes S. *Understanding Nutrition*. 7th ed. St. Paul, Minn: West Publishing Co; 1996.
15. Applegate L. Fad diets and supplement use in athletics. *Sports Sci Exch*. 1988;1(9).
16. Nuviala R, Castillo M, Lapieza M, Escanero J. Iron nutritional status in female karatekas, handball and basketball players and runners. *Physiol Behav*. 1996;59:449-453.
17. Kleiner S. The role of meat in an athlete's diet: its effect on key macro and micronutrients. *Sports Sci Exch*. 1995;8(5).
18. American College of Sports Medicine. Position paper on weight loss in wrestlers. *Med Sci Sports Exerc*. 1996;28:ix-xii.
19. Steen S, Oppliger R, Brownell K. Metabolic effects of weight loss and regain in adolescent wrestlers. *JAMA*. 1988;260:47-50.
20. Fogelholm G, Koskinen R, Laakso J, Ruokonen I. Gradual and rapid weight loss: effects on nutrition and performance in male athletes. *Med Sci Sports Exerc*. 1993;25:371-377.
21. Houston M, Marrin D, Green H, Thomson J. The effect of rapid weight loss on physiological functions in wrestlers. *Phys Sports Med*. 1981;9:73-78.
22. Department of Health and Human Services. Hyperthermia and dehydration-related deaths associated with intentional weight loss in three collegiate wrestlers—North Carolina, Wisconsin, and Michigan, November-December 1997. *MMWR Morb Mortal Wkly Rep*. 1998;47:105-108.

23. American College of Sports Medicine. Position stand on exercise and fluid replacement. *Med Sci Sports Exerc*. 1996;28:i-vii.

24. Clark N. *Nancy Clark's Sport Nutrition Guidebook*. 2nd ed. Champaign, Ill: Human Kinetics; 1997.

25. Daly P, Kreiger D, Dullo A, Young J, Landsberg L. Ephedrine, caffeine and aspirin: safety and efficacy for treatment of obesity. *Int J Obes*. 1993;17:S73-78.

26. Williams M. *The Ergogenics Edge*. Champaign, Ill: Human Kinetics; 1997.

27. The Centers for Disease Control and Prevention. Adverse events associated with ephedrine-containing products—Texas, December 1993-September 1995. *JAMA*. 1996;276:1711-1712.

28. Kleiner S, Greenwood-Robinson M. *Power Eating*. Champaign, Ill: Human Kinetics; 1998.

29. Kenshole A. Corridor consultations: chromium picolinate and polynicotinate. *Patient Care Canada*. 1998;9:7.

30. Clarkson P. Nutritional ergogenic aids: chromium, exercise, and muscle mass. *Int J Sport Nutr*. 1991;1:289-293.

31. Clarkson P. Nutritional supplements for weight gain. *Sports Sci Exch*. 1998;11(1).

32. Kreider R. Creatine supplementation: analysis of ergogenic value, medical safety, and concerns. *J Exerc Physiol*. 1998;1(1). http://www.css.edu/users/tboone2/asep/jan.htm. Accessed July 14, 1999.

33. Juhn M, Tarnapolsky M. Oral creatine supplementation and athletic performance: a critical review. *Clin J Sport Med*. 1998;8:286-297.

34. Juhn M, Tarnapolsky M. Potential side effects of oral creatine supplementation: a critical review. *Clin J Sport Med*. 1998;8:298-304.

The author would like to acknowledge Jason Su, MD, Sports Medicine Fellow, Department Family and Community Medicine, University of Toronto. Dr. Su is also a martial artist.

41

MILITARY TRAINING

Shirley Gerrior, PhD, RD

The Department of Defense (DoD) considers physical fitness an important component of the "general health and well-being" and readiness of military personnel. Physical fitness includes cardiorespiratory endurance, muscular strength, muscular endurance, and whole-body flexibility, as well as balance, agility, and explosive power. Military readiness consists of day-to-day productivity and the ability to deploy. It also requires a basic level of fitness for the health of individuals and a higher level of fitness for occupational performance. In June 1981, DoD mandated that all services have a physical fitness program for service members and a testing procedure to evaluate the efficiency of the program (1). The purpose of this directive was to ensure optimal body composition, military appearance, and performance of duty for all military personnel. Both the specific requirements of the program and fitness testing are left to each of the services, based on training and mission needs (2).

The emphasis on and the enforcement of leadership are important to effective military physical fitness programs and readiness goals. Military leaders must provide active-duty personnel with the time and resources to develop and participate in education and intervention programs on health and physical fitness. In 1993, the Department of the Army specified that as a first priority commanders will conduct physical fitness programs that enhance soldiers' ability to complete critical soldier tasks that support the unit mission, and of secondary importance prepare for the Army Physical Fitness Test (APFT) (3). In 1982, the Navy established a comprehensive Health and Physical Readiness (HAPR) program to promote health and physical fitness and set minimum standards for fitness and weight control, and emphasized the need for all active duty personnel to participate in lifestyle behaviors to promote good health (4). In 1992, the Air Force implemented the Cycle Ergometry Program to educate the active-duty population on its positive effects on aerobic exercise and impact on total health (2). Recent changes in military operations, including the downsizing of the active-duty force and greater reliance on the reserve force, shift the responsibility of military health and fitness from leadership to the individual service member who must meet physical fitness standards (see *Table 41.1*). Failure to meet these standards can result in denial to military schools, delayed promotion, or involuntary separation from the service.

TABLE 41.1   US Military Physical Fitness Standards

Policy	Army	Navy	Air Force	Marines
Fitness Test	Adjusted for age and gender	Adjusted for age and gender	Adjusted for age and gender	Adjusted for age and gender
Frequency of Assessment	Semiannual	Semiannual	Annual	Semiannual
Cardiovascular and Muscular Endurance*	2-mile run Sit-ups in 2 minutes Push-ups in 2 minutes	1.5-mile run or 500 yd swim Curl-ups in 2 minutes Push-ups in 2 minutes	Submaximal cycle ergometer test, percent of standard based on (VO_2 max) at maximum exercise	**Men:** 3-mile run Curl ups Push-ups Pull-ups in 2 minutes **Women:** 1.5-mile run Curl-ups Push-ups Bent-arm hang in 2 minutes
Flexibility		Sit-reach		Curl-ups
Duty Time Allowed for Physical Fitness Training	3 hours authorized	Commander's discretion	Commander's discretion	Part of weekly training day

Adapted from: Food and Nutrition Board Institute of Medicine. Committee on Body Composition, Nutrition, and Health of Military Women. *Assessing Readiness in Military Women: The Relationship of Body Composition, Nutrition and Health.* Washington, DC: National Academy Press; 1998.

*These events have specific criteria: Run must be completed within a specified amount of time, and a specific number of sit-ups and push-ups (or similar events) must be completed within the 2-minute period to achieve a passing score.

PHYSICAL FITNESS AND PERFORMANCE

Physical Fitness

Physical fitness is the ability to function effectively in physical work, training, and other activities and still have enough energy available to respond to emergency situations which may arise. Components of physical fitness are cardiorespiratory endurance, muscular strength, muscular endurance, flexibility, and body composition (5). Improving these three fitness components will have a positive impact on the service member's fitness level and body composition.

Levels of Fitness and Physical Training Protocols

A physical fitness program could consist of a preparatory, conditioning, and/or maintenance phase depending on individual and unit levels of fitness and the unit mission. Career-service members, especially those in infantry and military police units, who exercise regularly and are at a high fitness level and able to meet the physical demands of the job, may already be in the maintenance phase. Young, healthy persons may be able to start with the conditioning phase, while those who have been exercising regularly may already be in the maintenance phase. However, new recruits and reservists are very diverse as to age and fitness levels. New recruits are as young as 17 and have not reached full physical maturation. Initial Entry Training (IET) is a basic training program that brings the recruits up to the level of physical fitness needed to perform their mission. It permits lower minimum scores on fitness tests during occupational training, but by graduation the standard scores must met.

The reservist maintains a lifestyle separate from the military but must be able to meet physical fitness standards and to respond to the physical demands of occupational training. Failure to meet these standards is not uncommon across all age groups serving in the reserves. Physical training is much less a part of the daily life of the reservists, where recreational or weekend exercise may be the norm. The design of individual physical training protocols is instrumental to the physical health and military careers of these service members. Also, factors such as extended field training, time aboard ship or extended flight missions, leave time, and illness can cause a service member to drop from a maintenance to a conditioning phase. Persons who have not been active, as well as service members recovering from illness or injury, will probably fall into the preparatory phase category.

Four factors required for a successful physical training program are frequency, intensity, time, and type (FITT). When applied to four of the five components of fitness—cardiorespiratory endurance, muscular strength, muscular endurance, and flexibility—they provide the basis for the conditioning phase of a training program, but are important to the preparatory phase as well (see *Table 41.2*).

TABLE 41.2   FITT Factors Applied to Physical Conditioning Program

	Cardiorespiratory Endurance	Muscular Strength	Muscular Endurance	Muscular Strength and Muscular Endurance	Flexibility
Frequency = F	3-5 times/week	3 times/week	3-5 times/week	3 times/week	**Warm-up and cool-down:** Stretch before and after each exercise session. **Developmental stretching:** To improve flexibility, stretch 2-3 times per week.
Intensity = I	60%-90% HHR or 70%-90% MHR*	3-7 RM**	12+ RM	8-12 RM	Tension and slight discomfort, NOT PAIN
Time =T	20 minutes or more	The time required to do 3-7 repetitions of each exercise	The time required to do 12+ repetitions of each exercise	The time required to do 8-12 repetitions of each exercise	**Warm-up and cool-down stretches:** 10-15 seconds stretch
Type = T	Running Swimming Cross-country skiing Rowing Bicycling Jumping rope Walking Hiking Stair climbing	Free weights Resistance machines Partner-resisted exercises Body-weight exercises	Free weights Resistance machines Partner-resisted exercises Body-weight exercises	Free weights Resistance machines Partner-resisted exercises Body-weight exercises	**Stretching:** Static Passive

Adapted from: *Physical Fitness Training*. Washington, DC: Headquarters, Dept of the Army. Field Manual No. 21-20. September 30, 1992.

*HHR = heart rate reserve; MHR = maximum heart rate
**RM = repetition maximum

The preparatory phase benefits both the cardiorespiratory and muscular systems with a moderate workload. Initially, poorly conditioned service members should exercise three times per week at a comfortable pace that elevates heart rate to about 60% heart rate reserve (HRR) for 10 to 15 minutes. The duration and intensity of exercise should be gradually increased to reach 70% HRR for 20 to 25 minutes prior to beginning the next phase. Likewise, the preparatory phase for improving muscular strength and endurance through weight training should start easily with light weights to minimize soreness and progress gradually. Beginning weight trainers should select about 8 to 12 exercises that work all the body's major muscle groups, and based on 1-RM work towards 8 to 12 repetitions to muscle failure for each exercise before beginning the conditioning phase (5). A 1-RM is a repetition performed against the greatest possible resistance and the maximum weight a person can lift. A 8- to 12-RM is that weight which allows a person to do from 8 to 12 repetitions without fatigue.

In the conditioning phase the duration time of an event is increased. For example, the run time should be increased by 2 minutes each week until an individual runs continuously for 30 minutes before increasing the intensity of the event. For muscular endurance and strength, once an individual can do 12 repetitions of any weight-related exercise, the heaviness of the weight should be increased by about 5% or to a heaviness that allows 8 to 12 repetitions to be completed before muscle fatigue.

Once a service member is physically mission-capable and all personal, strength-related, and unit-fitness goals have been attained, the maintenance phase can begin. This phase sustains the high level of fitness achieved in the conditioning phase. The emphasis of this phase is no longer on progression, but rather on a well-designed 45- to 60-minute workout of appropriate intensity three times per week. While this program should be enough to maintain almost any appropriate level of physical fitness, more frequent training may be needed to reach and maintain peak fitness levels (5).

Physiological differences between military men and women influence physical performance. Physical training programs may need to be structured to account for these differences. Although women are able to participate in the same fitness programs as men, they must work harder to perform at the same absolute level of work or exercise. (The same is true for poorly conditioned soldiers performing with well-conditioned soldiers.) In general, men enter the military with lower percentages of body fat than women and are able to perform more sit-ups and push-ups and run faster than women. They also suffer fewer injuries than women because of their relatively higher level of endurance and possibly other associated factors such as body weight, bone thickness, cardiovascular fitness, and flexibility (6). In particular, women are more likely than men to suffer from stress fractures during basic training (2). To minimize such injury, consuming the recommended energy intake is essential to reduce fatigue, as is an adequate preparatory phase training with proper stretching, warm-up, and cool-down techniques.

Fitness Test

Service members with reasonable levels of overall physical fitness should easily pass the fitness test (see *Table 41.1*). Those individuals whose fitness levels are substandard will fail, and they should be provided with a special exercise program. Fitness trainers responsible for these programs must ensure that service members are not overloaded to the point where fitness training becomes counterproductive. To avoid this situation fitness trainers should place service members in a run "ability group." Ability groups are based on an individual's APFT run time for 2 miles. Individuals with similar run times (ie, 15:30 or 18:00) are grouped accordingly. This provides a positive training environment as the members of a particular group have similar running abilities and train accordingly. The "ability group" run in combination with a total-body strength-training program, including exercises designed for push-up and sit-up improvement, provides the best approach to remedial fitness training (5).

The Army has revised the APFT (7). Implementation of the new standards began in February 1999. Since 1984 when the APFT was first adopted, the overall level of fitness among soldiers, especially career-soldiers, has improved. Similarly, physical fitness scores were uniformly higher for the 1.5-mile run, push-ups, and sit-ups by Navy service members in 1993 than in 1983 (4). The new Army standards emphasize equity between the genders and among the age groups. Some maximum standards for both genders were relaxed because they were considered not attainable, but minimum standards are the same or higher for each of the three events. The 2-mile run is more challenging, and push-up minimums are increased for both male and female soldiers. Sit-ups have the same standard for both genders but generally higher minimums than the old test. The minimum score required for each event remains the same at 60 points; the maximum is 100 points. The new APFT standards are adjusted for age and gender differences and take into account age limitations and decline in physical performance (7).

FUEL UTILIZATION DURING PHYSICAL TRAINING

Military Dietary Reference Intakes (MDRIs) are used to establish food energy and nutrient needs. MDRIs are identical to the Food and Nutrition Board's 1989 Recommended Dietary Allowances, except as updated by the Food and Nutrition Board's 1997 Dietary Reference Intakes for calcium, phosphorus, magnesium, vitamin D, and fluoride and the 1993 Public Health Service recommendations for folic acid. However, MDRIs differ when known differences in the military population require adjustment of a particular nutrient (8). The energy needs of the service member vary by gender, activity level, and type of activity. MDRIs for food energy are established by activity level (see *Table 41.3*). Factors such as activity intensity and duration and the effects of prior physical conditioning and dietary intake as well as hormonal interactions influence the pattern of fuel utilization during activity (8).

While weightlifting and selected swimming events require anaerobic energy sources, the majority of training and physical fitness activities in the military require aerobic energy sources. For the most part military exercise routines are performed at greater than 60% of VO₂max, with muscles becoming progressively more dependent on glucose oxidation rather than on fatty acid oxidation. Generally, exercise training is less than 90 minutes, but military training is much longer and sustained. As this activity continues, free fatty acid concentrations in blood increase, and the muscle gradually shifts to burning more fatty acids and less glucose. Energy needs for the aerobic component of the physical fitness test are those required for activity at 75% to 85% of VO₂max, but duration is limited to 15 to 30 minutes.

TABLE 41.3 Military Dietary Reference Intakes (MDRIs) for Food Energy by Activity Level and Gender

Activity Level	Men	Women
Light*	3,000 kcal	2,200 kcal
Moderate**	3,250 kcal	2,300 kcal
Heavy†	3,950 kcal	2,700 kcal
Exceptionally heavy††	4,600 kcal§	3,150 kcal

*Light activity includes slow walking (≤2.5 mph) on hard surface, no load; driving a heavy truck; cleaning a rifle; dressing; showering; shooting pool.

**Moderate activity includes walking at moderate speed (3 mph), hard surface, no load; walking at 2.5 mph, hard surface with 66-lb load; marksmanship training, range firing; driving armored vehicle; airplane repair; noncompetitive weightlifting; walking at moderate speed (2.5 mph) on hard surface with 100-lb load; walking at 3.5 mph with no load; obstacle/endurance/confidence course; fast walking, bicycling at moderate speed.

†Heavy activity includes walking at 4 mph on hard surface, no load; foxhole digging; crawling with a full pack, regular road march; field assaults, fast uphill walking; walking at moderate speed (3.5 mph) with 66-lb load; emplacement digging; jogging (<11:30 minutes per mile), bicycling (10 mph); canoeing (3-5 mph); downhill skiing, swimming, weight training; fencing, wrestling.

††Vigorous activity includes walking at 3 mph with 100-lb load; assault course; forced road march; litter; carrying heavy load (75 to 99 lb), boxing (sparring), touch football, snowshoeing, hiking and mountain climbing, orienteering, swimming, basketball; running (8 to 9 minutes per mile), martial arts, canoeing/sculling, cross-country skiing, scuba diving.

§Military personnel doing heavy work or prolonged vigorous physical training have energy requirements that exceed 125 % of the MDRI for energy.

Source: *Power Performance: the Nutrition Connection*. Natick, Mass: Military Nutrition Division of the US Army Research Institute of Environmental Medicine; 1994. Modules 1-6.

NUTRITION FOR PHYSICAL FITNESS AND MILITARY TRAINING

The energy and macronutrient needs for service members 17 to 50 years of age engaging in high levels of physical activity are similar to general sports nutrition recommendations (see *Table 41.4*). Military personnel doing heavy work or involved in prolonged, vigorous, physical training may have energy requirements that exceed 125% of the MDRI for energy. Additionally, environmental factors can affect energy and macronutrient needs. Prolonged exposure to cold, even mildly cold temperatures of 32° to 57°F, can increase energy requirements 5% to 10%. For hotter temperatures in the 86° to 104°F range, energy requirements may increase 2.5% to 10%. Heat-acclimated individuals have less of an increase in energy requirement, but physical training and heat acclimatization can increase sweat rate by 10% to 20% or 200 to 300 mL per hour. Energy requirements for high-altitude operations greater than 10,000 feet are substantially increased with requirements for individuals performing extremely strenuous work or physical activity in high-mountain areas reaching 6,000 to 7,000 kcal per day, depending on body size, weight of load carried, the level of incline, walking surface features, and the ambient temperature (8).

TABLE 41.4   Recommended Daily Energy and Energy Nutrient Intake for Athletes and Service Members in Physical Training

Food Energy (kcal)	Carbohydrate (g)	Protein (g)	Fat (g)
2,500	344-438	75-94	56-69
3,000	413-525	90-113	67-83
3,500	481-613	105-131	78-97
4,000	550-700	120-150	89-111
5,000	688-875	150-188	111-139
% of Total Calories	55%-70%	12%-15%	20%-25%

Source: *Power Performance: the Nutrition Connection.* Natick, Mass: Military Nutrition Division of the US Army Research Institute of Environmental Medicine; 1994. Modules 1-6.

Micronutrient recommendations for service members 17 to 50 years of age engaging in high levels of physical activity are also similar to general sports nutrition recommendations (see *Table 41.5*). However, the MDRIs for calcium and phosphorus are higher for service members 17 to 18 years of age, as is the iron MDRI for males in this age group. Additionally, the magnesium MDRI is higher for older women. Adequate intakes of B vitamins, calcium, folate, iron, and magnesium are encouraged for optimal physical performance and recovery. With the emphasis on military training in a hot environment, the recommendation for sodium is higher than generally recommended for sports activities. Vigorous activity and hard physical work in a hot environment increase the amount of sodium lost in sweat. The need for extra sodium depends on the severity of sweat loss and the degree of acclimatization by the service member. When sodium replacement is required, it should be provided through food and beverages, and as salt added to foods, not salt tablets (see Chapter 6, Fluid and Electrolytes).

TABLE 41.5   Military Dietary Reference Intakes (MDRIs) for Protein, Vitamins, and Minerals, and Nutritional Standards for Operational Rations

Nutrient (unit)	Men	Women	Operational Rations
Food energy (kcal)			3,600[1]
Protein (g)	91 (63-119)	72 (50-93)	91[2]
Fat (g)			140 (maximum)[3]
Vitamin A (RE)	1,000	800	1,000
Vitamin D (µg)	5	5	5
Vitamin E (mg TE)	10	8	10
Vitamin K (µg)	80	65	80
Vitamin C (mg)	60	60	60
Thiamin (mg)	1.6	1.2	1.8
Riboflavin (mg)	2.0	1.4	2.2
Niacin (mg NE)	21	15	24
Vitamin B-6 (mg)	2.9	2.3	2.9
Folate (µg)	250	400	400
Vitamin B-12 (µg)	2.0	2.0	2.0

continued

TABLE 41.5   Military Dietary Reference Intakes (MDRIs) for Protein, Vitamins, and Minerals, and Nutritional Standards for Operational Rations (continued)

Nutrient (unit)	Men	Women	Operational Rations
Calcium (mg)[4]	1,000	1,000	1,000
Phosphorus (mg)[5]	700	700	700
Magnesium (mg)[6]	400	310	400
Iron (mg)[7]	10	15	15
Zinc (mg)	15	12	15
Sodium (mg)[8]	5,000 (4,550-5,525)	3,600 (3,220-3,910)	5,040
Iodine (μg)	150	150	150
Selenium (μg)	70	55	70
Fluoride (mg)	3.8	3.1	3.8
Potassium (mg)	3,500	3,500	3,500

Values are based on reference measures of military men of 174 lbs (79 kg) and of women 136 lbs (62 kg) at moderate activity levels.

Source: *Nutrition Standards and Education.* Washington, DC: AR 40-25/NAVMEDCOMINST 10110.1/AF 44-141. Draft, June 26, 1998.

[1]The average of moderate and heavy activity levels for the reference weight male
[2]Based on requirement level during intense activity (0.8 to 1.5 g/kg of body weight)
[3]Total energy from fat should not normally exceed 35% of total calories.
[4]The MDRI for men or women, 17 to 18 years of age, is 1,300 mg per day.
[5]The MDRI for men or women, 17 to 18 years of age, is 1,250 mg per day.
[6]The MDRI for men or women, 31 years or older, is 420 mg per day.
[7]The MDRI for men, 17 to 18 years of age, is 12 mg per day.
[8]The MDRI is based on 1,400-1,700 mg of sodium per 1,000 kcal of food served. May be inadequate in hot weather.

Fluid Needs

Service members must avoid dehydration to maintain optimal performance. Cool water (plain or flavored) is the beverage of choice for preventing dehydration. When training in hot environments or high altitudes, service members should consume approximately 4 to 6 quarts of beverage per day to avoid severe dehydration. More fluids are needed as physical work and temperatures increase and as sweating rates increase. In general, physically active service members should drink large quantities of water (20 oz) 1 to 2 hours before exercise to promote hyperhydration and keep pace with sweat losses, followed by drinking 3 to 6 oz of fluid every 15 to 30 minutes during exercise (5). Certain conditions merit the use of carbohydrate-electrolyte beverages. Continuous physical activity beyond 90 minutes and high loss of water and electrolytes not adequately replaced by diet are the most common. Carbohydrate-electrolyte beverages should provide a carbohydrate concentration of 6% to 8% sugar or starch, electrolytes as 20 to 30 mEq of sodium per liter and 2 to 5 mEq potassium per liter, and chloride as the only anion (8).

MILITARY TRAINING—A COMPETITIVE SPORT

The principles of physical fitness and sports nutrition are extremely relevant to the needs of many service members. The intense physical aspects of military training require endurance, strength, and quickness. Called upon to perform a number of different types of physical activities, the active-duty service member may participate in endurance activities such as forced marches and hikes, high-intensity moves such as obstacle courses, and anaerobic activities requiring the strength of a weightlifter to move and assemble large pieces of equipment.

Intense physical military training is encountered most often during field operations where energy expenditures are high (see *Table 41.6*). The operational ration, designed for military personnel in combat, provides the entire diet during sustained operations. The nutrition standards for operational rations are based on the MDRIs and are designed to support the special nutrient requirements for the various actual or simulated combat situations, and, in the case of B-vitamins, compensate for possible losses during storage (8). A nutritionally adequate ration composed of semiperishable and/or shelf-stable prepared food items, the operational ration includes the Meal, Ready-to-Eat (MRE), and B-ration and Unitized

TABLE 41.6   Energy Expenditure in Military Training during Field Operations and in Comparable Athletic Activities

Military Training	Calories Burned/Minute*	Athletic Activity	Calories Burned/Minute*
Grenade throwing	6.0	Calisthenics	5.8
Litter carry w/178-lb person	6.7	Hunting	6.7
Forward area foxhole digging	6.8	Baseball pitcher	7.0
Carrying boxes of ammunition	7.3	Nautilus	7.1
Trooping ridge position	7.3	Tennis	7.4
Forward area position digging	7.7	Walking treadmill, 4 mph	7.5
Rifleman in fire fight	7.9	Canoeing, fast	7.9
Walking 3.5 mph, 66-lb load	8.1	Soccer	8.9
Rapid marching w/rifle and pack	8.4	Football	9.0
Creeping and crawling in full gear	9.0	Skiing hard snow, moderate	9.2
Backpacking, general	9.0	Rowing machine, moderate	9.3
Loading and unloading trucks	9.0	Water skiing	9.4
Cross-country skiing, 55- to 77-lb pack, 3 mph	10.2	Backpacking, 11-lb load	9.9
Rock or mountain climbing	10.3	Swimming, crawl, fast	10.6
Digging trenches	10.9	Cross-country skiing	10.6
Climbing hills, 44 lb load	11.4	Basketball competition	11.4
Snowshoeing, soft snow, 2.5 mph	12.8	Cycling racing	12.0
Walking in loose snow, 44-kg load, 2.5 mph	20.2	Boxing, in ring, match	17.1

Source: *Power Performance: The Nutrition Connection.* Natick, Mass: Military Nutrition Division of the US Army Research Institute of Environmental Medicine; 1994. Modules 1-6.

*These figures are based on the energy expenditure of 170 lb men. Women burn about 10% fewer calories for the same event.

Group Rations (100 servings per pack for field kitchens). In operational rations total calories from fat should not exceed 35% of calories with a goal of no more than 30% of calories, but the nutrient-dense nature of this ration may result in varied fat content. Also, due to the concentration of some minerals, fluid needs are high and adequate intake of water before, during, and after physical activity is essential.

FOOD COMPONENTS AND PERFORMANCE

Basically, two food components—carbohydrate and creatine—are effective as ergogenic aids for physically active service members. The role of carbohydrate as a fuel source and the value of carbohydrate supplementation in extending physical performance are usually demonstrated after 60 to 90 minutes of continuous activity at 60% to 70% of VO_2max (9). Military training schedules generally preclude carbohydrate loading as training is often intermittent, and it is difficult to curtail activity 2 or 3 days before an event to effectively carbohydrate load. Therefore, the value of carbohydrates in extending physical performance is to replenish glycogen stores every day with a diet that is at least 55% to 60% carbohydrates.

Creatine supplementation has been shown to enhance muscular performance in repetitive exercise tests (10). A recent study suggests that creatine levels in skeletal muscle can be increased, performance of high-intensity exercise (military obstacle course tasks) enhanced, body mass significantly increased, and percent body fat decreased following a 5-day period of creatine supplementation and Such supplementation may be beneficial during repeated bouts of high-intensity exercise (11). See Chapter 7, Ergogenic Aids for more information on creatine.

CASE STUDY

SGT Moore is a 35-year-old reservist who is a medical unit supply sergeant. He is busy during most drills doing logistical paperwork and moving medical material. He has 4 months until his next APFT. He has noticed recently that he is easily fatigued by the physical demands of his job.

SGT Moore works from 9:00 AM to 5:30 PM 5 days a week as a computer specialist and spends 2 hours each day commuting to and from work. He has a fitness room available to him at his worksite, but does not like to stay after work to use it. In the evening he spends time with his wife and three children, ages 4 to 10 years. He is inactive on his job and does little recreational exercise; however, he likes to walk. Last year he passed the APFT with a score of 185, doing the minimum push-ups (33) and sit-ups (38) and making the run time by 30 seconds (17:30 min). SGT Moore tends to be on the stocky side, 210 lb and 72 in, and has a body fat of 24%. His diet includes daily servings of red meat or fried chicken, fried potatoes, and an occasional salad. He drinks whole milk and likes fresh fruit. A 1-week dietary recall indicates a total intake of 18,900 kcal (or 2,700 kcal per day), 47% carbohydrate, 38% protein, and 38% fat.

Physical Training Protocol

- SGT Moore should start out slowly and build up activity gradually in intensity and duration.
  - Initially he should walk or run three times a week at 60% heart rate reserve (HRR) for 10 to 15 minutes.
  - Gradually, he should lengthen his exercise session to 20 minutes and/or elevate his heart rate to 70% of HRR.
  - On alternate days he should lift weights for 8 to 12 RM (upper limit 12) using opposing muscle groups of the major muscle groups.
  - On weightlifting days he should practice crunches; sit-ups; and shoulder width, closed-hand, and wide-hand push-ups in sets of 10 each.
- At the end of the first month, SGT Moore should move into the conditioning phase of the program.
  - He should gradually increase the intensity of his run to 70% to 80% of VO_2max to score at least 80 points (16:00 minutes) on the APFT.
  - He should increase weight by 5% to do 12 repetitions without fatigue, especially of the upper body major muscle groups.
- Physical training protocol should consider, but not focus on, the APFT.

Diet Plan

- SGT Moore should follow the principles of the Food Guide Pyramid to achieve both a balanced diet and weight loss.
  - Complete a food and fitness diary for 1 week, watching for skipped meals, overeating, and low fluid intake.
  - Eat approximately 2,200 kcal daily with 55% to 60% of calories as carbohydrate, 12% to 15% calories as protein, and 20% to 25% of calories as fat.
  - Eat at least the daily number of food groups as recommended by the Food Guide Pyramid at 2,200 kcal: grains, 9; vegetables, 4; fruits, 3; milk, 2; and meat, 2.5 (or about 6 oz).
  - Limit use of fats and oils, substituting skim milk for whole milk and using low-fat cooking methods for meats (enroll he and his wife in a cooking class).
  - Daily eat fresh fruits and vegetables rich in vitamin C, vitamin A, and dietary fiber. Fruits make good snacks and when combined with a bagel and skim milk, a nutritious breakfast after his morning workout.
  - Receive instruction on reading and understanding the "Nutrition Facts" food label.
- SGT Moore should consider food energy and fluid sources to achieve optimal physical performance.
- He should be encouraged to consume carbohydrate-rich foods, such as fresh fruit, ready-to-eat cereals, and whole-grain breads after exercise (especially if done prior to his work day) to replace glycogen stores.
- He needs to replace fluids lost during exercise with about 3 to 6 oz of water every 15 to 30 minutes.

REFERENCES

1. *Physical Fitness and Weight Control Programs.* Washington, DC: US Dept of Defense; June 29, 1981. Dept of Defense Instruction 1308.1.
2. Food and Nutrition Board Institute of Medicine. *Assessing Readiness in Military Women: the Relationship of Body Composition, Nutrition, and Health.* Washington, DC: National Academy Press; 1998.
3. *Physical Fitness.* Washington, DC: US Dept of Defense; March 19, 1993. Army Regulation 350-41, Chapter 9.
4. Trent LK, Hurtado SL. Longitudinal trends and gender differences in physical fitness and lifestyle factors in career U.S. Navy personnel (1983-1994). *Mil Med.* 1998;163:398-407.
5. *Physical Fitness Training.* Washington, DC: Headquarters, Dept of the Army; September 30, 1992. Field Manual No. 21-20.
6. Moore J. Exercise, conditioning, and fitness as it relates to injury in active-duty women. *Women's Health Issues.* 1996;6:374-380.
7. *APFT Standards Changes.* Washington, DC: Secretary DCSOPS at MEDCOM7_FSHTX; October 24, 1997.
8. *Nutrition Standards and Education.* Washington, DC: AR 40-25/NAVMEDCOMINST 10110.1/AF 44-141; Draft, June 26, 1998.
9. *Power Performance: the Nutrition Connection.* Natick, Mass: Military Nutrition Division of the US Army Research Institute of Environmental Medicine; 1994. Modules 1-6.
10. Food and Nutrition Board Institute of Medicine. Committee on Military Nutrition Research. *Food Components to Enhance Performance: An Evaluation of Potential Performance-enhancing Food Components for Operational Rations.* Marriott BM, ed. Washington, DC: National Academy Press; 1994.
11. Warber JP, Patton JF, Tharion WJ, Montain SJ, Mello RP, Lieberman HR. Effects of creatine monohydrate supplementation on physical performance. *FASEB Abstracts.* 1998:6016.

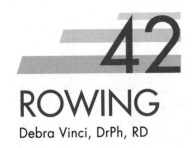

ROWING

Debra Vinci, DrPh, RD

Rowing is a dynamic sport that imposes great physiological demands on athletes. Elite rowers have exceptional aerobic and anaerobic capacities and high levels of muscular strength and power (1). In the sport of rowing, training involves a combination of strength development and endurance (2).

The sport of rowing is divided into two distinct categories: sweep rowing and sculling. Sweep rowing refers to an event in which each rower uses one long oar, whereas in sculling each rower uses two shorter oars. Sweep boats may include two, four, or eight rowers. The pairs and fours row without coxswains, while the eights always row with coxswains. Sculling includes single, doubles, and quadruple boats that are rowed without coxswains (1-4). Terminology associated with the sport is found in *Box 42.1*.

BOX 42.1 Definitions

Coxswain:	A member of the rowing team who steers the boat and calls out rowing commands to the crew (3,4,6)
Racing shell:	A slender, light, responsive, high-performance boat. The term "shell" is used in reference to boats since the hull is only about 1/8" to 1/4" thick to make the boats as light as possible. Weights and lengths differ between sculling boats and sweep boats (6).
Sculling:	An event that involves 1, 2, or 4 rowers. Only in rare cases do these boats have coxswains. Each rower uses two shorter oars (3 m), pulling on them simultaneously (4,6,8).
Sweep rowing:	An event that involves 2 or 4 rowers (with and without coxswains) or 8 rowers (with coxswain). Each rower uses a single long oar (3.9 m) on one side of the boat (4,6,8).
Weight classifications:	There are two weight classes for rowers—heavyweight (HWT) and lightweight (LWT). For men's LWT, there is a 72.5 kg individual maximum, and the boat must average (excluding coxswain) no more than 70 kg. The individual maximum for LWT woman is 59 kg, with the average weight of crew (excluding coxswain) no more than 57 kg (3,4,6).

Rowing is a recreational and competitive sport. Club rowing involves sweep rowing and sculling and ranges from the most competitive elite athletes to social participants. High school and collegiate teams compete primarily in sweep boats, whereas sculling races are contested at the club and international level. In international and collegiate rowing, the standard racing course is a distance of 2,000 meters and usually has six shells racing against each other. The course is 1,000 meters at the masters level and 1,500 meters for the junior division (high school) competition (3,5). These sprint races are usually in the spring and summer. Other competitive races include head races that are longer distances (2.5 to 3 miles) and generally take place in a time trail fashion during the fall and winter months (6). These races can be used to determine the effectiveness of fall and winter training programs that usually focus on endurance training (6).

Coxswains are members of the rowing team who steer the boat and call out rowing commands to the crew. The minimum weight is 55 kg for men's and junior men's coxswains and 56.8 kg for collegiate coxswains. The minimum weight for women's, junior women's, and mixed crew is 50 kg. If coxswains do not meet the minimum weight requirements, they are required to carry a maximum of 10 kg dead weight. In the United States female coxswains can compete in male events and male coxswains can compete in female events (3,4,6).

Rowers compete in age, weight, and skill classifications. Juniors are male and female rowers and coxswains who are no more than 18 years old. Masters men, women, and mixed events have a range of age categories. For example, Age Category A is a minimum of 27 years and Age Category H has an average age of 70 years (3).

Weight classifications exist for lightweight rowers. The average of men's crew (excluding coxswain) is no more than 70 kg with no individual oarsman weighing more than 72.5 kg. For women, the average weight of the crew (excluding coxswains) is no more than 57 kg with no individual oarswoman weighing greater than 59 kg (3). Competitions are also categorized by skills—intermediate, senior, and elite (3,4,6)

PHYSIOLOGY

Competitive rowing is one of the most physically demanding endurance-type sports, requiring an "all-out" effort for 2,000 meters lasting from $5^{1/2}$ to $8^{1/2}$ minutes depending on boat class, weather conditions, water current, physical condition, and the experience of the rowers (6). Studies have shown that maximal aerobic capacities of competitive rowers are among the highest recorded, with competitive male rowers having a VO_2max of approximately 6 L per minute and females rowers reaching about 4 L per minute (2).

The overall contribution of aerobic metabolism is 70% for males and 55% for females, and the anaerobic contribution is 30% in males and 45% for females. The aerobic response of rowers is related to the pattern of pacing that is used in 2,000-meter sprint racing. At the start, there is a brief moment requiring a tremendous burst of energy lasting 30 to 40 seconds, during which stroke cadence averages 40 to 50 strokes per minute. The stroke cadence is then reduced to 34 to 38 strokes per minute and maintained for approximately 4.0 to 4.5 minutes. The stroke cadence is increased again in the last minute of the race (7).

PHYSICAL CHARACTERISTICS

Top competitive heavyweight rowers are taller and heavier, and have longer arm spans and taller sitting heights as compared to other endurance athletes. *Table 42.1* profiles the physical characteristics of the 1992 US Olympic Rowing Team. While little has changed in heights and weights of elite rowers over the past 30 years, today's rowers have higher fat-free mass than in the 1960s (8).

TABLE 42.1 Average Physical Characteristics of 1992 US Olympic Team (8)

Team	n	Age	Height (cm)	Weight (kg)	Body Fat %
Heavyweight Women	25	24	178.6	73.6	15.4
Heavyweight Men	35	26	194.1	88.1	8.7

Since there is a wide gap in weight ranges between heavyweight and lightweight rowers, coaches are concerned that rowers selected for lightweight crews be naturally lean individuals (9). Cutting weight can result in disordered eating behaviors (fasting, vomiting, and bingeing) and decreased performance related to dehydration (9-11).

TOP NUTRITION CONCERNS

Due to the increased physiological demands in rowing, nutrition plays an important role in achieving optimal performance. Nutrition concerns for rowers include:

- Adequate energy intake
- Nutrient-dense diet
- Weight management
- Hydration

Adequate Energy Intake

Rowers undertake high-intensity training and require adequate caloric intake to meet their energy needs. Collegiate heavyweight male rowers may need over 6,000 kcal per day and collegiate heavyweight women rowers may need a minimum of 3,000 kcal per day. Due to the time demands of work, school, practice, and optional workouts, many heavyweight male rowers find it difficult to maintain or gain weight without the use of liquid supplements. This can also be true for male and female rowers who are vegetarians and have diets containing less than 20% of kcal as fat.

Nutrient-dense Diet

It has been recommended that endurance athletes derive 60% to 70% of kcal from carbohydrate, approximately 15% of kcal from protein (not to exceed 2 g/kg body weight), and less than 25% of kcal from fat (12-18). A study of female collegiate heavyweight rowers revealed an average carbohydrate intake of 51% (4.9 g/kg), which is lower than one would expect for an endurance athlete (19). Energy, carbohydrate, and protein needs of rowers are summarized in *Box 42.2*.

BOX 42.2 Energy, Carbohydrate, and Protein Needs of Rowers*	
Kilocalories (21)	45-87 kcal/kg per day
Carbohydrate (16)	8-10 g/kg per day
Protein (14,18)	1.4-1.7 g/kg per day

* Rowers' energy requirements vary with the intensity of training, with recreational rowers having lower energy needs than elite rowers. While some coxswains have energy and protein needs similar to rowers, others are not as active and have nutrient needs equivalent to the general population.

Some rowers consume a very high-carbohydrate intake (70% to 80% of kcal) while dietary intakes of protein and fat are low. This usually occurs in athletes who are vegetarian and have limited intake of dairy products and legumes. On the other hand, Eleanor McElvaine, University of Washington's Novice Women Coach, commented that when rowers discover they can eat more and not gain weight, they tend to eat foods that are higher in fat and simple carbohydrates (cookies, candy, fast foods) instead of increased amounts of whole grains, vegetables, fruits, and lean meats. Several studies have documented higher fat intake in female collegiate rowers (36% of kcal as fat) (19) and elite rowers (34% of kcal as fat) (18).

The use of liquid supplements and energy bars is a convenient way to increase caloric intake. For rowers who avoid meat and dairy products, liquid supplements are also a source of protein. Sports drinks, recovery carbohydrate beverages, and carbohydrate gels are products that can contribute to needed fluids and carbohydrate before, during, and after training (16,20). Iron and calcium supplements are recommended for many female rowers and coxswains, since dietary intakes of these nutrients are low compared to heavyweight female and male rowers (18,20,21).

While a nutrient-dense diet plays an important role in optimal performance for rowers, no sport is immune to the use of ergogenic aids. A recent study documented a positive relationship between increased whole-body creatine stores and higher, 1,000-m rowing performance with oral creatine supplementation, so it is reasonable to assume that these findings will stimulate an interest in creatine use in rowers (22). Bob Borberg, a competitive rower and founder of Elitefit.com, an internet site, shares his experience with creatine supplementation: "Working harder than ever, eating, sleeping, and training full time with creatine, my erg was the same. Was all the money on creatine a waste? I believe there is a better than average chance it was.... I think the bottom line, however, is that proper diet and training play a far greater role in improved performance than any supplement" (23).

Weight Management

Crew athletes engage in a number of dietary practices that influence weight regulation. Many heavyweight male athletes want to gain weight and need assistance with meal planning on a budget to meet their caloric needs of 5,000 kcal per day or more. While there are elite heavyweight women rowers who are interested in weight gain, many female heavyweight rowers, especially novice rowers, are interested in weight loss. At the collegiate level it is not uncommon for female rowers new to the sport to be concerned with the initial weight gain they experience early in the season. This weight gain is usually associated with weight training that is more intense than previous workout programs.

Male and female lightweight rowers and coxswains are also interested in assistance with weight loss. Clark (24) describes working with a coxswain who wanted to lose 16% of her body weight to qualify for a position on the national team. At 5'6" and 118 lb, her goal of 99 lb would place her at risk for nutritional deficiencies, amenorrhea, osteoporosis, and pathogenic eating behaviors.

This case illustrates the health concerns associated with dieting and weight loss in athletes. Sykora et al (9) evaluated the eating, weight, and dieting behaviors in 162 male and female lightweight and heavyweight collegiate rowers. It was determined that fasting, vomiting, binging, and weight fluctuations were not uncommon in male and female lightweight and heavyweight rowers. For example, 12% of the male and 20% of the female rowers reported binge eating at least twice a week. While 57% of males and 25% of females reported fasting, 2.5% of males and 13.2% of the females vomited as a weight loss method. Additionally, lightweight rowers reported fasting more frequently than heavyweight rowers, but did not have higher frequencies of binging or vomiting behaviors. Greater weight fluctuations were experienced by lightweight males during the season and greater offseason weight gain was experienced by lightweight males than by lightweight females and heavyweight males and females.

A sports nutritionist may be asked to evaluate the appropriateness of weight loss goals. In the case described above, Clark (24) commented on ethical concerns in working with athletes with weight goals that endanger health. By continued interaction with an athlete, the sports nutritionist can serve as a resource to reduce health risks while providing accurate sports nutrition information. The sports nutritionist can also play an important role in proactive sports education for coaches and athletic trainers. Strategies to reduce the risk of pathogenic eating behaviors include deemphasizing body weight, eliminating group weigh-ins, treating each athlete individually, and facilitating healthy weight management (25).

Hydration

Dehydration can cause fatigue and decreased performance. In addition to additional water intake, rowers can also benefit from the use of sports drinks with added carbohydrate and electrolytes (26). It is important to provide ongoing education on fluid requirements and the negative effects of dehydration on performance.

Anecdotal information indicates that lightweight rowers resort to dehydration practices approximately 24 hours prior to competition in order to "make weight" (11). This practice of making weight can be attributed to limited weight classifications in the sport of rowing. It is not unusual for a rower who is too small for the heavyweight division to try to lose weight to "make weight" to compete in the lightweight division. While the weight loss goal can result in a below-normal body weight, the alternative of not being able to compete can be devastating for an athlete (26).

The sports nutritionist can serve as a resource to reduce health risks associated with restricting food intake to cut weight. Hawley and Burke (26) contend that these practices will continue despite recommendations from medical, educational, and research bodies since they have been institutionalized within the sport. Hawley and Burke recommend that "athletes in weight-making sports receive individual expert advice about determining their optimal competition weight division and achieving it with minimal compromise to their success or health" (p. 243).

WORKING WITH COACHES

Generally, rowing coaches are very receptive to working with a sport nutritionist. Factors that contribute to a positive working relationship with coaches include understanding the many demands that athletes face during training and the competitive season, the ability to effectively interact with athletic trainers and athletes, the opportunity to work with athletes and provide nutrition interventions that improve athletic performance, knowledge of fundamental principles and training practices of the sport, and personal involvement in recreational or competitive sports.

Experienced coaches recognize that rowers need guidance in understanding the energy demands of the sport and translating them into food intake. A sports nutritionist can have a positive impact in assisting athletes in meal planning, grocery shopping, meal preparation, and the appropriate use of nutritional supplements.

CASE STUDY

Sam is a 19-year-old college sophomore competing in a Division I school as a heavyweight rower. At the beginning of October his weight was 89.5 kg. In January he had the flu and a cold for 3 days. He did not notice any drop in weight. However, by the end of February his weight dropped from 89.5 to 86.8 kg. He had never experienced weight loss before and was concerned since racing season started in 1 month. He made an appointment with the sports nutritionist to determine why he was losing weight.

Assessment

- Height = 196.85 cm
- Weight = 86.8 kg
- Percent body fat = 4.5%
- Analysis of a 3-day food record indicated Sam was consuming 3,380 kcal with 56% of kcal from carbohydrate, 12% of kcal from protein, and 32% of kcal from fat.

- His workout schedule included: indoor ergometer workout for 30 minutes, 1 hour before practice; on-water practice for $1^1/2$ hours, 6 days per week; weightlifting for 45 minutes, three times per week. Over winter and spring breaks, practice involved working out twice a day, early in the morning and again in the afternoon. By the end of March, Saturday workouts were replaced by competition.
- Estimated energy intake for weight maintenance at 86.8 kg was determined to be 6,007 kcal.
- Sam was living in the residence hall and eating in the cafeteria. The school meal plan was "a la carte" and typically cost a crew athlete with high-energy needs a minimum of $20 per day. Students received a meal card at the beginning of the quarter with a designated cash value. Sam ran out of money on his meal card in the sixth week of a 10-week quarter. He had been trying to prepare meals in his room since he planned to move out of the residence hall at the end of the quarter.

Recommendations

Sam's weight loss was related to decreased calorie intake when he began preparing meals in his room. The sports nutritionist intervened as follows:

- Discussed with Sam the option of adding money to his meal card since it was difficult for him to prepare meals in his room to meet his energy needs. Sam was concerned about having money left over on the card at the end of the quarter. It was suggested that he use the meal card for lunch and snacks during the spring quarter, while preparing dinner in his off-campus apartment.
- Explained the importance of eating three meals a day and planning snacks to meet energy needs
- Gave suggestions to increase calorie intake such as adding a sports drink at practice and consuming fruit juice as a beverage in between meals; using a liquid supplement such as instant breakfast with meals or as a snack; and carrying portable snacks in his day pack
- Encouraged the use of whole grains, fruits, vegetables, legumes, and lean meats to increase carbohydrate and protein intakes and decrease fat intake to less than 30% of kcal

Sam was able to add money to his meal card and started eating meals at on-campus cafeterias and eating snacks between meals. *Table 42.2* outlines a daily intake that would provide Sam with adequate energy for weight gain. Challenges to weight gain voiced by heavyweight male rowers include having money to afford the cost of food and beverages, needing to plan meals and snacks ahead of time, and constantly needing to eat and drink throughout the day.

Within 2 weeks, Sam had gained 1.8 kg. He was feeling better about his weight, strength, and competing in the upcoming racing season.

TABLE 42.2   Sample Dietary Intake for Heavyweight Male Rower*

7:30 AM	**Breakfast:**
	2 cups orange juice
	1 1/2 cups cornflakes
	1 cup granola
	2 cups 1% milk
	Peanut butter (2 T) and jelly (2 T) sandwich (2 slices whole-wheat bread) to eat on the way to class; water bottle with 16 oz cranberry juice to drink during the morning
10:00 AM	Fruit snack bar
11:30 AM	**Lunch:**
	6" roast beef grinder with 1 T mayonnaise
	1 1/2 oz bag of pretzels
	20 oz soft drink
	Banana
2:30 PM	30-minute erg workout
	Water bottle with 24 oz sport drink for afternoon practice
3:30 PM	On-water practice
6:00 PM	After practice: 16 oz cranberry juice and energy bar
7:00 PM	**Dinner:**
	2 cups spaghetti with meatballs (3 oz) and 1 cup tomato sauce
	1 cup broccoli
	2 dinner rolls
	2 t margarine
	2 cups lemonade
	1 1/2 cups frozen yogurt
	1 large chocolate chip cookie
10:00 PM	2 cups 1% milk with 1 packet instant breakfast
	Peanut butter (2 T) and jelly (2 T) sandwich (2 slices whole-wheat bread)

* Approximately 6,400 kcal; 65% carbohydrate, 11% protein, 24% fat. Estimated weight gain of 0.25 to 0.5 kg per week. Provides 4.6 L of energy-dense fluids, which contribute to fluid requirement estimated at 6.4 L (1 L for every 1,000 kcal).

REFERENCES

1. Hagerman FC. Applied physiology of rowing. *Sports Med.* 1984;1:303-326.

2. Secher N. Rowing. In: Reilly T, Secher N, Snell P, Williams C, eds. *Physiology of Sports.* Suffolk, NY: E & FN Spoon; 1990:259-286.

3. Federation Internationale des Societes d'Aviron (FISA). *FISA Rules of Racing.* 1997. http://www.fisa.org. Accessed September 7, 1998.

4. Human Kinetics with Hanlon T. *The Sports Rules Book: Essential Rules for 54 Sports.* Champaign, Ill: Human Kinetics; 1998.

5. Rower's World. *About Rowing:The Levels of Rowing.* http://www.rowersworld.com/ About-Rowing/rec.html. Accessed September 9, 1998.

6. Hofer H, Younger JW. *Rowing Frequently Asked Questions.* http://riceinfo.rice.edu/ ~hofer/Rowingfaq.html. Accessed September 9, 1998.

7. Hagerman FC, Connors MC, Gault JA, Hagerman GR, Polinski WJ. Energy expenditure during simulated rowing. *J Appl Physiol.* 1978;45:87-93.

8. Seiler S. *Physiology of the Elite Rower.* http://www.krs.hia.no/~stephens/ rowphs.htm. Accessed September 9, 1998.

9. Sykora C, Grilo CM, Wilfley DE, Brownell KD. Eating, weight, and dieting disturbance in male and female lightweight and heavyweight rowers. *Int J Eat Disord.* 1993;14:203-211.

10. Black DR, ed. *Eating Disorders and Athletes: Theory, Issues, and Research:* Reston, Va: American Alliance for Health, Physical Fitness, Recreation, and Dance; 1991.

11. Burge CM, Carey MF, Payne WR. Rowing performance, fluid balance, and metabolic function following dehydration and rehydration. *Med Sci Sports Exerc.* 1993;25:1358-1364.

12. Simonsen JC, Sherman WM, Lamb DR, Dernbach AR, Doyle JA, Strauss R. Dietary carbohydrate, muscle glycogen, and power output during rowing training. *J Appl Physiol.* 1991;70:1500-1505.

13. Harkins C, Carey R, Clark N, Benardot D. Protocols for developing dietary prescriptions. In: Benardot D, ed. *Sports Nutrition: A Guide for the Professional Working with Active People.* 2nd ed. Chicago, Ill: The American Dietetic Association; 1993:170-185.

14. Lemon, PWR. Effects of exercise on dietary protein requirements. *Int J Sport Nutr.* 1998;8:426-447.

15. Tarnopolsky MA, MacDougall JD, Atkinson SA. Influence of protein intake and training status on nitrogen balance and lean body mass. *J Appl Physiol.* 1988;64:187-193.

16. Coleman EJ. Carbohydrate—the master fuel. In: Berning JR, Steen SN, eds. *Nutrition for Sport and Exercise.* 2nd ed. Gaithersburg, Md: Aspen Publishers; 1998:21-44.

17. Snyder AC, Naik J. Protein requirements of athletes. In: Berning JR, Steen SN, eds. *Nutrition for Sport and Exercise.* 2nd ed. Gaithersburg, Md: Aspen Publishers; 1998:45-58.

18. Hagerman FC. Physiology and nutrition for rowing. In: Lamb DR, Knuttgen HG, Murry R, eds. *Perspectives in Exercise Science and Sports Medicine, Vol 7: Physiology and Nutrition for Competitive Sport.* Camel, Ind: Brown & Benchmark; 1994:221-302.

19. Steen SN, Mayer K, Brownell KD, Wadden TA. Dietary intake of female collegiate heavyweight rowers. *Int J Sport Nutr.* 1995;5:225-231.

20. Vinci DM. Effective nutrition support programs for college athletes. *Int J Sport Nutr.* 1998;8:308-320.

21. Paduda J. *The Art of Sculling.* Camden, Me: McGraw Hill; 1992.

22. Rossiter HB, Cannell ER, Jakeman PM. The effect of oral creatine supplementation on the 1,000-m performance of competitive rowers. *J Sports Sci.* 1996;14:175-179.

23. Borberg B. *What's Up with Creatine?* http://rowersresource.com/articles/elitefit/ creatine.html. Accessed August 23, 1998.

24. Clark N. Nutritional concerns of female athletes: a case study. *J Sport Nutr.* 1991;1:257-264.

25. Vinci DM. The female athlete triad: body image and disordered eating. *Athletic Therapy Today.* 1999;4:16-17.

26. Hawley H, Burke L. *Peak Performance: Training and Nutritional Strategies for Sport.* Sydney, Australia: Allen & Unwin; 1998.

43

SKIING: CROSS-COUNTRY, DOWNHILL, AND JUMPING

Charlene Harkins, MEd, RD, FADA

As a competitive and recreational sport, skiing—the use of flexible runners to traverse snowy terrain—has long been studied for its healthful benefits and potential for personal physical improvements. To make sound nutritional recommendations to both the competitive and recreational skier, the sports nutritionist needs to be familiar with the various types of skiing and understand the current research on its physiological impact on the body.

Snow skiing, the sport of sliding over snow on skis—long, narrow, flexible runners—has a history that stretches more than 4,000 years (1). Skiing was a vital form of transportation in 19th century Scandinavia, where military ability was judged by skiing acumen (2). Since the 1930s, downhill and cross-country skiing have enjoyed a tremendous boom in popularity as a recreational sport in the United States, possibly spurred on by the Winter Olympics at Lake Placid, New York in 1932 and 1988, and at Squaw Valley, California in 1960. Also, the advent of technology in the form of ski tows and ski lifts has made it possible for skiers to more fully enjoy their sport. Artificial snow-making machines and the construction of runs and trails have also served to increase participation in this cold-weather sport (1).

Skiing requires specific equipment. Once made of highly polished wood, skis are now made of polyethylene plastic that is continuously studied and modified to improve speed, agility, precision, and style. Skis come in different sizes and styles, depending on whether their intended use is cross-country, alpine (downhill), or ski jumping. Bindings, boots, and poles are also necessary equipment for participation. As the skis have become sport-specific, the bindings that attach the boots to the skis are also continuously undergoing technological refinement to assure proper fit, ability for control, efficiency of movement, and prevention of injury. The poles—hand rods consisting of wrist straps, pointed ends, and baskets—are the other mainstay of ski equipment. They are designed to assist the skier in maintaining balance, increasing power, and allowing for equilibrium-righting reactions in speed races. Ski poles are not used by ski jumpers. Concerns about head injuries have encouraged alpine and ski jumping to require the use of specially designed helmets (3).

Cross-country, downhill, and ski jumping, although all forms of skiing, are actually very different sports. This chapter discusses each type of snow skiing, addresses the nutritional concerns of each, explores the physiology of each type, and outlines issues important to the sports nutritionist working with athletes involved in each ski type. In addition, the nutritional concerns for recreational versus competitive skiing are discussed, as well as the relationship between nutrition and physical performance and current dietary recommendations and modifications.

PHYSIOLOGY

Muscle Fiber-type Composition

The three major groups of muscle fiber are identified histochemically as Types I, IIa, and IIb (4). Generally, Type I are slow-twitch fibers that have high capabilities for aerobic energy production. These fibers are recruited in endurance activities such as running and cross-country skiing. All of the biochemical characteristics that support aerobic metabolism are at high levels in these fibers. Dubovitz (5) reported that athletes who participated for long periods of time in endurance activities such as distance running have higher than expected percentages of Type I fibers. Cross-country skiers have a higher percentage of Type I fibers in both the lower and upper extremities than other types of skiers and the normal, nonskier population (6).

Type II are the fast-twitch fibers, which are classified into two subgroups: IIa (fast-twitch-oxidative-glycolytic) and IIb (fast-twitch-glycolytic). These fibers have high capabilities for producing energy anaerobically; however, Type IIa fibers also have the ability for aerobic energy production and are sometimes called the "super fiber" in terms of performance. Conditioning enhances the ability of this fiber type to use energy substrates by increasing the amount and activity of enzymes (4).

Generally, the slow-twitch Type I are larger fibers responsible for stability and are predominant in larger muscle groups. Type II fibers tend to be narrow and create speed and frequency of movement (5). While competitive alpine skiers are noted to have a greater percentage of Type II fibers in their lower extremities, cross-country skiers have a higher percentage of Type I fibers, possibly due to the varying terrain and nonsteady-state conditions (6).

Energy Systems

As the types of skiing are different, so are the energy requirements. The success of cross-country skiers depends largely on aerobic and anaerobic energy systems. These energy systems work together to provide fuel to working muscles (7). Ski jumping is an event of short duration and will depend mainly on anaerobic energy systems, and alpine skiing may be viewed as a cross between the endurance demands of cross-country skiing and the shorter completion interval of ski jumping.

The energy cost of skiing differs depending on the intensity and type of exercise. Depending on the demands of the sport, the range for total daily energy expenditure is highly variable (8). Activity level, age, gender, body size, weight, and body composition all contribute to differences in energy expenditure. The average daily energy expenditure for female and male cross-country skiers was studied by researchers at the University of Montana (9). They found the average daily caloric expenditures for female and male cross-country skiers in training to be 3,500 kcal per day for women and 5,000 kcal per day for men. When not in training, caloric expenditures were 2,700 kcal per day for women and 3,500 kcal per day for men (9). They compared this data to energy costs of other sports and found that tennis players expended 7.1 kcal per minute (male) and 5.5 kcal per minute (female); cross-country skiers use 24 kcal per minute (male) and 18 kcal per minute (female) (9).

DOWNHILL SKIING

Traditional downhill skiing is known as alpine skiing. Though a recreational sport for many, it is also a highly competitive sport that requires control of speed and precision. Competitive alpine skiers race in four types of events:

1. Downhill, a steep descent in a race against time
2. Slalom, raced on a sharply twisting course marked off by flags
3. Giant slalom, resembles slalom but uses longer, less twisted courses that permit faster speeds (10).
4. Supergiant, or super g, resembles giant slalom but uses longer courses

Though technique is crucial for success in this sport, endurance is not necessarily a focus. Thus the nutritional concerns of an alpine skier more resemble the dietary needs of a single-event athlete than those of an endurance-trained cross-country skier.

Physiologically, downhill skiing primarily uses the ATP-CP and lactic acid systems. Since ski runs are timed in minutes and partial seconds, training the specific muscles groups in motor planning methodology for appropriate reflex and timing, along with balance and equilibrium sequencing, is more important than training for maximal oxygen uptake (VO_2max) or strength training (4). The aerobic demands of competitive alpine skiing may approach 90% to 95% of the athlete's maximal aerobic power, with maximal heart rate achieved during the latter part of the race (11). Though elite skiers have a high VO_2max, this may be due more to their training programs than the actual demands of the sport (11). Alpine skiers depend on anaerobic metabolic power to aggressively turn and switch positions around corners. This type of muscular activity acts to impede blood flow and oxygen delivery.

The physiological profiles of elite alpine skiers reveal the importance of muscular strength, anaerobic power, aerobic endurance, coordination, agility, balance, and flexibility (11). Physical characteristics of elite skiers include average height and body mass, although today's successful skiers are taller and heavier than their predecessors. Slalom skiers tend to be leaner than skiers in the other events, while the downhill racers are the heaviest. Elite skiers have strong legs when peak torque is measured during isometric and isokinetic conditions involving knee extension; this may represent a specific adaptation since these skiers are in a crouched position for a prolonged period of time when racing (11).

Tesch (12), investigating the physiological demands of competitive alpine skiing, found maximal heart rates occur at the end of the four alpine ski events. The giant slalom, with the largest reliance upon aerobic energy, may increase oxygen uptake to 75% to 100% of maximal aerobic power. Further, anaerobic energy accounted for more than half of the total energy used. Accordingly, plasma and muscle lactate accumulation was substantial after a single race. Similarly, during skiing there is a high rate of glycogen utilization that eventually may result in depletion of muscle glycogen stores by the end of a day of intense skiing. Tesch (12) also found that alpine skiers did not possess a distinct muscle fiber-type composition, although a slight preponderance of slow-twitch fibers was noted. All muscle fiber types are used during slalom events. The most elite skiers had increased knee extensor strength, possibly due to their greater reliance on slow and forceful eccentric muscle action when performing turns in the slalom races (12).

CROSS-COUNTRY SKIING

A traditional Nordic type of skiing, cross-country enjoys popularity from the novice to the most experienced skier. This may be true because the sport is relatively inexpensive, the equipment is readily available, and the terrain can be as easy or as difficult as the participant chooses. Recreational skiers may be seen in their own backyards, local golf courses, snowed-over hiking trails, as well as specifically groomed cross-country trails. However, unlike alpine and ski jumping, cross-country skiing is an endurance sport (13). The elite skier is one who attains superiority through years of training; this has been demonstrated on Olympic levels where no junior skier has ever won an Olympic gold medal or World Championship in this event (14).

Because of the endurance nature of this sport, and the popularity and ease of participation for the novice, there is a great deal of research on the physiology of cross-country skiing. Most of it has been performed in Europe, the Scandinavian countries, and the United States. Other types of skiing associated with cross-country include telemarking and backcountry skiing. Telemarking is similar to downhill skiing in that the action is generally going down a hill. The equipment is heavier than cross-country equipment but similar in that the binding allows movement of the heel of the foot off the ski for a push-off stride motion. Backcountry skiing involves skiing on wide skis over areas that are not groomed, including deep snow. This is more like expedition travel and not a competitive endeavor.

Cross-country skiing, unlike the endurance sports of running and bicycling, places major demands on upper body musculature, including the latissimus dorsi, deltoids, and triceps groups (6). Due to the involvement of the upper body and the energy requirements of the sport, the maximal oxygen uptake (VO_2max) is the single most distinguishing factor between the novice skier and the elite athlete (15). The effect of VO_2max and cardiac conditioning is discussed later in this chapter.

Economy and Skiing Techniques

The many unique aspects of the sport of cross-country skiing include technique and style. Also, there are different ways to traverse the varied terrain of the sport, although generally the sport is divided into two styles with three varied techniques each: the traditional or classic style with skis placed horizontally in ruts includes the diagonal stride, double pole, and kick double pole; and the second style, skating, which includes the marathon skate, V2 skate, and V1 skate (16).

Cross-country skiing uses all of the major muscle groups. Studies at Montana State University (9) delineated several of the common ski patterns and the muscles used in order of greatest use, as shown in *Table 43.1*. This table provides information on the diagonal stride and double-poling technique of classic cross-country skiing, and skating. The most notable difference in comparing skating to classic is the heavy dependence on the lower extremities early in the skating event. The diagonal stride uses the sartorius muscle of the upper thigh more than other muscle groups. This muscle is not traditionally used in normal ambulation; thus, although the stride of classic is in diagonal, parallel patterns, development of this muscle requires a special training effort. Also, the gastrocnemius of the calf may also need development and may create Achilles-tendon problems, since it is used as both an agonist and antagonist in the stride, push-off, and glide nature of classic cross-country skiing. With double-poling the upper trunk and torso are involved. The pectorals and abdominals are used most heavily, followed by the deltoid of the upper arm and the latissimus muscles that span the back in a fan fashion from sacrum to lateral of the upper arm.

TABLE 43.1 Overview of Major Muscle Groups Used during Cross-Country Ski Patterns in Order of Use (9)

Diagonal Stride	Double-poling	Skating
• Sartorius	• Pectoralis major	• Gluteus maximus
• Rectus femoris	• Abdominal muscles	• Rectus femoris
• Triceps brachii	• Deltoid	• Biceps femoris
• Gastrocnemius	• Latissimus dorsi	• Sartorius
• Biceps brachii	• Biceps brachii	• Triceps brachii
		• Deltoid

According to the University of Montana research (9), although the classic double-poling technique is the most economical of the classic style, the skating technique is faster depending on temperature and snow conditions. Typically, skating races are 5% to 50% faster over the same distance when compared to classic skiing. Classic double-poling is more economical on level ground than skating; therefore, it is the most economical technique. However, double-poling involves a smaller muscle mass to generate work; the strain on the muscles initiated is higher and so is the perceived exertion of the skier. Researchers found that double-poling does not allow the athlete to use his or her maximal work capacity (9), so being energy efficient is not effective if too little power is generated. Thus, in the case of competitive cross-country skiers, the skier with the greatest VO_2max may be the winner (6).

The least economical style is the classic diagonal stride. Hoffman and Clifford (17) measured several physiological variables during skiing at a constant speed while using different techniques on level ground. The oxygen cost was 33% higher during the diagonal stride compared to double-poling on classic skis. Consequently, this technique is most frequently seen during hill climbing in classic races, when distributing the high workload over the largest muscle mass possible is important.

Heart rates, blood lactate concentrations, and perceived efforts elicited at a given oxygen uptake are similar between the diagonal stride and skating techniques. Therefore, the cardiorespiratory training benefits from classical skiing and ski skating will most likely be similar if performed at the same heart rates or perceived efforts (6).

Equipment design and use, as well as weather factors, also create variables for all skiers. How or if skis are waxed, with what kind of wax, and what part of the ski is waxed all play a role in the success of the athlete. Generally, wax is applied to the center part of the bottom of the ski in classic cross-country to provide a friction force to allow a kick motion to propel the skier forward. The wax is chosen based on the ambient air temperature, condition of the track (eg, cold, hard, slush) and skill of the participant. Since the skating technique requires an oblique angle of force to travel in a forward trajectory, wax is applied for glide and not friction (13).

SKI JUMPING

A traditional Nordic type of skiing, ski jumping is not for the faint of heart. This sport requires the participant to travel down a set track along a designed scaffold, jump off the edge, and travel through the air down a hill. Competition is based on the length of each jump, the style maintained during flight and landing, and the ability to stay upright to the end of the jump. It is a sport of strength and attempting to stay in the air longer and go farther than other competitors while airborne. It is also a sport of style. Jumpers are given style points awarded by judges. Jumpers have long been attracted to the sport because of the ability to fly (18). However, this is not a recreational sport or one that novices may dabble in.

The very nature of the sport, degree of difficulty, fear factor, and availability of ski jump facilities further limit participation. Common jumps are 70 to 90 meters high and designed with elongated S-shaped arcs to allow the jumpers to have in-air flights of 90 to 120 meters before touching ground. Speed is a factor with jumpers, hitting air speeds of 115 kilometers per hour (18).

Ski jumping is a sport that relies on a combination of biomechanics and aerodynamics. Physically, the jumper begins a run at the top of the ski jump in a crouched position with head tucked and arms drawn in a flexed pattern, along or within the body crouch. Upon initiation of movement down the jump, timing for maximal explosion of muscular power in the lower extremities, combined with a stretching out of the body in a linear fashion—a fluid motion to propel the skier through the air—is created. The single most significant training factor for this sport is lower-extremity, explosive extension from a crouched flexed position (18). This motion relies on the ATP-CP energy system and a coordinated movement of synergy quickly changing agonists to antagonists at the foot of the jump prior to airborne take-off. Strength and control of the synergists are demanded to maintain an upright posture to allow for the force of the landing. This is an explosive, single-episode type of sport and does not necessarily depend on cardiovascular fitness to perform a single jump (19). However, to train, climb the heights of the large jumps, and perform these amazing feats, physical fitness is necessary. Arstil and Rusco (19) noted the need for consecutive jumps during ski jump training that includes carrying heavy equipment up the steep slopes of the jumps. They calculated a rather high metabolic cost to ascending a jump at 2 L O_2 per minute, implying that cardiovascular fitness is important (19).

Ski jumping may be considered a power activity requiring that exercise is done in short periods of time. In power training, attention needs to be paid to the differences between muscular strength and muscular endurance (4).

Ski jumpers tend to have a lower mean body weight (61.9 kg) compared to a like group of controls (71.5 kg) and a lower body fat percentage (8.6% versus 16.1%). In a dietary study of Finnish ski jumpers, the mean energy intake was lower in ski jumpers than in a control group, whereas the percentage of energy derived from carbohydrates was higher in these athletes (20). The researchers suggested that despite the lower body weight and energy intake of the ski jumpers, their nutritional status was not compromised when compared with that of nonathletic controls (20).

As with all the ski sports, proper equipment and clothing play an important role in the success of the competitor. The ski's design and length, the type of ski wax used, and snow and weather conditions help determine the success of each jump.

FACTORS AFFECTING PERFORMANCE AND NUTRITION NEEDS

Multiple factors may affect the performance of individual skiing participants. These include cardiovascular factors, body composition and body mass, nutrient requirements (fat, carbohydrate, and protein), hydration, and immunity.

Cardiovascular Requirements

Cardiovascular fitness is a distinguishing factor for reaching the elite status for cross-country skiing (21). Though all sports require physical fitness to compete, cross-country skiing is one that requires total body fitness. Top cross-country skiers generally have exceedingly high maximal oxygen uptakes (VO2max).

Since more muscle groups are involved in skiing than in walking, the overall energy expenditure in transporting the body on skis from one place to another may be higher than the energy expenditure when moving the body the same distance on foot. Sharkey (22) compared runners to cross-country skiers and observed that highly trained runners have an arm VO2max that was only 60% of their leg or running VO2max, while highly trained skiers had observed arm VO2max of 85% of their leg VO2max (17). Kelly (15) reported that when trained runners were required to perform combined arm and leg work, their VO2max decreased by 6%. Kelly concluded that in athletes with poorly trained arms, the upper body demanded more blood than it could efficiently use while the legs may be deprived of available oxygen, thus resulting in early fatigue caused by inefficient distribution of oxygenated blood (15).

Cardiovascular conditioning is important for all athletes and especially for skiers. The competitive nature of skiing challenges coaches and sports nutritionists to identify factors limiting performance and to help the athlete delay or reduce them. Cardiovascular conditioning, when combined with nutritional support, may eliminate or reduce some of these factors.

Body Composition and Body Mass

The ideal body composition varies with different sports but, in general, the more desirable the body composition, the greater the performance. University of Montana researchers found that the average male Olympic cross-country skier is

25 years old, 5'10" tall, 165 lb, and has 5% body fat. The average female Olympic cross-country skier is 25 years old, 5'7" tall, 141 lb, and has 11% body fat (9).

The success of an athlete depends on body type. Body size, build, and composition can influence performance. Athletic performance relates to body type (body shape and size) and body composition (muscular development and amount of body fat). Body fat contributes no strength advantage and limits endurance, speed, and movement through space (23). Olympic cross-country skiers are extremely lean compared to average males and females (6).

Dietary Fat

At rest and during normal daily activities, fats are the primary energy source, providing 80% to 90% of energy (23). During exercise the proportion of this contribution will change.

During low-intensity aerobic activities, fats are the preferred substrate. Fatty acid use in aerobic metabolism results in far greater ATP production than that of carbohydrates. However, even when fats are the predominant energy source, carbohydrates must still be available to oxidize fatty acids. Therefore, fats are never an exclusive energy source. Even when large amounts of fats are available, or there are very low levels of carbohydrate to prime their oxidation, aerobic degradation of fat will be inefficient.

Fats are not converted to either protein or carbohydrate. Fat storage occurs within muscle cells for use during aerobic activity and within the adipocytes. Athletes benefit from having appropriate amounts of body fat in three ways: shock absorption, which is important in activities such as the landing of a ski jumper; thermal insulation, which is important in cold weather alpine and ski jumping; and fuel stores for aerobic endurance events such as cross-country skiing. Proper training can increase muscle mass and, when coupled with sound nutrition practices, can change body composition. Typically, cross-country skiers need to be muscular for energy demands and lean for good performance (24).

Carbohydrate

Pre-exercise diet. The importance of dietary carbohydrate to promote glycogen storage in the days preceding an exhaustive endurance event is well established (25). Endurance athletes and those who train exhaustively on successive days may require 65% to 75% of calories from carbohydrates to optimize performance (26). Glycogen depletion during training can be prevented by a high-carbohydrate diet and periodic rest days to allow muscles time to rebuild glycogen stores. Feelings of tiredness associated with overtraining could be partially related to lower glycogen stores (27).

A typical diet recommendation for a pre-exercise or preevent meal for alpine and ski jumpers would be one that is light, approximately 300 kcal, consists primarily of low-fiber carbohydrate-containing foods, and includes a moderate amount of protein (28). For prolonged exercise or events in cross-country skiing, a relatively large pre-exercise meal containing more than 200 g carbohydrate appears to improve performance by allowing the athlete to oxidize carbohydrates at a higher rate late in exercise (29). Consumption of the pre-exercise meal at least 2 to 3 hours prior to the exercise session typically allows for complete gastric emptying and minimizes the possibility of exercise-induced gastrointestinal upset.

Carbohydrate during exercise. Carbohydrate ingestion during low-intensity exercise increases blood glucose and insulin concentrations, which results in a two-fold increase in glucose uptake into skeletal muscle (30,31). Coggan and Coyle (31) found that endurance-racing cyclists using carbohydrate-enhanced drinks during moderate exercise improved their performance. Their research established that blood glucose can be oxidized at very high rates during low, moderate, and prolonged exercise, and that ingested carbohydrate makes a significant contribution to the energy substrate used by skeletal muscle (31). Applying this finding to skiers, it is important for the endurance cross-country skiers to consume adequate carbohydrates during exercise. However, due to the aerobic, short-time interval of alpine and ski jumping, carbohydrate ingestion during the activity is not feasible and probably not important for physical performance.

Both the timing and rate of carbohydrate ingestion during exercise can influence performance. Carbohydrate supplementation throughout prolonged endurance exercise or provided at least 35 minutes before the onset of fatigue is effective in delaying fatigue (31). Coggan and Coyle (31) suggest that ingesting carbohydrates throughout prolonged exercise may be of greater advantage because of the potential for glycogen resynthesis. They recommend that carbohydrate supplementation be sufficient to provide a minimum of 45 to 60 g of total carbohydrate for improvement of exercise performance (31). For skiers, this translates into 24 to 32 oz (3 to 4 cups) of a carbohydrate-containing beverage (eg, an appropriately formulated sports drink) throughout the event.

Postexercise diet. Replenishment of liver and muscle glycogen stores after strenuous physical activity is critical to perform subsequent endurance exercise. There appears to be an upper level of carbohydrate intake, ranging from 500 to 600 g per day, above which little additional contribution to glycogen storage or enhancement of athletic performance will occur (32). Carbohydrate intake recommendations that are based on a specific percentage of total energy intake can lead to daily intakes well above this recommended range, when overall energy intakes are particularly high. Therefore, the amount of carbohydrate consumed by athletes is more appropriately based either on total daily consumption (g/day) or, to account for athletes' differing body sizes, total daily consumption per unit body weight (g/kg/day).

Table 43.2 highlights the differing carbohydrate needs for skiers in different types of exercise formats from the single event and power needed for ski jumping, to the ongoing anaerobic and aerobic needs of the single-event alpine skier, to the ongoing endurance needs of the cross-country skier. However, all three types of competitive skiers are involved in training regimes in addition to the event participation. Therefore, this table outlines the training categories for carbohydrate intake for each type of skiing.

TABLE 43.2   Summary of Recommended Carbohydrate Intake Goals for Skiers (33)

Goal	Carbohydrate Intake Target
To participate in 5 to 6 hours of moderate-intensity exercise, extremely prolonged and intense. Very high total energy requirements, daily muscle glycogen recovery, and continued refueling during exercise. (Cross-country skiers for events >50 km)	10 to 12+ g/kg daily
To maximize daily muscle glycogen recovery in order to enhance prolonged daily training or "load" the muscle with glycogen before a prolonged exercise competition. (Cross-country skiers for events 20+ km)	7 to 10 g/kg daily
To meet fuel needs and general nutrition goals in a less fuel-demanding program. For example, <1 hour of moderate-intensity exercise or many hours of predominantly low-intensity exercise. (Short distance cross-country skiing of 6 to 15 km; alpine/ski jumping training)	5 to 7 g/kg daily
To enhance early recovery after exercise, when the next session is less than 8 hours away and glycogen recovery may be limiting. (Cross-country, alpine, and ski jumpers)	1 g/kg soon after exercise, with continued intake to meet a total of ~1g/kg every 2 hours. This is achieved in snacks or a large meal.
To enhance fuel availability for prolonged exercise session. (≥1 hour) (Cross-country skiers)	1 to 4 g/kg during the 1 to 4 hours pre-exercise
To provide an additional source of carbohydrate during prolonged moderate- and high-intensity exercise, particularly in hot conditions or where pre-exercise fuel stores are suboptimal. (Cross-country and during alpine and ski-jumping training)	30 to 60 g per hour in an appropriate fluid or food form

Dietary Protein

Protein supplementation to prolong endurance performance by acting as an accessory fuel is plausible because 5% to 10% of energy production during long-term endurance exercise is produced from protein catabolism (34). Several reviews also suggest that high-protein diets or protein supplements do not enhance long-term endurance performance (40); however, studies are sparse and not definitive. For athletes who consume high-protein diets, there has been a fear of adverse effects as well. However, there is no evidence that high-protein intake has any adverse effect on otherwise healthy individuals (40).

A consensus of research via different methodologies has found that endurance athletes have an intensity-dependent, dietary protein requirement of 1.2 to 1.4 g/kg per day (150% to 175% of the recommended daily requirement for sedentary people, which is 0.8 g/kg per day). This equates to a daily protein intake of almost 100 g for a 70-kg male (41). Due to the training needs of skiers, this protein intake seems to be a prudent recommendation.

Hydration

Adequate hydration is critical for temperature regulation and performance for athletes of all ages. It is an erroneous assumption that heat stroke occurs only in hot weather and that skiers, because they compete in cold weather, need not worry about this life-threatening condition. Sweating and heat loss do occur in cold weather sports. For skiers, it is important that body temperature regulation occurs through the maintenance of proper hydration (35).

Ideally, the volume of water intake during exercise should match its overall loss from sweat, urine, and respiration. Coaches and trainers should provide consistent encouragement for athletes to drink fluids prior to the onset of thirst and encourage an intake of at least 112 to 168 g of fluid every 20 to 30 minutes during exercise to optimize performance and prevent adverse health effects (36). For the skier in training, it is possible to simultaneously achieve fluid and carbohydrate requirements for endurance exercise with a wide choice of beverages containing up to 8% carbohydrate.

Postexercise, the athlete needs to consume sufficient amounts of fluid to reestablish water balance. The source of fluid may not be important, but sports drinks containing simple carbohydrates and sufficient electrolytes may be of benefit because they enhance rehydration, replace electrolytes, and provide carbohydrate for glycogen resynthesis. Several studies indicate that skiers generally have insufficient fluid intake practices to maintain adequate hydration (24,37). Thus, it is critical for the sports nutritionist working with skiers to emphasize proper hydration practices. For detailed information on fluid guidelines, see Chapter 6, Fluid and Electrolytes.

In consideration of hydration requirements particular to cold-weather sports, many researchers have studied the effects of lack of adequate water consumption as well as the temperature of the hydrating products. The lack of adequate water consumption (hypohydration) can reduce food consumption, efficiency of physical and mental performance, and resistance to cold exposure (38). While adequate fluid intake is paramount in preventing hypohydration in the cold, it is also prudent to consider the temperature of fluid and food provided for work in the cold. Warm fluids and heated food are generally recommended in cold weather whenever possible to impart a feeling of warmth and well-being (39). The warming effect of a hot beverage in the cold is probably related to its effect upon subsequent vasodilation and increased blood flow to cold extremities rather than to the actual quantity of heat contained in the ingested fluid.

Immunity

Epidemiological data suggest that endurance athletes are at increased risk for upper respiratory tract infections (URTI) during periods of heavy training and in the 1- to 2-week period following race events. However, moderate exercise training has been associated with a reduction in the incidence of URTI (42). Nieman (42) found that for several hours after heavy exertion, several components of both the innate and adaptive immune systems exhibit suppressed function. Further, the immune response to heavy exertion was transient (43).

Due to this apparent risk of URTI, several studies have been done with skiers to determine if there are chemical or nutritional means to attenuate the immune changes caused by intensive exercise. Nieman and Pedersen (44) studied the effects of nutritional supplements that included zinc, vitamin C, glutamine, and carbohydrate on the immune systems of endurance athletes. In addition, they attempted to quantify assertions by manufacturers that carbohydrate beverage ingestion diminished the frequency of infections. They found no convincing evidence that either nutritional supplements or carbohydrate beverages reduced the likelihood of URTI (44)

Vitamin C supplementation has been recommended for skiers (45). However, one study found that vitamin C supplementation did not alter the immune response of endurance runners who were involved in more than 2.5 hours of intensive training (46). Therefore, recommending vitamin C supplements to skiers is not based on adequate scientific study. However, consuming foods rich in vitamins is not harmful, and the simplest way to insure adequate vitamin C intake is through the inclusion of fresh fruits, vegetables, and citrus juice in the training diet. In addition, many juice products and energy bars are fortified with vitamin C.

ADDITIONAL FOOD CONSIDERATIONS

Snacks

Competitors may spend a long period of time on a hill, jump, or course. Therefore, in addition to regular meals, snacks should also be considered. Snacks that can be carried in a pocket or jacket pouch include hard candies, licorice or fruit-flavored snacks, energy bars, cheese or peanut butter crackers, dried fruits, and trail mix. In addition, fluids should be included with snacks. Hot beverages, sports drinks, and juice boxes are all good choices.

Meal Choices

Skiing is a great exercise for recreational and competitive athletes, but the food choices available at many ski resorts may not be the most healthful. A sports nutritionist can help the competitor review the menus at the ski resort facilities and make recommendations to help meet the energy and nutrient needs of the athlete. The appeal of food and the need for variety should be underscored for all types of skiers.

CASE STUDY

Joe is a 5'10", 160-lb collegiate cross-country skier. He trains 2 to 3 hours daily. In the off-season he weight trains, flexibility trains, roller skis, and runs. In season much of his training time is spent skiing 15 to 30 km per day along with weight training two times per week. He complains that his race time has not improved, even though his training is more intense and specific than it was in high school. He also complains of fatigue during weekend competition and lack of concentration in his classes.

The sports nutritionist asked Joe to maintain a diet record. This revealed that he eats a large breakfast on days when he does not have an early morning class. However, on the 3 days a week he has a morning class, he skips breakfast. His lunch consists of 2 cups of pasta salad from the deli and a piece of fruit. He finds it difficult to eat 2 hours before or after training, so his evening meal is consumed late in the evening and usually includes a convenience food item such as macaroni and cheese or frozen pizza. His dietary goal is to eat low-fat food, though he notes that he feels hungry but lacks the energy to make more food.

The nutritionist notes that Joe is not consuming adequate calories to support his energy expenditure.

Recommendations

- Suggest that Joe manage his training schedule by allowing for less rigorous workouts the day or two prior to weekend competition to allow muscles to adequately store glycogen.
- Increase calories to approximately 5,000 kcal/day (9) with 60% of calories as carbohydrates (3,000 kcal or 750 g), 10% to 15% of calories as protein (188 g), and 20% to 25% of calories as fat.
- Include at least 4 to 6 meals each day.
- Monitor weight to assure adequate hydration on a daily basis and encourage carrying a water bottle and consuming fluids throughout the day. Include sports drinks to provide carbohydrates as well as fluids.
- Develop a weight maintenance plan during the competitive season to insure a stable weight.
- Increase food intake and establish meal times. Suggest the purchase of a meal ticket for the campus dining hall.
- Encourage daily breakfast to include foods to meet at least 1/4 of his energy needs for the day.
- Plan nutrient-dense snacks—fruit, fruit juice, fruit or oatmeal cookies, sandwiches, and milk.

REFERENCES

1. *Columbia Encyclopedia.* 5th ed. New York, NY: Columbia University Press; 1993.
2. Jonas R, Masia S. Total skiing. *Ski Magazine.* 1987;13:232-238.
3. Barnett S. *Cross-Country, Downhill and Other Nordic Mountain Skiing Techniques.* Seattle, Wash: Pacific Search Press; 1998.
4. Jackson CG. Overview of human energy transfer and nutrition. In: Wolinski I, ed. *Nutrition in Exercise and Sport.* 3rd ed. New York, NY: CRC Press; 1998:159-175.
5. Dubovitz V. *Muscle Biopsy: A Practical Approach.* 2nd ed. Philadelphia, Pa: Bailliere Tindall; 1988.
6. Hoffman MD. Physiological comparisons of cross-country skiing techniques. *Med Sci Sports Exerc.* 1992;24:841-848.
7. Rusco HK. Development of aerobic power in relation to age and training in cross-country skiers. *Med Sci Sports Exerc.* 1992;24:1040-1047.
8. Guyton AC. *Textbook of Medical Physiology.* 8th ed. Philadelphia, Pa: W B Saunders Co; 1991.
9. Montana State University-Bozeman. *Physiology and Psychology: Performance Benchmarks.* http://btc.montana.edu/olympics/physiology. Accessed May 10, 1999.
10. McMurty JG. Biomechanics of alpine skiing. In: Casey MJ, Foster C, Hixson EG, eds. *Winter Sports Medicine.* Philadelphia, Pa: Davis Company; 1990:344-350.
11. Andersen RE, Montgomery DL. Physiology of alpine skiing. *Sports Med.* 1988;6:210-221.

12. Tesch PA. Aspects on muscle properties and use in competitive alpine skiing. *Med Sci Sports Exerc*. 1995;27:310-314.

13. Clifford PS. Scientific basis of competitive cross-country skiing. *Med Sci Sports Exerc*. 1992;4:1007-1009.

14. Seiler S. *The Physiology of Cross-Country Skiing. 1996.* http://www.krs.hia.no/~stephens/skiphysi.html. Accessed May 10, 1999.

15. Kelly JM. Physiology of cross-country skiing. In: Casey MJ, Foster C, Hixson EG, eds. *Winter Sports Medicine*. Philadelphia, Pa: Davis Company; 1990:277-283.

16. Maier S. *Cross-Country Skiing: Racing Techniques and Training Tips*. Woodbury, NY: Barrons Publishing; 1980.

17. Hoffman MD, Clifford PS. Physiological aspects of competitive cross-country skiing. *J Sports Sci*. 1992;10:3-27.

18. Harkins KJ. Physiology of ski jumping. In: Casey MJ, Foster C, Hixson EG, eds. *Winter Sports Medicine*. Philadelphia, Pa: Davis Company; 1990:308-314.

19. Arstil A, Rusco H. *Fitness Profiles of Elite Finnish Athletes*. Research Report #10. University of Jyvaskyla, Finland: Department of Biology of Physical Activity; 1976.

20. Rankinen T, Lyytikainen S, Vanninen E, Penttila I, Rauramaa R, Ususitupa M. Nutritional status of the Finnish elite ski jumpers. *Med Sci Sports Exerc*. 1998;30:1592-1597.

21. Bergh U, Forsberg A. Influence of body mass on cross-country ski racing performance. *Med Sci Sports Exerc*. 1992;24:1033-1039.

22. Sharkey BJ. *Coaches' Guide to Sport Physiology*. Champaign, Ill: Human Kinetics; 1986.

23. McArdle WE, Katch FI, Katch VL. *Exercise Physiology: Energy, Nutrition and Human Performance*. 3rd ed. Philadelphia, Pa: Lea & Febiger; 1991.

24. Parizkova J. Dietary intake and body physique in adolescent cross-country skiers. *J Sports Sci*. 1994;12:251-254.

25. Wilkinson JG, Liebman M. Carbohydrate metabolism in sport and exercise. In: Wolinsky I, ed. *Nutrition in Exercise and Sport*. 3rd ed. New York, NY: CRC Press; 1998:63-99.

26. Sherman W. Carbohydrates, muscle glycogen and muscle glycogen supercompensation. In: Williams MH, ed. *Ergogenic Aids in Sports*. Champaign, Ill: Human Kinetics; 1983:164-176.

27. Costill DL, Hargreaves M. Carbohydrate nutrition and fatigue. *Sports Med*. 1992;13:86-92.

28. Clark N. *Nancy Clark's Sports Nutrition Guidebook*. Champaign, Ill: Leisure Press; 1990.

29. Coyle EF. Substrate utilization during exercise in active people. *Am J Clin Nutr*. 1995;61(suppl):968S:12-16.

30. Burke LM, Claassen A, Hawley JA, Noakes TD. No effect of glycemic index of pre-exercise meals with carbohydrate intake during exercise. *Med Sci Sports Exerc*. 1998;30:3-12.

31. Coggan AR, Coyle EF. Carbohydrate ingestion during prolonged exercise: effects on metabolism and performance. *Exerc Sports Sci Rev*. 1991;19:1-40.

32. Lamb DR, Rinehardt KF, Bartels RL, Sherman WM, Snook JT. Dietary carbohydrate and intensity of interval swim training. *Am J Clin Nutr*. 1990;52:1058-1064.

33. Hawley JA, Burke LM. *Peak Performance: Training and Nutritional Strategies for Sport*. Sydney, Australia: Allen & Unwin; 1998.

34. Lemon PW. Do athletes need more dietary protein and amino acids? *Int J Sport Nutr*. 1995;(suppl):S39-S61.

35. Burke LM, Read RS. Sports nutrition: approaching the nineties. *Sports Med*. 1989;8:80-100.

36. Squire D. Heat illness: fluid and electrolyte issues for pediatric and adolescent athletes. *Sports Med*. 1990;37:1085-1093.

37. Iuliano S, Naughton G, Collier G, Carlson J. Examination of the self-selected fluid intake practices by junior athletes during a simulated duathlon event. *Int J Sports Nutr*. 1998;8:10-23.

38. Freund BJ, Sawka MN. Influence of cold stress on human fluid balance. In: Marriott BM, ed. *Nutritional Needs in Cold and in High-Altitude Environments*. Washington, DC: National Academy Press; 1996:69-103.

39. Young AJ, Roberts DE, Scott DP, Cook JE, Mays MZ, Askew EW. *Sustaining Health and Performance in the Cold. Environmental Medical Guidance for Cold Weather Operations*. Natick, Mass: US Army Research Institute of Environmental Medicine; 1992. No 92-2.

40. Lemon PW. Effects of exercise on dietary protein requirements. *Int J Sport Nutr*. 1998;8:426-447.

41. Bucci LR. Dietary supplements as ergogenic aids. In: Wolinsky I, ed. *Nutrition in Exercise and Sport*. 3rd ed. New York, NY: CRC Press; 1998:315-338.

42. Nieman DC. Exercise and resistance to infection. *Can J Physiol Pharmacol*. 1998;76:573-580.

43. Nieman DC. Immune response to heavy exertion. *J Appl Phys*. 1997;82:1385-1394.

44. Nieman DC, Pederson BK. Exercise and immune function: recent developments. *Sports Med*. 1977;27:73-80.

45. Case S, Evans D, Tibbets G, Case S, Miller D. Dietary intakes of participants in the IditaSport human powered ultra-marathon. *Alaska Medicine*. 1995;37:20-24.

46. Nieman DC, Henson DA, Butterworth DE, et al. Vitamin C supplementation does not alter the immune response to 2.5 hours of running. *Int J Sport Nutr*. 1997;7:173-184.

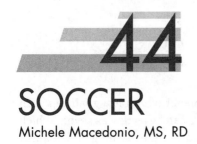

SOCCER

Michele Macedonio, MS, RD

Soccer, a very old team sport, is one of the most widely played sports in the world today and growing in popularity. Fédération Internationale de Football Association (FIFA) is the international governing body of soccer and considered the most powerful sports organization in the world. FIFA, founded in 1904 by delegates from France, Belgium, Denmark, the Netherlands, Spain, Sweden, and Switzerland, now has 190 member nations divided into confederations representing five continents and the Oceania region. American soccer can trace its origins to 1862 with the establishment of the Oneidas of Boston, the first organized football club formed in Boston, Massachusetts (1); but soccer did not enjoy wide popularity in the United States until the 1980s when interest skyrocketed.

Ranging from professional teams to recreational leagues, participation in soccer by men, women, adults, and children is steadily increasing. Evidence of soccer's increasing popularity in the United States is the burgeoning number of youth and women who are filling the soccer fields, the increasing number of and members in soccer associations (see *Box 44.1*), the growing number of college- and university-sponsored varsity soccer teams, and the expansion of professional soccer teams. Currently, soccer leads all United States team sports as the number one supervised activity for youth 18 and under. Among adults soccer play has increased 37% since 1990. More colleges and universities sponsor soccer than tackle football, and women's soccer at the college level has quadrupled since 1983 (2).

BOX 44.1   US Soccer Associations and Organizations

- US Soccer Federation
- US Soccer Federation Foundation
- US Soccer Amateur Division
- US Youth Soccer Association
- AYSO: American Youth Soccer Organization
- SAYUSA: Soccer Association for Youth, USA
- US Futsal Federation
- NSCAA: National Soccer Coaches Association of America
- US Paralympic Soccer
- The Soccer Industry Council of America publishes soccer participation statistics
- American Sports Participation Statistics from the Sporting Goods Manufacturing Association

---

More information on the associations and organizations listed above can be found on the web at http://www.sams-army.com/misc/associations/assocs.html

ELEMENTS OF SOCCER

A soccer team is usually made up of 11 players, one of whom is a goalkeeper. In age groups younger than 12, the number of players can be as few as seven, which gives the players more "touches" on the ball, enhancing the learning and acquisition of skills.

Soccer is most commonly played outdoors on a rectangular field 100 to 130 yards (90 to 117 meters) in length and 50 to 100 yards (45 to 90 meters) in width. A goal is positioned at each end of the length of the field. In the United States soccer is also played indoors on a smaller field and with different rules. A regulation outdoor game consists of two, 45-minute halves with a 15-minute half-time break. In groups under 12 years of age, soccer is generally played on a scaled down field for shorter lengths of time (3). Games for under 8 years of age (U-8) are generally divided into four, 12-minute quarters with 5-minute breaks and a 10-minute half-time. Under 10 (U-10) games usually have two, 25-minute halves increasing to 30-minute halves for U-12, and 45-minute halves at the U-19 level.

The four basic player positions in soccer are (4):

1. Goalkeeper
2. Defender, known as fullbacks, and includes sweeper
3. Midfielder or linkmen, known as halfbacks
4. Attackers, known as forwards, and includes wings and strikers

To address the nutrition needs of soccer players, it is important to understand the physiological demands of soccer and the energy systems involved. Soccer is a high-intensity, intermittent exercise. A soccer match entails periods of short, intense activity interspersed with periods of low-level, moderate-intensity exercise, as well as occasional rest periods during a 90-minute game (5-9). Reilly and Thomas (5), in scrutinizing individual play of an English soccer team throughout a 51-game season, were able to document specifics about the movements, speed, and distance involved in soccer.

Distance Covered in a Soccer Match

The average distance covered was 9 km, 60% of which was walking or jogging. Sprints totaled almost 800 meters averaging 10 to 40 meters in length. Bangsbo (9) compared Danish First and Second division players and concluded that the higher the level of performance, the more frequent and longer the periods of high-intensity exercise. For elite male soccer players, the total duration of high-intensity exercise is about 7 minutes, including 19 sprints, averaging 2 seconds per sprint, with high-speed running occurring every 70 seconds (9).

The total distance covered by any one player during a game varies with many factors including individual style of play and level of fitness. On average midfielders cover the most distance, between 9 and 11 km (5,7,10). Generally, midfielders are the most active players on the field, traveling farther than either defenders or attackers and covering a greater percentage of distance at a jog. They are expected to play both defense and offense and are the key to continuity among defenders and the forwards. Attackers may cover much of their distance as a sprint. Centerbacks cover the least distance, and a greater proportion of their distance is moving sideways and backwards.

Over the course of a soccer game, players are required to sprint, jog, stride, walk, and move sideways and backwards while tackling, jumping, accelerating, and turning. Regardless of position the greatest percentage of distance is covered at slower speeds (10,11). Kirkendall (11) estimates a change of speed or direction every 4 to 5 seconds.

ENERGY SYSTEMS

The nature of the activity in soccer taps both the aerobic and anaerobic energy systems. Soccer's specific energy demands have been estimated upon examination of the physiological response to participation. Bangsbo (12) estimated the relative levels of aerobic and anaerobic energy turnover and substrate utilization based on the cumulative results of various studies. (See *Figure 44.1*.)

FIGURE 44.1   Estimated Relative Aerobic and Anaerobic Energy Turnover and Corresponding Substrate Utilization during a Soccer Match

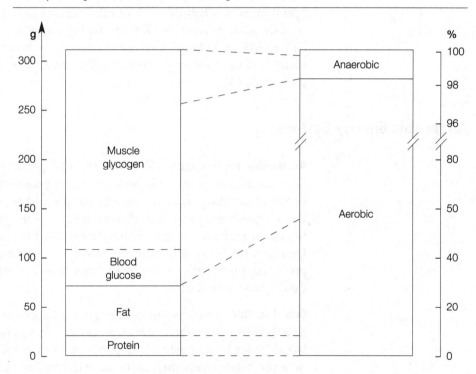

Used by permission: Taylor & Francis Ltd. Bangsbo J. Energy demands in competitive soccer. *J Sports Sci.* 1994;12:S10. http://www.tandf.co.uk/journals/jsp.htm

Aerobic Energy System

Heart rate. Attempts have been made to determine the aerobic energy contribution during soccer by measuring oxygen uptake. The procedure for collecting expired air, however, interferes with normal play and results are most likely imprecise. An alternative method of quantifying oxygen consumption during soccer is to estimate oxygen uptake based on heart rate. It must be noted, however, that heart rate (HR) does not always reflect the actual VO_2. Aside from its use in predicting oxygen uptake, heart rate provides a useful index of the overall physiologic demands of soccer (8).

During a match soccer players spend a significant amount of time working at heart rates above 160 beats per minute, 80% and often reaching 90% of maximum (7,13). Heart rate will be elevated beyond the HR-VO_2 relationship determined under laboratory conditions, but the overestimation of VO_2 is probably small (9). Several factors in a field situation contribute to this. High-intensity, dynamic exercise using large muscle groups will elevate oxygen consumption. Dribbling a soccer ball can elevate oxygen consumption 8% to 10%, costing 1.25 kcal per minute more than running without the ball (10,11). However, overall, the added cost of dribbling is small since the average player has the ball for less than 2 minutes or approximately 2% of the game. Intermittent exercise has an effect on oxygen consumption similar to submaximal, continuous running (9).

Although anaerobic activity is an important component of soccer, the greater demand is on aerobic metabolism. Considering total distance covered, the ratio of low-intensity to high-intensity activity is 2:1, while the relative time ratio is 7:1 (5). Sprinting occurs less than 1% of total playing time (14). Taking all factors into consideration, relative work rates during soccer have been estimated between 70% to 80% of VO_2max (7-9). Estimates of maximum oxygen uptake, based on many studies of soccer players over the years, suggest an average of 60 mL/kg per minute (10).

Anaerobic Energy System

Adenosine triphosphate (ATP) and creatine phosphate (CP). While the majority of the exercise in soccer is performed at submaximal intensities, high-intensity or all-out exercise plays a crucial role and players' ability to successfully carry out these high-intensity activities affects the result of the game. CP concentration fluctuates throughout a soccer match due to the intermittent nature of the game. Despite a small net utilization, CP plays an important role as an energy buffer, providing phosphate for the resynthesis of ATP during the rapid elevations in exercise intensity (9,12).

Blood lactate. Blood lactate concentrations have been measured and levels used as indicators of anaerobic energy production in soccer (7,9). The concentration of blood lactate levels fluctuates throughout a soccer match. Blood samples used to measure lactate levels are usually taken during half-time and at the completion of the match. Lactate is metabolized within the active muscle after high-intensity exercise. When high-intensity exercise is punctuated with low-intensity exercise, as in soccer, the rate of lactate metabolism increases. Furthermore, lactate released into the blood is taken up by the heart, liver, kidney, and other tissues. Evidence suggests that lactate is an important metabolic intermediate as a substrate for oxidative metabolism in cardiac and skeletal muscle and a precursor for gluconeogenesis (15). Thus, measurements of blood lactate concentration represent the balance of lactate released by muscle and taken up by blood, and will not fully reflect lactate production during a soccer match. It is reasonable to conclude that lactate production may be very high at points throughout a soccer game (7,9).

SUBSTRATE UTILIZATION AND MACRONUTRIENT NEEDS

The duration of exercise for soccer encompasses a 90-minute game plus 15- to 30-minutes of warm-up activities prior to match play. Aerobic and anaerobic energy demands over this period require significant amounts of substrates. Total energy expended during a soccer match is directly related to the distance covered during the 90 minutes of the game. The consensus in the literature indicates that soccer players cover between 8 to 12 km per game (5,7,12). For a 75-kg player, the average corresponding energy expenditure is estimated at 17 kcal per minute or 1,530 kcal per game.

Energy

Nutrition strategies designed for optimal performance should include adequate calories to support training and competition (16). (See Table 44.1.) Recommendations for energy intake should be based on the needs of each individual player. Clark (17) reports that intakes of professional male soccer players cover a range between 2,033 to 3,923 kcal per day. Data from a Major Indoor Soccer League team revealed that daily energy intakes of players averaged 2,662 kcal per day, with a maximum of 4,394 kcal per day and a minimum or 1,618 kcal per day (M. Macedonio, unpublished data, 1987).

TABLE 44.1   Macronutrient Needs of Adult Soccer Players—Training Nutrition Profile

	Males	Females
Energy	47-60 kcal/kg/day	45-50 kcal/kg/day
CHO	8-10 g/kg; 60%-70% calories	8-10 g/kg; 60%-70% calories
Protein	1.4-1.7 g/kg/day; 7%-12% calories	1.4-1.7 g/kg/day; 7%-12% calories
Fat	<30% calories	<30% calories
Postexercise Needs:		
CHO	2g/kg high glycemic index CHO	2g/kg high glycemic index CHO
	Solid or liquid	Solid or liquid

Specific information about the nutrition practices of female soccer players is limited and, thus, inferences have been made based on data gathered about "team sports." In a review of the literature examining the energy demands of soccer on female athletes and their dietary habits, Brewer (18) makes several observations:

- Female soccer players experience similar exercise intensity during a match yet expend less energy than male counterparts.
- Female players may have lower energy needs compared to males due to smaller body mass.

- An examination of female hockey players (19) reveals an energy intake less than expenditure, with eight of the nine players observed attempting to lose weight. In this group of athletes, iron and calcium intakes were 30% lower than the recommended levels.
- Several other observational studies reviewed by Brewer suggest similar trends in the diets of female athletes.

Economos et al (20) reviewed the dietary habits of elite athletes and made general recommendations. For endurance athletes training >90 minutes per day, the recommended energy intake ranges between 47 to 60 kcal/kg per day. A general guideline for males is 50 kcal/kg per day and for females 45 to 50 kcal/kg per day. Economos bases her recommendation for females on calculations using the profile of a "typical" elite female athlete weighing 55 kg, with a basal metabolic rate of 21.8 kcal/kg per day and an average training expenditure of 50.6 kcal/kg per day.

Carbohydrate (CHO) Metabolism

Muscle glycogen. The nature of the activity in soccer requires the use of both types of muscle fibers. A study by Jacobs et al (21) characterized soccer players' muscles by predominantly fast twitch (FT) fibers which have the greatest glycolytic potential. Tumility (10), however, summarized several studies and concluded that there is no pronounced dominance of either type. In a study by Gollnick et al (22), fast twitch fibers exhibited the greatest degree of glycogen depletion after "sprint-type" activities. Costill et al (23) showed that in distance running, glycogen was selectively depleted in slow twitch (ST) fibers but that FT fibers also bore some of the load. From these studies it appears that ST fibers are activated at lower workloads and that FT fibers are utilized under two conditions: when ST fibers are depleted of glycogen (24) and during high-intensity output (22).

It seems safe to conclude that the greater the muscle glycogen, the faster and farther players can run. Considering that soccer is a game of high-intensity, intermittent exercise spanning 90 minutes, with periods of short, intense activity of varying movements and longer periods of low-level, moderate-intensity work, it is no surprise that soccer is a glycogen-depleting activity. Glycogen depletion, a potential factor contributing to fatigue, may seriously limit players' ability to maintain high-intensity work output, particularly during the later stages of the game. Glycogen utilization in leg muscle is markedly increased during bouts of intense exercise. During periods of rest and low-intensity play, glycogen is resynthesized (25). In two separate studies (21,26) investigators found low levels of muscle glycogen upon completion of a soccer match and a greater use of glycogen in the first half compared to the second (26). The difference in muscle glycogen measured before and after a match represents the net glycogen utilization and does not fully reflect total glycogen turnover during play (9,12). Toward the end of a match, players experience fatigue and a decrease in performance. While an exact mechanism for this phenomenon has not been identified, low levels of muscle glycogen are likely a major factor. Saltin (26) observed that players with low levels of glycogen covered 24% less distance, 50% of which was covered by walking. Without sufficient muscle glycogen, exercise is fueled by fat and the intensity of that exercise is typically below 50% of capacity (27).

Blood glucose. Based on laboratory observations previously cited, it is reasonable to expect that a majority of the carbohydrate utilized during a soccer match is derived from endogenous sources, particularly muscle glycogen. While the stored glycogen in exercising muscle provides a major portion of carbohydrate used during a soccer match, blood glucose may also be utilized by exercising muscles (9) and may, in fact, spare muscle glycogen. As exercise duration increases carbohydrate from muscle glycogen declines while that from blood glucose rises (28). Blood glucose concentrations increase during high-intensity intermittent exercise as long as there is sufficient liver glycogen (7,9).

The specific energy demands of soccer make carbohydrate the predominant and most important source of fuel in the player's diet. Hypoglycemia and depletion of glycogen are associated with fatigue and reduced performance. In a series of studies Maughan et al (29) compared the effects of low-carbohydrate diets with high-carbohydrate diets on high-intensity exercise. A low-carbohydrate diet resulted in reduced endurance time, while the diet which provided 65% to 75% of kcal as carbohydrate increased exercise performance. Maughan also found that a high-protein diet, particularly in conjunction with a low-carbohydrate diet, will result in metabolic acidosis, which is associated with fatigue.

Hargreaves (30) presents an overview of the most relevant research results on the role of carbohydrate before, during, and after soccer. A training diet aimed at maximizing muscle glycogen and glucose availability needs to contain between 8 to 10 g CHO/kg body weight or 60% to 70% of total energy (31). To insure sufficient CHO availability and enhance performance during exercise, a high-carbohydrate meal (>200 g CHO) is recommended 3 to 4 hours prior to competition. Limited research suggests that low-glycemic solid carbohydrate may be best for the precompetition meal (32). As match time approaches Clark (17) recommends consuming 30 to 60 g CHO as solid or liquid up to 1 hour before competition.

A carbohydrate solution of up to 8% CHO consumed at the rate of 30 to 60 g CHO per hour during match play is recommended to delay the onset of fatigue and enhance performance (16,17,31,33). Since soccer is an activity of prolonged, variable-intensity exercise, soccer players should be encouraged to consume a dilute carbohydrate solution (see *Table 44.2*) prior to and during competition and training to minimize the depletion of muscle and liver glycogen.

TABLE 44.2 Fluid Replacement Solutions

Volume*	CHO**	Sodium†	Potassium
1 L	4%-8%; 60-70 g/L	20-30 mEq/L	2-5 mEq/L
	13-17 g/236 mL (8oz)	110-165 mg/8 oz	19-46 mg/8 oz

*Total volume of replacement fluid is recommended in *excess* of body fluid lost during exercise: at least a pint of fluid for every pound of body weight lost (34-36).

**A combination of high glycemic CHOs—sucrose, glucose, fructose, and maltodextrin—provides the most effective and acceptable blend from a sensory and physiological perspective (37).

†Sodium helps increase voluntary fluid intake and maintain both plasma volume and total body fluid balance (34-36).

Before adopting any eating and drinking strategies immediately prior to or during a match, players should be cautioned to experiment on training days to establish a comfortable routine and to avoid any unwanted consequences.

In spite of measures to minimize glycogen losses, match play drastically reduces glycogen stores. Aggressive attempts to restore muscle glycogen immediately after competition can result in supercompensation of glycogen stores. Research suggests that the consumption of high glycemic index (GI) foods shortly after exhaustive exercise yields maximum restoration of muscle glycogen (38). Burke et al (39) showed a greater glycogen storage, and greater postprandial glucose and insulin response, during 24 hours of postexercise recovery with high versus low GI carbohydrate foods. In a subsequent study, Burke et al (33) observed no difference in postexercise glycogen storage over 24 hours when a diet of high GI foods was consumed in small feedings or as large meals. Coyle (37) recommends ingesting 50 g per 2 hours of moderate- and high-GI carbohydrate foods immediately after exhaustive exercise to reach a total of 600 g in 24 hours. See the Tools section for the glycemic index of commonly consumed foods.

Protein

Studies have shown that amino acids can be oxidized for energy during exercise and that endurance training further enhances the oxidation, primarily that of the branched-chain amino acids (leucine, isoleucine, and valine). Data suggest that the absolute quantity of amino acids oxidized during endurance exercise can be significant, as much as 86% of the daily requirement for one amino acid after a 2-hour bout of exercise at 55% VO_2max (40), and that amino acids can serve as an auxiliary fuel during prolonged, moderate-intensity exercise such as soccer.

Amino acid oxidation is inversely related to muscle glycogen availability (41). During a soccer match muscle glycogen can be depleted depending on the intensity and duration of exercise and the pregame glycogen stores. The higher the intensity of exercise, the greater the glycogen usage and amino acid oxidation. If the amino acids are not replaced via diet, a net loss in amino acids can occur over time with losses in muscle strength and, possibly, performance.

Lemon (42) points to recent studies which indicate that a dietary intake of 0.86 to 1.4 g/kg of protein per day enhances protein synthesis in strength athletes, whereas no benefit was observed at protein intakes of 2.4 g/kg per day. These data indicate a plateau in protein synthesis at modest supplementation levels.

Protein recommendations for soccer players are made on the basis of research that shows the strength component of soccer and the use of protein as an energy source. Lemon (42) concludes that soccer players need more dietary protein than sedentary individuals and suggests a protein intake of 1.4 to 1.7 g/kg per day (175% to 212% RDA) for competitive soccer players. This recommended intake is an achievable amount of protein in a balanced diet of a variety of foods that supply adequate calories to maintain desirable weight, and it insures ample protein to maintain the amino acid pool. Lemon cautions against extremely high protein intakes (>2 g/kg per day), pointing to no evidence of performance advantage and possible health hazards.

Special considerations for protein. Children, because of their rapid growth, and individuals who severely limit calories or high-quality sources of protein pose a possible risk of inadequate protein intakes. Women, in particular, are more likely to restrict calories in attempting to reduce or lower body weight, and vegetarians generally consume lower quality protein sources. Careful attention to the protein intakes of these groups is highly recommended (see *Table 44.3*).

TABLE 44.3   Recommended Dietary Allowances for Protein Intakes of Children

Recommended Dietary Allowances (RDA) for protein intakes for children should be used as a guideline:

Age Group	Grams Protein/kg/day	Grams/day
7-10 year old boys and girls	1.0	28
11-14 year old boys and girls	1.0	45
15-18 year old boys	.9	59
15-18 year old girls	.8	44

Fat

Soccer involves both aerobic and anaerobic energy systems, with the greater demand being placed on aerobic metabolism. No data are available that specifically outline the contribution of fat as a substrate during soccer. Bangsbo (9) observed that free fatty acid (FFA) concentration increased during a soccer match, more so in the second half than the first. This pattern was attributed to a slower pace during the second half, allowing a greater blood flow to adipose tissue and possibly promoting a higher FFA release coupled with hormonal changes. Based on these observations a high uptake of glycerol in various tissues, primarily liver, is presumed, indicating that glycerol might be an important glucogenic precursor. Blood FFA concentration during soccer is the net result of the uptake of FFA in various tissue and the release from adipose tissue. Ketone bodies may also function as a minor fat source during exercise.

The mix of carbohydrate and lipid substrates used during exercise is primarily a function of the intensity and duration of exercise. Previous diet, level of fitness, and environmental factors also affect the substrate blend.

MICRONUTRIENT NEEDS

The energy demands of soccer training and competition are significant and require adequate intakes of all nutrients involved in energy production. There are no known micronutrient needs peculiar to soccer players and above the Recommended Dietary Allowances. Fogelholm (43) presents data on micronutrient status and the effects of micronutrient supplementation on exercise performance related to soccer and other team players.

In general, the micronutrient status of a soccer player is directly related to the quality of the dietary intake. Data collected from male and female team athletes as reported by Fogelholm (43) show some areas of concern. Low intakes of thiamin have been observed in the diets of male athletes. Among female athletes whose daily energy intakes were below 2,400 kcal, mineral and trace elements such as calcium, magnesium, iron, and zinc were suboptimal. This becomes particularly troublesome when athletes focus on weight reduction or the maintenance of a low body weight. Fogelholm recommends that nutrition education for soccer players start at an early age and focus on foods and macronutrients. Periodic dietary evaluation and nutrition education by a registered dietitian can detect early trouble signs, help prevent serious nutritional deficiencies, and screen for possible eating disorders (see *Box 44.2*).

BOX 44.2   Micronutrients to Monitor

- Micronutrients used in energy production, B vitamins, especially thiamin
- Calcium, magnesium, iron, zinc in the diets of young athletes, female athletes, and in those consuming diets lower than 2,400 kcal

---

FLUID NEEDS

The major causes of fatigue in endurance sports are depletion of muscle glycogen and problems associated with thermoregulation and fluid loss. Soccer requires that players exercise at high intensities for a prolonged period of time, often at elevated ambient temperatures and high humidity. The energy demands of soccer greatly reduce muscle glycogen stores and fluid reserves, which must be replenished before the next match. Repletion of muscle glycogen is dependent not only on carbohydrate intake but also on fluid intake, since each gram of muscle glycogen is stored with 2.7 g of water.

Under moderate temperatures (10°C or 50°F), the sweat losses of soccer players during a match may be as high as 2 L (39) with an average loss of 3 L or more in the heat (8). When the ambient temperature is higher than skin temperature, the body takes on additional heat. Soccer players who sweat profusely are likely to become dehydrated and fatigued toward the end of the game. Full rehydration after exercise requires replacement of fluid and electrolytes, primarily sodium, lost in sweat. A study by Shirreffs et al (34) suggests that full rehydration after intense exercise is best achieved when the replacement fluid contains sufficient sodium and is consumed at 150% of the fluid lost through exercise.

Following are the goals of hydration in soccer:

1. **Fluid ingestion before exercise**
   The objective of pre-exercise hydration is to maximize fluid intake during the 24 hours preceding training or competition (44). Research suggests that fluid consumed within an hour before exercise helps minimize elevations in heart rate and core body temperature during exercise (45). Soccer players should be encouraged to drink about 500 mL (about 17 oz) of cool fluid within the 2 hours prior to a match. This will provide adequate hydration and the excretion of excess water (44) with extra fluid consumed during the last 10 to 15 minutes before the game begins (46).

2. **Fluid ingestion during exercise**

   Voluntary fluid intake based on thirst is insufficient to meet the fluid demands of soccer. Players should be encouraged to consume fluid early and at regular intervals throughout exercise. Flavored fluids that are cooler than the ambient temperatures are more palatable. Due to the high intensity, intermittent nature, and duration of a soccer match, players may benefit from sports replacement beverages containing carbohydrate and electrolytes (44,47). Carbohydrates are recommended at the rate of 30 to 60 g per hour by consuming 600 to 1,200 mL (about 20 to 40 oz) of a solution containing 6% to 8% carbohydrates (glucose, sucrose, maltodextrin) and 0.5 to 0.7 g Na/L water (45). The total volume of fluid necessary is dependent upon the amount of sweat lost.

3. **Fluid ingestion after exercise**

   The strategy for fluid intake postexercise needs to focus on rapid and complete repletion of fluid, electrolyte, and carbohydrates used during training and exercise. Weight should be measured nude or in minimal clothing before and after exercise to quantify the amount of negative fluid balance and to insure full fluid replacement. Each pound of weight lost represents approximately 480 mL (about 16 oz) of fluid. Considering fluid needs for the storage of muscle glycogen and obligatory urine losses, players should be counseled to drink at least a pint of fluid for every pound of body weight lost through exercise (34-36).

It should be noted that alcohol is dehydrating and the consumption of alcoholic beverages would best be avoided within 72 hours before or after training or competition to minimize any additional dehydration. See *Table 44.4*.

TABLE 44.4   Fluid Intake Guidelines: before, during, and after Exercise

	Volume	Time Frame
Before	17oz/500mL	Within 2 hours of exercise
	8oz/240mL	15 minutes before exercise
During	20-40 oz/600-1,200 mL Solution containing 6%-8% CHO + 0.5-0.7 g Na/L	To equal sweat loss
After	24oz/720mL/lb weight loss*	Within 24 hours after exercise

*Players should be encouraged to weigh before and after exercise to assess fluid intake needs and to consume fluid in excess of body fluid lost (34-36).

Fluid Needs of Young Soccer Players

Special consideration and care should be paid to the fluid needs of young soccer players, particularly prepubescent youth. During exercise children produce more heat than adults yet have a greater relative surface area and a lower capacity for sweating, and take longer to acclimatize to warm weather. These factors place young athletes at increased risk for dehydration and heat illness. Given the heightened risk of hypothermia in children, the following precautions and practical measures should be taken:

- Fluids should be consumed at least every 15 to 20 minutes during training and exercise.
- Fluids should be cool and made as palatable as possible to encourage drinking. Grape has been reported to be the preferred flavor and the one that leads to the greatest rehydration following mild dehydration (48).
- Clothing should be lightweight and wick moisture away from the body. Cotton, which is very absorbent and traps moisture against the skin, is not recommended as a first layer. In warm weather goalkeepers should remove the team jersey when they wear the goalkeeper shirt while in the goal. Sweat-drenched clothing should be replaced with dry clothing when possible.
- When the relative humidity and ambient temperature are high, the intensity of exercise should be reduced, breaks should be taken more often, and extra fluid intake should be encouraged. When possible, players on the sidelines should be sheltered from direct sunlight during hot weather.

SPECIAL CONSIDERATIONS

The exercise intensity and duration of the game and the playing schedule of soccer give rise to several nutritional concerns for soccer players:

1. Soccer games can be scheduled close together, leaving little time for players to recover from exercise. Noting the glycogen depletion and heavy fluid losses sustained during soccer, players need to take calculated steps to insure that they begin subsequent games in positive fluid balance and with adequate nutrient levels. Travel and timing of matches can interfere with normal eating patterns and may limit food selection. Special consideration should be given to pregame meals, fluid replacement strategies, and postgame nutrition under these conditions.
2. Female soccer players attempting to lower or maintain weight need to carefully choose foods of high nutrient density and with sufficient calories and carbohydrates to support the high-energy and carbohydrate demands of soccer.
3. Children rely more heavily on fat than on carbohydrate utilization during moderate- to high-intensity exercise, yet the percentage of fat in their diets should be no higher than 30% of total calories, with saturated fat contributing no more than 10% of total calories (49).

WORKING WITH TRAINERS, COACHES, AND PLAYERS

There is more than one way to skin a cat or so the adage goes, and there is more than one way for a nutritionist to work with a sports team. Much of how you approach the team has to do with factors outside your control such as the players' and coaching staff's interest in nutrition, the previous exposure of players and staff to a nutrition professional, the current playing record, the fiscal state of the team, the presence of particular nutrition concerns, and the sports medicine staff.

A comfortable knowledge of the mechanics of the sport and the physiologic demands of each position are crucial to credibility as a nutrition expert. Before approaching a team, it is wise to learn as much about the team as possible and to assess the "climate" for nutrition support. It is also helpful to know something about the principal "players" on the coaching staff and their responsibilities. Generally, you will be interacting most closely with the head trainer or conditioning coach.

Several questions you may wish to investigate are:

- Is there any formal nutrition provision for the team? If so, exactly what is it and who is responsible for planning and providing it?
- Is there a common fluid replacement regime? If so, what is it and who is responsible for administering it?
- Is any attention given to nutrition assessment and body composition?
- Are there any special individual nutrition needs of players, such as weight management, eating disorders, diabetes, increasing muscle mass, gastrointestinal disturbances, or early fatigue during match play?
- Who provides the sports medicine care?

The answers to these questions give the sports nutritionist some valuable insight into the needs of the players and staff and how she or he might help meet those needs. Keeping in mind that the sport nutritionist's position is one of support, her or his specific involvement can take the form of nutrition consultant, educator, counselor, or therapist, depending on the needs of the team. And roles can change over time as players and staff become comfortable and begin to rely on your expertise.

CASE STUDY

A highly skilled soccer player is experiencing a noticeable decrement in performance toward the latter part of the second half of the game after a strong first half. A decline in accuracy and ability to execute a pass and a marked reduction in speed allow the opponent to gain ground. Tactical ability appears compromised. The team trainer has been concerned about the player's apparent loss of energy in the second half and asks you if there could be a nutrition-related contributing factor.

Assessment and Recommendations

- At an initial meeting to assess the player's needs and concerns, recommend that the player complete a 3-day food intake record for food selection and nutrient analysis.
- Screen dietary intake for nutrient inadequacies in total calories, percentage of calories from carbohydrate, protein intake, micronutrients, and fluid intake. Take note of sodium intake to insure sufficient replenishment of sodium lost in sweat.
- Measure fluid loss and intake during training and exercise.
- Attempt to examine and quantify carbohydrate, fluid, and sodium intakes within the first 24 hours after training and exercise.
- Review with the player the results of the dietary analyses:
  1. 3-day food intake record
  2. Fluid replacement
  3. Postexercise fluid and energy replacement
- Explain the effect of nutrient intake on performance. With the player, design a nutrition plan to meet performance demands according to the evaluative data collected. Provide education materials and recipes.
- Adjust the nutrition plan as needed.

REFERENCES

1. National Soccer Hall of Fame. *US Soccer History.* http://www.wpe.comm/~nshof/history/ushis.htm. Accessed November 19, 1998.
2. Briggs S. *Soccer in the USA.* Soccer Industry Council of America; 1995. http://www.sportlink.com/research/teamsports/soccer/soccerinusa95/index.html. Accessed October 20, 1998.
3. American Youth Soccer Organization. *By the Book.* ABCs of AYSO. http://www.soccer.org/abc/b_abc.htm. Accessed October 20, 1998.
4. Bradley G, Toye C. *Playing Soccer the Professional Way. Team Play and Systems of Play.* New York, NY: Harper & Row; 1973.
5. Reilly T, Thomas V. A motion analysis of work rate in different positional roles in professional football match play. *J Human Movement Studies.* 1976;2:87-97.
6. Withers RT, Maricic Z, Wasilewski S, Kelly L. Match analysis of Australian professional soccer players. *J Human Movement Studies.* 1982;8:159-176.
7. Ekblom B. Applied physiology of soccer. *Sports Med.* 1986;3:50-60.
8. Reilly T. Energetics of high-intensity exercise (soccer) with particular reference to fatigue. *J Sports Sci.* 1997;15:257-263.
9. Bangsbo J. The physiology of soccer. *Acta Physiol Scand Suppl.* 1994;619:1-155.
10. Tumility D. Physiological characteristics of elite soccer players. *Sports Med.* 1993;16:80-96.
11. Kirkendall D. The applied sport science of soccer. *Phys Sports Med.* 1985;13:53-59.
12. Bangsbo J. Energy demands in competitive soccer. *J Sports Sci.* 1994;12:S5-S12.
13. Smodlaka V. Cardiovascular aspect of soccer. *Phys Sports Med.* 1978;6:66-70.
14. Bangsbo J, Norregaard L, Thorsoe F. Activity profile of competition soccer. *Can J Sport Sci.* 1991;16:110-116.

15. Brooks G. Current concepts in lactate exchange. *Med Sci Sports Exerc.* 1991;23:895-906.
16. Williams C, Nicholas CW. Nutrition needs for team sport. *Sports Sci Exch.* 1998;11:70.
17. Clark K. Nutritional guidance to soccer players for training and competition. *J Sports Sci.* 1994;12:S43-S50.
18. Brewer J. Aspects of women's soccer. J Sports Sci. 1994;12:S35-S38.
19. Nutter J. Seasonal changes in female athletes' diets. *Int J Sport Nutr.* 1991;1:395-407.
20. Economos C, Bortz S, Nelson M. Nutrition practices of elite athletes. *Sports Med.* 1993;16:381-399.
21. Jacobs I, Westin N, Karlsson J, Rasmusson M, Houghton B. Muscle glycogen and diet in elite soccer players. *Eur J Appl Physiol.* 1982;48:297-302.
22. Gollnick P, Armstrong R, Saubert C IV, Shepherd R, Saltin B. Glycogen depletion patterns in human skeletal muscle fibers after exhausting exercise. *J Appl Physiol.* 1973;34:615-618.
23. Costill D, Gollnick P, Jansson E, Saltin B, Stein E. Glycogen depletion pattern in human muscle fibers during distance running. *Acta Physiol Scand.* 1973;89:374-384.
24. Gollnick P, Piehl K, Saubert C IV, Armstrong R, Saltin B. Diet, exercise, and glycogen changes in human muscle fibers. *J Appl Physiol.* 1972;33:421-425.
25. Nordheim K, Vollestad N. Glycogen and lactate metabolism during low-intensity exercise in man. *Acta Physiol Scand.* 1990;139:475-484.
26. Saltin B. Metabolic fundamental in exercise. *Med Sci Sports Exerc.* 1973;5:137-146.
27. Kirkendall D. Effects of nutrition on performance in soccer. *Med Sci Sports Exerc.* 1993;25:1370-1374.
28. Romijn J, Coyle E, Sidossis L, et al. Regulation of endogenous fat and carbohydrate metabolism in relation to exercise intensity and duration. *Am J Physiol.* 1993;265:E380-E391.
29. Maughan R, Greenhaff P, Leiper J, Ball D, Lambert C, Gleeson M. Diet composition on the performance of high intensity exercise. *J Sports Sci.* 1997;15:265-275.
30. Hargreaves M. Carbohydrate and lipid requirements of soccer. *J Sports Sci.* 1994;12:S13-S16.
31. Costill D, Hargreaves M. Carbohydrate nutrition and fatigue. *Sports Med.* 1992;13:86-92.
32. Coleman E. Update on carbohydrate: solid versus liquid. *Int J Sport Nutr.* 1994;4:80-88.
33. Burke L, Collier G, Davis P, Fricker P, Sanigorski A, Hargreaves M. Muscle glycogen storage after prolonged exercise: effect of the frequency of carbohydrate feedings. *Am J Clin Nutr.* 1996;64:115-119.
34. Shirreffs SM, Taylor AJ, Leiper JB, Maughan RJ. Post-exercise rehydration in man: effects of volume consumed and drink sodium content. *Med Sci Sports Exerc.* 1996;28:1260-1271.
35. Horswill CA. Effective fluid replacement. *Int J Sport Nutr.* 1998;8:175-195.
36. Burke LM, Hurley JA. Fluid balance in team sports. *Sports Med.* 1997;24:38-54.
37. Coyle E. Timing and method of increased carbohydrate intake to cope with heavy training, competition and recovery. *J Sports Sci.* 1991;9:29-51.
38. Rankin JW. Glycemic index and exercise metabolism. *Sports Sci Exch.* 1997;10:1.
39. Burke L, Hargreaves M, Collier G. Muscle glycogen storage after prolonged exercise. *J Appl Physiol.* 1993;74:1019-1023.
40. Evans W, Fisher E, Hoerr R, Young V. Protein metabolism and endurance exercise. *Phys Sports Med.* 1983;11:63-72.

41. Lemon P, Mullin J. Effect of initial muscle glycogen levels on protein catabolism during exercise. *J Appl Physiol*. 1992;48:624-629.
42. Lemon P. Protein requirements of soccer. *J Sports Sci*. 1994;12:S17-S22.
43. Fogelholm M. Vitamins, minerals and supplementation in soccer. *J Sports Sci*. 1994;12:S23-S27.
44. American College of Sports Medicine. Position stand on exercise and fluid replacement. *Med Sci Sports Exerc*. 1996;28:i-vii.
45. Greenleaf J, Castle B. Exercise temperature regulation in man during hypohydration and hyperthermia. *J Appl Physiol*. 1971;30:847-853.
46. Maughan R, Leiper J. Fluid replacement requirements in soccer. *J Sports Sci*. 1994;12:S29-S34.
47. Shi X, Gisolfi C. Fluid and carbohydrate replacement during intermittent exercise. *Sports Med*. 1998;25:157-172.
48. Meyer F, Bar-Or O, Salsberg A, Passe D. Hypohydration during exercise in children: effect of thirst, drink preferences and rehydration. *Int J Sport Nutr*. 1994;4:22-35.
49. Bar-Or O, Unnithan V. Nutritional requirements of young soccer players. *J Sports Sci*. 1994;12:S39-S42.

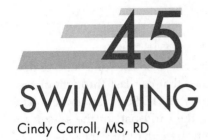

SWIMMING

Cindy Carroll, MS, RD

According to the National Sporting Goods Association's 1997 survey, swimming is second only to walking as America's most popular sport and fitness activity (1). Not only is it a popular sport but it is also one in which the United States has had great Olympic success (2). It could be argued that the successes of athletes such as Mark Spitz and Janet Evans have helped to propel the continued interest in swimming.

DEMOGRAPHICS

Swimming offers the opportunity for young and old to participate at various ages. Competitive swimming includes:

- Age group swimming which starts under age 10 and continues through high school
- National Collegiate Athletic Association (NCAA) swimming
- United States Swimming (USS) that includes national and international elite-level competition
- United States Master Swimming (USMS) that, unlike many sports, includes athletes starting at age 19 (3)

USMS alone has over 34,000 members (3). Many of the master teams are located in local YMCA pools or university pools. Master swimmers also can compete in national and world competition, which means that there are many swimmers ranging in age from 19 to over 80 years old who are training at a high intensity. Competitive swimming also extends beyond the pool to include open ocean and lake swimming, which offers its own challenges, but all providing the body with great physical benefits.

TRAINING DEMANDS

Competitive swimming has historically required its athletes to commit to long and strenuous training. Swimming requires a high degree of specificity of training, meaning swimmers cannot run to become faster swimmers; they must swim (4,5). The effectiveness of such long training is controversial but is still the standard of most swimming programs. Most elite competitive swimmers swim twice a day, totaling about 2 to 4 hours of swimming ranging from 6,000 to 16,500 meters per day (4,6-8). Many competitive master swimmers swim a minimum of 1 to 2 hours per day. Exercise intensities exceed 75% of VO_2max and frequently exceed 100% of VO_2max during interval training (6,7). In addition to the actual swim training in the pool, most competitive swimmers also use some kind of dry land resistance training, sometimes with weights, that can last throughout the entire season depending on coaching philosophy (9,11). Some swimmers use heavier weights with greater frequency during the early part of the season to build muscle and then continue lifting to maintain strength during the season.

Most competitive swimming seasons are long and strenuous, and are geared to maximize both the anaerobic and aerobic components that swimming requires (10). Swimming distances are measured in both yards and meters. The shortest race is 50 yards and at the elite level is swum as fast as 20 seconds and the longest race is 1,500 meters and swum in less than 16 minutes (1). Although swimming races are considered relatively short compared to many running races, tremendous aerobic training is needed. This is usually the focus of the early part of the swimming season, laying the foundation from which a swimmer can build on his or her specific races and strokes. Swimming consists of four strokes: butterfly, breaststroke, backstroke, and freestyle. All swimming strokes require use of all the major muscle groups, as well as requiring upper body strength, particularly for sprinting (9).

NUTRIENT REQUIREMENTS

Because competitive swimmers may swim at a high intensity up to 4 hours a day, weight train to build and maintain muscle several times a week, and also continue with activities of daily living, their energy expenditure is high. It is not uncommon for competitive swimmers to require 6,000 kilocalories per day (6,12-15). With such high-energy needs and repetitive daily workouts, muscle and liver glycogen stores can be quickly depleted, making it imperative that swimmers eat regular meals and snacks with adequate carbohydrate to maximize glycogen stores.

Carbohydrates

Carbohydrates provide quick energy to muscles, which is necessary for interval workouts and sprinting. Carbohydrate recommendations typically are 55% to 65% of total kilocalories, providing energy intake is adequate (12). However, this may not be appropriate for all swimmers. Because energy needs are high, it is recommended that swimmers calculate carbohydrate needs according to body weight instead of using a percentage of total kilocalories (6). Eating at least 500 g of carbohydrate per day (8 to 10 g/kg per day) with a calorie intake equal to energy expenditure is recommended (6,12,16). The body can synthesize only a certain amount of glycogen in a 24-hour period, so eating more than this may be unnecessary (6,17,18). Swimmers who do not keep up with daily energy and carbohydrate needs have poorer performance in practice, presumably because of lower glycogen stores and inadequate energy, particularly when training is intensified (7).

Protein

Protein intakes ranging from 1.2 to 1.7 g/kg per day with intakes on the high end during the initial training weeks will provide optimal amino acids for growth, maintenance, and repair of all tissue, providing calories are adequate. Research shows that many swimmers, both male and female, are easily meeting their protein needs, some eating as much as 2 g/kg per day (12,19,20). However, vegetarians, weight-conscious athletes, and female athletes have shown potential for inadequate protein intake (12). These population groups should be carefully monitored.

Fat

Recommended fat intakes are 25% to 30% of total energy (21). Some swimmers may need to eat 30% of kilocalories from fat to maintain an optimal weight. Eating fat within the range of 20% to 30% of kilocalories will also help swimmers adhere to the American Heart Association and American Cancer Society's low-fat guidelines to help prevent various chronic diseases (22,23). Studies show that some swimmers eat much greater than 30% fat, at the expense of adequate carbohydrate (12).

Vitamins and Minerals

Eating a balanced diet of 55% to 65% carbohydrate, 12% to 15% protein, and 25% to 30% fat, including all groups on the Food Guide Pyramid, helps ensure adequate intake of vitamins and minerals. If calorie intake is adequate to meet needs, athletes are probably getting a good balance of vitamins and minerals. However, because no one eats perfectly and everyone has personal taste preferences, taking a daily multivitamin-mineral supplement with 100% of the RDA will help ensure a safe intake of all nutrients (12).

Some studies have shown that a deficiency of B vitamins may negatively affect physical performance (24,25). Female swimmers may be at risk for inadequate iron (26), which may need to be prescribed under medical supervision (12,26). Women who are unable to obtain adequate dietary calcium and especially if amenorrheic should consider taking a calcium supplement (27). Lukaski et al (28) examined dietary intakes and blood levels of iron, copper, magnesium, and zinc and hypothesized that adequate intake of these nutrients reflected faster 100-yard sprint times.

Some research suggests that athletes who exercise intensely may have less than adequate immune function (29-31). High-intensity endurance training, as occurs with swimming, may suppress the immune system and place athletes at risk for more frequent infectious diseases (31). Some researchers, as well as The United States Olympic Committee, have recommended additional intakes of some of the antioxidant vitamins, including vitamin C, vitamin E, and beta carotene for some athletes (30-33).

Fluids

It could be argued that maintaining adequate fluids is the single most important nutrition principle for any athlete to follow. Despite the irony that exercising in water poses, the greatest risk to a swimmer's performance is fluid loss (34). Dehydration can occur within 30 minutes of swimming. Poor environmental conditions, such as warm pool water, warm air temperatures, or high humidity, can further add to the risk of dehydration and can be detrimental to the performance of even the fittest and fastest swimmers (35). Dehydration of as little as 2% of body weight can impair performance. Sports drinks are beneficial for swimming bouts lasting longer than 1 hour and for shorter practices at high intensity. Sports drinks increase the drive to drink as well as the body's ability to absorb fluid. Water alone may not be able to replace fluid losses and cannot maintain blood glucose levels.

The guidelines in *Box 45.1* will help swimmers maintain optimal hydration (36,37). Also see *Table 45.1*.

BOX 45.1   Fluid Guidelines for Swimmers

- Drink at least 2 cups of fluid for every pound of weight lost. Weigh in immediately before and after training. If weight loss occurs during practice, aim to replace weight within 24 hours.
- Check urine color. Darker-colored urine may indicate dehydration. Drink more fluids.
- Keep a log of how many cups you drink until it becomes a habit. Carry a fluid bottle to work, to class, and to the pool.
- Keep a fluid bottle at the pool and drink between sets and immediately before and after practice. Drink 4 to 8 oz every 20 minutes.
- Choose a sports drink that contains 6% to 8% carbohydrate with a flavor to your liking, and use it during practices.
- Avoid alcohol; it contributes to fluid loss. Avoid excessive caffeinated beverages (≤2 cups per day).

TABLE 45.1   Summary of Nutrient Needs for High-intensity Swimming (6,12,19,33-37)

Total Kilocalories Per Day	CHO g/kg/day	Protein g/kg/day	Fat % of Total Kilocalories	Fluids	Vitamin and Mineral Supplementation
3,000-6,000	8-10	1.2-1.7	25-30	2 cups/lb weight lost	Multivitamin-mineral supplement with 100% of RDA
				4-8 oz every 20 min during training	Consider vitamin C and vitamin E supplements.
				Drink to maintain clear urine.	Consider additional supplements such as calcium for women, as needed.

NUTRITION NEEDS

During Training

Swim workouts usually consist of continuous repeating sets, making it difficult to eat during practice. Using sports drinks during practice can help maintain blood glucose levels. Although eating during practice is not always an option, some athletes can tolerate energy bars or gels in between sets.

Postexercise

Obtaining adequate energy and carbohydrates after practice is crucial for glycogen repletion. At least 1.5 g/kg of carbohydrate within 30 minutes after a workout is recommended followed by an additional 1.5g/kg for every 2 hours thereafter (16). This will help ensure adequate synthesis of muscle glycogen before the next workout. Because calorie needs may be quite high for some swimmers, it may be difficult for them to maintain their optimum weight. High-calorie, high-carbohydrate supplements such as energy bars or carbohydrate-rich liquid supplements may be helpful as snacks to meet energy needs.

Before, during, and after Swim Meets

Swim meets can last 1 day, 2 days, or several days. Some international competitions last 7 to 10 days (2). In a typical swim meet, swimmers may have events scattered throughout the day. Adequate nutrition every day for optimum storage of glycogen is important during training because poor eating patterns cannot be replaced by a good pre-event meal. By race time muscles should be glycogen-filled and pre-event meals should be used to top off glycogen stores and help to raise blood glucose. The amount of exercise that actually occurs during a swim meet includes a warm up and, if available, cool down in a separate pool. An athlete may swim several races at a high intensity but total yardage for the day will not be as high as in practice. There is time to eat during swim meets, but the timing of food intake is important. The simple rules in *Box 45.2* can help.

BOX 45.2   Guidelines for Eating during Swim Meets

- Eat high-carbohydrate, easy-to-digest foods that are familiar when there is a short time between races (less than 1 hour). Try bananas, crackers, or sports drinks.
- Add more carbohydrate (500 to 1,000 kilocalories) for longer times between races (2 to 4 hours). Choose bagels, English muffins, jelly, high-carbohydrate energy bars, gels, or raisins (16).
- Add small amounts of protein with the added carbohydrate, such as low-fat yogurt, low-fat milk with graham crackers, turkey or chicken sandwiches, or energy bars containing 7 to 14 g of protein if greater than 4 hours between events.
- Maintain adequate fluids. Air temperatures during swim meets can be warm and humid. A conscious effort should be made to increase fluid consumption throughout the day to maintain a pale urine color.

ERGOGENIC AIDS

Manipulation of diet and use of dietary supplements are popular practices among swimmers. Three practices of particular interest in swimming are the use of creatine, the Zone Diet, and the more traditional carbohydrate-loading to improve performance.

Creatine

Creatine monohydrate has become popular for swimmers hoping to increase power, strength, and speed (see Chapter 7, Ergogenic Aids) (38). Many of the studies on creatine have been conducted on swimmers, although results of effectiveness are equivocal (38-41). Some studies have shown faster swim times in repeat performances, while other studies have shown no improvement in single effort sprints (39). One study showed improved times in three 100-meter sprint efforts with a 60-second rest in between (40). The benefits of creatine supplementation are thought to occur because of its ability to recharge muscle cells for faster recovery, with optimal benefits occurring between 1 to 3 minutes (38). Theoretically, creatine supplementation could improve interval training. Whether this increase in power and strength could transfer from interval training and be applied to individual swimming efforts is still unknown. Weight gain is also a side effect of creatine supplementation (38). If the weight gain is from fluid, it may hinder stroke efficiency.

Zone Diet

The Zone Diet (see Chapter 2, Carbohydrate and Exercise) has gained some of its popularity because the author claims that it is responsible for the success of some collegiate swimmers (42). The benefits of the Zone Diet have been anecdotal and no clinical studies have been completed to show if it improves athletic performance (16). Given the tremendous aerobic training that swimming entails, the scientific literature still supports carbohydrate as the key nutrient to fuel muscle contraction (16). Inadequate carbohydrate stores for swimmers result in poorer performance (7). The Zone Diet recommends 40% of kilocalories from carbohydrates, which is less than the 55% to 65% carbohydrates recommended by other sport nutrition experts (42). If swimmers adhered to the Zone Diet recommendation of 30% protein while meeting their energy needs on a 5,000-kilocalorie diet, they would get 375 g of protein, well over the recommended amount for this nutrient.

Carbohydrate-loading

Carbohydrate-loading is still practiced among some endurance athletes. It helps with exercise that is 90 minutes or longer, which includes competitive swim training where practices may be 2 to 4 hours long, but not competitive pool races which are all less than 30 minutes for the more elite swimmers (16). For longer, continuous swimming events such as a lake or ocean event, carbohydrate-loading may be effective. For competitive pool events, maintaining adequate daily carbohydrate intake to meet training needs while decreasing training before a swim race will allow for optimal glycogen storage (see Chapter 2, Carbohydrate and Exercise).

WEIGHT CONTROL

Some studies have suggested that swimming is not a good exercise for weight loss (43,44). However, these published studies have been criticized for their design. Specifically, using body weight and not body fat to assess body composition; using recreational swimmers who exercised at a low intensity compared to competitive swimmers; and not controlling for dietary intake have been pointed out as flaws in study design (43).

Intensity of Effort

Regardless of the type of activity performed, energy expended in exercise is a function of intensity of effort, which can be measured by oxygen consumption. Monitoring heart rate gives an indirect indication of effort and oxygen consumption (45). The higher the heart rate, the more energy expended during the exercise. Because swimming requires appropriate technique to swim efficiently, the average person with fair swimming skills is not able to exercise for any significant length of time, compared to the same effort for a dry-land exercise. Exercise books categorize swimming expenditure as either fast or slow, whereas running is measured in miles per hour. A fast crawl burns about 11 kilocalories per minute and a slow crawl burns 9 kilocalories per minute (46). What constitutes a slow swimming speed is unclear, especially if compared to the same speed of running (46). Equalizing intensity of effort when comparing different sports has been key to recognizing the weight loss benefits of swimming. Lieber et al (47) studied sedentary men who exercised for 1 hour per day for 3 months. Half of the men jogged and half swam. Each man exercised at about 75% of his VO_2max. All the subjects lost weight and body fat, with the swimmers losing slightly more. Dietary intakes were not measured but presumably if the subjects' diets were calorie restricted, then weight loss would probably have been even greater.

CHRONIC ATHLETIC FATIGUE

Because swimming training is long and strenuous, swimmers may be a risk for "chronic athletic fatigue."

The diagnosis of "chronic athletic fatigue" is controversial (6,48). It is sometimes used interchangeably with overtraining and burnout but is thought to include psychological and physiological components (6,48,49). Signs and symptoms include loss of appetite, weight loss, insomnia, muscle joint pain, and soreness without apparent cause, frequent respiratory infections, irritability, and anxiety sometimes accompanied by depression (6). Inadequate glycogen stores are believed to be a major contributing factor to this condition. *Box 45.3* delineates factors that may contribute to chronic athletic fatigue.

BOX 45.3   Factors Contributing to Chronic Athletic Fatigue

- Excessive training
- Insufficient recovery
- Improper nutrition

Nutrition Recommendations

- Aim for a minimum of 500 g carbohydrate/kg per day with adequate total calories.

For rapid glycogen synthesis:

- Eat 0.35 to 1.5 g carbohydrate/kg between multiple daily training sessions.

Or try a more frequent feeding schedule:

- Eat 0.4 g carbohydrate/kg every 15 minutes during the first 4 hours after exercise (6).

Other Recommendations to Prevent "Chronic Athletic Fatigue"

- Allow adequate recovery time between sessions of intense training.
- Obtain adequate sleep every night.
- Minimize other potential stresses.

Box 45.4 suggests ways coaches and trainers can best work with swimmers.

BOX 45.4   Tips for Coaches (gathered from collegiate swimmers, coaches, and author's experience)

- Believe in the power of nutrition. Coaches must value proper nutrition just as they value interval training.
- Be a role model. What is eaten in the coach's office or at swim meets may influence a swimmer's behavior.
- Keep healthy and adequate amounts of food and fluid available at swim meets and practices.
- Avoid food as a reward for swimming efforts, particularly for younger swimmers.
- Involve the parents of younger swimmers in nutrition education programs.
- Reinforce the importance of fluid replacement. Carry a bottle of fluids during practice to reinforce the desired behavior.
- Be aware of carbohydrate repletion guidelines and which foods contain adequate carbohydrate, especially immediately after practices.
- Notice changes in an athlete's swimming performance and consider inadequate nutrition as a potential cause.
- If athletes are involved in weight training, include this activity when calculating energy and protein needs.
- Recognize and help athletes choose optimum weights for performance. Energy must not be compromised because performance will suffer. Despite the high energy needs of many swimmers, some female swimmers may have a hard time controlling their weight. Do not encourage rigid dieting practices.
- Provide structure, education, and guidelines for college athletes but avoid being overbearing. It is a delicate balance. The transition from age-group swimming to NCAA training can be overwhelming. During age-group swimming, athletes often have structure provided by parents. The transition to a college environment offers freedoms, but the freedom to eat whatever is desired without support or structure can contribute to undesirable weight changes and poor eating patterns.
- Use the services of a dietetics professional to advise your swimmers.

AREAS FOR FURTHER RESEARCH

- Swimming uses a larger amount of carbohydrate as fuel than running (50). Since swimming uses more of the body's musculature than many other sports, does it promote a lower postexercise blood glucose level than other sports, if intensity and duration are equal? Anecdotal observations show swimmers may eat more after exercise than other athletes, but it is unclear if this is related to blood sugar level.
- Some claim that a swimmer's body fat level is higher than other athletes' and is often attributed to exercising in water. Most elite swimmers have body fat levels that are classified as low to normal (51). Anecdotal observations suggest swimmers' kilocalorie intakes are closer to their energy expenditure than runners. Perhaps a runner's body fat level is lower than a swimmer's body fat level because runners are not eating enough kilocalories to equal expenditure. It may not be the sport that determines body fat, but rather, calorie consumption.
- Future studies on swimming and weight control should consider all components—equalizing intensity of effort, energy intake, and appropriate methods for measuring body fat—to assess body composition.

CASE STUDY

Kim is a 19-year-old junior in college, competing on a Division I NCAA swim team. She swims twice a day, from 5:30 to 7:30 AM, and again in the afternoon from 5:30 to 7:00 PM. She is taking four classes. She does some weight training and other dry land resistance exercises three times per week; her routine takes her 1 1/2 hours. When she is not swimming or in class, she is usually studying. She complains that she is constantly tired, particularly during her early morning workouts. She admits that she studies late into the evening and her average weekday bedtime is 11 PM. Weekends she stays up much later to attend parties and socialize.

- Height: 5 ft 7 in
- Weight: 135 lb
- Body fat: 17%

She would like to lose 5 lb. Her energy needs are estimated to be 3,500 to 4,000 kilocalories per day. Kim's dietary patterns include:

- 16 oz water during morning swim practice
- 9:00 AM: Breakfast before her first class—one bagel and 8 oz orange juice
- 2:00 PM: Lunch—salad with either a ham and cheese sandwich or two slices of cheese pizza, one apple
- Snack: Frozen yogurt and diet soda
- 5:30 PM: Swim practice—24 oz water during practice
- 8:30 PM: Dinner—usually 2-3 cups of cooked pasta with spaghetti sauce and a salad, or hamburger, fries, and diet soda

While Kim is studying, she drinks coffee or diet soda and snacks on pretzels. She eats cookies and ice cream four to five times per week. She drinks six beers per week, usually on weekends.

Assessment

- Kim's weight and body fat are appropriate and her swimming may not improve if she compromises energy to lose weight.
- Kim is drinking inadequate fluids and is dehydrated, particularly if drinking alcohol and excess caffeinated beverages.
- Her morning blood sugar may be low going into her workout, and most certainly becomes low as she starts swimming because she does not eat until after practice. Hypoglycemia has been shown to result in increased fatigue and may be related to decreased motivation, desire, and performance (16,52).

- Kim is not replacing carbohydrates soon enough after her exercise. Her breakfast is inadequate and is eaten too long after her workout. She then waits 5 more hours before eating lunch. This does not allow for optimal glycogen repletion.
- Lunch and dinner choices are high in fat and low in carbohydrate. She also gets inadequate calcium. Her energy intake meets her needs on some days but not on all, and carbohydrate intake is inadequate. On some days her energy intake is only 2,500 kilocalories. Protein needs are 1.2 to 1.7 g/kg, which is 74 to 104 g per day. She is not meeting this every day.
- Kim's fatigue is probably a combination of dehydration, inadequate energy and carbohydrate intake, inadequate glycogen stores, and lack of sleep. Drinking coffee and alcohol late at night may also hinder her sleep.

Recommendations

- Drink water and sports drinks during practices, especially if not eating before the morning workout. This will help prevent dehydration and elevate blood sugar.
- Consider eating a small breakfast before morning practice, such as toast with jelly and juice.
- Eat small snacks immediately after practice, such as sports drinks, energy bars, bagels, bananas, and raisins, to help quickly replenish glycogen stores. Eat at least 1.5 g/kg (92 g of carbohydrate) within the first 30 minutes after swimming.
- Limit alcohol.
- Choose protein sources lower in saturated fat such as chicken, fish, peanut butter, or low-fat yogurt, and eat protein foods every day to meet needs of 74 to 104 g per day.
- Take a multivitamin-mineral supplement with 100% of the RDA as well as a calcium supplement if unable to increase dietary calcium. Ask a physician to evaluate for iron-deficiency anemia.
- Consider adding antioxidants vitamin C and vitamin E supplements with high training levels, after consulting with a physician or registered dietitian (33).
- Increase intake of fruits, vegetables, and low-fat dairy products, while decreasing frequency of high-fat snacks.
- Focus on maintaining weight, not losing weight.

REFERENCES

1. National Sporting Goods Association. *Sports Participation. National Sporting Goods Association Survey 1997*. http://www.nsga.org. Accessed September 26, 1998.
2. United States Swimming. Top 16/Top 100. http://www.usswim.org. Accessed September 25, 1998.
3. United States Master Swimming. http://www.usms.org. Accessed September 26, 1998.
4. Neufer PD, Costill DL, Fielding RA, Flynn MG, Kirwan JP. Effect of reduced training on muscular strength and endurance in competitive swimmers [abstract]. *Med Sci Sports*. 1987;19:486-490.
5. International Center for Aquatic Research. Interval training design [abstract]. *The Coaches' Newsletter of United States Swimming*. 4(5).
6. Sherman MW, Maglischo EW. Minimizing "chronic athletic fatigue" among swimmers: special emphasis on nutrition. *Sports Sci Exch*. 1991;4(35).
7. Costill DL, Flynn MG, Kirwan JP, et al. Effects of repeated days of intensified training on muscle glycogen and swimming. *Med Sci Sports Exerc*. 1988;20:249-254.
8. Hawley JA, Williams MM. Dietary intakes of age-group swimmers. *Br J Sports*. 1991;25:154-158.
9. Hawley JA, Williams MM. Relationship between upper body anaerobic power and freestyle swimming performance. *Int J Sports Med*. 1991;12:1-5.
10. International Center for Aquatic Research. Training response and adaptations. Training for swimming; The Coaches' Newsletter of United States Swimming. *Swimming Science Journal*. http://www-rohan.sdsu.edu/dept/coachsci/swimming/abstract/training/table.html. Accessed September 26, 1998.
11. Hsu TG, Hsu KM, Hsieh SS. The effects of shoulder isokinetic strength training on speed and propulsive forces in front crawl swimming [abstract]. *Med Sci Sports Exerc*. 1997;29(5 suppl):713.
12. Maglischo EW. *Nutritional Guidelines for Swimmers*. Gatorade Sports Science Institute. Coaches' Corner; 1996.
13. Trappe TA, Gastaldelli A, Jozsi AC, Troup JP, Wolfe RR. Energy expenditure of swimmers during high volume training. *Med Sci Sports Exerc*. 1997;29:950-954.
14. Jones PJ, Leitch CA. Validation of doubly labeled water for measurement of caloric expenditure in collegiate swimmers. *J Appl Physiol*. 1993;74:2909-2914.
15. Berning JR, Troup JP, Van Handel PJ, Daniels J, Daniels N. The nutritional habits of young adolescent swimmers. *Int J Sport Nutr*. 1991;1:240-248.
16. Coleman EJ. Carbohydrate—the master fuel. In: Berning JR, Steen SN, eds. *Nutrition for Sport and Exercise*. 2nd ed. Gaithersburg, Md: Aspen Publishers; 1998:21-44.
17. Costill DL, Sherman WM, Fink WJ, Maresh C, Witten M, Miller JM. The role of dietary carbohydrates in muscle glycogen resynthesis after strenuous running. *Am J Clin Nutr*. 1981;34:1831-1836.
18. Lamb DR, Rinehardt KF, Bartels RL, Sherman WM, Snook JT. Dietary carbohydrate and intensity of interval swim training. *Am J Clin Nutr*. 1990;52:1058-1063.
19. Butterfield G. Amino acids and high protein diets. In: Lamb D, Williams M, eds. *Perspectives in Exercise Science and Sports Medicine*. Carmel, Ind: Cooper Publishing Group; 1991:87-122.
20. Lemon PW. Is increased dietary protein necessary or beneficial for individuals with a physically active lifestyle? *Nutr Rev*. 1996;54(suppl):169-175.
21. Economos CD, Bortz SS, Nelson ME. Nutritional practices of elite athletes. Practical recommendations. *Sports Med*. 1993;16:381-399.
22. American Heart Association Science Advisory and Coordinating Committee. *Dietary Guidelines for Healthy American Adults*. Dallas, Tex: American Heart Association; 1996.

23. American Cancer Society. *Guidelines on Diet, Nutrition and Cancer Prevention*. Atlanta, Ga: American Cancer Society; 1996.

24. Soares MJ, Satyanarayana K, Bamji MS, Jacob CM, Ramana YV, Rao SS. The effect of exercise on the riboflavin status of adult men. *Br J Nutr*. 1993;69:541-551.

25. Belko AZ, Obarzanek E, Kalkwarf HJ, et al. Effects of exercise on riboflavin requirements of young women. *Am J Clin Nutr*. 1983;37:509-517.

26. Brigham DE, Beard JL, Krimmel RS, Kenney WL. Changes in iron status during competitive season in female collegiate swimmers. *Nutrition*. 1993;9:418-422.

27. Otis C. Too slim, amenorrheic, fracture-pone: the female triad. *ACSM Health Fitness J*. 1998;2:20-25.

28. Lukaski HC, Siders WA, Hoverson BS, Gallagher SK. Iron, copper, magnesium and zinc status as predictors of swimming performance. *Int J Sports Med*. 1996;17:535-540.

29. Shephard RJ, Shek PN. Heavy exercise, nutrition and immune function: is there a connection? *Int J Sports Med*. 1995;16:491-497.

30. Kanter M. Free radicals, exercise and antioxidant supplementation [abstract]. *Proc Nutr Soc*. 1998;57:9-13.

31. Clarkson PM. Vitamin nutrition for physically active people. *Vitamin Nutriton Informaton Service*. 1996;6(1):1-8.

32. USOC Sports Medicine Committee. *Guidelines on Dietary Supplementation*. Colorado Springs, Col: United States Olympic Committee; 1996.

33. Kanter M. Antioxidant supplementation for persons who are physically active. In: Berning JR, Steen SN, eds. *Nutrition for Sport and Exercise*. 2nd ed. Gaitherburg, Md: Aspen Publishers; 1998:45-55.

34. Taimura A, Sugahara M, Lee JB, Matsumoto T. Effect of fluid intake on plasma volume, osmolality, body temperature, and performance during swimming training [abstract]. *Med Sci Sports Exerc*. 1997;29(suppl):764.

35. Neilsen B. Physiology of thermoregulation during swimming [abstract]. In: Eriksson B, Furberg B, eds. *Swimming Medicine IV—Proceedings of the Fourth International Congress on Swimming Medicine*. Baltimore, Md: University Park Press; 1997.

36. Murray R. Fluids needs of athletes. In: Berning JR, Steen SN, eds. *Nutrition for Sport and Exercise*. 2nd ed. Gaithersburg, Md: Aspen Publishers; 1998:143-153.

37. Murray B. Fluid Replacement: The American College of Sports Medicine Position Stand. *Sports Sci Exch*. 1996;9(4).

38. Volek J, Kraemer WJ, Bush JA, et al. Creatine supplementation enhances muscular performance during high-intensity resistance exercise. *J Am Diet Assoc*. 1997;97:765-776.

39. Burke LM, Pyne DB, Telford RD. Effect of oral creatine supplementation on single-effort sprint performance in elite swimmers. *Int J Sport Nutr*. 1996;6:222-233.

40. Grindstaff PD, Kreider R, Bishop R, et al. Effects of creatine supplementation on repetitive sprint performance and body composition in competitive swimmers. *Int J Sport Nutr*. 1997;7:330-346.

41. Mujika I, Chatard JC, Lacoste L, Barale F, Geyssant A. Creatine supplementation does not improve sprint performance in competitive swimmers. *Med Sci Sports Exerc*. 1996;28:1435-1441.

42. Sears B. *The Zone*. New York, NY: Harper Collins; 1995.

43. Gwinup G. Weight loss without dietary restriction: efficacy of different forms of aerobic exercise. *Am J Sports Med*. 1987;15:275-279.

44. Avlonitou E, Georgiou E, Douskas G, Louizi A. Estimation of body composition in competitive swimmers by means of three different techniques [abstract]. *Int J Sports Med*. 1997;18:363-368.

45. Astrand P, Rodahl K. *Textbook of Work Physiology*. 3rd ed. New York, NY: McGraw-Hill Book Co; 1986.

46. Katch FI, McArdle WD. *Introduction to Nutrition, Exercise and Health*. 4th ed. Philadelphia, Penn: Lea & Febiger; 1993.
47. Lieber DC, Lieber RL, Adams WC. Effects of run-training and swim-training at similar absolute intensities on treadmill Vo$_2$ max. *Med Sci Sports Exerc*. 1989;21:655-661.
48. Parker J. Wiping your swimmers out. *Swimming Technique*. 1989;May-July:10-16.
49. Theriault D, Richard D, Labrie A, Theriault G. Physiological and psychological variables in swimmers during a competitive season in relation to the overtraining syndrome [abstract]. *Med Sci Sports Exerc*. 1997;29(suppl):1237.
50. Flynn MG, Costill DL, Kirwan JP, et al. Fat storage in athletes: metabolic and hormonal responses to swimming and running. *Int J Sports Med*. 1990;11:433-440.
51. Houtkooper LB. Body composition assessment and relationship to athletic performance. In: Berning JR, Steen SN, eds. *Nutrition for Sport and Exercise*. 2nd ed. Gaithersburg, Md: Aspen Publishers; 1998:155-166.
52. Davis M. Carbohydrates, branched-chain amino acids and endurance: the central fatigue hypothesis. *Int J Sport Nutr*. 1995;5(suppl):29-38.

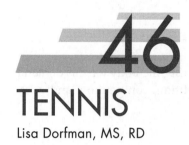

TENNIS

Lisa Dorfman, MS, RD

Tennis is a sport that requires energy to support speed; strength for short, explosive, intermittent bursts; and endurance for training and matches that can last more than 4 hours in various climates and temperatures (1,2). In addition, the professional and/or recreational player requires a high degree of flexibility and agility and an adequate aerobic training base (3).

For professional tennis players, training often exceeds 6 hours a day with a minimum of two or three strength-training sessions a week (2). Weight training has been shown to decrease body fat, increase muscle mass, and improve serve velocity and forehand and backhand strokes (2-4). Recreational players frequently spend several hours playing in singles or doubles matches. Frequently, these social players cross-train with a variety of aerobic-based activities including dance classes, power-walking, swimming, jogging, and/or weight training (2).

Tennis players must also manage fluid and electrolyte balance (1,5). Bergeron et al (1) note that even though an individual's on-court performance is dependent on many factors including environmental conditions, intensity of play, acclimatization, aerobic fitness, age, and gender, fluid intake must match sweat loss or a significant body water deficit can develop which can impair temperature regulation and athletic performance (1).

Another challenge for professional tennis players is maintaining an adequate food intake to meet energy and nutrient needs for training and competing while traveling the world. Regardless of a player's normal eating habits, it is difficult to maintain an adequate diet and training program on the road, in the air, or while venturing on foreign territory. Complicating this issue even further is the young age at which players begin competing (6). Sports nutritionists can help tennis players select nutritious foods that can positively affect their performance (7).

ENERGY UTILIZATION

Although it is difficult to quantify the energy demands of tennis, the sport relies on both aerobic and anaerobic systems (2). Most points in tennis last less than 10 seconds. On a hard court, one point between two equally matched players lasts about 5 seconds (2). A player may have 300 to 500 short bursts of effort during a match (2). The energy systems used for singles and doubles matches are primarily anaerobic; however, since there are approximately 25 seconds of rest between points and 90 seconds between games, maintaining a strong aerobic base enables a tennis player to recover more quickly between points and games (2).

The ability of the athlete to access long-term energy fuel such as fat for longer matches could ultimately determine the winner of the match, set, and perhaps some of the world's most prestigious events. Preparing the body for this demand requires nutritious foods and fluids in precompetition, competition, and post-competition meals (8).

ENERGY AND NUTRIENT NEEDS

In determining energy needs, two important factors should be considered:

1. Basal energy expenditure (BEE)
2. Tennis training and other activity energy expenditure

To calculate basal energy needs, it is desirable to know the player's weight, height, and fat-free mass. A goal weight and desirable percent of body fat should be based on the individual's age, weight history, and health (7).

Several authors (9,10) have described the body fat composition of elite and recreational tennis players. Berning and Steen (11) describe body fat percentages for competitive tennis players as 10% to 20% for females and 6% to 15% for males. For elite male tennis players, Forsyth (12) estimates body fat to be 15.2%.

Love (9) and Vodak (10) have also provided estimates of body fat percentages on tennis players. Love described the body composition of female elite-level junior tennis players as averaging 19.4% body fat (64 in tall and 114.9 lb). Males averaged 7.5% body fat (65.6 in tall and 118.3 lb) (9). Vodak et al (10) measured body composition on middle-aged tennis players and found a 42-year-old male with 16.3% body fat (77.1 kg and 179.6 cm or 170 lb and 71 in). Recreational female players (average age 39 years) were 20.3% body fat, weighed 55.7 kg (122.5 lb), and were 163.3 cm (64.3 in) tall (10). Roetert and Ellenbecker (2) suggest body fat percentages for tennis players should fall between 8% to 18% for men and 15% to 25% for women. The sports nutritionist can use these guidelines to evaluate a player's current body composition and prescribe an appropriate nutrition plan to help the player reach his or her goals.

After calculating the basal energy needs, one must add the energy expenditure for playing tennis and other activities. Age, gender, level of intensity, body composition, and weight will affect the amount of calories used for playing. Formulas for calculating energy expenditure can be found in Chapter 27, Managing Body Weight.

Research on tennis players during singles practice and match play have consistently rated tennis as a prolonged, moderate-intensity exercise activity (2). The exercise intensity levels range from 60% to 90% maximum heart rate during play (2). According to Dawson and Pyke (13), heart rates of players measured during work and recovery periods were approximately 80% of maximum for a full 60 minutes of play. It is estimated that 60% of that energy is derived from anaerobic sources (2,3). The calorie expenditure for singles recreational tennis ranges from 5 to 11 kcal per minute, 3.4 to 7.7 kcal per minute for doubles, and 6.4 to 14.4 kcal per minute at the competition level (11).

Carbohydrates

Carbohydrates are essential for maintaining adequate glycogen stores and should provide about 60% of total calories or at least 6 g/kg body weight (BW) daily and 7 to 10 g/kg BW when playing time exceeds several hours at 70% of VO_2max (12). Vergauwen et al (15) demonstrated that carbohydrate feedings could improve stroke quality in the final stages of prolonged tennis play. Groppel (8) suggests a minimum of 400 kcal of carbohydrates within 30 minutes of playing and an additional 200 calories within the next 2 hours.

Complex carbohydrates provide a nutrient-dense form of energy for maintaining glycogen stores and managing blood sugar levels and energy on the court. Appropriate food choices include whole-grain pasta, brown rice, beans, legumes, peas, apples, pears, sweet potatoes, yogurt, and low-fat milk. Complex carbohydrate foods will also provide a greater selection of vitamins, minerals, fiber, and phytochemicals (7).

Energy bars can help active players increase carbohydrates and calories. Energy bars can provide additional carbohydrates, vitamins, and minerals, and some contain protein. They can be a good snack choice for training and traveling. Frozen fruit smoothies, sports drinks, and frozen yogurt shakes are also court favorites (7).

Protein

Protein recommendations for the tennis player range from 1.2 to 1.4 g protein/kg BW (11). Slightly higher recommendations for competitive players of up to 1.6 g protein/kg BW may be warranted since amino acid oxidation, specifically branched-chain amino acids (BCAAs), have been shown to decline by 14% during continuous tournament play (16).

The protein needs of tennis players should be individualized, and food choices should include low-fat animal sources (lean red meat, poultry, fish, eggs, reduced-fat cheeses, and low-fat dairy foods). In addition, energy bars and shakes can help the players meet their protein needs (7). According to Bergeron (1), these products are especially helpful to junior players who have difficulty meeting their energy and protein needs while competing and traveling.

Some players consume excesses of protein. They believe extra protein in the form of BCAA supplements, shakes, or bars will build muscle mass and strength and prevent fatigue. None of these products or the use of extra protein in the well-nourished tennis player has been found to be helpful (7).

Fat

During prolonged exercise for more than 2 hours, fat is the major fuel source; however, carbohydrates are the predominate fuel for high-intensity exercise bouts (11). Since tennis has no clear dietary fat prescription, no more than 30% of total calories from fat is recommended. Saturated fat should provide 10% of calories or less since it has been linked to an increased risk of coronary heart disease.

Healthy food choices include polyunsaturated or monounsaturated fats from vegetable oils, wheat germ, salad dressings, margarine, and trail mix that includes soy nuts, seeds, raisins, apricots, and/or other dried fruits (7). Energy bars and shakes also can provide a source of fat if included in the bar or shake's formulation.

Fluids

Fluid needs must be met consistently throughout the training period. According to Bergeron (1), tennis players are at risk for premature fatigue, compromised performance, and an increased potential for heat illness during training and competition. As little as 1% fluid loss can cause discomfort and affect sport performance (11). Sweat rates in male and female tennis players can range between 0.5 and 2.5 L per hour (2). Bergeron (5) described a 17-year-old nationally ranked player who lost 2.5 L of fluid per hour. The combined effects of excessive and repeated fluid and sodium losses predisposed this player to heat cramps (5). His on-court sweat sodium losses of 89.8 mmol per hour of play exceeded his daily average dietary intake of 87 to 174.0 mmol per day and caused severe cramps (5). Salting foods and using an electrolyte replacement beverage were recommended (5).

For tennis matches lasting longer than 1 hour, a carbohydrate-containing sports drink is recommended (1,2,15,17). Vergauwen et al (15) demonstrated that carbohydrate feedings before and during matches produced more powerful and more precise shots, reduced net-error rate, reduced shuttle run performance, and reversed fatigue in more stressful defensive rallies.

In addition to daily fluids from water, tea, juice, and sports drinks, fresh fruits and vegetables are recommended to meet fluid and carbohydrate needs (7). Sport drinks are helpful for carbohydrate and fluid replacement during and after the match and for electrolyte replacement during hot, humid conditions (2,8,9,11,15). The sports nutritionist needs to discourage the use of herbal teas, coffee, and alcoholic beverages for fluid replacement since these beverages can act as diuretics, affect performance, and may even contain substances illegal to competition (7,14).

Vitamins and Minerals

Love (9) described inadequate dietary intakes of iron, riboflavin, magnesium, calcium, and vitamin A in junior elite tennis players, although the diet analyses were limited to 1-day food records. Ensuring adequate intakes of vitamins and minerals can be achieved through consumption of a balanced intake of whole-grains, lean meats, poultry, fish, low-fat dairy foods, fruits, and vegetables.

When the player finds it challenging to eat nutritious meals on the road, energy bars, shakes, and drinks can fill the vitamin/mineral gap since many products are fortified. If necessary, a multivitamin/mineral supplement can be recommended to players when dietary consumption is not adequate. Multivitamin supplements should not exceed 100% of the RDAs for vitamins and minerals (7).

SUPPLEMENT USE

Although the use of supplements by tennis players has not been described in the literature, Roetert reports the most popular supplements consumed by competitive tennis players include creatine, multivitamins, B-vitamins, antioxidants (specifically vitamins E and C), and protein (2). Since creatine has not been shown to enhance performance in tennis, such supplementation is ill advised.

A multivitamin/mineral supplement may help certain players who have limited time for the preparation and consumption of nutritious foods. Eating on the road can be a challenge to balanced eating and consuming an adequate intake of vitamins, minerals, and protein, particularly for the younger player (9,14).

Multiple and/or singular forms of B-vitamins are also used by tennis players. Some believe that extra B-vitamins will help carbohydrates and fats to be used more efficiently. Since research has not demonstrated the need for extra B-vitamin supplementation in athletes unless a deficiency exists, this is not a sound recommendation.

When whole foods are difficult to find or consume, the next best "supplemental" alternative for vitamins and minerals can be fortified shakes, energy bars, and drinks (7). Since competitive athletes tend to overdo even a good thing, the trainer, coach, or sports nutritionist should monitor the intake of heavily fortified products.

PRECOMPETITION, COMPETITION, AND RECOVERY MEALS AND SNACKS

Players can benefit from manipulating the amount of carbohydrate and fluid they consume to prepare for competition, training, and recovery from their activities (2,11,14,17). An overview of the amounts, foods, and timing of these "ergogenic" meals and snacks are described in *Table 46.1*.

TABLE 46.1   Tennis Foods and Fluids: Competition and Performance Meals and Snacks

Event	Carbohydrates	Fluids
Pretraining/Competition	Moderate to low glycemic index foods; 1 to 4 g carbohydrate/kg BW 1 to 4 hours before training and competition, respectively (3,7,17)	12 to 16 oz water before playing time Prepare 2 quarts to drink during play.

- **Precompetition foods:** Energy bars; sports drinks; high-carbohydrate, low-fat shakes; apples, pears, oranges, or grapes; low-fat yogurt; multigrain bread or cereal (hot or cold); sweet potatoes; fruit smoothies; low-fat, whole-grain waffles; low-fat granola with yogurt; low-fat frozen yogurt; low-fat bran/raisin muffin

Competition/Training	25 to 30 g every half hour of playing time for matches; after warm up and after every hour of play	4 to 8 oz (4 to 8 normal "gulps") every changeover

- **Training drinks and meals:** Energy bars; sports drinks; high-carbohydrate, moderate-protein, low-fat shakes; apples, pears, oranges, or grapes; low-fat yogurt or frozen yogurt; baked potato; chips or pretzels; fruit smoothies; rice cakes

continued

TABLE 46.1   Tennis Foods and Fluids: Competition and Performance Meals and Snacks (continued)

After Training/Competition	400 calories carbohydrates high glycemic index within 30 minutes of playing. Continue consuming a carbohydrate-rich diet of 7 to 10 g/kg BW per day to replenish glycogen stores (5,17).	150% of fluids lost At least 16 oz for every lb lost Add salt to food if sweat loss is excessive.

- **Posttraining drinks and meals:** Energy bars; sports drinks; frozen yogurt or fruit smoothie shakes; baked potatos; pasta; cheese pizzas; burritos

TIPS FOR COACHES AND TRAINERS

1. Encourage the intake of adequate complex carbohydrates, protein, and moderate fat by recommending small, frequent meals and snacks throughout the day. When preferred foods are difficult to find or consume, be prepared to provide sports drinks, shakes, or energy bars.
2. Help the player maintain adequate hydration by making fluids available at all times.
3. Encourage players to consume sports drinks during training so when they consume them at tournaments they will be better tolerated.
4. Discourage the use of unnecessary dietary supplements. Think food first.
5. Facilitate discussion about training and tournament stress to prevent over-training syndrome and eating disorders, all of which can affect a balanced nutritional intake.

CASE STUDY

Competitive Female Tennis Player on the Pro Tour

Age: 19
Height: 5'4"
Weight: 138 lb (63 kg)
Desired body weight: 135 to 138 lb
Percent body fat: 18.5%
Medical problems: amenorrhea
Medications/supplements: birth control pills to regulate menstrual cycle
Training: 6 to 8 hours court time daily plus weight training two
    to three times per week

Food Intake:

Morning: Hot chocolate, banana, and two frozen waffles with syrup
Lunch: Baked chips, 4 oz turkey on pita bread, diet soda, and pear

Evening: White rice, canned beans, sweet potato, apple, and diet soda
Snacks: 6 pieces of gum daily

Dietary Analysis:
Kcal: 1,675
Protein: 68 g (16%)
Carbohydrate: 310 g (73%)
Sugar: 87 g (24 t)
Fat: 21 g (11%)
Fiber: 26 g
Vitamin D, calcium, biotin, zinc, copper <50% of the RDAs

Recommendations

- Include more calories. Using the basal energy expenditure (BEE), this player needs a minimum of 1,630 kcal for BEE alone. Using the values provided by Vodak et al (11) for the estimation of calorie expenditure by competitive tennis playing, this player would use about 9.1 kcal per minute, an additional 546 kcal per hour for activity. After calculating her approximate daily needs of 2,393 kcal (BEE + energy expenditure + TEF [thermic effect of food]), conservatively her current calorie intake is almost 1,000 kcal less than her estimated needs.
- Suggested foods and snacks:
  — High complex carbohydrate, moderate protein, and low-fat whole foods and snacks
  — Less processed foods, foods designed for convenience, and diet sodas
  — Energy bars, shakes, smoothies, vegetable soups, brown rice, whole-grain cereals, waffles, and breads to meet recommended levels of carbohydrates, protein, fat, vitamins, and minerals
- Carbohydrates: To ensure adequate energy with carbohydrate-rich foods, based on her body weight of 63 kg, approximately 441 to 630 g (7 to 10 g/kg BW per day) is recommended for the maintenance of glycogen stores, energy levels, and the ability to recover from training and competition.
- Protein: She needs a minimum of 75 g of protein per day to meet her needs.
- Vitamins and minerals: In addition to providing additional calories, protein, carbohydrates, and fat, the addition of foods rich in calcium and trace minerals is recommended and can easily be included by eating more whole grains, fortified cereals, fruits and fruit juices, vegetables, energy bars, shakes, and fortified beverages. A multivitamin is not necessary if usual intake contains a wider variety of foods.
- Fluids: Encourage the liberal consumption of fluids, including sport drinks and fruit juices.

REFERENCES

1. Bergeron M, Armstrong LE, Maresh CM. Fluid and electrolyte losses during tennis in the heat. *Clin Sports Med.* 1995;14:23-32.
2. Roetert P, Ellenbecker TS. *Complete Conditioning for Tennis.* United States Tennis Association. Champaign, Ill: Human Kinetics; 1998.
3. Roetert P, Piorkowski P, Woods R, Brown S. Establishing percentiles for junior tennis players based on physical fitness testing results. *Clin Sports Med.* 1995;4:1-21.
4. United States Tennis Association. Research grants reveal strength training makes better tennis players. *Sport Science for Tennis* [newsletter]. Key Biscayne, Fla: United States Tennis Association; Spring 1993:6.
5. Bergeron M. Heat cramps during tennis: a case report. *Int J Sport Nutr.* 1996;6:62-68.
6. Otis C. A review of the age eligibility commission report. *Sport Science for Tennis* [newsletter]. Key Biscayne, Fla: United States Tennis Association; 1994.
7. Dorfman L. *The Vegetarian Sports Nutrition Guide: Peak Performance for Everyone from Beginners to Gold Medalists.* New York, NY: John Wiley & Sons; 1999.
8. Groppel J. Ask the professor. Refuel after workout with carbs, fuel and rest. *USPTA ADDvantage Magazine Online.* http://www.uspta.org. Accessed March 17, 1999.
9. Love P. Nutrition assessment of junior elite tennis players: body composition assessment and nutritional intake evaluation [abstract]. *USTA Coaches Workshop.* 1996.
10. Vodak PA, Savin WM, Haskell WL, Wood PD. Physiological profile of middle-aged male and female tennis players. *Med Sci Sports Exerc.* 1980;12:159-163.
11. Berning J, Steen S. *Nutrition for Sport & Exercise.* 2nd ed. Gaithersburg, Md: Aspen Publishers; 1998.
12. Forsyth HL, Sinning WE. The anthropometric estimation of body density and lean body weight of male athletes. *Med Sci Sports Exerc.* 1973;5:174-180.
13. Dawson E, Pyke F. The energetics of singles tennis. *J Human Movement Studies.* 1985;11:11-20.
14. Steen S. Eating on the road: where are the carbohydrates? *Sports Sci Exch.* 1998;11:4.
15. Vergauwen L, Brouns F, Hespel P. Carbohydrate supplementation improves stroke performance in tennis. *Med Sci Sports Exerc.* 1998;38:1289-1295.
16. Struder HK, Hollman W, Duperly J, Wber K. Amino acid metabolism in tennis and its possible influence on the endocrine system. *Br J Sports Med.* 1995;29:28-30.
17. Williams C, Nicholas C. Nutrition needs for team sport. *Sports Sci Exch.* 1998;11:3.

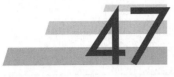

TRACK AND FIELD EVENTS

Debra Vinci, DrPH, RD

Track and field events include a wide range of short-duration and long-duration activities that vary in intensity from a 100-meter dash, to the throw of a shot put, to the 10,000-meter run. USA Track and Field is the national governing body for the sport, with competitive classifications for youth (under age 19), senior, submasters (ages 30 to 39), and masters (age 40 and over) (1,2).

Running events take place on a track, and field events compete on the field inside a track or in a field away from the track. Races are run counterclockwise on an indoor or outdoor track with a runner's left hand always toward the inside of the track. Outdoor events are held around a 400-meter oval track that has six to nine lanes; indoor tracks vary in size with many 200 meters in length. Sprinters who compete in races of 400 meters or less run in the same lane during the whole race. In an 800-meter race, racers run in lanes until they complete the first turn and then they move to the inside lane. Races are not run in lanes in events beyond 800 meters (1). *Tables 47.1* and *47.2* provide an overview of events in which track and field athletes compete from the local to the elite level (1).

TABLE 47.1 Championship Track Events

Event	Indoor	Outdoor	Men	Women
60-meter dash	x		x	x
100-meter dash		x	x	x
200-meter dash	x	x	x	x
400-meter dash	x	x	x	x
800-meter run	x	x	x	x
1,500-meter run		x	x	x
1-mile run	x		x	x
3,000-meter run	x		x	x
3,000-meter walk	x			x
3,000-meter steeplechase		x	x	x
5,000-meter run		x	x	x
5,000-meter walk	x		x	x
10,000-meter run		x	x	x
10,000-meter walk		x		x
20,000-meter walk		x	x	x
60-meter hurdles	x		x	x
100-meter hurdles		x		x
110-meter hurdles		x	x	x
400-meter hurdles		x	x	x

continued

TABLE 47.1   Championship Track Events (continued)

Event	Indoor	Outdoor	Men	Women
400-meter relay		x		x
800-meter relay		x		x
1,600-meter relay	x		x	x
1,600-meter relay	x			x
3,200-meter relay	x		x	
3,200-meter relay		x		x

Source: Human Kinetics with Hanlon T. *The Sports Rules Book: Essential Rules for 54 Sports*. Champaign, Ill: Human Kinetics; 1998. Used with permission.

TABLE 47.2   Championship Field Events

Event	Indoor	Outdoor	Men	Women
High jump	x	x	x	x
Pole vault*	x	x	x	x
Long jump	x	x	x	x
Triple jump	x	x	x	x
Shot put	x	x	x	x
Discus throw		x	x	x
Javelin throw		x	x	x
Hammer throw		x	x	x
Weight throw	x		X	X

*In 1999, women's indoor pole vaulting was added to championship field events.

Source: Human Kinetics with Hanlon T. *The Sports Rules Book: Essential Rules for 54 Sports*. Champaign, Ill: Human Kinetics; 1998. Used with permission.

FUELING PEAK PERFORMANCE

Peak performance for the track and field athlete ultimately depends on the body's capacity to provide power to meet the demands of exercise of varying intensity and duration (3,4). A comprehensive understanding of the physiology of anaerobic and aerobic exercise provides the sports nutritionist with the knowledge to provide nutrition recommendations that match the physiological demands of track and field athletes. *Table 47.3* provides a brief overview of the distinct power systems that supply energy for selected track and field events (3-6). Anaerobic and aerobic exercise are reviewed in more detail in Chapter 1, Physiology of Anaerobic and Aerobic Exercise.

TABLE 47.3 Major Power Systems and Principal Fuels that Supply Energy for Selected Track and Field Events

Event Duration	Major Power System	Principal Fuel(s)	Track & Field Events
6 seconds or less	Phosphagen	ATP and CP	Development of explosive power: • Sprint starts • Initiation of jump or throw
30 seconds or less	Phosphagen Anaerobic glycolytic	ATP and CP Muscle glycogen	100-meter dash (10.18)* 200-meter dash (20.50) *
15 minutes or less	Anaerobic glycolytic Aerobic glycolytic	Muscle glycogen Blood glucose	400-meter dash (45.40) * 800-meter run (1:47.20) * 1,500-meter run (3:41.30) *
15 to 60 minutes	Aerobic glycolytic	Muscle glycogen Blood glucose	5,000-meter run (13:48.00) * 10,000-meter run (29:10.00) *

*1999 Division I Men's Outdoor Track and Field Automatic Qualifying Standards (7)

Adapted from: Hawley H, Burke L. *Peak Performance: Training and Nutritional Strategies for Sport.* Sydney, Australia: Allen & Unwin; 1998.

TOP NUTRITION CONCERNS

The nutrition concerns of track and field athletes are as varied as the events in this sport. The top nutrition concerns of track and field athletes include:

- Adequate energy and nutrient intakes
- Weight and body composition
- Nourishment before and during events
- Recovery after training and competition
- Hydration

Adequate Energy and Nutrient Intakes

Track and field athletes have a range of energy needs that are influenced by age, gender, specialty event, level, intensity, and frequency of training. Track athletes may struggle with problems of fatigue and poor workouts and seek nutrition counseling after the athletic trainer or team physician has ruled out any medical causes for these problems. Nutrition assessment frequently reveals an underestimation of energy needs for the level of training required for the event. For example, a 21-year-old, 70-kg male's resting energy expenditure (REE) is approximately 1,750 kcal. His daily energy expenditure without sport training would be approximately 2,365 kcal. If this individual trained competitively as a distance runner, his daily energy expenditure would increase to approximately 3,500 kcal. Factors that can contribute to inadequate energy intake include overcommitted lifestyle, vegetarian diet, limited meal planning and preparation skills, frequent travel related to competitive events, and reliance on energy bars and sports beverages for a significant source of energy (3).

In addition to inadequate calorie intake, an athlete's fatigue and lethargy could also be due to inadequate carbohydrate (CHO) intake to fuel training or competition. Studies on nutrient intakes reveal that it is not unusual for athletes' diets to be lower in carbohydrate than the recommended 7 to 10 g/kg per body weight (BW) (8-12).

Weight and Body Composition

For some athletes decreased energy intake is related to the desire to lose weight and body fat to improve performance. While low body mass and/or low body fat may assist in improved performance since athletes must move their own body mass against gravity, many athletes have misconceptions about ideal body weight and body composition (13-15). This is especially true for female distance runners where the normative body type is perceived as a svelte athletic figure (16). In reality, there is significant variability in lean body weight and body fat among athletes in any sport. Wilmore et al (17) presented data on 70 elite women distance runners and found their average body fat was 16.8% (5.5% with ranges of 6% to 35.8%). One of the leanest athletes, at 6% body fat, had established several national running records including the best time in the world for the marathon. At the other extreme the woman with the highest body fat (35.8%) had the best time in the world in the 50-mile run (17).

The variability in body composition could reflect an individual's natural weight, genetics, and the influence of diet and training necessary for the sport. Many female athletes have a tendency to view minimal weight as optimal weight and struggle to lose weight below what is natural for them. This can place female athletes at risk for developing a triad of interrelated health problems: disordered eating, amenorrhea, and premature osteoporosis. These are referred to as the female athlete triad (13,18).

Male athletes also have weight concerns that influence eating behaviors and energy intake. Many are interested in bulking up by increasing muscle mass and decreasing fat stores (19). Frequently, for nutrition information they rely on popular muscle magazines that usually encourage the use of supplements and ergogenic aids. Although usually thought of as a female's domain, male athletes also have body image disturbances and disordered eating behaviors (20). Assessment of energy requirements, eating disorders, and healthful weight management strategies, and the use of ergogenic aids are discussed in more detail in other chapters in this book.

Nourishment before and during Events

While athletes understand the importance of a well-planned training program for peak competitive performance, many lack the knowledge and skills necessary to develop a sport nutrition "game plan." Several factors influence athletes' food choices prior to and during an event.

Travel schedule. During the competitive season, track and field athletes often travel to events. Each competition provides a nutritional challenge since food resources are often unknown to the athlete. While some coaches or athletic trainers plan meals for the traveling team, others leave that responsibility to the athlete who most likely lacks solid nutrition knowledge. While sports nutritionists may not travel with the team, they can provide practical tips for the athlete when he or she is eating on the road (3,21).

Limited money and time. Many athletes have limited food budgets and are trying to save money and time by eating at fast-food restaurants. While athletes perceive these meals to be good because they are less expensive, they are high in fat and can result in inadequate carbohydrate intake prior to competition (21).

Such occurrences provide the sports nutritionist with an excellent opportunity to review the benefits of high-carbohydrate, low-fat preevent meals. It is also important to recognize that many coaches assume that their athletes are making sound food choices. Many become more open to a sports nutritionist's involvement when they discover the less-than-ideal eating habits of their athletes.

Competing in multiple events at a track meet. Track and field athletes may compete in multiple events over the course of several hours. While some athletes will compete in one event, others can be competing in up to four events. The exceptions are decathlon for men, which consists of 10 events over 2 days, and the heptathlon for women, which consists of seven events over 2 days.

While guidelines for preevent and during-event nourishment focus on high-carbohydrate, low-fat foods, there is individual variability in what athletes can tolerate prior to and during competition (11). For example, during a 1-day track meet, one female athlete at a NCAA Division I university raced in the 100-meter hurdle, 400-meter hurdle, 400-meter relay, and the 1,600-meter relay, with only 20 minutes to 1 hour between events. Since precompetition stress made it difficult for her to eat a large breakfast, she would rely on sport drinks when she only had 20 minutes between events and four to six crackers or 1/2 banana and sports drinks when she had up to 1 hour between events.

It is not unusual for track and field athletes to find themselves hungry during a track meet and yet be too nervous to eat. One way to decrease hunger is to encourage athletes to have a high-carbohydrate dinner and bedtime snack the night before a track meet.

Recovery after Training and Competition

Increasingly, competitive athletes are becoming more aware of the benefits of carbohydrate intake after exercise to restore the body's glycogen stores and to refuel for the next day's training or competition. However, many athletes delay the intake of carbohydrate for recovery. Some are too busy trying to juggle school, jobs, training, and competing. Many lack time-management and meal-planning skills and need encouragement to pack high-carbohydrate foods such as fruit, fruit juice, sports drinks, cereal bars, crackers, and bagels in their gym bags.

The restoration of muscle glycogen is especially important for athletes who train several times a day. Recommended levels of carbohydrate include 1.0 to 1.5 g/kg/BW within 30 minutes after exercise and continued intake of carbohydrate over several hours for a total of approximately 1 g/kg/BW. Daily carbohydrate intake should be 7 to 10 g/kg/BW (3). For example, a 66-kg female hurdler would need a daily intake of 462 to 660 g carbohydrate (CHO) with 66 to 99 g CHO within 30 minutes after a workout. Sample snacks of 66 g CHO include:

- 16 oz sports drink and banana
- 8 oz cranberry juice and cereal bar
- 15 saltine crackers and 12 oz can soft drink (not diet)
- 8 oz sports drink and large bagel

Hydration

The relationship between optimal performance and hydration status is well documented (22,23). Despite this fact, mild to severe dehydration commonly occurs among athletes (3,24). For track and field athletes, factors contributing to dehydration include:

- Unsupervised workouts, placing the responsibility for hydration on the athlete
- Limited availability of fluids at the training location
- Travel from cooler environments to warmer, humid locations without adequate time to acclimate
- Increased fluid loss from the body during air travel
- A competitive psyche that pushes athletes to continue exercising despite dehydration

Strategies for adequate hydration include working with coaches and athletic trainers to provide cool fluids at workouts and to give athletes time to drink at frequent intervals throughout the training period (25). It may be helpful for athletes, especially those training in hot environments or those who are chronically dehydrated, to monitor weight before and after exercise and match fluid intake with sweat loss (3,25). It is important to remember that often signs of thirst are not immediate or strong enough for the athlete to properly rehydrate (3). A complete discussion on fluid needs before, during, and after exercise is presented in Chapter 6, Fluid and Electrolytes.

WORKING WITH COACHES AND ATHLETES

Because there are different events within track and field, the sports nutritionist may work with several coaches. This is an exciting opportunity and it is important for the sports nutritionist to be knowledgeable about the sport and to be aware of the coaches' and athletes' attitudes about nutrition and performance. Use of supplements, ergogenic aids, and illicit anabolic steroids is a reality within the track and field world since the margin between winning and losing is down to fractions of seconds (5,26,27).

Additionally, an athlete who competes in two events, such as sprint and long jump, may work with more than one coach with different beliefs about nutrition and performance. For example, a heptathlon athlete may work with three different coaches. While two coaches may stress the importance of adequate energy intake for her level of training and remind her that improved performance will come with maturity in the sport, the third coach may focus on her need to lose weight and body fat as a measure of improved performance. In this situation the sports nutritionist plays an important role in assisting the athlete to acquire accurate sports nutrition information. A situation such as this may also provide the sports nutritionist with an opportunity to educate athletic administrators and sports medicine physicians on the role of nutrition in performance and the dangers associated with the female athlete triad.

CASE STUDY

"I am so tired. I started training hard in September and competed in the indoor season during the winter months. Now that it's March and the outdoor season has started, I am really worried that I won't be competitive since I barely have enough energy."

Sharma, a 20-year-old African American track and field athlete, is a sprint and long jump specialist at a NCAA Division I university. She is ranked third on the team in the 100- and 200-meter events and was the second best long jumper on the team the previous year. Her goal for the spring outdoor season is to qualify for the NCAA championships; however, her fatigue is preventing her from feeling strong and capable of performing at her best. *Box 47.1* illustrates Sharma's typical day during the outdoor competitive season.

BOX 47.1   Sharma's Typical Day during the Outdoor Competitive Season

8:00 AM	Wakes and showers
8:30 AM	1 cup dry cereal with 3/4 cup skim milk and 2 cups lemonade
9:30 AM	In class until 10:20 AM
10:30 AM	In class until 11:20 AM
11:30 AM	Break between class: bagel with 1 oz cheese and 2 cups lemonade
12:30 PM	In class until 1:20 PM
1:30 PM	Walks from class to workout facilities and gets ready for practice
2:00 PM	Practice until 5:00 PM; occasionally drinks water during practice
5:30 PM	Walks back to dorm after practice
6:00 PM	2 cups lemonade
6:30 PM	3 cups broccoli, 1 cup angel hair pasta with 1/2 cup tomato sauce, 2 cups lemonade
8:00 PM	Studying; 1 cup tea with 1 heaping tablespoon sugar
10:00 PM	Visiting friends
12:00-1:00 AM	Usual bedtime

Assessment

- Height: 171.5 cm (67.5")
- Weight: 59.5 kg (131 lb)
- Body fat: 11%
- Analysis of a 3-day food record estimates energy intake at 1,910 kcal, 83% carbohydrate or 396 g, 10% protein or 48 g, and 7% fat or 15 g.

- Laboratory tests were within normal limits and anemia was ruled out.
- She has regular menstrual cycles.
- Sharma trains year-round. Over the summer months, her workouts are less formal and lower in intensity. She trains 5 days either running, biking, or swimming for 45 to 60 minutes and lifts weights three times a week for 2 hours. When school starts in the fall, Sharma returns to formal workouts with the team 5 to 6 days a week. These practices require approximately 3 hours of running and 2 hours of strength development. The running training includes overdistance training and tempo running to develop an endurance base, along with interval training, hills, and fartlek (speed play). The strength-development program involves resistance-training with heavy weights (85% of maximum weight) with four to six sets of 8 to 10 repetitions. Sharma also long jumps so she does plyometics to develop leg strength and resilience for explosive power. Winter quarter marks the start of the indoor season which runs from January to the beginning of March. Sharma continues training during the week with a shift from running training to more sprint training, track workouts, and technique work. On the weekends she races in the 55- or 60-meter and/or 200-meter and long jump events. Once the outdoor season starts, Sharma's workouts enter the competition phase and involve more explosive workouts that focus on speed and technique for 100-meter, 200-meter, and long jump events. She continues to train 5 days a week with shorter workouts and competes on the weekends until the end of May.
- Sharma's energy requirements are influenced by her training cycle. Higher energy needs occur in the fall as she builds her fitness base, and lower energy is required in early summer as she lowers her training intensity to recover from the competitive season. Additionally, it is not unusual for Sharma to lose weight by the end of the outdoor track season.
- Sharma states that it is difficult for her to eat a variety of foods since she lives in an on-campus apartment and shares kitchen facilities with five roommates. On the weekends that she competes, coaches provide money for food. Sharma states that it is not unusual for college athletes to eat at fast-food restaurants in order to save money. Sharma finds that when she eats hamburgers and french fries, she gets an upset stomach so she avoids meat during the week. She does not report lactose intolerance with dairy products. However, she does not like the taste of milk but will eat yogurt and cheese.

Recommendations

Sharma realized that she needed to make changes in her daily routine and eating patterns. While she knew that it was necessary for her to go to bed earlier, she found it helpful to understand why sleep was important for a competitive athlete.

Dietary recommendations include increasing total energy, protein, and fat in her daily diet and providing her with tips for precompetition and postcompetition meals.

- While 3-day food records estimated Sharma's caloric intake at 1,910 kcal, her energy needs were determined to be 2,500 to 2,750 kcal during the competitive season. Suggestions to increase energy intake included having a larger breakfast and planning a snack between breakfast and lunch.
- Sharma's current intake was high in carbohydrates (396 g or 83% of kcal) and low in protein. A significant source of carbohydrates in her diet was from lemonade. While juices and fruit drinks can contribute to proper hydration, they were providing calories from carbohydrates at the expense of foods that would be good sources of protein and fat. Sharma was given guidelines to increase her caloric intake to approximately 2,700 kcal with 405 to 439 g CHO (60% to 65% carbohydrate) which is based on 7 to 10 g CHO/kg/BW (3).
- Protein requirements for athletes are 1.2 to 1.7 g of protein/kg/BW (11,28,29). Sharma needs to increase her daily protein intake from 48 g (0.8 g/kg/BW) to approximately 71 to 101 g/kg/BW. This could be accomplished by adding 8 oz low-fat yogurt for a morning snack, 2 oz lean meat to the bagel at lunch, and 3 oz ground turkey or beef in the tomato sauce at dinner. By adding these protein sources, Sharma will also increase her energy and fat intake. (See *Box 47.2*.)

BOX 47.2	Recommended Nutrient Intakes	
Energy (45 kcal/kg/day)	2,678 kcal	
Carbohydrate (7-10 g/kg/day) (3)	416 - 439 g	62% - 65% of total kcal
Protein (1.2-1.7 g/kg/day) (11,28,29)	71 - 101 g	11% - 15% of total kcal
Fat (minimum 1 g/kg/day)	60 - 81 g	20% - 27% of total kcal

- For optimal performance during weekend competition, Sharma was encouraged to consider alternatives to hamburgers and fries. Her upset stomach may be related to the high fat in fast-food meals and precompetition stress. Eventhough she needed to add protein and fat to her diet, Sharma's precompetition meals should be higher in carbohydrate and lower in fat. Alternatives include making lower-fat food choices at fast-food restaurants and stopping instead at a sandwich shop or grocery store where she can order a sandwich made with lean meats. Grocery stores also provide the opportunity to purchase yogurt, string cheese, fruits, juices, and snacks such as pretzels, low-fat crackers, and granola bars.

Sharma's referral to the sports nutritionist provided her with increased knowledge and skills to make the dietary changes to decrease her fatigue and boost her confidence to perform well during the outdoor track season. Another benefit was that Sharma's success encouraged her teammates also to consult with the sports nutritionist.

REFERENCES

1. Human Kinetics with Hanlon T. *The Sports Rules Book: Essential Rules for 54 Sports.* Champaign, Ill: Human Kinetics; 1998.
2. USA Track & Field (USATF). *About USATF.* http://www.usatf.org/about/staff.shtml. Accessed September 20, 1998.
3. Hawley H, Burke L. *Peak Performance: Training and Nutritional Strategies for Sport.* Sydney, Australia: Allen & Unwin; 1998.
4. McArdle WD, Katch FI, Katch VL. *Sports and Exercise Nutrition.* Baltimore, Md: Lippincott Williams & Wilkins; 1999.
5. Williams C, Gandy G. Physiology and nutrition for sprinting. In: Lamb DR, Knuttgen HG, Murry R, eds. *Perspectives in Exercise Science and Sports Medicine, Vol. 7: Physiology and Nutrition for Competitive Sport.* Carmel, Ind: Cooper Publishing Group; 1994:55-98.
6. Maughan R. Physiology and nutrition for middle distance and long distance runners. In: Lamb DR, Knuttgen HG, Murry R, eds. *Perspectives in Exercise Science and Sports Medicine, Vol. 7: Physiology and Nutrition for Competitive Sport.* Carmel, Ind: Cooper Publishing Group; 1994:329-371.
7. National Collegiate Athletic Association. *1999 Division I Men's Outdoor Track and Field Qualifying Standards.* http://www.ncaachampionships.com/sports/motrx/i_99qualifying.html. Accessed July 14, 1999.
8. Tanaka JA, Tanaka H, Landis W. An assessment of carbohydrate intake in collegiate distance runners. *Int J Sport Nutr.* 1995;5:206-214.
9. Van Erp-Baart AMJ, Saris WHM, Binkhorst RA, Vos JA, Elvers JWH. Nationwide survey on nutritional habits in elite athletes: part I. Energy, carbohydrate, protein, and fat intake. *Int J Sports Med.* 1989;10:S3-S10.
10. Coleman EJ. Carbohydrate—the master fuel. In: Berning JR, Steen SN, eds. *Nutrition for Sport and Exercise.* 2nd ed. Gaithersburg, Md: Aspen Publishers; 1998:21-44.
11. Harkins C, Carey R, Clark N, Benardot D. Protocols for developing dietary prescriptions. In: Benardot D, ed. *Sports Nutrition: A Guide for the Professional Working with Active People.* 2nd ed. Chicago, Ill: The American Dietetic Association; 1993:170-185.
12. Williams C. Macronutrients and performance. *J Sports Sci.* 1995;13:S1-S10.
13. Burke L. Practical issues in nutrition for athletes. *J Sports Sci.* 1995;13:S83-S90.
14. Brownell KD, Steen SN, Wilmore JH. Weight regulation practices in athletes: analysis of metabolic and health effects. *Med Sci Sports Exerc.* 1987;19:546-556.
15. Clarkson P, Manore M, Oppliger B, Steen SN, Walberg-Rankin J. Roundtable: methods and strategies for weight loss in athletes. *Sports Sci Exch.* 1998;9:1-5.
16. Committee on Sports Medicine. Amenorrhea in adolescent athletes. *Pediatrics.* 1989;84:394-396.
17. Wilmore JH, Brown CH, Davis JA. Body physique and composition of the female distance runner. *Ann N Y Acad Sci.* 1977;301:764-776.
18. Benson JE, Engelbert-Fenton KA, Eisenman PA. Nutritional aspects of amenorrhea in the female athlete triad. *Int J Sport Nutr.* 1996;6:134-145.
19. Cox G, Frail H, Leech K. Nutrition for speed and endurance. In: Reaburn P, Jenkins D, eds. *Training for Speed and Endurance.* Sydney, Australia: Allen & Unwin; 1996:140-170.

20. Thompson JK. Introduction: body image, eating disorders, and obesity—an emerging synthesis. In: Thompson JK, ed. *Body Image, Eating Disorders, and Obesity: An Integrative Guide for Assessment and Treatment*. Washington, DC: American Psychological Association; 1996:1-20.

21. Steen SN. Eating on the road: where are the carbohydrates? *Sports Sci Exch*. 1998;11:1-5.

22. Pivarnik JM, Palmer RA. Water and electrolyte balance during rest and exercise. In: Wolinsky I, Hickson JF, eds. *Nutrition in Exercise and Sport*. 2nd ed. Boca Raton, Fla: CRC Press; 1994:245-262.

23. Kleiner SM. Water: an essential but overlooked nutrient. *J Am Diet Assoc*. 1999;99:200-206.

24. Murray R. Fluid needs in hot and cold environments. *Int J Sport Nutr*. 1995;5:S62-S73.

25. Murry R. Fluid needs of athletes. In: Berning JR, Steen SN, eds. *Nutrition for Sport and Exercise*. 2nd ed. Gaithersburg, Md: Aspen Publishers; 1998:143-153.

26. Lamb DR. Abuse of anabolic steroids in sport. *Sports Sci Exch*. 1989;2:1-4.

27. Radford PF. Sprinting. In: Reilly T, Secher N, Snell P, Williams C, eds. *Physiology of Sports*. Edmunds, Suffolk, England: E & FN Spoon; 1990:71-99.

28. Lemon PWR. Effects of exercise on dietary protein requirements. *Int J Sport Nutr*. 1998;8:426-447.

29. Snyder AC, Naik J. Protein requirements of athletes. In: Berning JR, Steen SN, eds. *Nutrition for Sport and Exercise*. 2nd ed. Gaithersburg, Md: Aspen Publishers; 1998:45-58.

48

ULTRAENDURANCE SPORTS

Ellen Coleman, MA, MPH, RD

The increased popularity of marathon runs, triathlons, and cycling events has allowed many athletes to further challenge themselves by competing in ultraendurance events. Single-day ultraendurance events involve races that last from 4 to 24 hours and include running ≥30 to 100 miles, cycling ≥100 to 300 miles, and triathlons ranging from the half-Ironman distance to the full Ironman distance: a 2.4-mile swim, 112-mile bike ride, and 26.2-mile marathon run. Multistage ultraendurance events involve competing over consecutive days, such as the Tour de France bicycle race (2,500 miles over 22 days), Tour of Spain (2,250 miles over 21 days), the Race Across America (RAAM) individual and 4-member team cycling event (3,000 miles), and the Australian Sydney to Melbourne foot race (628 miles within 9 days).

ENERGY NEEDS

The predominant energy system for ultraendurance athletes is aerobic with brief, intermittent involvement of anaerobic energy systems. The athlete's actual energy expenditure depends on the intensity, duration, and type of activity. Exercise intensities may range between 50% and 90% VO_2max for events lasting 4 to 24 hours, with total energy expenditures ranging between 5,000 and 10,000 kcal per day (1).

In a typical ultraendurance event such as the individual RAAM, the exercise intensity averages about ≤65% VO_2max, and lipid is the primary fuel source. However, in a high-intensity ultraendurance event such as the team RAAM, the exercise intensity is often ≥75% VO_2max, and carbohydrate is the primary fuel source (2).

Burke and Reed (3) reported that elite male ultraendurance triathletes consumed an average of 4,079 kcal per day during a weekly training schedule of 8.1 miles of swimming, 202 miles of cycling, and 47 miles of running.

Saris et al (4) calculated a mean daily energy expenditure of 6,069 kcal and a mean daily energy intake of 5,785 kcal in five male cyclists competing in the Tour de France. Gabel et al (5) reported a mean energy intake of 7,125 kcal per day for two elite male cyclists during a 10-day, 2,050-mile ride on the original Pony Express Trail. Garcia-Roves et al (6) reported a mean energy intake of 5,595 kcal per day for 10 elite male cyclists during the Tour of Spain. Laursen and Rhodes (2) calculated a mean daily energy expenditure of 8,200 kcal for the RAAM team cycling event. Eden and Abernathy (7) reported a mean energy intake of 5,952 kcal per day for a male ultradistance runner who completed the Australian Sydney to Melbourne foot race in 8.5 days.

Lindeman (8) reported a mean energy intake of 8,429 kcal per day for a male cyclist competing in the RAAM. The male cyclist finished the race in 10 days, 7 hours, and 53 minutes after riding as much 22 hours per day. Clark et al (9) reported a mean energy intake of 7,950 kcal per day for a female cyclist who competed in and won the RAAM. She finished the race in 12 days, 6 hours, and 21 minutes after riding as much as 20 hours per day.

NUTRIENT NEEDS

Training for an ultraendurance event involves hours of prolonged exercise that may include daily multiple training sessions. The stress of such rigorous training can decrease appetite, resulting in reduced consumption of calories and carbohydrate. Inadequate energy and carbohydrate intake can lead to chronic fatigue, weight loss, and impaired performance (10). *Box 48.1* provides dietary recommendations for training.

BOX 48.1 Dietary Recommendations for Training

7 to 10 g of carbohydrate/kg per day:

   7 g/kg for 1 hour of training per day

   8 g/kg for 2 hours of training per day

   l0 g/kg for 3 to 4 hours of training per day

≥1.2 to 1.4 g of protein/kg per day

≥1 g of fat/kg per day

Above all, ultraendurance athletes should match energy intake to energy expenditure during training (4,10). To meet energy demands ultraendurance athletes often need to eat meals and snacks continuously throughout the day. Athletes who have difficulty eating enough regular food may consider incorporating liquid meals and high-carbohydrate liquid supplements into their diet (4).

Consuming adequate energy and carbohydrate during training enables the athlete to maintain a desirable training intensity. In addition, testing specific foods and fluids before, during, and after training sessions allows the athlete to determine effective nutrition strategies for competition.

Burke and Reed (3) found that male ultraendurance triathletes (average weight 67.5 kg) consumed 9 g of carbohydrate/kg (60% of energy intake), 2 g of protein/kg (13% of energy intake), and 1.8 g of fat/kg (27% of energy intake) during training. The researchers noted that this group of athletes had adopted eating habits that met the recommendations of sports nutritionists for an optimal diet.

Nutrient needs for competition are higher than during training, especially for multiple-day events. During competition ultraendurance athletes should consume 12 to 22 g of carbohydrate/kg per day (≥60% of energy intake), 1.5 to 3.0 g of protein/kg per day (≥12% of energy intake), and 1 to 3 g of fat/kg per day (20% to 30% of energy intake) (3-8).

A study of Tour de France male cyclists (average weight 69.2 kg) by Saris et al (4) found that the cyclists consumed an average of 12 g of carbohydrate/kg (62% of energy intake), 3.1 g of protein/kg (15% of energy intake), and 2.1 g of fat/kg (23% of energy intake) each day during the race. Nearly half (49%) of the daily calories were consumed during the race, resulting in a carbohydrate intake of 94 g per hour. About 30% of the total carbohydrate consumed came from high-carbohydrate beverages (eg, high-carbohydrate drinks, sports drinks, soft drinks, and liquid meals).

A study of Tour of Spain male cyclists (average weight 66.9 kg) by Garcia-Roves et al (6) found that the cyclists consumed an average of 12.6 g of carbohydrate/kg (60% of energy intake), 3.0 g of protein/kg (14.5% of energy intake), and 2.3 g of fat/kg (25.5% of energy intake) each day during the race. Only 14% of the daily calories were consumed during the race, resulting in a carbohydrate intake of 25 g per hour. The cyclists consumed two meals following competition that provided 1.1 g of carbohydrate/kg per hour in the first 6 hours following the race. The first postrace meal, an hour after the race, was semisolid food (eg, milk, condensed milk, yogurt, muesli, cereals) and the second postrace meal 3 to 4 hours after the race was conventional carbohydrate-rich foods (eg, pasta or rice, bread, vegetables, biscuits, and confectionery).

A case study of two male cyclists (average weight 63.9 kg) during a 10-day, 2,050-mile ride by Gabel et al (5) found that the cyclists consumed an average of 18 g of carbohydrate/kg (63% of energy intake), 2.7 g of protein/kg (10% of energy intake), and 3.5 g of fat/kg (27% of energy intake). The cyclists consumed about 60 to 75 g of carbohydrate per hour of cycling and obtained about 24% of their total energy intake from high-carbohydrate beverages (eg, sports drinks, fruit juices).

Lindeman (8) reported that a male cyclist (79 kg) who competed in the RAAM consumed an average of 22.6 g of carbohydrate/kg (78% of energy intake), 3.6 g of protein/kg (13% of energy intake), and 1 g of fat/kg (9% of energy intake). The cyclist obtained the majority of his total energy intake from a high-carbohydrate liquid supplement (23% carbohydrate) that also provided protein and free amino acids (13% protein).

Clark et al (9) reported that a female cyclist (67 kg) who won the RAAM consumed an average of 420 kcal per hour (predominately from high-carbohydrate beverages and a liquid meal) during the race.

Eden et al (7) reported that a male ultradistance runner (55.5 kg) competing in the Australian Sydney to Melbourne foot race consumed an average of 17 g of carbohydrate/kg (62% of energy intake), 2.9 g of protein/kg (11% of energy intake), and 3.2 g of fat/kg (27% of energy intake). The runner consumed approximately 39 g of carbohydrate per hour and utilized a combination of high-carbohydrate solid foods and a sports drink during running to meet his energy requirements.

The nutrient density of the diet during training and competition is important to ensure adequate micronutrient intake. Burke and Reed (3) found that male ultraendurance triathletes had adequate intakes of the major micronutrients during training. Lindeman (8) noted that a male cyclist had an adequate intake of micronutrients during training for the RAAM.

Gabel et al (5) found that vitamin and mineral intakes were two to three times the RDA for most vitamins and minerals for two male cyclists during a 10-day, 2,050-mile ride. Eden and Abernathy (7) found that all of the micronutrients except riboflavin were met in the diet of a male ultradistance runner competing in the Australian Sydney to Melbourne foot race.

Saris et al (4) found that the high-calorie intake of the Tour de France cyclists resulted in a high iron and calcium intake. In spite of a high-calorie intake, the cyclists had a low intake of thiamin due to their heavy consumption of refined carbohydrate foods such as sweet cakes and soft drinks. The researchers conceded that any questions and concerns about food quality and nutrient density became immaterial after consideration of the intake of micronutrients from pills and injections. Although the supplemental intake of vitamins and minerals far exceeded that derived from food, the researchers also noted that the dosages were unlikely to cause harm.

Clark et al (9) noted that ultraendurance athletes may jeopardize their micronutrient status during training by emphasizing convenient, familiar, high-carbohydrate foods (eg, bagels and pasta made from refined flour, commercial sports drinks, high-carbohydrate liquid supplements) that are low in fiber and lack nutrient density. Adding unrefined, nutrient-dense, high-carbohydrate foods such as whole-grain breads, marinara sauce with vegetables (on pasta), and juices and fruit (such as bananas, dried apricots, raisins) can significantly improve the nutritional quality of the training diet.

FLUID NEEDS

To prevent dehydration ultraendurance athletes should closely match their fluid intake to their fluid loss from sweating. Dehydration of as little as 2% of body weight impairs both cardiovascular function and temperature regulation. Proper hydration enhances endurance and helps to protect against heat injury (11).

The ultraendurance athlete should weigh in before and after training in simulated race conditions to determine the amount of fluid lost per hour. A 1-lb weight loss is equivalent to 16 oz (480 mL) of fluid. The athlete should follow a fluid replacement schedule that is based on the hourly amount of fluid lost during exercise (1,11). For example, if the athlete loses 2 lb per hour, he or she should drink 8 oz (240 mL) of fluid every 15 minutes.

Consuming adequate fluids during training enables the athlete to maintain a desirable exercise intensity and protects against heat illness. It also allows the athlete to practice proper hydration techniques for competition. Therefore, two hours before exercise, the ultraendurance athlete should hyperhydrate by drinking 16 oz (500 mL) of fluid. During exercise, the athlete should drink at least 5 to 10 oz (150 to 300 mL) of cool fluid every 15 to 20 minutes to replace sweat losses. The actual amount of fluid consumed during exercise will depend on the athlete's rate of fluid loss from sweating (11).

Following exercise, athletes are often advised to drink 16 oz for every pound lost (11). However, this amount does not consider the obligatory urine losses that occur during the period of rehydration. Since such losses can represent 25% to 50% of the ingested fluid, the athlete should consume at least 20 oz for every pound lost (12). *Box 48.2* summarizes fluid replacement guidelines.

> **BOX 48.2**   Fluid Replacement Guidelines
>
> Before exercise—16 oz (500 mL)
> During exercise—5 to 10 oz (150 to 300 mL)
> After exercise—20 oz (600 mL) for every pound lost

A gradual weight loss during hot weather training may be caused by chronic dehydration rather than fat loss (1). Urine that is of small volume and dark in color, and has a strong odor may also indicate a dehydrated state (12).

Consuming beverages that contain sodium following exercise may help to restore plasma volume and thereby enhance rehydration. Drinking only plain water tends to decrease plasma osmolality, which decreases thirst and increases urinary water losses. However, drinking beverages that contain sodium helps to retain water in the extracellular space, which reduces urine production without decreasing thirst (12).

Ultraendurance athletes should also consume adequate electrolytes (particularly sodium) through food and/or sports drinks during training and competition. A sodium deficit may occur during ultraendurance events when acclimating to a hot environment and following successive days of exercise in hot weather. During exercise the athlete's fluid replacement beverage should contain 500 to 700 mg of sodium/L to enhance palatability, promote fluid retention, and prevent hyponatremia (11). The loss of 1 g of sodium (which occurs with a 2-lb sweat loss) can easily be replaced by moderate salting of food. One-half teaspoon of salt supplies 1 g of sodium.

The Tour de France researchers (4) recorded individual fluid intakes of more than 10 L per day. Mean intake during the July race was 6.7 L but varied considerably throughout the race. The runner in the Sydney to Melbourne foot race consumed an average of 11 L per day (7). The two male cyclists drank an average of 10.5 L per day (approximately 620 mL per hour of exercise) during their 10-day, 2,050-mile ride (5). The male RAAM cyclist (8) drank an average of 15.7 L per day (approximately 677 mL per hour of exercise). The Tour of Spain researchers recorded an intake of only 3.29 L per day during the April race (6).

COMPETITION CONSIDERATIONS

The ultraendurance athlete may utilize the carbohydrate-loading technique (tapered training combined with a carbohydrate-rich diet) the week before competition to maximize muscle glycogen stores (13). Consuming a low-fiber, low-fat, carbohydrate-rich meal (1 to 4 g of carbohydrate/kg) 1 to 4 hours before competition may also enhance endurance (14,15).

Garcia-Roves et al (6) noted that the Tour of Spain cyclists consumed a conventional breakfast that provided 4.5 g of carbohydrate/kg 3 hours before competition. The pre-exercise meal contained about 12% of calories from protein and 23% from fat and was well tolerated. Some ultraendurance athletes prefer liquid meals before competition due to their shorter gastric emptying time.

Consuming 1.5 g of carbohydrate/kg immediately after exercise promotes muscle glycogen storage and enhances recovery (16,17). An additional 1.5 g of carbohydrate/kg feeding is recommended 2 hours later (if the athlete is awake) (17). Replenishing muscle glycogen stores as much as possible during rest periods is especially important for athletes participating in multiple day events (2,6,9). *Box 48.3* summarizes carbohydrate recommendations.

BOX 48.3   Summary of Carbohydrate Recommendations

Consume 1 to 4 g of carbohydrate/kg, 1 to 4 hours before exercise.

Consume 30 to 60 g of carbohydrate every hour during exercise.

Consume 1.5 g of carbohydrate/kg immediately after exercise followed by an additional 1.5 g of carbohydrate/kg feeding 2 hours later.

Garcia-Roves et al noted that the carbohydrate intake of the Tour of Spain cyclists following competition (1.1 g of carbohydrate/kg per hour for 6 hours) may have helped promote muscle glycogen restoration. The carbohydrate/ protein ratio of 3:1 (1.1 g of carbohydrate/kg:0.35 g of protein/kg) for the postexercise meals may have further enhanced glycogen repletion. Both of these feeding patterns could have a positive impact on performance during multiple-day events (6).

The importance of proper refueling and rehydrating during ultraendurance events cannot be overemphasized (1,2,10). For ultraendurance athletes the food and fluid consumed during the event are more important than what was consumed several days prior to the event. The two primary nutrition goals during ultraendurance events are to maintain adequate hydration and normal blood glucose levels (2,9,10).

Proper hydration is the major concern during prolonged competition as the athlete can have adequate muscle glycogen stores and blood glucose levels and still collapse from a heat injury. Athletes will perform at their best when their fluid intake closely matches their fluid loss from sweating. Fluid intake must be regulated by drinking according to a set schedule (eg, 5 to 10 oz every 15 to 20 minutes), rather than in response to thirst (11,12).

Consuming carbohydrate during ultraendurance events improves performance by maintaining blood glucose levels and promoting carbohydrate oxidation (18,19). The athlete should consume at least 30 to 60 g of carbohydrate per hour (18,19). This amount can be obtained from carbohydrate-rich foods (eg, grain products, fruit, energy bars), fluids (eg, sports drinks, high-carbohydrate liquid supplements, fruit juices, liquid meals), or carbohydrate gels (20).

Each carbohydrate form (liquid and solid) has advantages and drawbacks (20). Sports drinks are a practical source of carbohydrate because they also replace fluid losses. Sports drinks containing 6% to 8% carbohydrate provide the right proportion of water to carbohydrate to provide energy and replace fluid losses (11).

Saris et al (4) reported that consuming large quantities of carbohydrate-rich fluids (eg, high-carbohydrate drinks, sports drinks, soft drinks, and liquid meals) was an appropriate strategy to optimize performance during the Tour de France. Laursen and Rhodes (2) indicated that consuming carbohydrate-rich fluids (eg, liquid meals and sports drinks) was effective for maintaining both energy and fluid balance during the team RAAM event. However, the team RAAM cyclist may have as little as 30 to 240 minutes to rest and refuel, compared to 18 hours for the Tour de France cyclist, even though both ride about 6 hours a day.

In the 1996 team RAAM, the winning team's nutrition strategy attempted to optimize carbohydrate absorption during exercise periods and glycogen repletion during rest periods (2). When gut blood flow was low, as during a 30-minute ride, the cyclist consumed a sports drink to promote rapid gastric emptying and carbohydrate absorption. When gut blood flow was moderate, as during a 30-minute rest, the cyclist consumed a sports drink and liquid meal. During a 2-hour rest period when gut blood flow was near normal, the cyclist consumed a liquid meal.

High-carbohydrate liquid supplements containing 20% to 24% carbohydrate may be utilized during the event to help increase carbohydrate and energy intake. However, they are too concentrated in carbohydrate to be used as the sole fluid replacement beverage and may cause gastrointestinal distress when consumed in large volumes. Lindeman (8) noted that the male RAAM cyclist's reliance on a 23% carbohydrate solution to meet the majority of his energy needs contributed to gastrointestinal distress during the race. Despite consistent dilution to a 17% carbohydrate solution, the carbohydrate content was apparently too high to allow adequate gastric emptying.

Carbohydrate-rich foods can be easily carried and provide both variety and satiety, which help to prevent a boredom-related decline in energy intake (20). Gabel et al (5) reported that the two ultraendurance cyclists who cycled 2,050 miles in 10 days achieved an optimal intake due to the variety and palatability of foods that were available during the event. Eden and Abernathy (7) noted that the foods eaten during the Sydney to Melbourne race were based on what the male ultradistance runner had enjoyed eating during training and what he could tolerate while competing.

Fiber-rich foods should be limited during the event to avoid gastrointestinal distress (eg, abdominal bloating, cramping, bathroom breaks). Lindeman (8) noted that the male RAAM cyclist's high-fiber intake (57 g per day from consuming 5.4 fiber-rich energy bars and 11 pieces of fruit) may have contributed to his gastrointestinal distress during the race.

Above all, the athlete should consume familiar, well-tolerated, and palatable foods and fluids. In addition, the athlete should consume modest amounts of food and/or fluid according to a schedule (eg, every 15 to 20 minutes) to promote hydration, maintain proper blood glucose levels, and avoid gastrointestinal upset (7).

The following pointers are also helpful:

1. The food plan should be built around the athlete's food preferences and include a variety of foods rather than a limited number of items (5,7,9).

2. Food and fluid intake should be closely monitored (5,7-9). The crew should be prepared to enforce an eating and drinking schedule during multiple-day events. If necessary, separate timers can be set for both liquid and solid feedings (9).

3. Weighed food records are recommended to assess dietary intake (5). Ideally, body weight should be assessed daily during multiple-day events (5). By tracking the athlete's food and fluid intake and body weight, the crew can take immediate corrective action if the athlete starts to fall behind on fluid or energy intake (5,9).

4. Solid food should be easy to handle, chew, and digest. Beverages should promote rapid gastric emptying so that fluids and nutrients are quickly absorbed. Concentrated supplements such as high-carbohydrate liquid supplements or liquid meals may be offered immediately before a scheduled rest (2,8,9).

5. New foods and fluids should never be tested during competition. The result may be severe indigestion and/or impaired performance.

TOP NUTRITION CONCERNS

1. Match energy intake to energy expenditure with a carbohydrate-rich diet to maintain carbohydrate stores and lean tissue.

2. Match fluid intake with fluid loss to promote optimum athletic performance and protect against heat injury.

3. Drink and eat according to a schedule during exercise to promote hydration, maintain proper blood glucose levels, and avoid gastrointestinal upset.

In an ultraendurance event adequate nutrition can mean the difference between successfully completing the event or dropping out of it. The expertise of a registered dietitian is essential to determine the ultraendurance athlete's nutritional requirements and develop an individualized dietary plan. The dietitian can also help to monitor the athlete's nutrition during multiple-day events and enforce programmed food and fluid intake when necessary (5,7-9).

CASE STUDY

Rob's goal was to complete the Hawaii Ironman triathlon (2.4-mile ocean swim, 112-mile bike ride, 26.2-mile marathon) in less than 11 hours. His weekly training consisted of running 40 to 50 miles, cycling 100 to 150 miles, and swimming 8,000 to 10,000 yards. He weighed 160 lbs (62.7 kg) and consumed approximately 4,500 kcal per day while training.

Rob tapered his training the week before the event. The day before the Ironman, he emphasized high-carbohydrate, low-residue foods such as GatorPro and mangoes. On the morning of the race, Rob drank 1 can of GatorPro (58 g of carbohydrate) and 16 oz of Gatorade (28 g of carbohydrate) an hour before the swim; this provided 1.3 g of carbohydrate/kg. He completed the 2.4-mile swim in about 1 hour.

During the bike ride Rob set his watch to beep every 15 minutes as a reminder to drink fluids. He drank approximately 8 oz (240 mL) of Gatorade every 15 minutes on the bike, which provided 56 g of carbohydrate and 32 oz (960 mL) of fluid per hour. In addition, he consumed 1/4 to 1/2 of an energy bar every 30 minutes, which provided an additional 20 to 40 g of carbohydrate per hour. He completed the 112-mile bike ride in about 5 hours and 45 minutes.

During the run Rob drank approximately 5 oz of Gatorade every mile, which provided 56 g of carbohydrate and 32 oz (960 mL) of fluid per hour. He ran the first 16 miles in an 8-minute/mile pace but was forced to slow down for the last 10 miles. Rob completed the 26.2-mile run in about 4 hours. His total time for the Ironman was 10:46 minutes, a remarkable achievement for his first finish.

In review, Rob noted that he would have benefited from a higher carbohydrate and calorie intake during the race, particularly during the bike stage. He felt that consuming more carbohydrate and calories from gels or sports bars while on the bike would have enabled him to maintain a faster pace during the last 10 miles of the run.

REFERENCES

1. Kreider RB. Physiological considerations of ultraendurance performance. *Int J Sport Nutr*. 1991;1:3-27.
2. Laursen PB, Rhodes EC. Physiological analysis of a high-intensity ultraendurance event. *Strength Conditioning J*. 1999;21:26-38.
3. Burke LM, Reed RSD. Diet patterns of elite Australian male triathletes. *Phys Sports Med*. 1987;15:140-155.
4. Saris WHM, van Erp-Baart MA, Brouns F, Westerterp KR, ten Hoor F. Study of food intake and energy expenditure during extreme sustained exercise: the Tour de France. *Int J Sport Med*. 1989;10(suppl):26-31.
5. Gabel KA, Aldous A, Edgington C. Dietary intake of two elite male cyclists during a 10-day, 2,050-mile ride. *Int J Sport Nutr*. 1995;5:56-61.
6. Garcia-Roves PM, Terrados N, Fernandez SF, Patterson AM. Macronutrient intakes of top-level cyclists during continuous competition—change in feeding pattern. *Int J Sport Med*. 1998;19:61-67.
7. Eden BD, Abernathy PJ. Nutritional intake during an ultraendurance running race. *Int J Sport Nutr*. 1994;4:166-174.
8. Lindeman AK. Nutrient intake of an ultraendurance cyclist. *Int J Sport Nutr*. 1991;1:79-85.
9. Clark N, Tobin J, Ellis C. Feeding the ultraendurance athlete: practical tips and a case study. *J Am Diet Assoc*. 1992;92:1258-1262.
10. Applegate EA. Nutritional considerations for ultraendurance performance. *Int J Sport Nutr*. 1991;1:118-126.
11. American College of Sports Medicine. Position stand: exercise and fluid replacement. *Med Sci Sports Exerc*. 1996;28:i-vii.
12. Murray R. Fluid needs of athletes. In: Berning JR, Steen SN. *Nutrition for Sport and Exercise*. 2ⁿᵈ ed. Gaithersburg, Md: Aspen Publishers; 1998:143-153.
13. Sherman WM, Costill DL, Fink WJ, Miller JM. The effect of exercise and diet manipulation on muscle glycogen and its subsequent use during performance. *Int J Sport Med*. 1981;2:114-118.

14. Sherman WM, Brodowicz G, Wright DA, Allen WK, Simonsen J, Dernbach A. Effects of 4 hour pre-exercise carbohydrate feedings on cycling performance. *Med Sci Sports Exerc.* 1989;12:598-604.

15. Sherman WM, Peden MC, Wright DA. Carbohydrate feedings 1 hour before exercise improve cycling performance. *Am J Clin Nutr.* 1991;54:866-870.

16. Ivy JL, Katz AL, Cutler CL, Sherman WM, Coyle EF. Muscle glycogen synthesis after exercise: effect of time of carbohydrate ingestion. *J Appl Physiol.* 1988;6:1480-1485.

17. Ivy JL, Lee MC, Broznick JT, Reed MJ. Muscle glycogen storage after different amounts of carbohydrate ingestion. *J Appl Physiol.* 1988;65:2018-2023.

18. Coyle EF, Hagberg JM, Hurley BF, Martin WH, Ehsani AA, Holloszy JO. Carbohydrate feeding during prolonged strenuous exercise can delay fatigue. *J Appl Physiol.* 1983;55:230-235.

19. Coyle EF, Coggan AR, Hemmert WK, Ivy JL. Muscle glycogen utilization during prolonged strenuous exercise when fed carbohydrate. *J Appl Physiol.* 1986;61:165-172.

20. Coleman E. Update on carbohydrate: solid versus liquid. *Int J Sport Nutr.* 1994;4:80.

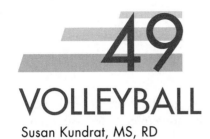

49

VOLLEYBALL

Susan Kundrat, MS, RD

Volleyball is a game of explosive power, quickness, strength, and precision. Volleyball players burst very short distances, start and stop quickly, jump often, dive swiftly, and change directions frequently during play. In addition, in a competitive tournament a match may be won or lost by the team that possesses the endurance required to stay strong for the last match of the day. Pregame nutrition, intermatch fueling, and consistent glycogen-building are all very important to the success of volleyball players.

ENERGY SYSTEMS

During match play volleyball players rely most heavily on the anaerobic energy system for fuel. In fact, the anaerobic system supplies roughly 90% of the energy required in typical volleyball play. In a study of junior men's competition, approximately 18% of rallies were 3 seconds or less, 54% lasted 5 to 7 seconds, and 15% lasted 9 to 10 seconds. An elite male volleyball player who was monitored closely in the study executed 250 to 300 high-power motor acts per five-game match, most of which were jumps and quick dashes for the ball. In addition, the average number of rallies per game in junior men's competition was 53, and the average number of rallies in senior women's competition was 47 (1).

The energy system used primarily for strength, power, and speed, such as a serve, spike, block, or dig, is supplied by the ATP-CP (adenosine triphosphate creatine phosphate) system. For short-term muscular work such as a rally lasting 15 seconds to 2 minutes, the lactic acid system supplies energy. The aerobic system supplies energy for infrequent and longer endurance rallies, training sessions, and recovery periods (2,3). Although volleyball players may not require extensive endurance capacity, they do need adequate aerobic fitness as the critical resynthesis of phosphagens and replenishment of oxygen stores take place between high-power performances and during heavy training periods (4). Setters have been found to have the highest postgame blood lactate levels, indicating that setters require more endurance than other players on the team (2). See *Table 49.1* for a review of energy systems utilized for volleyball activities.

TABLE 49.1 Energy Systems Utilized for Volleyball Activities

Energy Systems Utilized	Volleyball Activity
ATP-CP system	Serve, spike, block, dig, roll
Lactic acid system	Long rallies
Aerobic system	Very long rallies, training sessions, rest and recovery periods

ENERGY AND MACRONUTRIENT NEEDS

Macronutrient needs for volleyball do not differ greatly from general sports nutrition recommendations. A diet high in carbohydrate (60% to 65%) and moderate in fat (20% to 30%) and protein (12% to 20%) will supply players with a balance of needed macronutrients. A consistently well balanced diet based on whole-grain carbohydrates will provide energy for training and competition as well as quick energy and glycogen for refueling muscles. Fat needs vary depending on the individual goals of each player. For athletes in need of body fat loss, limit dietary fat to 20% of total kilocalories. However, adequate dietary fat is needed to provide energy and supply essential fatty acids. It is important for the volleyball player to obtain adequate protein to aid in tissue development and repair. Most volleyball players eat adequate amounts of protein (12% to 20%). A protein intake of 1.2 to 1.7 g/kg of body weight is sufficient to meet needs (5,6).

Energy needs are determined from the individual athlete's body weight, goals (weight loss or gain), and average kilocalories burned during exercise. See *Table 49.2* for estimations of caloric expenditure per minute for competitive volleyball play.

TABLE 49.2   Estimated Energy Expenditure per Minute of Vigorous Volleyball

Body weight in lbs	100	130	160	190	220
Kcal burned	6.5	8.4	10.4	12.4	14.4

Source: Williams MH. *Nutrition for Health, Fitness, and Sport.* 5th ed. Dubuque, Ia: WBC-McGraw Hill; 1999.

MICRONUTRIENT NEEDS

Micronutrients of particular concern for the volleyball player include sodium, potassium, calcium, and iron. During heavy workouts and excessive sweating, sodium and potassium must be replaced to avoid electrolyte imbalances. Generally, these minerals can be obtained in a balanced diet. Sports drinks may also be used to supply small amounts of sodium and potassium. During most intermittent exercise activities such as volleyball, plasma sodium levels probably remain within a normal range, but it is important to include sodium in a rehydration solution during exercise and recovery (7).

Health professionals should monitor the diets of female teenage and college volleyball players for a low calcium or iron intake. A diet consistently low in calcium can contribute to stress fractures. Good sources of calcium include milk, yogurt, cheese, calcium-fortified juices and grain products, calcium-fortified soy products such as tofu, and greens. Since iron is essential for the formation of hemoglobin which transports oxygen from the lungs to the working muscles, a low iron intake can lead to a deficiency exhibited as low energy and endurance in practice and competition. Teenage girls in particular may be susceptible to low iron stores. Foods high in iron include lean red meats, dark-meat chicken or turkey, iron-fortified breads and cereals, and dried beans and peas. A multivitamin preparation with 100% iron is recommended for teenage and/or vegetarian female players. Female players should obtain yearly physical exams with blood work to detect low iron stores.

Antioxidant supplements such as vitamin E and vitamin C have been shown to favor decreased free radical formation in competitive athletes, thus aiding in tissue repair. Although research is unclear as to the recommended amount of supplementation at this time, players are encouraged to review their individual requirements with a sports nutritionist.

ERGOGENIC AIDS

Volleyball players are most interested in ergogenic aids marketed to enhance power, quickness, mental acuity, and fat loss (8). Because over-the-counter ergogenic aids are not currently regulated in the United States, the use of an ergogenic aid should be thoughtfully considered and monitored closely. Ergogenic aids and their reported benefits for volleyball players are found in *Table 49.3*.

TABLE 49.3   Ergogenic Aids and Possible Benefits for Volleyball Players

Ergogenic Aid	Reason for Use	Comments
Caffeine	Mental stimulation	May cause dehydration; banned by NCAA in large amounts; may cause nervousness and anxiety if not habituated to caffeine
Creatine	Enhance muscular power	May add excess weight; unsure of long-term safety
HMB	Enhance power, strength	High cost; research still in preliminary stages; weight gain

Caffeine has been found to enhance performance by stimulating the central nervous system, thus increasing psychological arousal. In addition, caffeine may enhance cardiovascular function and fuel utilization by stimulating the release of epinephrine from the adrenal gland. Caffeine may also act to facilitate free fatty acid metabolism and enhance the release of calcium from muscle cells, stimulating muscle contraction more effectively (8).

Research on creatine has focused on the supplement's ability to resynthesize ATP in the body, aiding in short bursts of activity and muscle-building. Improvement in jumping height has also been observed after creatine ingestion (9).

Beta-hydroxy beta-methylbutyrate (HMB) supplementation may also be of interest to volleyball players, as it has been found to decrease stress-induced muscle protein breakdown and may enhance muscle increases in both size and strength when combined with a resistance training program (6). This may result in greater power on the court. (See Chapter 7, Ergogenic Aids for more detailed information).

FLUID NEEDS

Hot and humid conditions increase the need for fluids among volleyball players. Heavy training periods including multiple practices also increase fluid needs. Sand volleyball players should pay special attention to fluid needs as the hot sun and humidity combine for large fluid losses. Studies indicate that sweat loss during intermittent exercise such as volleyball is at least comparable to loss during continuous exercise for a similar period of time (7). Volleyball players often monitor their weight fluctuations and thus may avoid drinking adequate fluids in hopes of keeping additional weight down. Since adequate hydration is key to top performance, these athletes need education regarding their individual fluid needs, how their body responds to different fluids, and how this affects their performance. Encourage athletes to weigh themselves before and after practice to ensure appropriate rehydration in warm, hot, and cool environments.

Although volleyball matches involve intermittent activity, a 6% to 8% carbohydrate beverage can be beneficial for this type of short-term, high-intensity intermittent exercise as well as for longer endurance exercise (7). These beverages help maintain blood volume, assist in thermoregulation, reduce the risk of injury, provide exogenous energy, and enhance performance during prolonged exercise. Sports drinks are especially critical during tournament play when only short breaks are provided, limiting solid food intake. See *Table 49.4* for a review of fluid recommendations.

TABLE 49.4   Fluid Recommendations for Volleyball Players

Timing	Recommendations
2 hours before practice or match	At least 2 cups of water or sports drink
During warm-up	5 mL/kg of fluid as tolerated
During practice/match	1/2-1 cup of water/sports drink every 15 minutes
After practice/match	2 cups of water/sports drink for every pound lost in sweat

TOP NUTRITION CONCERNS

Maintaining Maximal Strength and Weight

Of special challenge to volleyball players is the need to increase muscle strength, improve vertical jump, gain power, and achieve peak performance while at the same time limiting excess weight to maximize jumping ability and quickness on the court. These goals may be contradictory problems for players who may be resistant to maintaining the weight needed to maximize power. In fact, in one study of NCAA Division I female basketball, softball, and volleyball players, significantly more volleyball players (71%) than softball players (32%) or basketball players (11.3%) reported using weight-reducing products, diuretics, or laxatives. A total of 23.6% of the volleyball players reported using diuretics and 18.8% reported using laxatives to keep weight down particularly during the season (10).

Thus, it is imperative to educate female volleyball players about the physiological needs of their sport and encourage sensible weight management practices.

Fueling during All-day Tournaments

Obtaining appropriate nutrition during a day-long volleyball tournament is a challenge. Play may begin early in the morning, last until evening, and involve as many as five or more matches. In addition, subsequent match times are not always known until the previous match is completed. Therefore, having appropriate food available at tournaments is key. Players should know the foods they can digest easily within shortened time constraints and have immediate access to these foods for quick recovery. The following snacks are quick and easy-to-transport foods to have available when time is short between matches.

- Sports drinks
- 100% fruit juices
- Fresh fruit
- Dried fruit
- Granola bars
- Trail mix
- Cereal
- Energy bars or gels
- Yogurt
- Crackers
- Low-fat sandwiches

Preseason Training Needs

Preseason training often includes 2- or 3-a-day practices with high nutritional demands placed on the athletes. This is an important time to enhance strength, build muscle, increase glycogen storage capabilities, and improve fitness. Pre- and postworkout fueling must be a priority for coaches and athletes during this crucial time. Consistently eating high-carbohydrate meals and snacks, particularly before and after workouts, is essential to the success of the athlete. See *Table 49.5* for a sample 3,500-kilocalorie plan for a typical two-a-day heavy training schedule.

TABLE 49.5   Sample 3,500-Kilocalorie Plan for Heavy Training

7 AM	Breakfast	1 cup oatmeal with skim milk
		1 cup low-fat yogurt
		Banana
9 to 11 AM	Workout	4 cups sports drink
11:30 AM	Lunch	Tuna sandwich
		1 cup watermelon
		1 oz pretzels
		2 cups orange juice
		2 cookies
2 to 4 PM	Workout	4 cups sports drink
4:30 PM	Snack	1 cup dry cereal with skim milk
		1 cup grape juice
6:30 PM	Supper	4 oz grilled chicken breast
		1 cup rice pilaf
		1 cup broccoli
		1 cup salad with dressing
		1 piece cornbread with margarine
		1 cup skim milk
9 PM	Snack	4 graham cracker squares with 1 T peanut butter
		1 peach

Totals: 3,500 Kcals, 574 g carbohydrate (66%), 119 g protein (13%), 81 g fat (21%)

CASE STUDY

Trina, captain and setter of her team, has been training very hard during the off-season and preseason. The first tournament is coming up, and she wants to be prepared to handle the nutritional demands of the day without running out of energy. Trina is 5'10" and weighs 150 lb. How can she best lead the team through an all-day tournament?

Nutrition Goals

- Maintain a high-carbohydrate (7 to 10 g/kg of carbohydrate or 477 to 682 g per day), high-performance diet to enhance glycogen storage.
- Eat high-carbohydrate dinners (ie, pasta and bread, stir-fry with rice, sandwiches with fruit) and drink plenty of fluids for several days before the tournament.
- Get up 2 hours early on the tournament day to get in a high-powered breakfast (ie, oatmeal, banana, toast, and juice) including 2 extra cups of fluid.
- Drink additional fluids (5 mL/kg during the warm-up period as tolerated).

- Drink water and a sports drink during breaks between matches ($1/2$ cup every 15 minutes as tolerated).
- Carry easy-to-digest foods to the tournament to eat between matches.

REFERENCES

1. Belyaev AV. Methods of developing work capacity in volleyball. *Soviet Sports Rev.* 1985;20:35-38.
2. Black B. Conditioning for volleyball. *Strength Conditioning.* 1995;17:53-55.
3. Biddle S, deLooy A, Thomas P, Youngs R. *Volleyball Training.* 2nd ed. Marlborough, Great Britain: The Crowood Press Ltd; 1995.
4. Viitasalo JT, Rusko H, Pajala O, Rahkila P, Ahila M, Montonen H. Endurance requirements in volleyball. *Can J Sport Sci.* 1987;12:194-201.
5. Clark N. *Nancy Clark's Sports Nutrition Guidebook.* 2nd ed. Champaign, Ill: Human Kinetics; 1997.
6. Berning JR, Steen SN. *Nutrition for Sport and Exercise.* 2nd ed. Gaithersburg, Md: Aspen Publishers; 1998.
7. Shi X, Gisolfi CV. Fluid and carbohydrate replacement during intermittent exercise. *Sports Med.* 1998;25:157-172.
8. Williams MH. *The Ergogenics Edge: Pushing the Limits of Sports Performance.* Champaign, Ill: Human Kinetics; 1998.
9. Bosco C, Tihanyi J, Pucspk J, et al. Effect of oral creatine supplementation on jumping and running performance. *Int J Sports Med.* 1997;18:369-372.
10. Martin M, Schlabach G, Shibinski K. The use of nonprescription weight loss products among female basketball, softball, and volleyball athletes from NCAA Division I institutions: issues and concerns. *J Athl Train.* 1998;33:41-44.

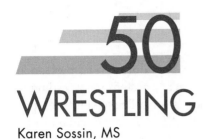

50

WRESTLING

Karen Sossin, MS

Wrestling is a high-intensity and exhausting sport demanding both physical and mental stamina. To achieve their desired certification weight, wrestlers may develop a mindset that can lead to dangerous weight-loss methods. A common belief within the wrestling community is that to gain a competitive edge wrestlers should compete at a weight category lower than their preseason weight. Consequently, nutritional status and athletic performance may be compromised.

In 1998, three college wrestlers died in their pursuit of rapid weight loss (1). Since then the National College Athletic Association has approved significant changes in the guidelines for identifying a weight classification for each wrestler; the rationale is to prevent dehydration and dangerous weight control practices and to implement penalties for noncompliance (2). Similarly, over the past few years several state high school athletic associations, including Wisconsin, Michigan, and New York, have developed and implemented programs to safeguard wrestlers (3). *Box 50.1* describes the New York State Public Health High School Athletic Association's Wrestling Minimum Weight Certification Program.

BOX 50.1   New York State Public High School Athletic Association (NYSPHSAA) Wrestling Minimum Weight Certification Program

- Percentage of body fat and minimum wrestling weight are determined from skinfold measurements. All wrestlers must be assessed within 2 weeks from the first day of the season.
- Hydration status is monitored by the specific gravity of urine. Specific gravity shall be 1.025 or lower. If the wrestler is dehydrated (above 1.025), skinfold measurements will not be completed and testing must be rescheduled for a different time when the wrestler will be hydrated.
- Minimum wrestling weight is set at 7% body fat. (The minimum wrestling weight is not established as the athlete's best weight but rather the minimum weight at which the athlete will be allowed to compete.)
- Only NYSPHSAA-approved measurers may perform the measurements to determine body fat and state of hydration.
- Sports, Cardiovascular, and Wellness Nutritionists (SCAN) provide nutrition education seminars and resource materials to all coaches throughout New York State.

ENERGY AND MACRONUTRIENT NEEDS

The energy demands placed on a wrestler during a match shift and overlap. The match is interspersed with explosive movements, which place a high demand on the ATP-CP system (adenosine triphosphate-creatine phosphate), yet the wrestler must have an aerobic system that allows quick recovery during brief periods of rest or low-intensity sparring. The predominant energy system for wrestling is the anaerobic or lactic acid system. Energy demands for collegiate and freestyle wrestling have been hypothesized to be 70% to 90% ATP-CP/lactic acid and 10% to 30% aerobic (4). High school wrestling bouts consist of three 2-minute sessions and college bouts are three sessions, with the first lasting 3 minutes and the second and third lasting 2 minutes each. This is a high-intensity sport and, as such, caloric intake must match energy demands. The minimal caloric intake for wrestlers of high school and college age should range from 1,700 to 2,500 kcal per day, and rigorous training may increase the requirement up to an additional 1,000 kcal per day (5). *Box 50.2* gives the American College of Sports Medicine (ACSM) recommendations for body composition for wrestlers.

BOX 50.2   Wrestlers, Body Composition, and Calories

The American College of Sports Medicine recommendations for weight loss in wrestlers:

- The body composition of each wrestler is assessed prior to the season using valid methods for this population.
- Males 16 years of age and younger with a body fat below 7% or those over 16 years of age with a body fat below 5% need medical clearance before being allowed to compete.
- A lower limit of 5% to 7% body fat is proposed as the lowest acceptable level for safe wrestling competition.

A wrestler's macronutrient needs—55% to 60% carbohydrate, 25% to 30% fat, and 15% to 20% protein—are the same as for most athletes and healthy individuals. Further research shows that high-intensity power can be maintained in wrestlers undergoing weight loss if carbohydrate intake is 65% or greater, possibly by minimizing the loss of muscle glycogen (6-9). One study found that total power and average power produced on the Wingate test (a test measuring anaerobic exercise performance) were impaired by 7 days of negative energy balance in male wrestlers consuming a 55% carbohydrate diet; however, no adverse effects were seen in those consuming 70% of kcal as carbohydrate (9). Since a wrestler's training protocol can vary throughout the year, macronutrient recommendations for the wrestler should be based on individual needs considering maturity level, weight history, and training regime. Carbohydrate should provide at least 6 g/kg of body weight daily to support glycogen synthesis, and with intense training of several hours or more each day, 7 to 10 g/kg body weight would be appropriate (10).

Adequate caloric consumption is essential for high power performance. See *Table 50.1* for an explanation of caloric requirements. Two factors that must be accounted for when determining protein requirements on an individual basis are carbohydrate and energy intake. When adequate calories are consumed to support energy needs, protein can be used for muscle growth and enhancement; therefore, the body does not need to rely on it as a significant source of energy. Similarly, sufficient carbohydrate intake can also strengthen muscle synthesis. Depending on the individual needs listed above, protein requirements can be met by consuming anywhere from 1.2 to 1.7 g/kg of body weight.

TABLE 50.1   Basal Caloric Requirements for High School Wrestlers

Weight (lb)	Basal Calories
98	1,544
107	1,674
115	1,728
123	1,781
130	1,824
137	1,910
145	1,952
155	2,017
165	2,081
175	2,100
185	2,206

To estimate additional calories needed for wrestling practice and daily school activities, multiply body weight by 11.3 kcal per hour/kg for wrestling practice and 1.5 kcal per hour/kg for school activities.

Adapted from: Tipton CM, Making and maintaining weight for interscholastic wrestling. *Sports Science Exchange.* 1990;2:22.

MICRONUTRIENT NEEDS

Wrestlers' micronutrient needs remain the same as the general adolescent and young adult population; however, their nutritional profile can be compromised. One study found that the calorie and micronutrient content of college wrestlers' diets during the season fell short of the Recommended Dietary Allowances (RDA) for energy, protein, thiamin, iron, zinc, magnesium, and vitamins A, C, and B-6 (10). Wrestlers typically return to a healthier nutrient profile out of season.

Special attention should be paid to iron and calcium. Adolescent athletes are at increased risk for iron deficiency due to their rapid growth and elevated energy requirements. Wrestlers will typically forego red meat when they are trying to lose weight. They must be taught about heme and nonheme food iron sources and how to healthfully incorporate them into their diet during the season.

The wrestler must also learn how to balance meals and stabilize energy and nutrient intake throughout the season. During the zealous attempt to achieve a specific weight in order to compete in a desired weight class, food intake during the week can be more restricted than on the weekend or after a match or tournament. Wrestlers have described "diets" that include no more than 800 kcal per day. Once the competition is over and restricted eating habits cease, the wrestler will revert to overconsumption of calories and fat. This is a scenario that is typical of restricted eating patterns.

While current studies suggest that calcium intake among adolescent males is slightly greater than the RDA (11), one must be aware that the wrestler is not always an average teenager or typical athlete. He can be a teenager struggling with weight loss issues and restricting foods such as dairy products that may be perceived as fattening. This is of concern due to bone growth that occurs at this age and the window of opportunity to establish peak bone mass. It is especially important to encourage the consumption of high quality calcium sources such as low-fat dairy products. Some athletes believe that all dairy foods are high in fat and that milk causes "cotton mouth." Athletes must become educated as to the value of a well-balanced diet and its influence on bone health.

FLUID NEEDS

Dehydration has long been a concern for wrestlers. In their quest for rapid weight loss to achieve a specific weight class, wrestlers have succumbed to drastic weight-loss methods. The most common is dehydration through excessive sweating, fluid restriction, rubber suits, and sauna use (12). For each pound of weight lost through sweat, the wrestler should be advised to consume at least 20 oz of fluid to make up for obligatory urine losses (13). Some wrestlers believe that they can weigh in for a match, then immediately drink water to rehydrate. Even when adequate amounts of fluids are consumed, at least 6 hours are required to achieve normal hydration levels (14). *Box 50.3* highlights tips for preventing dehydration.

BOX 50.3   Guidelines to Avoid Dehydration

- Drink before thirst sets in.
- Weigh in before and after every workout.
- Drink enough fluid to have pale yellow urine.
- Avoid caffeine and alcohol; both act as diuretics.
- Replace sweat loss with at least 20 oz of water for each pound lost.
- Drink 2 to 3 cups of water 2 hours before practice or a match.
- Drink 1 to 2 cups of water 15 minutes before practice or a match.
- When possible, drink 1/2 cup water or sports drink during practice every 15 to 20 minutes.

The time of weigh-in is very important in the wrestling community and is governed by varying rules and regulations throughout the country. Examples of this time frame include an honor weigh-in, which must be completed within 1 hour of the start of the regular school day, allowing a 3-lb allowance at matside, or matside weigh-ins that use limits of a maximum of 1 hour and a minimum of a half hour before a meet is scheduled to begin. These regulations vary from state to state and differ at the high school and college levels. Check the rules for an individual state athletic association for further details.

To promote rehydration, fluid choices should include water, sports drinks, and fruit juices. Caffeine and alcohol should be avoided due to their diuretic properties. Athletes need to be reminded that iced tea and soft drinks contain caffeine, as does coffee. Foods consumed after training or the weigh-in will also provide fluid as well as sodium that will help contribute to rapid rehydration. Refer to *Box 50.4* for foods containing a high water content.

BOX 50.4   Foods that Contribute to Rehydration

- Grapes
- Blueberries
- Cantaloupe
- Cherries
- Apples
- Asparagus
- Celery
- Green peppers
- Tomatoes
- Peaches
- Strawberries
- Honeydew
- Oranges
- Grapefruit
- Cucumber
- Lettuce
- Zucchini

COMPETITION DAY

The day of competition the wrestler should consume an easily digested, low-residue meal. Liquid carbohydrate meals such as a commercially prepared or a homemade-liquid meal might be suitable. The goal of this meal is to prevent hunger, stabilize blood glucose levels, and provide adequate fluids. Because of the relatively short duration of a wrestling match, it is likely that energy requirements the day of competition are not as great as during intense training days. However, in tournament settings energy requirements will be just as high as those during daily training.

There are no unique fluid or fuel requirements *during* the match because it is so short. However, on tournament days between matches, wrestlers should consume water or a sports drink and easily digested carbohydrate foods such as bagels, English muffins, cereals, crackers, graham crackers, pretzels, fruit (as tolerated), or fat-free yogurt.

WORKING WITH WRESTLERS

Coaches and trainers should consider these points:

- Emphasis must be placed on the overall training diet, not on weight loss in order to make weight.
- Consider this new paradigm: Rather than the traditional approach of losing weight rapidly in order to compete in a lower weight class, wrestlers compete in the next higher weight class because of a sound nutrition plan and an appropriate strength-training program.
- Establishing a healthy body weight prior to the season should be given top priority. Instead of seeking an unrealistic weight which encourages weight cycling throughout the season, base weight class on a wrestler's body composition and educate the wrestler how to maintain that weight during the season.
- Some wrestlers become discouraged with the sport because they experience symptoms of hunger which can also affect schoolwork and even relationships with friends and family. With a different approach participation in wrestling can be a great opportunity to learn about the role that nutrition plays in athletic performance and

healthy eating and on maintaining a healthy body composition and weight.
- Become aware of signs and symptoms of eating disorders as well as disordered eating patterns and their implications on athletic performance and psyche. One study discovered that 43% of high school wrestlers exhibit signs of bulimia (15). Another study concluded that 20% of high school wrestling coaches suspected that one of their wrestlers might actually have an eating disorder (16).

The challenges of working with wrestlers often center around the attitude of the athlete. For many years a common belief among the wrestling community has been that weight loss by any means will enable wrestlers to achieve a competitive edge over their opponent by competing in a lower weight class. More and more states throughout the country are diligently working to dispel this belief at the high school level. Wisconsin, Michigan, and New York are just a few that have implemented aggressive programs designed to promote health and wellness. The Nutrition Game Plan as reviewed in *Box 50.5* shaped the nutrition education component of the New York State Public High School Athletic Minimum Weight Certification Program.

BOX 50.5   Nutrition Game Plan for Wrestlers

- Eat a high complex carbohydrate, moderate protein, and low-fat training diet.
- Drink to stay hydrated.
- Consume a high-carbohydrate, easily digested prematch meal.
- Eat or drink carbohydrates to replenish glycogen after exercise.
- Maintain lean body mass.

Working with wrestlers can be a challenge for the sports nutritionist. Sue Travis, lecturer at Cornell University in New York and SCAN member, shares this tip for effective communication with wrestlers. "Involve an experienced wrestler with appropriate nutrition background in the planning and presentation of workshops for coaches and wrestlers at the high school or college level. We involved a former New York State high school wrestling champion and Cornell wrestler who is a nutrition major in a nutrition education workshop for 60 coaches. This enhanced interest and credibility and provided valuable educational experience for the students."

With some patience, flexibility, and understanding of the mindset of wrestlers, the savvy nutritionist can turn this challenge into an achievement.

ERGOGENIC AIDS

Creatine supplementation has become popular among athletes seeking to increase muscle mass. Wrestlers are vulnerable to experimentation with creatine as they search for opportunities to increase strength and power. Some research has suggested that at least part of the increase in body mass associated with creatine supplementation may be due to water retention with a decrease in urinary volume. Other research has indicated that creatine supplementation increased peak power but did not significantly change percent body fat or fat-free mass as measured by hydrostatic weighing (17). These observances are of interest to the wrestler because wrestlers are often in a dehydrated state, yet creatine supplementation requires proper hydration to avoid serious health risks. Additionally, while the wrestler may be seeking to increase peak power, research has not yet definitively established that creatine supplementation will do so. On the contrary, one study showed that during rapid weight loss, creatine may adversely affect muscular endurance during short-duration, high-intensity intermittent exercise (18). There have been no studies on the effects of long-term creatine supplementation.

TOP NUTRITION CONCERNS

Weight Loss and Weight Maintenance

In a study of high school wrestling coaches, it was reported that when attempting to make weight, it is appropriate to lose an average of 1.9 lb per day. The same coaches understood that rapid weight loss could have a negative effect on endurance, strength, performance, and health (16). Athletes rate coaches as an important source of weight control and training information. One study discovered that 64% of high school wrestlers considered coaches to be an important influence on their decision to lose weight (19). Seventy-six percent of high school wrestlers felt that coaches dispense accurate information about muscle development (20). Coaches, therefore, must become educated as to appropriate weight loss and training methods, healthy rate of weight loss, and nutrient needs for proper growth and development.

Dehydration and Inappropriate Weight-loss Methods

Wrestlers and their coaches seem to have a common lack of regard for the value of hydration. They are not fully aware of the stages of dehydration and how even a 1% weight loss from fluid loss can negatively impact performance. These athletes try to resist the need as well as the desire for fluids, believing that water will add unnecessary weight. Based on experiences with the New York State Public High School Athletic Association nutrition education training for wrestling coaches throughout the state, Sports, Cardiovascular, and Wellness Nutritionists (SCAN) found that there is some confusion among this population between weight loss from body fat and weight loss from dehydration. Refer to *Box 50.1* to review the details of the New York State Minimum Wrestling Weight Loss Program designed to safeguard wrestlers throughout the state. Coaches often do not consider the significant implications of dehydration on health and athletic performance. Wrestling coaches must become more aware of the hazards associated with dehydration so that they do not underestimate the consequences.

Prematch and Tournament Eating

Wrestlers ask, "What should I eat before a competition?" Craig Horswill, PhD, senior research scientist, Gatorade Exercise Physiology Laboratory, believes that "there is a misconception among wrestlers that no matter what they do to lose weight, they can repair everything in the interval between the weigh-in and the competition. A better approach would be to view *every* meal during the season as if it were a prematch meal" (21). This is precisely correct, especially when one considers that wrestling practice is much more intense than the match itself, and the energy required to improve skills and technique during practice must come from a sound training diet throughout the season. The purpose of the meal before competition is simply to stabilize glucose levels so that the wrestler does not become hungry and to assure optimal hydration. Prematch meals should consist of primarily carbohydrates and very little or no protein or fat. Liquid meals, as illustrated in *Box 50.6*, can also prove to be beneficial. During a tournament and between bouts, sports drinks containing 6% to 8% carbohydrate solution would be effective. These drinks will help elevate blood glucose levels and delay the onset of dehydration and therefore support the goals of the prematch meal (22).

BOX 50.6   Benefits of Liquid Prematch Meals for the Wrestler

- Low stool residue; therefore, will keep weight gain after the meal to a minimum
- Can be consumed close to competition and after weigh-in
- Provide calories as well as fluids
- Convenient to carry for all-day tournaments

CASE STUDY

A 16-year-old wrestler, Paul has been referred by his athletic trainer for nutrition counseling before the wrestling season. The trainer noticed that during the prior season Paul was often moody and irritable and had trouble concentrating. While usually a good student, his performance in school began to suffer and one of his teachers expressed concern to Paul's parents. Paul is a motivated and talented athlete yet seems to run out of energy during the last 2-minute bout of a wrestling match. He was frustrated and becoming disenchanted with the sport. Last season he wrestled at 112 lb and was hoping to compete in the same weight class this season. Based on measurements by the trainer using skinfold calipers and a computerized scale, his current weight is 121 lb and body fat is 14%. Paul felt that since the minimum percent body fat he could achieve was 7%, he could lose 9 lb and have an advantage over his opponents. He agreed to meet with a sports nutritionist because he was looking for a weight loss program that would enable him to lose the weight but still have energy to compete.

The counseling session revealed that Paul's weight fluctuated 6 to 9 lb throughout the prior wrestling season. He always seemed to make weight just before weigh-in, but it was always a struggle to do so. During the week he restricted his fat intake, ate one egg white each day, and ate only fruits and vegetables if he was "really starving." During the week he felt the need to "make up" for his poor eating on the weekends, which included pizza, fried chicken, French fries, and cheeseburgers—the foods he really liked. Paul was in a vicious cycle of weight loss and weight gain and didn't know how to break. He never allowed himself to drink enough fluid during the week and waited until the weekend to rehydrate.

Paul is spending too much time and energy focusing on his weight loss, at the expense of learning skills and conditioning himself adequately to be a successful wrestler.

Recommendations

- Consider moving up to the next weight class of 119 lb. He should initiate a strength-training program, three times per week in the summer and two times per week in-season. With increased strength and more muscle mass, Paul can gain the confidence to compete in the 119-lb weight category.
- Attend summer wrestling camps to advance technical skills in the sport.
- To condition the energy systems as needed during the season, train (running, cycling, etc) with an emphasis on the aerobic system in the summer and early fall and concentrate on the anaerobic system in-season by doing interval training and sprint work.
- Maximize performance by following a training diet that stabilizes weight and energy levels. This can be accomplished by consuming a minimum of 2,500 kcal daily and eating four to six small meals throughout the day.
- Stabilize glucose levels by consuming an adequate breakfast that contains both low-fat protein and carbohydrate and eating every 3 to 4 hours.
- Maintain hydration and weigh-in before and after each workout. Drink at least 20 oz of fluid for each pound lost.
- Replenish glycogen after wrestling practice in order to have optimal energy levels for daily wrestling practices. Paul should consume 1.5 g of carbohydrate per kg body weight (82 g) within 30 minutes, followed by an additional 1.5 g/kg feedings every 2 hours thereafter. An example of a meal containing 80 g of carbohydrate would be 1 bagel, 1 whole banana, 1 T of raisins, and an 8-oz container of yogurt.

REFERENCES

1. Center for Disease Control and Prevention. Hyperthermia and dehydration-related deaths associated with intentional rapid weight loss in three collegiate wrestlers—North Carolina, Wisconsin, and Michigan, November-December 1997. *MMWR Morb Mortal Wkly Rep.* 1998;47:105-108.

2. National College Athletic Association. *NCAA Wrestling Rules.* Overland Park, Kan: 1999.

3. New York State Public High School Athletic Association. *Scholastic Athletics.* 1996-97;7:2.

4. Bellenger S. Wrestling with wrestling. *Training Conditioning.* 1997;7:50-55.

5. American College of Sports Medicine. Position stand on weight loss in wrestlers. *Med Sci Sports Exerc.* 1996;28:ix-xix.

6. Horswill CA, Hickner RC, Scott JR, Costill DL, Gould D. Weight loss, dietary carbohydrate modifications, and high-intensity physical performance. *Med Sci Sports Exerc.* 1990;22:470-476.

7. Walberg J, Ocel J, Craft LL. Effect of weight loss and refeeding diet composition on anaerobic performance in wrestlers. *Med Sci Sports Exerc.* 1996;28:1292-1299.

8. Walberg J, Leidy MK, Sturgill DJ, Hinkle DE, Rithcey SJ. Macronutient content of a hypoenergy diet affects nitrogen retention and muscle function in weight lifters. *Int J Sports Med.* 1988;9:261-266.

9. McMurray RG, Proctor CR, Wilson Wl. Effect of caloric deficit and dietary manipulation on aerobic and anaerobic exercise. *Int J Sports Med.* 1991;12:167-172.

10. Steen SN, McKinney S. Nutrition assessment of college wrestlers. *Phys Sports Med.* 1986;1411:100-116.

11. US Dep of Agriculture, Agriculture Research Service. 1997 data tables: results from USDA's 1994-96 Continuing Survey of Food Intakes by Individuals and 1994-96 Diet and Health Knowledge Survey. http://www.nal.usda.gov/fnic/usda.html. Accessed May 9, 1999.

12. Woods E, Wilson C, Masland R. Weight control methods in high school wrestlers. *J Adolesc Health Care.* 1988;9:394-397

13. Berning JR, Nelson-Steen S. *Nutrition for Sport and Exercise.* 2nd ed. Gaithersburg, Md: Aspen Publishers; 1998:143-153.

14. Shirreffs S, Taylor AJ, Lieper JB, Maughan RJ. Post-exercise rehydration in man: effects of volume consumed and drink sodium content. *Med Sci Sports Exerc.* 1996;28:1260-1271.

15. Oppliger RA, Landry GL, Foster SW, Lambrecht AC. Bulimic behaviors among interscholastic wrestlers: a statewide survey. *Pediatrics.* 1993;91:826-831.

16. Sossin K, Gizis F, Marquart LF, Sobal J. Beliefs, attitudes and resource of high school wrestling coaches. *Int J Sport Nutr.* 1997;7:219-228.

17. Zoeller ZF. Creatine supplementation and exercise performance. *ACSM Certified News.* 1998;8(2):1-4.

18. Oopik V, Paasuke M, Timpmann S, Medijainen L, Ereline J, Smirnova T. Effect of creatine supplementation during rapid body mass reduction on metabolism and isokinetic muscle performance capacity. *Eur J Appl Physiol.* 1998;78:83-92.

19. Marquart L, Sobal J. Weight loss beliefs, practices and support systems for high school wrestlers. *J Adolesc Health.* 1994;15:410-415.

20. Marquart L, Sobal J. Beliefs and information sources of high school athletes regarding muscle development. *Pediatrics.* 1993;5:377-382.

21. Roundtable: physiology and nutrition for competitive sport. *Sports Sci Exch.* 1993;4:1-4.

22. American College of Sports Medicine. Position stand on exercise and fluid replacement. *Med Sci Sports Exerc.* 1996;28:i-vii.

SECTION 5 TOOLS AND RESOURCES FOR THE SPORTS NUTRITIONIST

Today's sports nutritionist must be properly equipped with the tools needed to counsel athletes, coaches, trainers, parents, and other health professionals. This Tools section offers examples of screening forms and questionnaires used successfully by sports nutritionists. Useful reference information and electronic resources are also provided.

Much of the material in this section was researched and compiled by the 1998-1999 Georgia State University Dietetic Internship class. Under the direction of Barbara Hopkins, MMSc, RD, the interns played an important role in completing this section. Special thanks to the interns: Marcia Berlin, Susi Bracknell, Lauren Goldman, Jennifer Hutchings, DeAnna Jorgensen, Julie Merry, Abigail Mueller, Wendy Pippin, Yvonne Portelli, Ruth Quintero, Dawn Reppucci, Leslie Rodriguez, Darrin Seybold, Sherri Siorek, Olivia Thomas, Karen Wahl, and Angela Westbrook.

SECTION 5 CONTENTS

1. SAMPLE MEDICAL HISTORY QUESTIONNAIRE

Please read and complete this form carefully. This form is intended to reveal a complete medical history. All information will be kept confidential.

Date: _____ Sport: _____ Eligibility Year: _____
(years participating in this college sport)

Name: _____

Birth date: _____ Age: _____ Social Security #: _____

Local Address: _____ Local Phone #: _____

Permanent Address: _____ Phone #: _____

Person to notify in case of emergency (parent/guardian/spouse):

Name: _____ Relationship: _____ Phone #: _____

Address: _____

MEDICAL HISTORY

Please answer every line and be as specific as possible.

I. Personal Disease and Illness History

Please indicate if you have or have ever had any of the following medical conditions:

Disease/Illness	No	Yes	Date(s)	Disease/Illness	No	Yes	Date(s)
Chest pain during exercise				Fainting during exercise			
Attention deficit disorder				Appendicitis			
Osteoarthritis				Cardiomyopathy			
Rheumatoid arthritis				Anaphylaxis			
Iron deficiency anemia				Osteomyelitis			
Diabetes				Rheumatic fever			
Epilepsy				Scarlet fever			
Hay fever				Frequent headaches			
Hepatitis				Migraines			
Asthma				Heart murmur			
Chronic cough				Heat exhaustion			
Malaria				Heat stroke			
Hernia				Significant weight gain			
Pneumonia				Significant weight loss			
Pernicious anemia				Mononucleosis			
Sickle cell anemia				Seizures			
Anorexia nervosa				Abdominal pain			

continued

Personal Disease and Illness History (continued)

Disease/Illness	No	Yes	Date(s)	Disease/Illness	No	Yes	Date(s)
Bulimia nervosa				Kidney problems			
Thyroid disease				Ulcer			
Bladder infection				Chest tightness			
Fainting "spells"				Colitis			
Vertigo				Irritable bowel syndrome			
Polio				Crohn's disease			
Lyme disease				Sleep disturbances			
Wheeze/cough after exercise				Bloody stools			

II. Allergies

Please indicate if you are allergic to or have experienced a reaction to any of the following:

	No	Yes	Specify		No	Yes	Specify
Aspirin				Ice			
Acetaminophen (eg, Tylenol)				Ibuprofen (eg, Advil/Motrin)			
Sulfa				Ointments			
Penicillin				Adhesive tape			
Other antibiotics				Tape adherent			
Other drugs				Insect stings/bites			

III. Dental/Optical/ENT

Please indicate if you have or have had any of the following:

	No	Yes	Date(s)		No	Yes	Date(s)
Corrected vision				Gum disease			
Detached retina				Bridge			
Partial blindness				False tooth			
Hard contacts				Implants			
Soft contacts				Bite plate			
Glasses				Mouthguard to play			
Other eye disorders				Ear trouble			
Broken nose				Poor hearing			
Braces				Punctured ear drum			
Crown				Ear infection			
Retainer				Ringing in ear			
Partial denture				Swimmer's ear			
Full denture				Throat irritation			

IV. Optical Wear

	No	Yes
Do you wear glasses during activity?		
If you wear glasses, are they safety glasses or goggles?		
Do you wear your lenses for activity?		
Do you own an extra pair of lenses?		
Are you farsighted?		
Do you have astigmatism?		

V. Medication

A. *Please list any prescription medication that you are currently taking:*

Medication	Length of Use (weeks)

B. *Please indicate if you are taking or have taken any of the following medications:*

Medication	Past Use	Current Use	Medication	Past Use	Current Use
Aspirin			Diet pills		
Ibuprofen			Caffeine pills (Vivarin, etc)		
Acetaminophen			Menstrual cramp medication		
Acne medication			Allergy medications		
Antihistamines			Antacids		
Asthma medication			Nasal sprays		
Other					

VI. Orthopedic - General

Please indicate if you have or have ever had any of the following:

Condition	No	Yes	Right	Left	Date(s)	Please Specify
Concussion						
Skull fracture						
Hospitalized for head injury						
Ruptured disk						
Whiplash						
Pinched nerve						

continued

Orthopedic - General (continued)

Condition	No	Yes	Right	Left	Date(s)	Please Specify
Osgood-Schlatter Disease						
Chondromalacia						
Bone graft						
Spinal fusion						
Stress fracture						
Osteopenia						
Have you worn a brace, sleeve, etc, on either knee?						
Do you have pins, screws, staples, or other metal implants in your body?						
Have you seen a chiropractor for any injury?						
Do you use orthotics?						
Other						

VII. Orthopedic - Specific

*Please indicate if you have injured any of the following body parts (please note **left** or **right**):*

	No	Yes	Date(s)	Type of Injury (sprain, strain, fracture, etc)
Foot/arch				
Ankle				
Shin/lower leg				
Knee				
Thigh/groin				
Hip				
Upper back				
Lower back				
Shoulder				
Elbow/forearm				
Wrist				
Hand/fingers				
Neck				

VIII. Orthopedic - Surgery

*Please indicate if you have had surgery on any of the following body parts (please note **left** or **right**):*

	No	Yes	Right	Left	Date(s)	Surgery Type	Physician
Foot/arch							
Ankle							
Shin/lower leg							
Knee							
Thigh/groin							
Hip							
Upper back							
Lower back							
Shoulder							
Elbow/forearm							
Wrist							
Hand/fingers							
Neck							
Other surgeries:							

IX. Family History

Please indicate if anyone in your immediate family (parents, brothers, sisters, grandparents, uncles, or aunts) has a history of any of the following:

Condition	No	Yes	Family Member	Age at Onset
Heart attack before age 50				
Heart disease before age 50				
Nontraumatic sudden death				
Seizures				
Marfan syndrome				
Mitral valve prolapse				
Cardiomyopathy (enlarged heart)				
Type 2 diabetes mellitus				
Hypertension (high blood pressure)				
Stroke before age 50				
Osteoporosis				
Any other heart problems before age 50 (please list)				

X. Gynecological/Menstrual History

The following questions concern problems that are unique to women.

1. Have you ever had a menstrual period? _____ yes   _____ no (skip to #12)
2. How old were you when you had your first menstrual period? _____
3. How many menstrual cycles have you had in the last 12 months? _____
4. How many days are there between your cycles? _____
5. How many days do your periods (bleeding) last? _____
6. Use your response to question #4 to determine the regularity of your cycle:
   _____ I am very regular (within 3 days)
   _____ I am somewhat irregular (4- to 10-day variation)
   _____ I am very irregular (variation > 10 days)
7. When was you last period? (date): _____
8. Do your periods change with changes in your training regimen? _____ yes _____ no
9. Have you ever gone for more than 2 months without having a menstrual period? _____
   • If yes, how old were you when you first missed ≥2 periods? _____
   • How long did you go without menstruating? (months): _____
   • Did you see a physician? _____ yes _____ no
    – If yes, what were the diagnosis and treatment? _____
10. Do you currently take birth control pills or hormones? _____ yes _____ no
    • If yes, describe type and length of use: _____
11. Have you ever taken medication for menstrual pain? _____ yes _____ no
    • If yes, describe type and length of use: _____
12. Have you ever experienced pain during ovulation? _____ yes _____ no
13. Have you had a pelvic exam? _____ Date of last exam: _____
14. Have you had a Pap smear? _____ Date of last Pap smear: _____
15 Have you had any type of gynecological surgery? _____ yes _____ no
    • If yes, describe: _____
16. Has a physician ever prescribed any type of hormonal medication? _____ yes _____ no
    • If yes, describe: _____
17. Please describe any other menstrual irregularities or problems not already covered in the above questions.

   _____
   _____

XI. Nutrition and Weight History

1. Height: _____ 2. Weight: _____ 3. Length of time at current weight: _____ (months)
4. Highest weight since age 18: _____ 5. Lowest weight since age 18: _____
6. How many times has your weight fluctuated by at least 5 lbs in the last year? _____
7. What is your "ideal" weight? _____ 8. Have you ever been at your ideal weight? _____
9. If you did not consciously control your weight, what do you think it would be? _____

10. Over the past year have you used any of the following methods to control your weight?

Method	Yes	No	Number of Times Used
Commercial weight-loss programs (eg, Jenny Craig, Weight Watchers)			
Over-the-counter diet pills (eg, Dexatrim)			
Fasting			
Liquid diet supplements (eg, Slim Fast)			
Very-low-calorie diet (<800 calories/day)			
Laxatives			
Diuretics			
Vomiting			
Skipping meals			
High-protein/low-carbohydrate diets			
Nutritional counseling with a health care professional (dietitian)			
Additional exercise beyond regular training			
Other (please describe)			

11. Which of the following are you currently trying to do about your weight?
    a. lose weight   c. stay the same weight
    b. gain weight   d. I am not doing anything about my weight.

12. Circle the average number of hours per day you exercise for pleasure or weight control:
    a. 0   b. less than 1   c. 1- 1.5   d. 2   e. more than 2

13. Are you or have you ever been diagnosed or treated for an eating disorder? _____ yes _____ no

14. Do you think you might have an eating disorder? _____ yes _____ no

15. How many meals (ie, breakfast, lunch, dinner) do you eat per day?
    a. 1-2   b. 3-4   c. 5-6   d. more than 6

16. How many snacks (ie, candy bars, energy bars, piece of fruit) do you eat per day?
    a. 1-2   b. 3-4   c. 5-6   d. more than 6

17. Do you frequently skip meals? _____ yes _____ no

18. Please circle any of the following foods that you avoid:
    a. red meat   g. breads
    b. poultry (chicken, turkey)   h. grains (pasta, rice)
    c. fish   i. fast foods
    d. dairy (milk, cheese)   j. sweets (candy, desserts)
    e. vegetables   k. fats/oils (mayonnaise, salad dressings, butter)
    f. fried foods   l. fruits

19. Circle the average number of dairy products you eat:
    a. 0   c. 3-5 per day   e. 3-5 per week
    b. 1-2 per day   d. 1-2 per week   f. 5-7 per week

20. Check the statement that best describes your typical eating behavior.

___ I always eat whatever I want, whenever I want.

___ I often eat whatever I want, whenever I want.

___ I only sometimes eat whatever I want, whenever I want.

___ I often refrain from eating what I want but often "give in" and eat it anyway.

___ I often refrain from eating what I want and rarely "give in" and eat it anyway.

___ I often refrain from eating what I want and never "give in" and eat it anyway.

21. Do you take vitamin or mineral supplements?

a. yes, daily   b. yes, but not every day   c. no (skip to #23)

22. Please indicate the type(s) of supplement(s) you use. **(Check all that apply.)**

___ multivitamin	___ iron
___ multivitamin/mineral	___ zinc
___ vitamin C	___ magnesium
___ vitamin E	___ calcium
___ B-complex vitamins	___ chromium
___ other (please describe): _____	

23. Do you use nutritional supplements or sports products?

a. yes, daily   b. yes, but not every day   c. no (skip to #25)

24. Please indicate the type(s) of supplement(s) you use. **(Check all that apply.)**

___ protein powder/drink	___ energy bars (eg, Power Bar, Clif Bar)
___ amino acids	___ sports drinks (eg, Gatorade, Powerade)
___ glutamine	___ liquid meals (eg, Ensure, Boost)
___ HMB	___ "fat burners"
___ branched-chain amino acids	___ pyruvate
___ creatine	___ hormones (androstendione, DHEA)
___ other (please describe): _____	

25. Do you think your diet is nutritionally adequate? ____ yes ____ no

26. Please rate your satisfaction with the following factors (ie, how satisfied are you with...):

	Very Satisfied	Somewhat Satisfied	Neutral	Somewhat Dissatisfied	Very Dissatisfied
Your overall physical fitness					
Your muscular strength					
Your cardiovascular endurance					
Your muscle tone and appearance					
Your body weight					
Your body fat percentage					
Your overall athletic ability					
Your ability to be successful in your sport					
Your body shape					
Your overall physical appearance					

This form was developed by Katherine A. Beals, PhD, RD and is used at Ball State University.

2. SAMPLE NUTRITION SCREENING FORM FOR COLLEGIATE ATHLETES

1. Name: _____

2. Sport: _____ 3. Position:_____

4. Age: _____ years   5. Gender: ____ Male ____ Female

6. Which one of the following best describes your ethnic background? **(Check one.)**

    a.____White/Caucasian   c. ____Hispanic   e.____Other; specify_____

    b.____Black/African-American   d. ____Asian or Pacific Islander

7. What year in college are you? **(Check one.)**

    a.____Freshman   c. ____Junior   e.____5th year senior

    b.____Sophomore   d. ____Senior

8. How would you describe your eating habits? **(Check one.)**

    a.____Good   b. ____Fair   c.____Poor

9. How many times a day do you eat? _____

10. How often do you eat out? _____ (number of times per week)

11. When you go out to eat, what are the three most common places you go?

    a. _____

    b. _____

    c. _____

12. Do you avoid any of the following foods? **(Check all that apply.)**

    a.____Red meat   f.____Fruits   k.____Sweets (candy, desserts)

    b.____Poultry (chicken, turkey)   g.____Fried foods   l.____Alcohol

    c.____Fish   h.____Breads   m.____Fats/oils

    d.____Dairy (milk, cheese)   i.____Grains (pasta, rice)   (mayo, salad dressing, butter)

    e.____Vegetables   j.____Fast foods

13. Do you currently take any dietary supplements? ____Yes ____No

    If yes, which ones? **(Check all that apply.)**

    a. ____Creatine   e.____Vitamins   i.____Pyruvate

    b. ____Protein shakes   f.____Minerals   j.____Energy boosters

    c. ____Amino acids   g.____Herbs   (eg, Ephedra, Ma Huang)

    d. ____HMB   h.____"Andro"/DHEA   k.____Other; specify_____

14. Do you know which dietary supplements are banned or restricted by the NCAA?   ____Yes   ____No

15. In a typical workout, about how many cups of water, juice, sports drink, or noncaffeinated beverages do you drink before or during exercise? **(Check one.)**
    a.____None   c. ____3-5 cups
    b.____1-2 cups   d. ____More than 5 cups

16. Overall, how satisfied are you with the physical appearance of your body? **(Check one.)**
    a. ____Very satisfied   c. ____Somewhat dissatisfied
    b. ____Somewhat satisfied   d. ____Very dissatisfied

17. How easy or difficult is it for you to maintain your in-season weight? **(Check one.)**
    a. ____Very easy   c. ____Somewhat difficult
    b. ____Somewhat easy   d. ____Very difficult

18. Do you have any personal goals for body composition?   ____Yes   ____No
    If yes, which ones? **(Check all that apply.)**
    a.____Gain lean mass/weight gain
    b.____Decrease body fat
    c.____Lose weight
    d.____Maintain current body composition
    e.____None

19. Do you use the nutrient analysis cards that are posted on the training table to help you make food selections?
    a.____Yes
    b.____No
    c.____Freshman, have not eaten on campus
    d.____Do not regularly eat at the training table

20. Do you read the table tents that are placed on the dining tables?
    a.____Yes
    b.____No
    c.____Freshman, have not eaten on campus
    d.____Do not regularly eat at the training table

21. Please indicate the topics you would like to learn about by checking "Yes." If you are not interested in learning about a topic, mark "No."
a. Nutrition programs for peak performance	____Yes	____No
b. Weight control	____Yes	____No
c. Weight gain	____Yes	____No
d. Eating disorder counseling	____Yes	____No
e. Exercise and fitness programs	____Yes	____No
f. Grocery store tour	____Yes	____No
g. Cooking demonstrations/meal preparation	____Yes	____No
h. Tips on eating out	____Yes	____No

Please indicate whether you agree or disagree with the following statements by placing a check (✓) in the appropriate column.

	Agree	Disagree	Don't Know
22. Carbohydrates and fats are the main source of energy for muscles.			
23. Protein is the primary source of energy for muscles.			
24. Sweets should not be eaten prior to an athletic event.			
25. Fluids should be replaced before, during, and after athletic events.			
26. Sports drinks are better than water for replacing fluid losses.			
27. Protein supplements are needed in addition to diet for muscle growth and development.			
28. Eating carbohydrates makes you fat.			
29. Meals high in fat should be consumed 2 to 3 hours before training or competition.			
30. Athletes can rely on thirst to ensure fluid replacement during and after competition.			
31. Dehydration decreases athletic performance.			
32. Vitamin and mineral supplements increase energy level.			

3. SAMPLE NUTRITION HISTORY FORM

NAME _____   DATE _____

SPORT and POSITION _____

HEIGHT _____

PRESENT WEIGHT _____

BODY FAT % _____

> To be completed by dietitian
>
> GOAL WEIGHT _____ BMI _____

1. How would you generally describe your eating habits?   Good ❏   Fair ❏   Poor ❏

2. Has your appetite changed recently?   Yes ❏   No ❏

3. How many times a day do you eat? _____

4. How long does it usually take you to complete a meal? _____

5. When you chew your food, do you   _____ take your time?
                                      _____ chew a few times, then swallow?

6. Do you chew gum?   Yes ❏   No ❏   How often? _____

7. Number of carbonated beverages daily? _____

8. Number of caffeinated beverages daily (coffee, regular colas, tea)
   _____ Cups of coffee (regular)
   _____ Cans of soda (regular, diet, Mellow Yellow, Mountain Dew)
   _____ Cups of tea (regular)

9. Do you take any vitamin/mineral/herbal/sports supplements? _____
   If yes, please list _____
   _____

10. List any foods that you do NOT tolerate: _____
    _____

11. Are you now or have your ever followed any special diet? _____
    If yes, what type of diet? _____

12. How often do you eat out? _____ times per week
    What types of restaurants? _____

Adapted from: *Medical Nutrition Therapy Across the Continuum of Care*. Chicago, Ill: The American Dietetic Association; 1996.

4. SAMPLE FOOD FREQUENCY RECORD

Please indicate which foods you eat.

	Less than once a week	Not daily but at least once a week	Daily	Never/Rarely
Milk, yogurt				
Cheese				
Red meat				
Poultry				
Fish				
Eggs				
Mixed dishes				
Dried beans, legumes				
Peanut butter				
Nuts				
Breads, cereal				
Potatoes, pasta, rice				
Fruits, juices				
Vegetables				
Margarine, butter				
Cooking oil				
Sour cream, salad dressing				
Ice cream				
Cookies, cake, pie				
Candy				
Soft drinks				
Coffee				
Tea, iced tea				
Alcohol				

Source: *Medical Nutrition Therapy Across the Continuum of Care.* Chicago, Ill: The American Dietetic Association; 1996.

5. SAMPLE 3-DAY DIET RECORD INSTRUCTIONS AND FORM

The Homer Rice Center for Sports Performance
Sports Nutrition Center

In order to assist you in reaching your goals with respect to body composition and fueling athletic performance, it is important for us to know your current eating patterns. On the following page(s) write down everything you eat and drink for 3 consecutive days. Try to pick 3 days (preferably 2 weekdays and 1 weekend day) that are somewhat "typical" of the way you eat. Do not try to change your eating habits during the days of record keeping.

Remember to include all the information about your choices. Your dietary analysis will be valid only if you provide complete and truthful information.

Helpful hints on filling out the form:

1. Record what you have eaten as soon as possible after meals. This makes it much easier to remember what (and how much) you consumed.

2. When you record the foods you have eaten, it is important to be as specific as possible. Remember to specify the following:

• **Preparation:** How was the food cooked: Was it fresh, frozen, or canned? Was it fried, baked, steamed, boiled, or grilled? If you prepared a mix, did you add water or milk?

• **Canned foods:** If you had a canned product, was it packed in water, in oil, in juice, or in syrup? Include the brand name of the food item.

• **Portion size:** Indicate how much you had of each food using standard measures. Cups, ounces, teaspoons, or tablespoons. Avoid terms such as "one bowl" or "a handful" where possible. To measure meats, remember that 3 oz is about the size of a deck of cards or the size of your palm.

• **Condiments:** Indicate what was added to foods and how much was added. Include mustard, ketchup, mayonnaise, cream or sugar, steak sauce, salsa, etc.

• **Other:** If you had bread, was it white bread, multigrain, whole-wheat, french, etc? Was your milk whole milk, 2%, or fat-free? Was your coffee or tea decaffeinated, sweetened, etc?

3. Be sure to complete the section pertaining to exercise/physical activity.

4. Include your telephone number and e-mail address. If the record is incomplete, you may be called to provide more information.

The Homer Rice Center for Sports Performance
Sports Nutrition Center

Name: _____   Date: _____

Age: _____   Sex: _____   Height: _____   Weight: _____

Desired body weight (if different from current weight): _____

Body fat % (if known): _____   Desired body fat %: _____

Phone number: _____   E-mail address: _____

Exercise/Physical Activity:

Type: _____

Duration: _____

Times/Week: _____

Type: _____

Duration: _____

Times/Week: _____

Time	Food Item and Method of Preparation	Amount Eaten

Source: Used with the permission of the Georgia Tech Athletic Association.

continued

Time	Food Item and Method of Preparation	Amount Eaten

6. SAMPLE PERFORMANCE CONTRACT

Sports Nutrition Center

PERSONAL PERFORMANCE CONTRACT FOR

_____

Student-Athlete

My current data in the area of

Sports Nutrition

Reflects a significant opportunity for me to improve my athletic performance. Jointly with

Rob Skinner, RD, CSCS
Chris Rosenbloom, PhD, RD

I have established a _____ month goal of _____.

In order to accomplish this goal I commit to:

1. _____

2. _____

3. _____

Athlete's Signature:_____

I verify the above noted data and commit to support _____ in realizing his/her goal by:

1. _____

2. _____

3. _____

HRCSP Staff Signature: _____

Source: Used with permission of The Georgia Tech Athletic Association

7. NUTRIENT CONTENT OF POPULAR ENERGY BARS

Name and Manufacturer	Size	Flavor*	Calories	Carbohydrate (g)	Protein (g)	Fat (g)	Calcium (mg)	Iron (mg)
Balance Bar Bio Foods, Inc Santa Barbara, CA	1.76 oz (50 g)	Toasted crunch	180	19	14	6	250	3.6
BumbleBar (organic) BumbleBar Vashon, WA	1.58 oz (45 g)	Chocolate crisp	230	20	6	15	200	5.4
Clif Bar Clif Bar, Inc Berkeley, CA	2.4 oz (68 g)	Apple cherry	250	52	4	2	40	1.45
Harvest Bar PowerBar, Inc Berkeley, CA	2.3 oz (65 g)	Cherry crunch	240	45	7	4	150	2.7
Met-Rx High Protein Food Bar Met-Rx USA, Inc Irvine, CA	4.41 oz (125 g)	Chocolate roasted peanut	380	57	30	7	1,000	9
Mountain Lift Energy Bar Optim Nutrition Salt Lake City, UT	2.1 oz (60 g)	Chocolate	220	34	12	5	350	6.3
PowerBar PowerBar, Inc Berkeley, CA	2.3 oz (65 g)	Chocolate	230	45	10	2	300	6.3
PR Bar PR Nutrition, Inc San Diego, CA	1.76 oz (50 g)	Granola crunch	180	21	14	6	250	7.2
ProPortion Rexall Boca Raton, FL	1.4 oz (40 g)	Chocolate peanut butter	160	17	12	6	100	9
Source One Met-Rx USA, Inc Irvine, CA	2.2 oz (62.5 g)	Peanut butter and jelly sandwich	190	22	15	3	500	4.5
Zone Perfect Eicotech Corporation Beverly, MA	1.76 oz (50 g)	Honey peanut	200	22	14	7	400	2.7

*For most brands, several flavors are available. Nutrient content may vary by flavor.

Source: Manufacturer data

8. CALCULATING THE ENERGY COST OF PHYSICAL ACTIVITY USING METs

The following table may be used to estimate the energy expended during activities ranging from planned exercise (eg, walking, cycling, running) to leisure/home activities (eg, fishing, home repair, yardwork) in kilocalories (kcals) per kilogram (kg) body weight per minute. Multiplying this value by the amount of time spent performing the activity provides an estimate of the *total caloric cost* of the activity. These tables use MET values. A MET is a unit of energy relative to the energy cost of sitting quietly (1 MET). For example, a 5-MET activity requires five times the amount of energy expended as sitting quietly. For the average adult, 1 MET requires approximately 3.5 mL of oxygen/kg body weight per minute (mL/kg/min). The values in this table were derived from previously published energy expenditure lists from a variety of sources. Consult the reference for specific information, such as limitations of this method, and additional listings for activities not listed here.

How to use this table:

1. Information you need: Body weight in kg (or lb, multiplied by 2.2)
                                    Description of the activity performed
                                      Intensity of the activity (eg, miles per hour, "vigorous" or "moderate" effort)
                                      Duration of the activity (eg, minutes, hours)
2. Using the description and reported intensity of the activity, determine the MET value from the table.
3. Multiply the MET value by *body weight* (in kg).
4. To determine the *total energy cost* of the activity, multiply this number by the number of *hours* spent performing the activity (or minutes/60).

Example: A 70-kg individual reports cycling at about 15 miles per hour ("vigorous" effort) for 45 minutes (45/60 = 0.75 hour)

                  10 METs x 70 kg x 0.75 hour = 525 total kcals

Note: The accuracy of this method may be improved if an individual's actual resting metabolic rate (RMR) is known. Multiply the RMR (in kcals/hr or kcals/min) by the MET value listed for that activity to provide an estimate of energy expended during the activity.

Example: An individual's measured RMR is 1,500 kcals/day, or 62.5 kcals/hour (1,500 kcals/24 hours). Using the same activity information as the previous example:

                  10 METs x 62.5 kcals/hour x 0.75 hour = 469 total kcal

If the intensity of the activity is not known, the "general" MET value should be used. Activities performed at a health club that are not specifically listed in the table may be categorized as "Health club exercise, general."

Activity (description)	Intensity (METs)
Aerobic dance, teaching	6.0
Aerobic dance, ballet or modern	6.0
Aerobic dance, general	6.0
Aerobic dance, low impact	5.0
Aerobic dance, high impact	7.0
Cycling, BMX or mountain	8.5
Cycling, <10 mph, general, leisure	4.0
Cycling, 10-12 mph, leisure, slow, light effort	6.0
Cycling, 12-14 mph, leisure, moderate effort	8.0
Cycling, 14-16 mph, racing or leisure, fast, vigorous effort	10.0
Cycling, 16-19 mph, racing, very fast, racing general	12.0
Cycling, >20 mph, racing, not drafting	16.0
Conditioning exercise, cycling, stationary, general	5.0
Conditioning exercise, cycling, stationary, very light effort	3.0
Conditioning exercise, cycling, stationary, light effort	5.5
Conditioning exercise, cycling, stationary, moderate effort	7.0
Conditioning exercise, cycling, stationary, vigorous effort	10.5
Conditioning exercise, cycling, stationary, very vigorous	12.5
Calisthenics (eg, push-ups, pull-ups, sit-ups), heavy, vigorous effort	8.0
Calisthenics, home exercise, light or moderate effort, general	4.5
Circuit training, general	8.0
Dancing, general	4.5
Dancing, fast (disco, folk, square)	5.5
Dancing, ballroom, slow	3.0
Fishing, general	4.0
Fishing, from riverbank and walking	5.0
Fishing, from boat, sitting	2.5
Fishing, from riverbank and standing	3.5
Fishing, in stream, in waders	6.0
Health club exercise, general	5.5
Home activities, sweeping floors	2.5
Home activities, sweeping garage or outside of house	4.0
Home activities, cleaning, heavy or major, vigorous effort	4.5
Home activities, cleaning, general	3.5
Home activities, cleaning, light (dusting, vacuuming), moderate effort	2.5
Home activities, putting away groceries	2.5
Home activities, walking-shopping (not groceries)	2.3
Home activities, moving furniture, household	6.0
Home activities, moving household items, carrying boxes	7.0
Home activities, scrubbing floors, on hands and knees	5.5
Home repair, automobile body work	4.5
Home repair, automobile repair	3.0

continued

Activity (description)	Intensity (METs)
Home repair, carpentry, general	3.0
Home repair, carpentry, outside house	6.0
Home repair, painting outside house	5.0
Home repair, painting, papering, plastering, remodeling	4.5
Home repair, roofing	6.0
Hunting, large game	6.0
Hunting, general	5.0
Hunting, small game	5.0
Lawn and garden, chopping wood	6.0
Lawn and garden, digging, spading	5.0
Lawn and garden, using heavy power tools, tilling, shoveling	6.0
Lawn and garden, mowing lawn, general	5.5
Lawn and garden, riding mower	2.5
Lawn and garden, walking, hand mower	6.0
Lawn and garden, power mower	4.5
Lawn and garden, raking	4.0
Lawn and garden, gardening, general	5.0
Occupational work, building road	6.0
Occupational work, carrying heavy loads such as bricks	8.0
Occupational work, construction, outside	5.5
Occupational work, farming, baling hay, cleaning barn	8.0
Occupational work, firefighting, general	12.0
Occupational work, forestry, general	8.0
Occupational work, masonry, concrete	7.0
Occupational work, shoveling, digging ditches	8.5
Rowing, stationary ergometer, general	9.5
Rowing, stationary ergometer, light effort	3.5
Rowing, stationary ergometer, moderate effort	7.0
Rowing, stationary ergometer, vigorous effort	8.5
Rowing, stationary ergometer, very vigorous effort	12.0
Running, jogging, general	7.0
Running, 5 mph (12 min/mile)	8.0
Running, 6 mph (10 min/mile)	10.0
Running, 7 mph (8.5 min/mile)	11.5
Running, 8 mph (7.5 min/mile)	13.5
Running, 9 mph (6.5 min/mile)	15.0
Running, 10 mph (6 min/mile)	16.0
Running, 10.9 mph (5.5 min/mile)	18.0
Running, cross-country	9.0
Running, general	8.0
Running, up stairs	15.0
Running, on a track, team practice	10.0

continued

Activity (description)	Intensity (METs)
Sitting, desk work	1.8
Sitting, reading	1.3
Sitting, typing, computer	1.5
Skating, ice, 9 mph or less	5.5
Skating, ice, general	7.0
Skating, ice, rapidly, >9 mph	9.0
Skating, speed, competitive	15.0
Skiing, general	7.0
Skiing, cross-country, 2.5 mph, slow or light effort	7.0
Skiing, cross-country, 4-5 mph, moderate speed and effort, general	8.0
Skiing, cross-country, 5-8 mph, brisk speed, vigorous effort	9.0
Skiing, cross-country, >8 mph, racing	14.0
Skiing, downhill, light effort	5.0
Skiing, downhill, moderate effort, general	6.0
Skiing, downhill, vigorous effort, racing	8.0
Ski machine, general	9.5
Snowshoeing	8.0
Sports, badminton, competitive	7.0
Sports, basketball, game	8.0
Sports, basketball, nongame, general	6.0
Sports, basketball, wheelchair	6.5
Sports, bowling	3.0
Sports, boxing, in ring, general	12.0
Sports, boxing, sparring	9.0
Sports, coaching: football, soccer, basketball, baseball, swimming	4.0
Sports, fencing	6.0
Sports, football, competitive	9.0
Sports, frisbee, ultimate	3.5
Sports, golf, general	4.5
Sports, golf, carrying clubs	5.5
Sports, golf, using power cart	3.5
Sports, gymnastics, general	4.0
Sports, handball, general	12.0
Sports, handball, team	8.0
Sports, hockey, field	8.0
Sports, hockey, ice	8.0
Sports, horseback riding, general	4.0
Sports, judo, karate, kick boxing, taekwondo	10.0
Sports, lacrosse	8.0
Sports, polo	8.0
Sports, racquetball, competitive	10.0
Sports, racquetball, casual, general	7.0

continued

Activity (description)	Intensity (METs)
Sports, rock climbing, ascending	11.0
Sports, rock climbing, rappelling	8.0
Sports, rope jumping, fast	12.0
Sports, rope jumping, moderate, general	10.0
Sports, rugby	10.0
Sports, soccer, competitive	10.0
Sports, soccer, casual, general	7.0
Sports, softball or baseball, general	5.0
Sports, squash	12.0
Sports, table tennis, ping pong	4.0
Sports, Tai Chi	4.0
Sports, tennis, general	7.0
Sports, tennis, doubles	6.0
Sports, tennis, singles	8.0
Sports, volleyball, competitive, in gymnasium	4.0
Sports, volleyball, noncompetitive, general	3.0
Sports, volleyball, beach	8.0
Sports, wrestling	6.0
Stair-treadmill ergometer, general	6.0
Stretching, hatha yoga	4.0
Walking, backpacking, general	7.0
Walking, hiking, cross-country	6.0
Walking, marching, rapidly (military)	6.5
Walking, race walking	6.5
Walking, 2 mph, level ground, firm surface, slow pace	2.5
Walking, 3 mph, level, firm surface, moderate pace	3.5
Walking, 4 mph, level, firm surface, very brisk pace	4.0
Walking, 4.5 mph, level, firm surface, very, very brisk pace	4.5
Walking, for pleasure, work break, walking the dog	3.5
Walking, grass track	5.0
Walking, to work or class	4.0
Water activities, canoeing, rowing, 2-4 mph, light effort	3.0
Water activities, canoeing, rowing, 4-6 mph, moderate effort	7.0
Water activities, canoeing, rowing, >6 mph, vigorous effort	12.0
Water activities, canoeing, rowing, for pleasure, general	3.5
Water activities, canoeing, rowing, in competition, crew or sculling	12.0
Water activities, diving	3.0
Water activities, kayaking	5.0
Water activities, sailing, in competition	5.0
Water activities, skiing, water	6.0
Water activities, scuba diving, general	7.0
Water activities, surfing, body or board	3.0

continued

Activity (description)	Intensity (METs)
Water activities, swimming, laps, freestyle, fast, vigorous effort	10.0
Water activities, swimming, laps, freestyle, slow, moderate or light effort	8.0
Water activities, swimming, backstroke, general	8.0
Water activities, swimming, breaststroke, general	10.0
Water activities, swimming, butterfly, general	11.0
Water activities, swimming, crawl, fast, vigorous effort	11.0
Water activities, swimming, crawl, slow, moderate or light effort	8.0
Water activities, swimming, lake, ocean, or river	6.0
Water activities, swimming, leisurely, not lap swimming, general	6.0
Water activities, swimming, sidestroke, general	8.0
Water activities, swimming, synchronized	8.0
Water activities, swimming, treading water, fast, vigorous effort	10.0
Water activities, swimming, treading water, moderate effort, general	4.0
Water activities, water polo	10.0
Water activities, water volleyball	3.0
Water aerobics, water calisthenics	4.0
Weightlifting (free, Nautilus, or universal-type), light or moderate effort, general	3.0
Weightlifting (free weights, Nautilus, or universal-type), power lifting or bodybuilding, vigorous effort	6.0

Source: Ainsworth BA, Haskell WL, Leon AS, et al. Compendium of physical activities: classification of energy costs of human physical activities. *Med Sci Sports Exerc.* 1993;25:71-80.

9. GLYCEMIC INDEX OF COMMONLY CONSUMED FOODS

The Glycemic Index (GI) is defined as the response of blood glucose to a 50-g carbohydrate portion of a food expressed as a percentage of the response to the same amount of carbohydrate from a standard or comparison food, usually white bread or glucose. There is large variability for a GI for each group of foods. The form of the food, how the food is processed, how the food is cooked, how the food is chewed, the rate of emptying from the stomach, and the response of the individual can all affect the GI of a food.

In sports nutrition, generally the GI has been used in two ways. The first is the inclusion of foods with a low GI pre-exercise for those athletes who are subject to hypoglycemia during exercise. The second is the use of high-GI foods after exercise to help restore muscle glycogen stores. The GI is only a tool for food selection for athletes. There are limitations to using this tool and athletes should use the information as a guideline, not as an absolute.

High Glycemic Index (>85)	Medium Glycemic Index (60-85)	Low Glycemic Index (<60)
glucose	rice cakes	brown rice
carrots	vanilla wafers	white rice
white potatoes	bagel	plums
honey	saltine crackers	most dairy products
potato	white bread	yogurt
corn flakes	soda	apple
most breads	angel food cake	chick-peas
most breakfast cereals	high-fiber cereals	most pastas
corn chips	wheat bread	lentils
sports drinks	sucrose	peaches
	ice cream	kidney beans
	oatmeal	fructose
	most cookies	nuts
	sweet potatoes	
	potato chips	

For a more complete listing (over 600 GI for the most common Western foods), see Foster-Powell K, Miller JR. International tables of glycemic index. *Am J Clin Nutr.* 1995;62:871S-893S.

10. USDA RECOMMENDED WEIGHT RANGES

Healthy Weight Ranges for Men and Women of All Ages

Height	Weight (in pounds)	Height	Weight (in pounds)
4'10"	91-119	5'9"	129-169
4'11"	94-124	5'10"	132-174
5'0"	97-128	5'11"	136-179
5'1"	101-132	6'0"	140-184
5'2"	104-137	6'1"	144-189
5'3"	107-141	6'2"	148-195
5'4"	111-146	6'3"	152-200
5'5"	114-150	6'4"	156-205
5'6"	118-155	6'5"	160-211
5'7"	121-160	6'6"	164-216
5'8"	125-164		

Source: *Report of the Dietary Guidelines Advisory Committee on Dietary Guidelines for Americans*, Washington, DC: US Dept of Agriculture, Agriculture Research Service, and Dietary Guidelines Advisory Committee; 1995. Available at http://www.nalusda.gov/

11. RECOMMENDED DIETARY ALLOWANCES

	Age	Protein (g)	Vitamins				Minerals			
			A (mcg RE)	E (mg)	K (mcg)	C (mg)	Iron (mg)	Zinc (mg)	Iodine (mcg)	Selenium (mcg)
Infants	0-6 mos	13	375	3	5	30	6	5	40	10
	7-12 mos	14	375	4	10	35	10	5	50	15
Children	1-3 yrs	16	400	6	15	40	10	10	70	20
	4-6	24	500	7	20	45	10	10	90	20
	7-10	28	700	7	30	45	10	10	120	30
Males	11-14 yrs	45	1,000	10	45	50	12	15	150	40
	15-18	59	1,000	10	65	60	12	15	150	50
	19-24	58	1,000	10	70	60	10	15	150	70
	25-50	63	1,000	10	80	60	10	15	150	70
	51+	63	1,000	10	80	60	10	15	150	70
Females	11-14 yrs	46	800	8	45	50	15	12	150	45
	15-18	44	800	8	55	60	15	12	150	50
	19-24	46	800	8	60	60	15	12	150	55
	25-50	50	800	8	65	60	15	12	150	55
	51+	50	800	8	65	60	10	12	150	55
Pregnant		60	800	10	65	70	30	15	175	65
Lactating	1st 6 mos	65	1,300	12	65	95	15	19	200	75
	2nd 6 mos	62	1,200	11	65	90	15	16	200	75

mcg RE = microgram Retinol Equivalents   mcg = micrograms   mg = milligrams   g = grams

Adapted with permisssion from *Recommended Dietary Allowances,* 10th ed. Washington, DC: National Academy Press.
© 1989 by the National Academy of Sciences.

12. DIETARY REFERENCE INTAKES: RECOMMENDED INTAKES FOR INDIVIDUALS

Food and Nutrition Board, National Academy of Sciences — Institute of Medicine (1997-1998)

Age/Life-stage	Calcium (mg)	Phosphorus (mg)	Magnesium (mg)	Vitamin D a,b (mcg)	Fluoride (mg)	Thiamin (mg)	Riboflavin (mg)	Niacin (mg) c	Vitamin B6 (mg)	Folate (mcg) d	Vitamin B12 (mcg)	Pantothenic Acid (mg)	Biotin (mcg)	Choline (mg) e
Infants														
0-6 months	210*	100*	30*	5*	0.01*	0.2*	0.3*	2*	0.1*	65*	0.4*	1.7*	5*	125*
7-12 months	270*	275*	75*	5*	0.5*	0.3*	0.4*	4*	0.3*	80*	0.5*	1.8*	6*	150*
Children														
1-3 years	500*	460	80	5*	0.7*	0.5	0.5	6	0.5	150	0.9	2*	8*	200*
4-8 years	800*	500	130	5*	1*	0.6	0.6	8	0.6	200	1.2	3*	12*	250*
Males														
9-13 years	1,300*	1,250	240	5*	2*	0.9	0.9	12	1.0	300	1.8	4*	20*	375*
14-18 years	1,300*	1,250	410	5*	3*	1.2	1.3	16	1.3	400	2.4	5*	25*	550*
19-30 years	1,000*	700	400	5*	4*	1.2	1.3	16	1.3	400	2.4	5*	30*	550*
31-50 years	1,000*	700	420	5*	4*	1.2	1.3	16	1.3	400	2.4	5*	30*	550*
51-70 years	1,200*	700	420	10*	4*	1.2	1.3	16	1.7	400	2.4 f	5*	30*	550*
>70 years	1,200*	700	420	15*	4*	1.2	1.3	16	1.7	400	2.4 f	5*	30*	550*
Females														
9-13 years	1,300*	1,250	240	5*	2*	0.9	0.9	12	1.0	300	1.8	4*	20*	375*
14-18 years	1,300*	1,250	360	5*	3*	1.0	1.0	14	1.2	400 g	2.4	5*	25*	400*
19-30 years	1,000*	700	310	5*	3*	1.1	1.1	14	1.3	400 g	2.4	5*	30*	425*
31-50 years	1,000*	700	320	5*	3*	1.1	1.1	14	1.3	400 g	2.4	5*	30*	425*
51-70 years	1,200*	700	320	10*	3*	1.1	1.1	14	1.5	400	2.4 f	5*	30*	425*
>70 years	1,200*	700	320	15*	3*	1.1	1.1	14	1.5	400	2.4 f	5*	30*	425*
Pregnancy														
≤18 years	1,300*	1,250	400	5*	3*	1.4	1.4	18	1.9	600 h	2.6	6*	30*	450*
19-30 years	1,000*	700	350	5*	3*	1.4	1.4	18	1.9	600 h	2.6	6*	30*	450*
31-50 years	1,000*	700	360	5*	3*	1.4	1.4	18	1.9	600 h	2.6	6*	30*	450*
Lactation														
≤18 years	1,300*	1,250	360	5*	3*	1.5	1.6	17	2.0	500	2.8	7*	35*	550*
19-30 years	1,000*	700	310	5*	3*	1.5	1.6	17	2.0	500	2.8	7*	35*	550*
31-50 years	1,000*	700	320	5*	3*	1.5	1.6	17	2.0	500	2.8	7*	35*	550*

mg = milligrams   mcg = micrograms

*Note: This table presents Recommended Dietary Allowances (RDAs) and Adequate Intakes (AIs). (AI values are followed by an asterisk.) RDAs and AIs may both be used as goals for individual intake. RDAs are set to meet the average daily needs of almost all (97% to 98%) healthy individuals in a life-stage group. The AI is believed to cover the daily needs of most healthy people, but lack of data or uncertainty in the data prevents clear specification of an RDA.

a As cholecalciferol (1mcg cholecalciferol = 40 IU vitamin D)

b In the absence of adequate exposure to sunlight

c As niacin equivalents: 1mg of niacin = 60 mg of tryptophan

d As dietary folate equivalents (DFE): 1 DFE = 1 mcg food folate = 0.6 mcg of folic acid (from fortified food or supplement) consumed with food = 0.5 mcg of synthetic (supplemental) folic acid taken on an empty stomach.

e Although AIs have been set for choline, there are few data to assess whether a dietary supply of choline is needed at all stages of the lifecycle.

f Since 10% to 30% of older people may malabsorb food-bound B12, it is advisable for those older than 50 years to meet their RDA mainly by taking foods fortified with B12 or a B12-containing supplement.

g It is recommended that all women capable of becoming pregnant consume 400 mcg of folic acid from fortified foods and/or supplements in addition to intake of food folate from a varied diet.

h Women should continue taking 400 mcg of folic acid until their pregnancy is confirmed, at which time the recommended daily intake increases.

Adapted with permission from the National Academy of Sciences; 1998.

DIETARY REFERENCE INTAKES: TOLERABLE UPPER INTAKE LEVELS (ULa) FOR CERTAIN NUTRIENTS AND FOOD COMPONENTS

Food and Nutrition Board, Institute of Medicine—National Academy of Sciences

Life-stage Group	Calcium (g/day)	Phosphorus (g/day)	Magnesium (mg/day)[b]	Vitamin D (µg/day)	Flouride (mg/day)	Niacin (mg/day)[c]	Vitamin B$_6$ (mg/day)	Synthetic Folic Acid (µg/day)[c]	Choline (g/day)
0-6 months	ND[d]	ND	ND	25	0.7	ND	ND	ND	ND
7-12 months	ND	ND	ND	25	0.9	ND	ND	ND	ND
1-3 years	2.5	3	65	50	1.3	10	30	300	1.0
4-8 years	2.5	3	110	50	2.2	15	40	400	1.0
9-13 years	2.5	4	350	50	10	20	60	600	2.0
14-18 years	2.5	4	350	50	10	30	80	800	3.0
19-70 years	2.5	4	350	50	10	35	100	1,000	3.5
> 70 years	2.5	3	350	50	10	35	100	1,000	3.5
Pregnancy									
≤ 18 years	2.5	3.5	350	50	10	30	80	800	3.0
19-50 years	2.5	3.5	350	50	10	35	100	1,000	3.5
Lactation									
≤ 18 years	2.5	4	350	50	10	30	80	800	3.0
19-50 years	2.5	4	350	50	10	35	100	1,000	3.5

[a]UL = the maximum level of daily nutrient intake that is likely to pose no risk of side effects. Unless otherwise specified, the UL represents total intake from food, water, and supplements. Due to lack of suitable data, ULs could not be established for thiamin, riboflavin, vitamin B$_{12}$, pantothenic acid, or biotin. In the absence of ULs, extra caution may be warranted in consuming levels above recommended intakes.

[b]The UL for magnesium represents intake from a pharmacological agent only and does not include intake from food and water.

[c]The ULs for niacin and synthetic folic acid apply to forms obtained from supplements, fortified foods, or a combination of the two.

[d]ND: Not determinable due to lack of data of adverse effects in this age group and concern with regard to lack of ability to handle excess amounts. Source of intake should be from food only to prevent high levels of intake.

13. GUIDELINES FOR EVALUATING SPORTS NUTRITION INFORMATION ON THE INTERNET

It can be a challenge to determine the reliability of information presented on the Internet. Everyone has the ability to broadcast his or her opinion or belief on the Internet, and it becomes increasingly difficult to determine what is fact and what is fiction. The following criteria can help determine the reliability of a sports nutrition Web site.

Author
- Is the author listed?
- What are the credentials of the author? What is the author's occupation or position? What is the author's experience in sports nutrition? Who employs the author? Will the author gain financially from the information presented on the Web site?
- If no author is identified with the electronic document, back up to see if another part of the file contains the information. Look for name and E-mail address. Write and ask for more background information on the author of the Web site.

Type of Publication or Information
- Is the information an electronic version of a newspaper, magazine, journal, or book? If so, how reliable is the original source? What institution (company, government, or university) supports the information?
- Is the information an abstract or summary from another source? If so, can you locate the original document?
- Is the information presented as opinion or a presentation of referenced facts?
- Is the information representative of an institution, organization, or personal Web page?

Content
- Is the intent of the content to inform, explain, or persuade?
- How current is the information? When was it last updated?
- Do the links lead to other reliable/accurate sources?

Source
The final three letters in a URL (uniform resource locator) indicate the type of Web site. For example:
- *.com* indicates a commercial site (frequently trying to sell a product)
- *.edu* indicates an educational site (a university or college)
- *.gov* indicates a government site
- *.org* indicates an organization site (nonprofit, not for profit, or for profit)

14. GUIDELINES FOR EVALUATING ERGOGENIC AIDS

Using the SOAP format, ask these questions when evaluating an ergogenic aid:

SUBJECTIVE
- What claims are being made for the supplement?
- Who is making the claims?
- What is the motivation behind the claims?
- How is the supplement marketed?
- Does the claim make sense?

OBJECTIVE
- What are the ingredients and how much of each ingredient is in the supplement?
- What is the recommended dosage of the supplement?
- What is (are) the physiological role(s) of the ingredients?
- Are the ingredients legal (ie, not banned or restricted by a sport-governing body)?
- Are the ingredients safe?
- Are the ingredients effective?

ASSESSMENT
- Based on subjective and objective data, what is your assessment of the supplement's claims?
- What is the risk/benefit ratio to the athlete of using the supplement?
- Would you recommend the supplement?

PLAN
- If the supplement is to be used, determine guidelines for monitoring supplement use.
- Decide for what length of time the product should be used.
- Ascertain whether the athlete will be able to make the appropriate diet or training modifications necessary to see the desired results.
- Document your recommendations, both pros and cons, about the supplement in a written record.

Adapted with permission. *SCAN'S PULSE*, 1996; Fall,17(4). Official publication of Sports, Cardiovascular, and Wellness Nutritionists (SCAN), The American Dietetic Association, Chicago, Illinois.

15. SELECTED SPORTS NUTRITION-RELATED POSITION STATEMENTS

American College of Sports Medicine (ACSM)

"The Recommended Quantity and Quality of Exercise for Developing and Maintaining Cardiorespiratory and Muscular Fitness and Flexibility in Healthy Adults," © 1998 American College of Sports Medicine (*Med Sci Sport Exer*. 1998;30(6):975-991)

"Exercise and Physical Activity for Older Adults," © 1998 American College of Sports Medicine (*Med Sci Sport Exer*. 1998;30(6):992-1008)

"The Female Athlete Triad," © 1997 American College of Sports Medicine (*Med Sci Sport Exer*. 1997;229(5):i-ix)

"Heat and Cold Illnesses During Distance Running," © 1996 American College of Sports Medicine (*Med Sci Sport Exer*. 1996;28(12):i-x)

"The Use of Blood Doping as an Ergogenic Aid," © 1996 American College of Sports Medicine (*Med Sci Sport Exer*. 1996;28(6):ix-xii)

"Exercise and Fluid Replacement," © 1996 American College of Sports Medicine (*Med Sci Sport Exer*. 1996;28(1):i-vii)

"Osteoporosis and Exercise," © 1995 American College of Sports Medicine (*Med Sci Sport Exer*. 1995;27(4):i-vii)

"Exercise for Patients with Coronary Artery Disease," © 1994 American College of Sports Medicine (*Med Sci Sport Exer*. 1994;26(3):i-v)

"Physical Activity, Physical Fitness, and Hypertension," © 1993 American College of Sports Medicine (*Med Sci Sport Exer*. 1993;25(10)i-x)

"The Use of Anabolic-Androgenic Steroids in Sports," © 1984 American College of Sports Medicine (*Med Sci Sport Exer*. 1987;19(5):534-539)

"Proper and Improper Weight-Loss Programs," © 1983 American College of Sports Medicine (*Med Sci Sports Exer*. 1983;15(1):ix-xiii)

"The Use of Alcohol in Sports," © 1982 American College of Sports Medicine (*Med Sci Sport Exer*. 1982;14(6)x-xi)

Joint Position Statements

"Recommendation for Cardiovascular Screening, Staffing, and Emergency Policies at Health/Fitness Facilities," American College of Sports Medicine and American Heart Association, © 1998 (*Med Sci Sport Exer*. 1998;30(6):109-1018)

"Diabetes Mellitus and Exercise," American College of Sports Medicine and American Diabetes Association, © 1997 (*Med Sci Sport Exer*. 1997;29(12)i-vi)

Opinion Statement

"Physical Fitness in Children and Youth," © 1988 American College of Sports Medicine (*Med Sci Sport Exer.* 1998;20(4):422-423)

American Dietetic Association

The American Dietetic Association publishes position papers that are available on the Web at http://www.eatright.org. The following is not a list of all position papers, but includes those that may be useful for the health professional working with active people.

"ADA: Women's Health and Nutrition" (published in 1995, reaffirmed)

"ADA: Nutrition Education for the Public" (published in 1996, expires in 2000)

"ADA: The Role of Nutrition in Health Promotion and Disease Prevention Programs" (published in 1998, expires in 2001)

"ADA: Vitamin and Mineral Supplementation" (published in 1996, reaffirmed)

"ADA: Weight Management" (published in 1997, expires in 2000)

"ADA: Food and Nutrition Misinformation" (published in 1995, expires in 2000)

"ADA: Phytochemicals and Functional Foods" (published in 1995, reaffirmed)

"ADA: Nutrition for Athletic Adults" (published in 1993, expired in 1998)

"ADA: Vegetarian Diets" (published in 1997, expires in 2001)

"ADA: Eating Disorders" (published in 1994, reaffirmed)

16. SPORTS NUTRITION-RELATED WEB SITES

Professional Associations/Organizations

Aerobics and Fitness Association of America
www.afaa.com

Amateur Athletic Union
www.aausports.org

American Alliance for Health, Physical Education,
Recreation, and Dance
www.aahperd.com

American College of Sports Medicine
www.acsm.org

American Council on Exercise
www.acefitness.org

American Dietetic Association, The
www.eatright.org

American Fitness Professionals and Associates
www.astafitness.com

American Society of Exercise Physiologists
www.vacumed.com/links.htm

American Sport Education
www.ASEP.com

American Sports Education Institute/Booster Club
of America
www.sportlink.com

Canadian Association for Health, Physical Education,
Recreation, and Dance
www.activeliving.canperd/index.html

ECA Fitness
www.ecaworldfitness.com

Exercise & Sport Research Institute
www.asu.edu/clas/espe

Gatorade Sports Science Institute
www.gssiweb.com

IDEA (The International Association for Fitness
Professionals)
www.ideafit.com

International Health, Racquet, and Sportsclub Association
www.ihrsa.org

International Institute for Sport & Human Performance
http://darkwing.uoregon.edu/-micropub

International Olympic Committee
www.olympic.org

International Sports Sciences Association
www.issa-usa.com

National Association of Collegiate Directors of Athletics
www.nacda.com

National Association for Girls and Women in Sports
c/o American Alliance for Health, Physical Education,
Recreation, and Dance
www.aahperd.org/nagws/nagws.html

National Association for Sport and Physical Education
www.aahperd.org/naspe/material.html

National Collegiate Athletic Association
www.ncaa.org

National Dance Association
www.aahperd.org

National Employee Services and Recreation Association
www.nesr.org

National Federation of State High School Associations
www.nsshsa.org

National Fitness Leaders Association
http://wellness.uwsp.edu/nfla

National Fitness Trainers Association
www.icnweb.com/nfta

National Recreation & Park Association
www.nrpa.org

National Sporting Goods Association
www.nsqa.org

National Strength and Conditioning Association
www.nsca-lift.org

Special Olympics International
www.specialolympics.org

Sporting Goods Manufacturers Association
www.sportlink.com

Sports Safety Board of Quebec
www.rssq.gouv.qc.ca

United States Association of Blind Athletes
www.usaba.org

United States Olympic Committee
www.olympic-usa.org/

Veggie Sports Association
www.veggie.org/

Weight Control Information Network
www.niddk.nih.gov/NutritionDocs.html

Wellness Council of America
www.welcoa.org

Women's Sports Foundation
www.lifetimetv.com/WoSport

Sports Organizations

America Running and Fitness Association
www.arfa.org

American Volkssport Association
www.ava.org/index.htm

American Youth Soccer Organization
www.soccer.org

Bicycle Federation of America
www.bikespeed.org

Jazzersize, Inc.
www.jazzersize.com

League of American Bicyclists
www.bikeleague.org

Road Runners Club of America
www.rrca.org

Runners World
www.runnersworld.com/nutrition

United States Squash Racquets Association
www.us-squash.org/squash

United States Swimming
www.usswim.org

United States Weightlifting Federation
www.usysa.org

Other Web sites

Body Basics Creative Instructor Training
www.theriver.com/bodybasics

Covert Bailey's Fitness Homepage
http://www.covertbailey.com/

Dietitians of Canada
www.dietitians.ca

Dietsite
www.dietsite.com

Healthtouch Online
www.healthtouch.com

Human Kinetics Journals
www.humankinetics.com/infok/journl.htm

International School of Aerobics Training
www.ata.fitness

Sportscience News
www.sportsci.org

The Physician and Sports Medicine
www.physsportsmed.com

Tufts University Nutrition Navigator
www.navigator.tufts.edu/sportsnut.html

Note: This list includes Web sites that might be valuable to the sports nutritionist. The inclusion of the Web site addresses listed in this section does not constitute an endorsement of any one site. At the time of publication, all Web sites were operable.

INDEX